The Silk Route and The Diamond Path

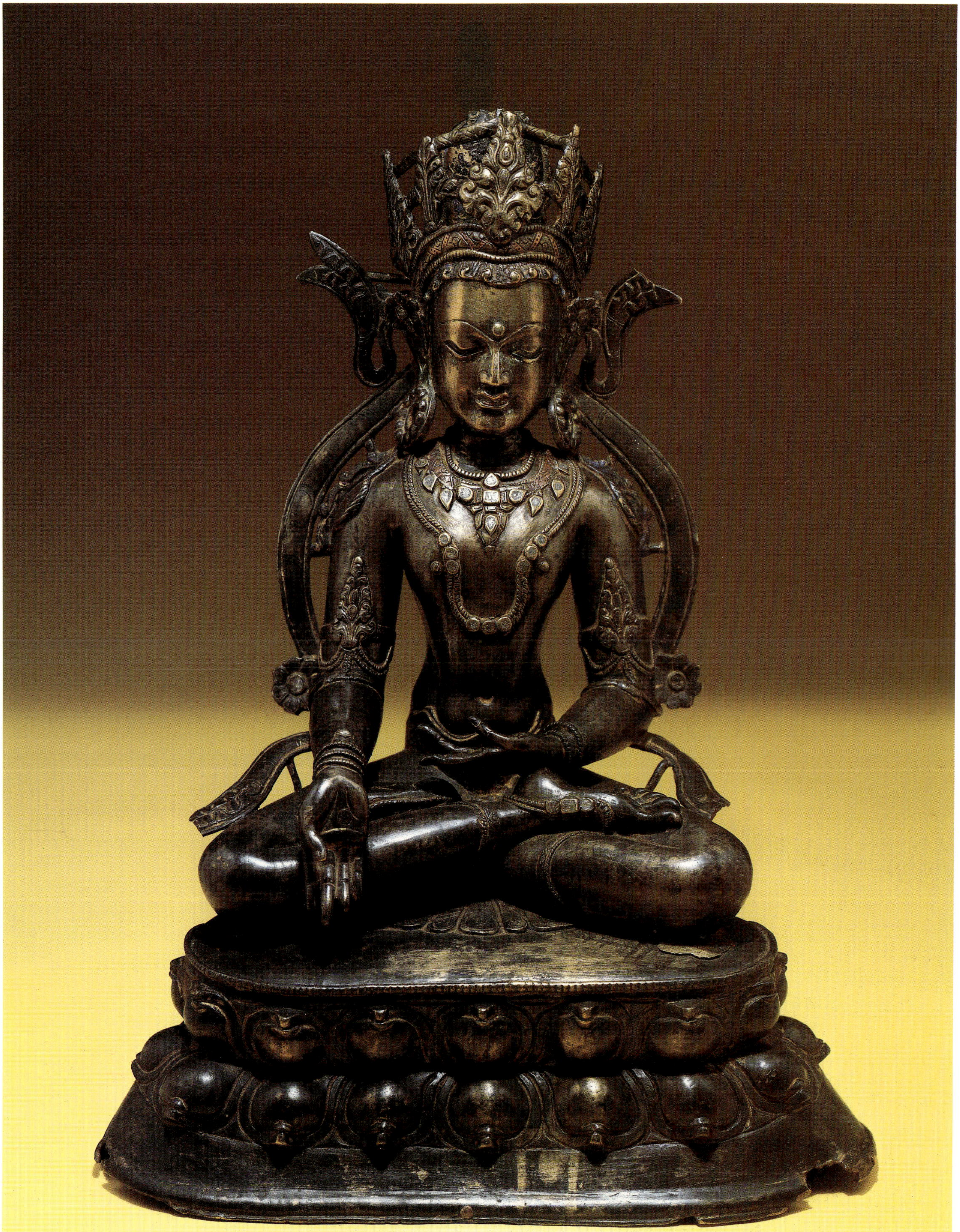

To the memory of my Grandparents and

His Holiness the Sixteenth Gyalwa Karmapa, Rangjung Rikpe Dorje

List of Lenders

The Asia Society
George P. Bickford
The Trustees of the British Museum, London
The Brooklyn Museum
The Cleveland Museum of Art
Professor Samuel Eilenberg
Mr. and Mrs. Walter Eisenberg
Robert H. Ellsworth Limited
Field Museum of Natural History, Chicago
Istituto Italiano per il Medio e Estremo Oriente (ISMEO), Rome
Kreitman Gallery, Los Angeles
Neil Kreitman, Los Angeles
Los Angeles County Museum of Art
Metropolitan Museum of Art, New York
University of Michigan Museum of Anthropology
Musée Guimet, Paris
Museo Nazionale d'Arte Orientale, Rome
Museum für Volkerkunde, Vienna
National Museum of American Art, Smithsonian Institution
National Museum, New Delhi
Navin Kumar Inc. , New York
William Rockhill Nelson Gallery and Atkins Museum of Fine Arts, Kansas City, Missouri
The Newark Museum
Österreichisches Museum für Angewandte Kunst, Vienna
Pacific Asia Museum, Pasadena
Michael Phillips
Mr. and Mrs. Robert L. Poster
Mrs. John D. Rockefeller 3rd
The St. Louis Art Museum
Shey Art Collection
Jerry Solomon, Los Angeles
Marie-Hélène and Guy Weill
Doris Wiener Gallery, New York
and
Four private collections

The Silk Route and The Diamond Path

Esoteric Buddhist Art on the Trans-Himalayan Trade Routes

Published
under the sponsorship
of the
UCLA Art Council

Deborah E. Klimburg-Salter

Essays by

Maximilian Klimburg

David L. Snellgrove

Fritz Staal

Michel Strickmann

Chögyam Trungpa, Rinpoche

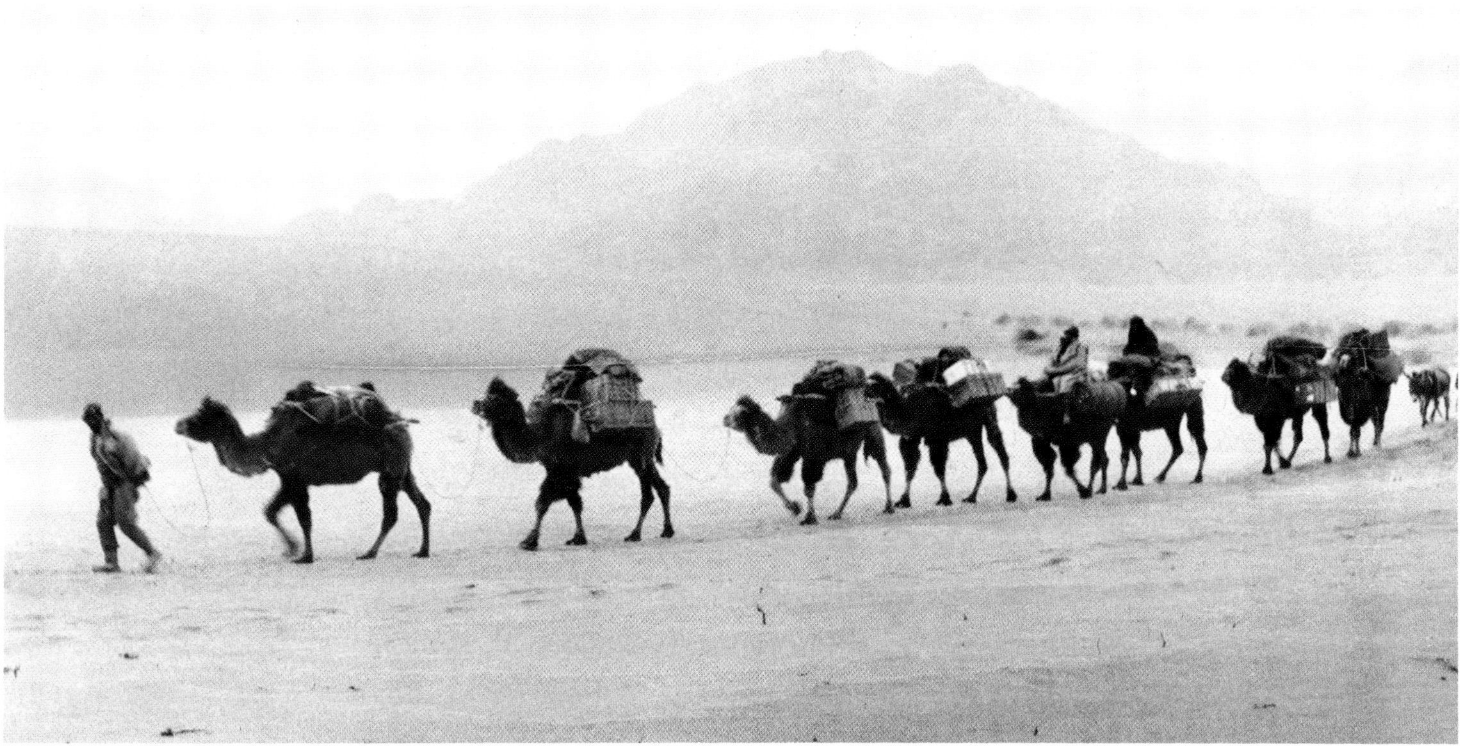

The exhibition, THE SILK ROUTE AND THE DIAMOND PATH, has been supported by a grant from the National Endowment for the Arts and the National Endowment for the Humanities, Washington, D.C., federal agencies created by an Act of Congress, 1963.

Cover: detail from Pl. 62
Frontispiece: Pl. 84, page 172

Camel Caravan
Alashan Desert
Inner Mongolia, China
Frederick Roelker Wulsin, 1923
Courtesy Peabody Museum, Harvard

Exhibition dates

Frederick S. Wight Art Gallery
University of California, Los Angeles
November 7, 1982 — January 2, 1983

Asia Society Gallery
New York City, New York
February 6 — April 3, 1983

National Museum of Natural History
National Museum of Man
Smithsonian Institution
Washington, D.C.
April 28 — June 30, 1983

Library of Congress Catalogue Card Number 82-620035
Printed in the United States of America

Contents

List of Plates 8
List of Figures 10
Foreword 11
Preface 12
Editor's Note 14

Section One—Introductory Essays

I. Introduction: The Art of the Western Himalaya in Historical Perspective 18

II. The Setting: The Western Trans-Himalayan Crossroads 24
Maximilian Klimburg

III. The Himalayas and the Fall of Religion 38
Frits Staal

IV. India in the Chinese Looking-Glass 52
Michel Strickmann

V. Buddhism in North India and the Western Himalayas — Seventh to Thirteenth Centuries 64
David L. Snellgrove

Section Two—Art and Ritual

VI. Esoteric Buddhist Art of the Western Himalayas 82

(a) The Early Phase: Northwest India — Seventh to Tenth Centuries 82
Catalogue: Entries 1–45 91

(b) Reflections from along the Silk Route — Seventh to Tenth Centuries 112
Catalogue: Entries 46–77 120
With entries by Chhaya Bhattacharya (nos. 55, 57, 58, 62–67 and 71–77) and Roderick Whitfield (nos. 56 and 69)

(c) Monastic Art of the Western Trans-Himalayas — Seventh to Seventeenth Centuries 152
Conservation Work at Ta-Pho Monastery — R. Sengupta 168
Catalogue: Entries 78–127 169

(d) Epilogue: Vajrayāna Ritual and Art, a Contemporary Example 205
Catalogue: Entries 128–140 209

VII. Sacred Outlook: The Vajrayoginī Shrine and Practice — *Chögyam Trungpa, Rinpoche* 226

Glossary of Sanskrit and Other Names and Terms 243
Bibliography 245

List of Plates

The plates have been arranged in four parts. The sequence varies in some instances because of printing considerations.

Part I. This section follows page 90.

1 Reliquary *Stūpa,* Gandhāra; undetermined date
2 Buddha Śākyamuni, Kāpiśa, Afghanistan; 6th century
3 Buddha Śākyamuni, Sahri Bahlol, Pakistan; 6th–7th century
4 Buddha Plaque, Afghanistan; 6th–7th century
5 Buddha, Pakistan; 7th century
6 Seated Buddha, Afghanistan or Pakistan; 9th century
7 Buddha with Female Attendants, Swat Valley; 7th–8th century
8 Seated Buddha, Pakistan; 9th century
9 Jeweled Śākyamuni (The Consecration of Śākyamuni), Northern Pakistan; 8th–early 9th century
10 Buddha Akṣobhya, North Pakistan; 8th century
11 Vairocana, Northern Pakistan; 9th century
12 Maitreya, Pakistan; 5th–6th century
13 Avalokiteśvara or Padmapāni, Northern Pakistan; 7th–8th century
14 Seated Maitreya, Pakistan; 7th century
15 Avalokiteśvara, Pakistan; 7th–8th century
16 Detail of Pl. 56 Iconographical Painting, Dunhuang, Qianfodong; 7th–8th century
17 Seated Bodhisattva, Swat Valley; 7th–8th century
18 Four-armed Brahmā, Swat Valley; 7th century
19 Vajradharma Lokeśvara, Swat Valley; 9th century
20 Hayagriva Lokeśvara, Swat Valley; 8th–9th century
21 Sūrya, Pakistan; 7th century
22 Face from *Liṅga,* Afghanistan; 8th century
23 Mahiṣāsuramardinī, Afghanistan; 8th century
24 Ekamukha-*liṅga* (One-faced *Liṅga*), Pakistan; 9th century
25 Female Head, Afghanistan; 7th century
26 Mirror Handle, Kashmir; 8th century
27 Buddha, Kashmir; 10th–11th century
28 Seated Avalokiteśvara, Kashmir; 8th century
29 Arapacana Mañjuśrī, Kashmir; 11th century
30 Bodhisattva, Kashmir; 9th century
31 Six-armed Lokeśvara, Kashmir; 10th–11th century
32 Eleven-headed Avalokiteśvara (Ekadaśamukha), Kashmir; 10th century
33 Bhairava, Kashmir; 8th–9th century
34 Śaṃvara, Kashmir; 10th century
35 Vighnāntaka, Kashmir; 10th century
36 Yama or Yamāri, Kashmir; 10th century
37 Guhya-Mañjuvajra, Kashmir; 10th–11th century
38 Vajrasattva and Consort, Kashmir; 11th century
39 Sūrya, Kashmir; 8th century
40 *Ekamukha-liṅga (One-faced Liṅga)*, Kashmir; 7th–8th century
41 Umā-Maheśvara, Kashmir; 7th–8th century
42 Durgā Mahiśāsuramardini, Kashmir; 8th century
43 Parvati, Kashmir; 8th century
44 Female Head, Northwest India; 7th century
45 Male Head, Northwest India; 7th–8th century

Part II. This section follows page 119.

46 Three Heads; Kizil (Turfan); 625–650 A.D.
47 Assembly Listening to the Buddha Preaching, Kizil (Turfan); 625–650 A.D.
48 Standing Monk in Patched Robe; Group of Heavenly Attendants; Kizil (Turfan), 625–650 A.D.
49 Hermit in Cave, Kizil (Turfan); 625–650 A.D.
50 Head of Devatā, Kizil (Turfan); 625–650 A.D.
51 Central Asian Male Head, Kucha; 6th–7th century
52 Central Asian Female Head, Kucha; 6th–7th century
53 Finial with Nine Buddhas, Central Asia; 6th–7th century
54 Traveling Shrine, Central Asia; 9th century
55 Buddha, Dunhuang, Qianfodong; 7th–8th century
56 Iconographic Painting/Representations of Famous Buddha Images, Dunhuang; 8th century
57 Copies of Buddha and Bodhisattva Images from India, Dunhuang; 7th–8th century
58 Mañjuśrī, Dunhuang; 9th–10th century
59 Vaiśravana, Dunhuang; 9th–10th century
60 Indra, Dunhuang; 9th century
61 Maṇḍala of Avalokitésvara (Guanyin), Dunhuang; 10th century
62 and
63 Fragment of a Maṇḍala with Bodhisattva Figures, Dunhuang; 8th–9th century
64 and
65 "Child-Protecting" Maṇḍala, Dunhuang; 8th–9th century
66 Deity with Five Buddhas on Crown, Dunhuang; 8th–9th century
67 Deity with Five Buddhas on Crown, Dunhuang; 8th–9th century
68 Maṇḍala of the Five Jinas (The Five Buddhas), Dunhuang; 9th century
69 The Five Dhyāni Buddhas, Dunhuang; 9th century
70 Amoghapāśa, Dunhuang; 9th century
71 Two Buddha Figures, Dunhuang; 7th–8th century
72 Maṇḍala with Healing Scene, Dunhuang; 9th–10th century
73 Diagram for Maṇḍala of Uṣṇīṣavijayā, Dunhuang; 9th–10th century

74 Bodhisattva Padmapāni, Dunhuang; 8th century
75 Mudrās of the Thousand-armed Avalokiteśvara, Dunhuang; 8th–9th century
76 Avalokiteśvara, Dunhuang; 7th–8th century
77 Riders on Horse and Yak, Karakhoto; 11th–12th century

Part III. This section follows page 168.

78 Head of a Divinity, Himachal Pradesh; 8th–9th century
79 Head of a God, Himachal Pradesh/Masrur, Kangra; 8th century
80 Chörten, West Tibet; 13th century
81 Seated Buddha, Western Himalayas; 10th–11th century
82 Buddha, Western Himalayas, perhaps Ladakh; 12th–13th century
83 Amoghasiddhi, Ladakh or Northern Pakistan; ca. 10th century
84 Ratnasaṃbhava, West Tibet; 13th–14th century
85 Amitābha, Lahul, Kyelong Monastery; 10th century
86 Wood Crown, Tibet; 13th–14th century
87 Wood Crown, Tibet; 13th–14th century
88 Avalokiteśvara, Western Himalayas or Kashmir; 8th century
89 Avalokiteśvara, West Tibet (Kashmir style) or Western Himalayas; 10th–11th century
90 Standing Mañjuśrī on Lion Throne, Western Himalayas; 11th–12th century
91 Bodhisattva, West Tibet; 13th century
92 Bodhisattva Vajrapāṇi, Western Trans-Himalayas; 11th–12th century
93 Mañjuśrī with Inscription, Central or Southwest Tibet; 13th century
94 Eleven-headed Avalokiteśvara, Tibet; ca. 8th century
95 Eleven-headed Avalokiteśvara, or Unidentified Bōn Deity, Western Trans-Himalaya; 11th–12th century
96 Dhanadā-Tārā, Himachal Pradesh; 9th–10th century
97 Usnīsavijayā, Spiti; 10th–11th century
98 Vajrakīla, Western Trans-Himalaya; 11th century
99 Kālacakra and Consort, (Spiti/Guge?) Western Himalayas; 11th century
100 Padmasambhava, West Tibet; 14th century
101 Prajñāpāramitā Manuscript, p. 56, T 'oling; 11th century
102 Prajñāpāramitā Manuscript, p. 36 of Vol. "gam," T'oling; 11th century
103,103a, 103b Kālacakra-tantra Manuscript, West Tibet; 14th century
104 Vajradhara Manuscript Cover, West Tibet; 14th century
105 Fragment of Wall Painting, Luk Monastery, West Tibet; 14th century
106 Fragment of Wall Painting, Luk Monastery, West Tibet; 14th century
107 Fragment of Wall Painting, Luk Monastery, West Tibet; 14th century
108 Vairocana, Spiti, Po Monastery, Himachal Pradesh (T'angka); 13th century
109 Buddha Ratnasaṃbhava, Western Trans-Himalaya; 12th century
110 Vajrasattva and Consort, Western Trans-Himalaya; 12th century
111 Śaṃvara and Prajñā, Western Trans-Himalaya; 13th century
112 Vajravārāhī (the Adamantine Sow), Western Trans-Himalaya; 13th century
113 Vairocana, Western Trans-Himalaya; 15th century
114 Vajrayoginī, West Tibet or Tibet; 14th century
115 Ma-chik Drönma, West Tibet or Tibet; 14th century
116 Stūpa t'sa t'sa, Ladakh; data undetermined
117 T'sa-t'sa Śākyamuni with Attendants, Ladakh; date undetermined
118 T'sa T'sa Cakraśaṃvara, Ladakh; date undetermined
119 Buddha, Ladakh (Lamayuru) Western Trans-Himalaya; 15th century
120 Buddha, West Tibet; 15th century
121 Śākymuni, Luk Monastery, West Tibet; 16th century
122 Lokeśvara, T'saparang Style; West Tibet; 14th–15th century
123 Padmasaṃbhava, Tibet; 17th century
124 Guardian Deity, Ladakh; 16th century
125 Maṇḍala of Kurukullā, Ngor Monastery, Tsang, Tibet; 16th century
126 Kālacakra Maṇḍala, Tibet; 16th century
127 The Kingdom of Shambala, Tibet; 17th–18th century

Part IV. This section follows page 208.

128 Vajrayoginī, Tibet; 19th century
129 Offering Bowls, Tibet; 19th century or earlier
130 Pair of Wall Hangings, Monastery in Lhasa; 18th–19th century
131 Skull Cup with Stand and Lid, Tibet; 19th century or earlier
132 Skull-shaped Cup with Cover, Eastern Tibet; 19th century or earlier
133 Offering Bowls, Eastern Tibet; 19th century
134 Bell and rDor-je, Tibet; 19th century
135 Five Butter Lamps, Eastern Tibet; 19th century or earlier
136 Set of Seven Offering Bowls, Tibet; 20th century
137 Set of Two Butter Lamps, Tibet; 20th century
138 Bell and rDor-je with Carrying Case, Tibet; 20th century
139 Altar Table; Vajrayoginī Maṇḍala, Tibet, 20th century
140 Chopper, Tibet; 19th century

List of Figures

Lists of maps, plans, illustrations, and a diagram also appear at the end of this list. The sequence of page numbers varies in some instances because of printing considerations.

1. The Indus Valley between Kandai and Besham, Pakistan *20*
2. Standing Buddha, rock engraving above Skyok River *20*
3. *Stūpas,* rock engraving near Chilas, Indus Valley *21*
4. Standing Buddha, rock sculpture at Nanpur near Gilgit *22*
5. Seated Buddha, rock sculpture at Shakorai, Swat Valley; 7th-8th century *22*
6. Jewelled Buddha, rock engravings near Chilas *29*
6a. Rock engravings of Tiger Jātaka near Chilas *30*
7. Bardun Gompa Monastery, Zangskar *130*
7a. Chemre Monastery, Ladakh *41*
8. Fire Ceremony, Zangskar *48*
9. Reliquary *Stūpa,* Peshawar Museum, Pakistan *54*
10. Cave temple (2nd century B.C.) *stūpa,* Bhaja *65*
11. *Stūpa* cave temple, Bhaja *65*
12. A freestanding *stūpa,* identified with one built by Kuṣāṇa Emperor Kaniska, Sani; 1st–2nd centuries A.D. *66*
13. Image of Buddha preaching, identifiable as Buddha Vairocana; before 13th–14th centuries *67*
14. Śākyamuni Buddha wall painting, Lhakhang Soma, Alchi, 12th–13th centuries *69*
15. One of 16 wall paintings, Sani Monastery, Zangskar; probably 17th century *69*
16. Rock carving of Bodhisattva Maitreya, Mulbek Ladakh; 9th century *70*
17. Wall painting of Bodhisattva Maitreya, Lhakhang Soma, Alchi; 12th–13th centuries *70*
18. Portrait of Rin-chen bZang-po in the "Translator's Temple," Alchi; probably 13th century *72*
19. Ruins of Nyar-ma Monastery, Ladakh; founded 1000 A.D. *72*
20. Alchi Monastery, Ladakh; second half of 11th century *73*
20a. Facade, Sum-tsek Chapel, Alchi *73*
21. Image of Bodhisattva Avalokiteśvara, Sum-tsek Temple, Alchi; 12th century *74*
21a. Image of Maitreya, Sum-tsek Temple, Alchi; 12th century *74*
22. Wall painting, Maṇḍala of Sarvavid Vairocana, Sum-tsek Temple, Alchi; 12th century *75*
23. Wall painting, Vairocana Maṇḍala in the *'du-khang* at Alchi, 12th century *75*
24. Rock carving of the Five Buddhas near Shey, Ladakh; prior to 10th century *76*
25. Images of Nāropa with Buddha Vajradhara behind him, Dzong-khul, Zangskar *79*
26. Mural of Atīśa and Padmasaṃbhava, Lhakhang Soma, Alchi; probably 13th century *80*
27. Maitreya, Cave "K," Bāmiyān, Afghanistan *85*
28. 38 meter Buddha donor figures, Bāmiyān *28*
29. Niche "E" Bodhisattva, Bāmiyān *87*
30. Gilgit manuscript covers, Institute for Central Asian Studies, Srinagar, Kashmir *88*
31. Gilgit manuscript covers, Institute for Central Asian Studies, Srinagar, Kashmir *88*
32. Gilgit manuscript covers; the Bodhisattva blessing a donor *88*
33. Gilgit manuscript covers; two Sāhī donors kneel before a Bodhisattva *88*
34. Central Asian ruins *112*
35. Central Asian caravan *113*
36. Bust of Śiva, Karakhoto, Fogg Museum *113*
37. Sculpture of Buddha, Karakhoto, Fogg Museum *114*
38. Sculpture of Bodhisattva, Karakhoto, Fogg Museum *114*
39. Sculpture of guardian figure, Karakhoto, Fogg Museum *115*
40. Drawing from Hatt Chörten, Newark Museum *115*
40a. Drawing from Hatt Chörten, Newark Museum *116*
41. Wall painting of Buddha, *'du-khang,* Ta-pho *116*
42. Clay sculptures after earthquake, *'du-khang* apse, Ta-pho *117*
43. Clay sculpture, *'du-khang* apse, Ta-pho *117*
44. Lamayuru Monastery, Ladakh *118*
45. Wall painting, Lhakhang, Soma, Alchi; 12th–13th centuries *118*
46. Wall painting of crowned Buddha, Alchi *153*
47. *'Du-khang,* Sarvavid Vairocana, sculpture, Ta-pho *155*
48. *'Du-khang,* sculpture, Ta-pho *155*
49. *'Du-khang,* sculpture, Ta-pho *156*
50. *Chos-'khor,* Ta-pho *157*
51. Wall painting, *mgon-khang,* Ta-pho *158*
52. Masks, *mgon-khang,* Ta-pho *159*
53. *'Du-khang,* Ta-pho *160*
54. Wall painting, *'du-khang,* Ta-pho *160*
54a. Wall painting, *'du-khang,* legend of Sudhana, Ta-pho *161*
55. Wall painting, *'du-khang,* Jātaka story, Ta-pho *161*
56. Sculpture of guardian statue, *'du-khang,* Ta-pho *161*
57. Sculpture of Amitābha, *'du-khang,* Ta-pho *162*
58. Wall painting, blue Bodhisattva, *'du-khang* ambulatory, Ta-pho *162*
59. Wall painting, green Bodhisattva, *'du-khang* ambulatory, Ta-pho *163*
60. Buddha, Foladi, Afghanistan *163*
61. Performance of *Vajrayoginī Sādhana, Rumtek Monastery, Sikkim* *231*
62. Chögyam Trungpa, Rinpoche, performing initiation of Vajrayoginī *232*
63. *Vajrayoginī Sādhana* practitioners, Dorje Dzong, Boulder, Colorado *233*

Diagram

1. Construction and repair of sculpture, *'du-khang,* Ta-pho *159*

Illustrations

1. 38 meter Buddha, Pāñcavarṣika, Bāmiyān *23*
2. Five-Buddha Families Diagram *70*
3. Vajrayoginī *234*
4. Shrine of Vajrayoginī *237*

Maps

1. The Western Trans-Himalaya and Surrounding Regions *16–17*
2. Historical Northwest India *26*
3. Central Asia *33*
4. The Western Trans-Himalaya *35*

Plans

1. Ta-pho Monastery *158*
1a. *'Du-khang,* Ta-pho Monastery *159*
2. Alchi Monastery Complex *166*

Foreword

This book-catalogue has been published on the occasion of the exhibition *THE SILK ROUTE AND THE DIAMOND PATH: ESOTERIC BUDDHIST ART ON THE TRANS-HIMALAYAN TRADE ROUTES* for the UCLA Frederick S. Wight Art Gallery through the generosity of the UCLA Art Council.

Approximately three years ago the project's curator, Dr. Deborah Klimburg-Salter, and I introduced her project to the UCLA Art Council with the intent that it be their annual exhibition for 1982. With the Art Council's financial contribution and much needed support, both the National Endowment for the Arts and the National Endowment for the Humanities were persuaded to fund the planning and also the implementation stages of the exhibition. We would also like to thank the Smithsonian Foreign Currency Program for providing travel funds to visiting Indian scholars, and the Hyatt Corporation for their generous contribution.

This is the first major exhibition of Vajrayāna art from the western Himalayas to be organized. We are confident that it will open avenues of research and provide opportunities for a later generation of scholars on the subject.

We are honored that two distinguished American institutions are participating with us and we wish to thank Alan Wardwell, Director, Asia House Gallery, New York City; Paul N. Perrot, Assistant Secretary for Museum Programs; and Gene Behlen, Chief, Office of Exhibits, National Museum of Natural History, Smithsonian Institution, Washington, D.C. For his support of the idea we also thank Charles Blitzer, Assistant Secretary for History and Art at the Smithsonian Institution.

We are grateful to Ted M. G. Tanen, American Executive Director, Indo-U.S. Subcommission on Education and Culture, for providing invaluable assistance in negotiating the loans from the National Museum in New Delhi, as well as financial support; to His Excellency, Ambassador K. B. Narayanan, Indian Embassy, Washington, D.C.; and to the Honorable Ishrat Aziz, Consul General, Consulate General of India, San Francisco.

We are deeply indebted to Dr. Elwin V. Svenson, Vice-Chancellor, Institutional Relations, UCLA, for his continued advice and support, and also to Dr. Robert H. Gray, Dean of the College of Fine Arts, UCLA and his staff for their many and varied contributions to the administrative management of the project.

As the Acting Director of the Frederick S. Wight Art Gallery during the planning and production of this project, I want to thank Dr. Klimburg-Salter for bringing an unusual, stimulating, and exciting exhibition to our campus and sharing with us her knowledge and expertise on the subject.

The 140 objects in the exhibition came from 37 institutions and private lenders from Europe, Asia, and the United States. Without the involvement and assistance of all these individuals and organizations this project could not have been initiated and carried to completion. We want to express our thanks to all.

Jack Carter
Project Director

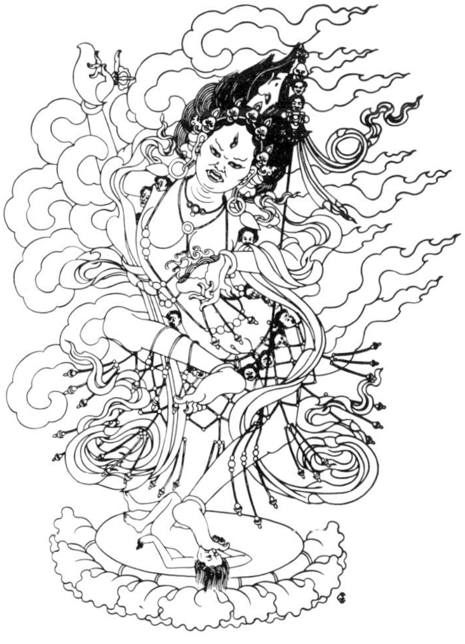

Preface

It is our intention in this exhibition and catalogue to suggest theoretical perspectives for the study of the Buddhist arts of the western Himalayas and, through the collaborative efforts of scholars in different disciplines, to place the arts within their historical, ideological, and aesthetic contexts. The title of the exhibition, *The Silk Route and the Diamond Path,* may be thought to imply an emphasis on Central Asia. But as the subtitle, *Esoteric Buddhist Art on the Trans-Himalayan Trade Routes* indicates, the focus of this study is the monastic art that developed along the trade routes which traversed the Himalayas connecting ancient northwest India and the western Himalayas with Central Asia. It is not our intention, nor indeed would it have been possible, to present a comprehensive survey of the Buddhist arts of Central Asia, northern India, or even the western Himalayas. The scope of the material is too vast, on the one hand, and our knowledge concerning its origins and development is too limited, on the other. The available archaeological record furnishes only a fragment of the great artistic treasures produced during this period; furthermore, the extant scholarship on mediaeval Buddhism and history provides us with insufficient documentation. The basic questions of provenance, chronology, and iconography must first be resolved before undertaking critical studies of the culture. This exhibition and study seek to further these goals.

It is indeed in order to advance this preliminary research that the present volume presents a variety of viewpoints derived from different disciplines and stemming from different cultural perspectives. The fascination and difficulty of the study of the arts of the western Himalayas result precisely from the rich interweave of cultural elements derived from China, Tibet, and Iran into the fabric of Indian Buddhist culture. Thus, the study of the arts of India's Inner Asian frontiers ultimately depends on a knowledge not only of Indian artistic traditions but also of those other arts and cultures with which the Buddhist arts interacted during the long period discussed here.

This study presents a variety of methods as well as viewpoints. Hopefully, it will provoke scholarly debate and lead to diverse directions for future study; and carry forward the proposed method for the study of the arts of the Trans-Himalaya as a regional historical phenomenon. Thus Dr. Maximilian Klimburg has analyzed the geographic and ethnographic settings and described the network of trade routes during relevant historical periods. Professor Frits Staal's essay deals with aspects of culture and philosophy in the western Himalayas, ranging from the Vedic to the contemporary periods within this region. Professor Michel Strickmann reviews the important cultural counterpoint provided by Chinese Buddhism. Professor David L. Snellgrove discusses Indo-Tibetan Buddhism in the western Himalayas, from its Indian roots up to the thirteenth century. The Ven. Vajracarya, Chögyam Trungpa, Rinpoche, explains the contemporary approach to and practice of Vajrayāna Buddhism in the west, from the perspective of his traditional Tibetan training.

The idea of the exhibit evolved during planning sessions with Professor Frits Staal and Professor Lewis Lancaster for an interdisciplinary symposium at the University of California, Berkeley, which was intended to explore the cultural interaction between northern India, the western Himalayas, and Central Asia. Both scholars also served as project consultants and I am grateful for their initial support and continued advice. During this early stage Dr. Pratapaditya Pal, Los Angeles County Museum of Art, also acted as a consultant and provided encouragement and useful suggestions, including the evocative title of the exhibition.

These scholarly explorations would have remained in the realm of discussion alone, however, had it not been for the active support and encouragement of Professor Jack B. Carter, then Acting Associate Director of the Frederick S. Wight Art Gallery, UCLA and the UCLA Art Council, particularly Mrs. Judy Riley, President; Mrs. Arlette Crandall, Vice President; Ms. Linda Brownridge, Docents Chairman; Mrs. Judith Murphy, Exhibitions Chairman; and Mrs. Nancy Berger, Past President. Thanks to the initial grant from the UCLA Art Council, I was able to travel to major collections in Europe and Asia, and consult with curators and scholars.

There is a special sense of adventure and commitment on the part of those who study and collect Vajrayāna art, in particular the little-known early arts of the western Himalayas. As a result, discussions with curators and collectors invariably led to new insights, which eventually found their way into this study. In particular I should like to thank Dr. Chhaya Bhattacharya of the National Museum, New Delhi, my companion in field research, who also wrote the entries (Nos. 55, 57, 58, 62–67, and 71–77) for the objects from the National Museum, New Delhi; Dr. S. P. Gupta, Curator, Central Asian Department, National Museum, New Delhi; Dr. Donatello Mazzeo, Director of the National Museum of Oriental Art, Rome; Professor John Rosenfield, Acting Director, Fogg Art Museum; David Kamansky, Director of the Pacific Asia Museum; Alan Wardwell, Director and Sarah Bradley, Assistant Director, The Asia Society Gallery; Dr. Robert Mowry, Curator, John D. Rockefeller 3rd Collection; Madame Krishna Riboud, Dr. Robert Jéra Bezard, and Gilles Béguin of the Musée Guimet; Martin Lerner, Curator of Indian and Southeast Asian Art, Metropolitan Museum of Art; Stan Czuma, Curator of Indian and Southeast Asian Art, The Cleveland Museum of Art; Valrae Reynolds, Curator of Oriental Collections, The Newark Museum; A. H. N. Verwey, National Museum of Ethnology, Leiden; and from the British Museum Dr. Wladimir Zwalf, Curator Indian Section, and Dr. Roderick Whitfield, Assistant Keeper, Oriental Antiquities, who wrote the entries (Nos. 56 and 69) for the Dunhuang objects from the British Museum Collections; Dr. Alfred Janata and Professor Dr. Hans Manndorff, Director, Museum für Volkerkunde, Vienna; and Professor Dr. Herbert Fux, Director, Österreichisches Museum für Angewandte Kunst, Vienna. We should also like to acknowledge the contributions of other scholars who assisted us: Hugh Richardson, Dr. Tadeuz Skorupski, Professor Martin Powers, Professor John Huntington, Professor Marilyn Rhie and Professor Akira Fujieda. We also would like to thank Richard Ravenal, Navin and Vinit Kumar, Doris Wiener, Robert Ellsworth, Tom and Margo Pritzker, and particularly Neil Kreitman, who generously shared his knowledge of the arts at every stage of this exhibition.

An exhibition and book that sought to bring together masterworks of Indian, Chinese, and Tibetan inspiration from some of the great collections of Europe, Asia, and the United States—and to present these within a meaningful historical context—would have been a difficult task under any circumstances. For a small university art galley it was indeed formidable. This project never could have been accomplished without the support and encouragement of Dean Robert Gray, Dean of the College of Fine Arts, UCLA and the "team" he provided, particularly: Dr. Sarah Handler, Assistant Curator, who at the last minute generously consented to coordinate the symposium held at UCLA on the occasion of the opening of the exhibition; Mrs. Etsu Garfias, Administrative Assistant, who graciously worked countless long hours whenever needed and at whatever task was necessary; and Glynn Davies, Fiscal Officer. Greatly appreciated was the unflagging enthusiasm of the students who worked as Research Assistants and Museum Interns—Molly Alexander, Elizabeth Goldblatt, Chandra Reedy, Elsie Ritchie, Audrey Spiro, and Vickie Lockwood Joralemon, who from the very inception of the project was tireless in her efforts to assist us in fulfilling our goals.

The audiovisual and graphic components of the exhibition were prepared under the direction of Dr. Maximilian Klimburg; the maps were compiled by him and drawn by Mrs. Roberta Roberts. We should also like to thank Anthony W. Scott and Ramesh Sharma for their assistance on the film which Dr. Klimburg, with the assistance of Nina Toumanoff, prepared for the exhibit. In addition to this exhibition staff, the permanent Gallery staff, and in particular Jan Keller, always provided cheerful assistance. I should also like to thank Robert Woolard, Anne Bomeisler Farrell, and Dr. Charles Speroni, Dean Emeritus of the College of Fine Arts.

The realization of this exhibition also owes much to the patient assistance of the Indo-U.S. Subcommission, particularly Ted Tanen. In addition, I should like to thank the Government of India; I. D. Mathur, Assistant Director of the National Museum, New Delhi; Dr. Kapila Vatsyayana, Joint Educational Advisor, Department of Culture; and Mrs. Pupul Jayakar for their support.

This study derives not only from the several decades of field research conducted by my husband, Dr. Maximilian Klimburg and myself, but also from many fruitful discussions and seminars held in the UCLA Department of Art with consultants Klimburg, Professor Timothy Earle, and Professor Shiva Bajpai. As a result of these seminars a number of students made important contributions to the catalogue: Elizabeth Goldblatt (page 225) in the field of ethno-musicology, who also recorded in Rumtek Monastery, Sikkim, the liturgy of Vajrayoginī used in the exhibition: in the fields of art history and archaeology, Molly Alexander (no. 24); Eve Dambra (no. 3); Barbara Paulson (no. 7); Chandra Reedy (no. 75); Elsie Ritchie (no. 102); Cheryl Snell (no. 122); and Audrey Spiro (no. 179), who also researched a chronology for the Trans-Himalayan research project in consultation with Professor Shiva Bajpai.

The catalogue also benefited from the patience and expertise of Kim Lockard, Ruth Hoover, and Professor Jack Carter, who was responsible for the design of both the catalogue and the exhibit. Several friends and scholars read sections of the manuscript and I gratefully acknowledge their suggestions: Professor Don McCallum; Professor David Kunzle; Professor Hans-Peter Schmidt; Francine Farr; Jared Rhotan; Vickie Joralemon; Carolyn Gimian, who edited and coordinated both the essay by Chögyam Trungpa, Rinpoche and the construction of the Vajrayoginī Shrine used in the exhibition. I benefited from the substantial criticism of my husband, as well as from Professor Frits Staal and Professor Shiva Bajpai, who also consulted on other aspects of the project, and from Professor David L. Snellgrove, all of whom read large portions of the manuscript. As always in these cases, the errors that may remain despite their criticism are mine alone.

Archaeological field work has provided the basis for the study of the arts of the western Himalayas. During the past century, however, any scholar who has attempted this research has had to battle different bureaucracies in order to study sites of the same culture located even a relatively short distance from each other. These difficulties could never have been surmounted without the collaboration and scholarly commitment of colleagues in Afghanistan, Pakistan, and India. I should particularly like to acknowledge the generosity and enthusiasm of many friends in the Archaeological Survey of India (ASI) and the support of M. N. Deshpande, former Director General of Archaeology, and R. Sengupta, Director, Dept. of Conservation, who also contributed to this study. Since the nineteeth century it has been the role of the ASI to brave the hardships of these inaccessible regions in order to study and conserve the historical treasures of India. During the last two decades I visited ASI "camps" in Bāmiyān, Kashmir, Ladakh, and Himachal Pradesh, where Indian colleagues always provided much welcomed hospitality. I should also like to thank Mr. Bahn, Director of the Museum of the Institute of Central Asian Studies in Srinagar, and Mr. Sehrai, Director of the Peshawar Museum, for permission to photograph and publish photographs of objects in their collections.

In Afghanistan, during the years when field work and multinational collaboration were still possible, my husband and I benefited from the generosity of many friends, among them Dr. Rawan Ferhadi; Mr. and Mrs. A. A. Motamedi; Dr. Zemaryalai Tarzi; Dr. and Mrs. Chaibai Moustamandi; and Said Mohammad Dao'ud Eqbali Balkhi.

The Ven. Vajracarya Chögyam Trungpa, Rinpoche, contributed many essential components to this exhibit: above all, throughout my studies his teachings have provided access to the meaning and function of the sacred arts. I am also indebted to the Ven. Thartse Khenpo, Rinpoche, for his Tibetan translations and research and the many hours he spent with us explaining Buddhist texts. We are also grateful to H. H. Jetsun Kusho, who came to teach in the Drögon Sakya Center, Los Angeles, in 1981–82. Jared Rhotan, Columbia University, contributed to the catalogue in countless ways, particularly related to the Tibetan transcriptions, glossary, and some of the translations.

This study and the exhibition which it accompanies is only one part of an ongoing research project on the western Trans-Himalaya. Scholarly monographs, because of their very specialized nature, have only a limited audience. It has been my hope, through the more popular format of this exhibition, to promote more widespread appreciation for the unique cultural achievements of this region and thus to encourage not only further study but also international assistance in the preservation of the living cultures. It is not only a question of the massive investment necessary for the preservation of the artistic monuments but more importantly the preservation of these cultures—now threatened by the displacement and dislocation of many of the peoples of this region. The Afghan refugees are certainly among the most desperate of the many refugee groups. Less publicized is the present state of Tibetan culture. Substantial efforts are being made by the Indian government to assist the Tibetan refugees in their losing battle to preserve their cultural traditions while in exile. Also, there is the different problem of the culturally Tibetan population native to India in Ladakh and Himachal Pradesh, whose educational and religious institutions have decayed as a result of the separation from and destruction of the once great Buddhist centers in Tibet. The plight of these geographically isolated people is seldom acknowledged by the international community; yet the humanity and power of their arts, philosophy, and literature have reached far beyond the boundaries of their mountain home. Buddhist monuments and teachings (*dharma*) survive in many corners of the world, only one of which is the western Trans-Himalaya. But they are not merely relics suited only to antiquarian inquiry. For many, these monuments, material reflections of the Buddhist *dharma*, continue to inspire both a greater metaphysical vision and a practical approach to everyday life.

Deborah E. Klimburg-Salter
New Delhi, September 1982

Editor's Note

Buddhist names and terms appear here in transliteration from Sanskrit, Tibetan, or Chinese according to the context. It has not been possible to adopt a uniform system of orthography, due to the differences in sources and scholarly traditions as well as to the discrepancy between the spellings of place names in the premodern and modern periods. The transliteration systems employed here are intended to be both intelligible to the general reader and also readily understood by the specialist.

In the transcription of Tibetan words, which appear in italics, we have provided both a phonetic and a transliterated version; e.g., *chöd (gCod).* The first corresponds to present-day pronunciation in the standard Central Tibetan dialect, while our system of transliteration, given in parentheses, follows that adopted by the Vienna Congress of Orientalists and observed by Sarat Chandra Das in his *Tibetan-English Dictionary.* Exceptions will be noted in our substitution of *ṅa* for *ṅa, dza* for *dsa, ź̇a* for *sha,* ' for *ha,* and *śa* for *ca.* Popularized spellings of familiar names of people and places have been generally retained in Roman type; e.g., Milarepa, Ta-pho. In certain cases where the transliterated form of a historical name commonly appears in western literature, individual authors have retained their customary usage: *e.g.,* Rin-chen bzang-po for Rinchen Zangpo; Ye-śes 'Od for Yeshe Ö. Variations in the spellings of the most frequently used proper names are noted in the Glossary.

Sanskrit words have been transliterated throughout according to the system employed by M. Monier-Williams in his *Sanskrit-English Dictionary.* Our use of diacritical marks differs from his only in the case of two letters: *ś* for *ṡ;* and *ṣ* for *sh.* Words from foreign languages are transliterated according to their usage in Sanskrit, hence Śāhī. Popular spellings for modern place names have been retained; *e.g.,* Kashmir for Kāsmīra, Benares for Vārāṇasī, etc.

The transliteration of Chinese characters into the Latin alphabet follows the *pinyin* system. But in order to reduce confusion for the reader, the more familiar transliteration for well-known names and places is given in parentheses after the *pinyin* wherever the word first occurs in each chapter: hence Xuanzang (Hsüan Tsang); Faxian (Fa Hsien). Words frequently encountered in English, such as Tao, remain in their familiar form.

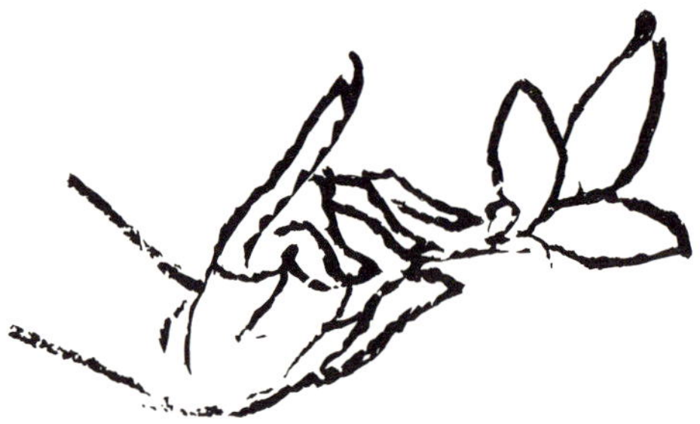

Section One

Introductory Essays

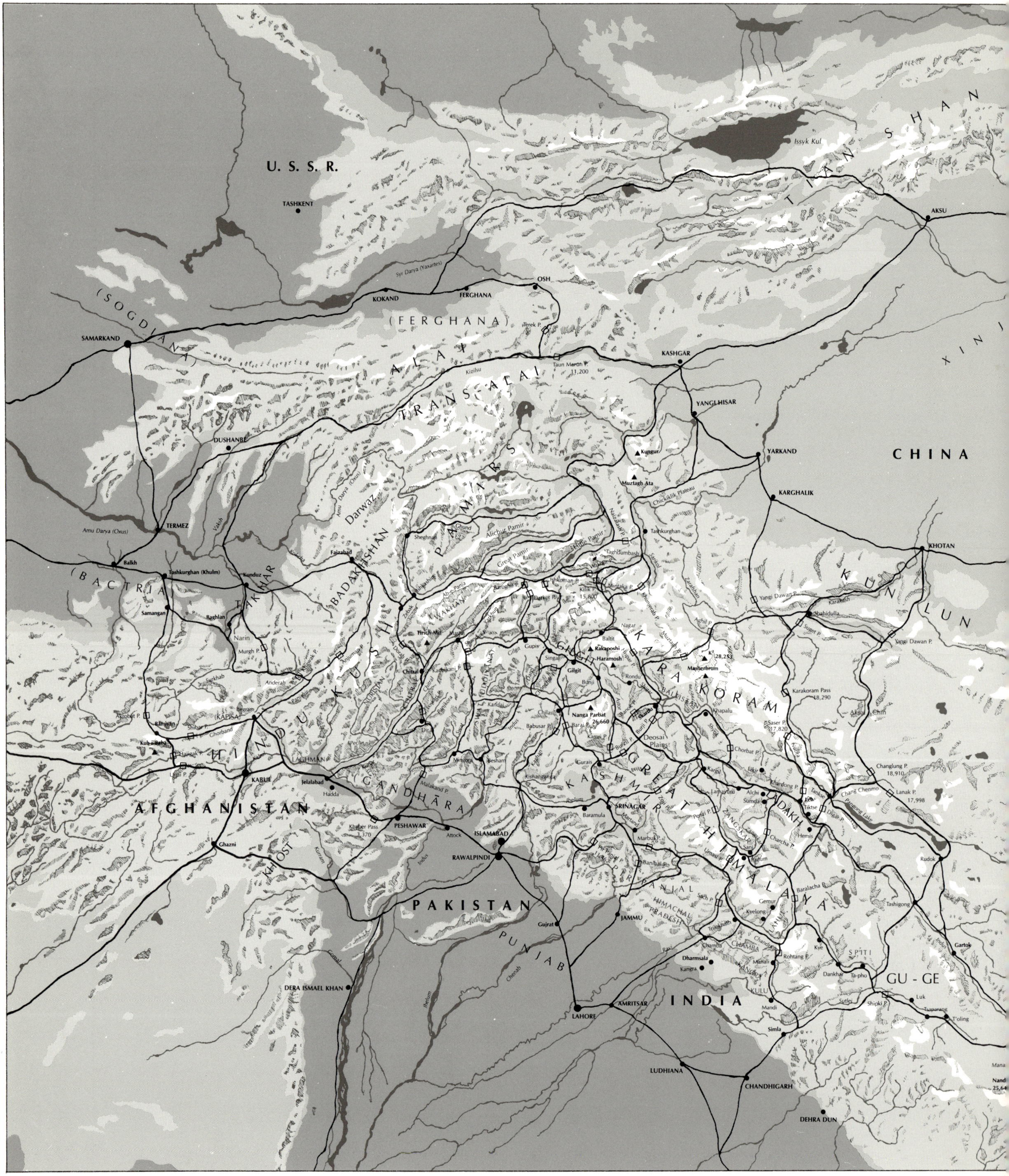
U. S. S. R.
TASHKENT
TIAN SHAN
Issyk Kul
AKSU
(SOGDIANA)
KOKAND
FERGHANA
OSH
(FERGHANA)
SAMARKAND
ALAI
TRANS-ALAI
KASHGAR
YANGI HISAR
YARKAND
CHINA
DUSHANBE
PAMIRS
KARGHALIK
TERMEZ
Amu Darya (Oxus)
KHOTAN
Balkh
Faizabad
(BACTRIA)
TAKHAR
BADAKHSHAN
KUN LUN
HINDU KUSH
KARAKORAM
Gilgit
Nanga Parbat
Karakoram Pass
KABUL
AFGHANISTAN
GANDHARA
KASHMIR
SRINAGAR
GREAT HIMALAYA
LADAKH
PESHAWAR
ISLAMABAD
RAWALPINDI
Ghazni
PAKISTAN
JAMMU
PUNJAB
Gujrat
DERA ISMAEL KHAN
LAHORE
AMRITSAR
INDIA
GU - GE
Simla
LUDHIANA
CHANDHIGARH
DEHRA DUN

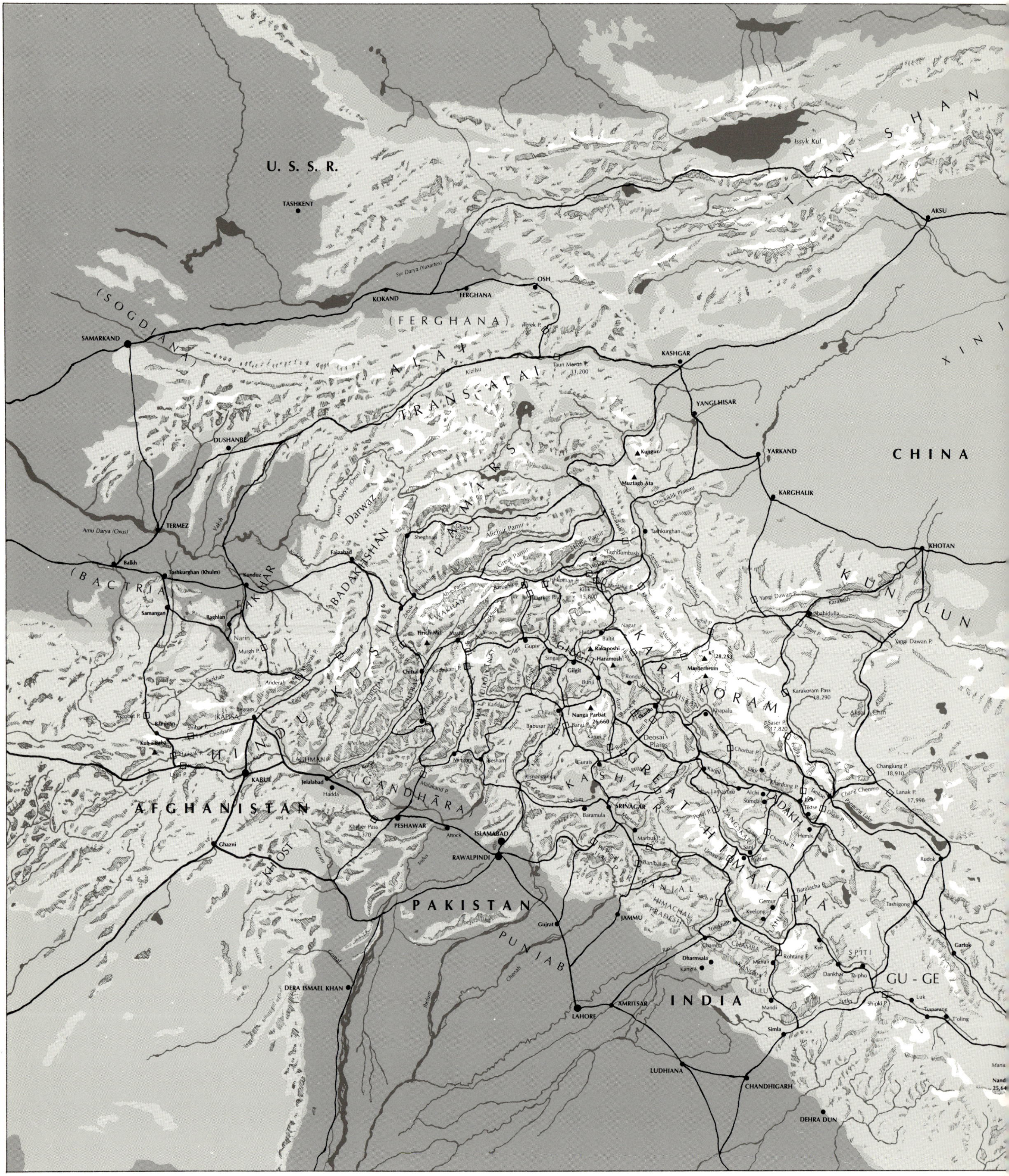

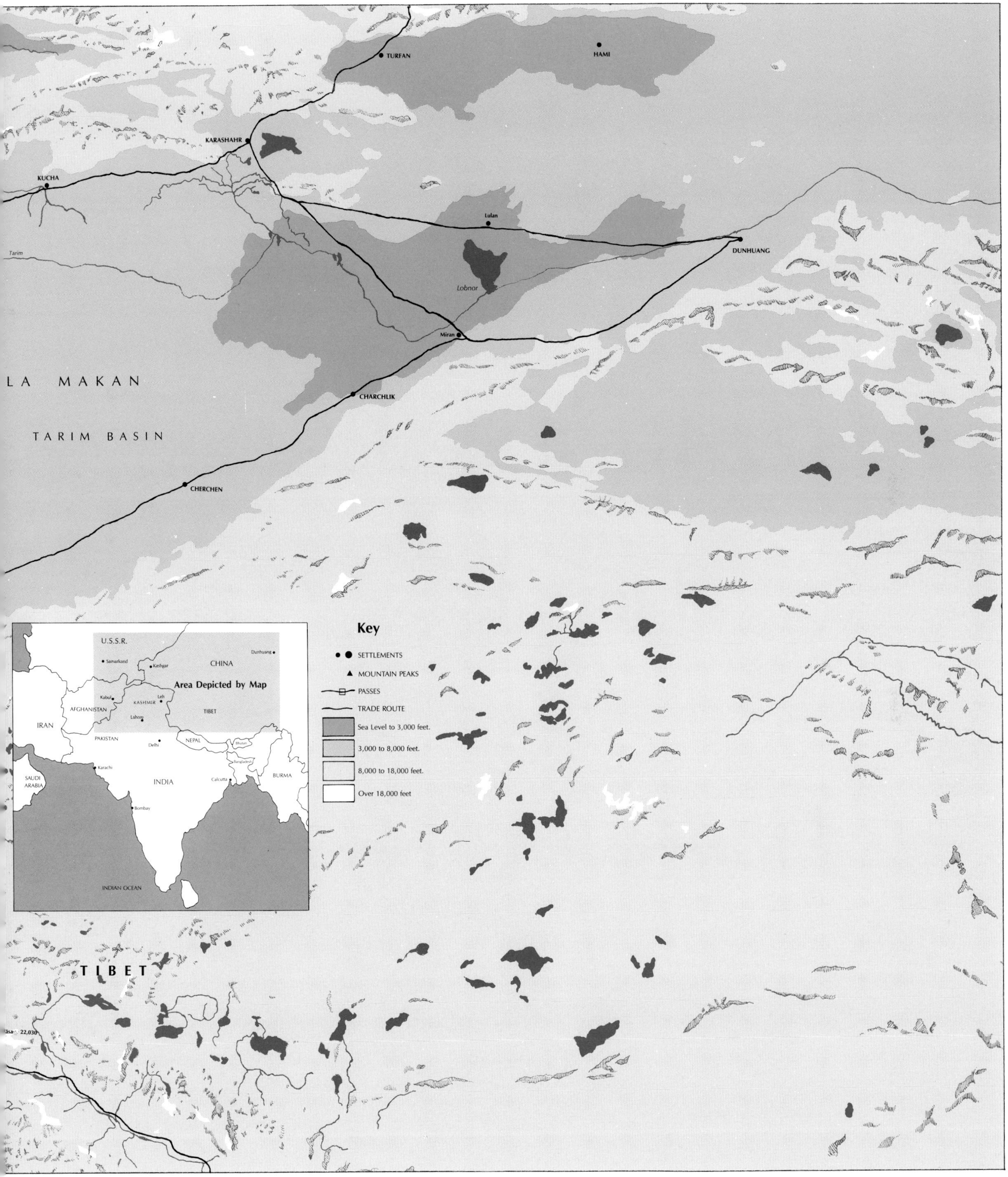

Map 1 The Western Trans-Himalaya and Surrounding Regions

1

Introduction:

The Art of the Western Himalayas in Historical Perspective

Deborah Klimburg-Salter

Four important cultures of the Asiatic mainland—the Indian, Chinese, Iranian, and Tibetan—converge in the Trans-Himalayan region; consequently, this area has played an important role in history. Extreme geographic conditions and ongoing strategic concerns have conspired to keep the region one of the last frontiers on earth. In almost every way it is a land of contrasts. Snow and ice-covered mountain peaks give way to vast uplands and deserts, interspersed with fertile valleys and oases, and the climate ranges between similar extremes. The population is also very diverse, belonging to several ethnic and linguistic groups.

Renewed political conflicts, the culmination of nineteenth-century geopolitical struggles, have again focused international attention on this little-known region (Fisher, Rose and Huttenback 1963: 5–10). Today the Trans-Himalaya may appear to be an inhospitable, isolated corner of the world, but in the first millennium A.D., when trade between the great civilizations of Asia flourished and the "silk routes" were important avenues of commerce, this region gave birth to distinctive artistic and intellectual achievements. In this heterogeneous environment Buddhism developed syncretic and esoteric features.

This is the first time an exhibition has focused on the distinctive art of the western Trans-Himalaya—an art that vividly reflects the varied lifestyles and cultural complexity of the area. By contrast, the arts of the central and eastern Himalayas (Tibet, Nepal, Sikkim, and Bhutan) have been the subject of several exhibitions and numerous studies. Even though this study focuses on the extreme northwest of the Indian subcontinent, that does not imply that this particular region has been preeminent in the development of Tantric Buddhist art. Rather, this emphasis has developed as a result of recent archaeological finds which stimulated the examination of the art within its cultural and historical contexts. The most significant development has occurred in the Trans-Himalayan region where the oldest, continuously-existing Buddhist monasteries in India have preserved later Mahayāna art within its original architectural settings for almost one thousand years. To relate the art of this region to other important centers of Esoteric Buddhist art would be the logical next phase of this inquiry.

The term "Trans-Himalaya" refers to the regions directly north of the Himalayan range. Elsewhere this term has been used to refer broadly to Central and Western Tibet (Tucci 1973:9). We have used the term "western Trans-Himalaya" to refer to the regions north of the western end of the great Himalayas: the Pamirs, Gilgit, Baltistan, Ladakh, and adjacent areas of Himachal Pradesh, and western Tibet (see Maps 1 and 3). The eastern boundary of this region is Mount Kailāsa, the source of the Indus River and the mythic home of the gods.

PREVIOUS STUDIES

Only recently has archaeological and scholarly research enabled us to understand the genesis and diversity of the art of the western Trans-Himalaya. Political changes in the region following World War II permitted increased exploration of the area; at the same time, interest in the translation and study of Vajrayāna Buddhist texts intensified. Some of the events that produced this burst of scholarly activity were: the exodus of an educated elite from Tibet after the Chinese takeover; the opening of Indian border regions to field study; the increased activity of the Archaeological Survey of India (see Sengupta); and, most recently, the Chinese government's willingness to allow foreigners to visit Chinese Central Asian sites.

Descriptions of the early mediaeval monasteries of the western Trans-Himalaya have come down to us in the travel accounts of the Chinese pilgrims and scholars who braved incredible hardships in order to visit these religious centers famous for their sacred relics and painted paradises (see Klimburg; also F. de Filippi 1934, C. Wessels 1924, and Petech 1952–56).

The extent of the artistic and philosophical genius of these cultures only became known at the beginning of the twentieth century as the result of archaeological exploration by a group of men from several nations. Most important among them was Sir Aurel Stein, born Hungarian, but later a subject of the "Queen-Empress" of England. The other leading explorers were Albert Grünwedel and Albert von Le Coq (Germany), Paul Pelliot (France), Sven Hedin (Sweden), Langdon Warner (U.S.A.), Count Otani (Japan), and Kozlov and Oldenburg (Russia). Although today some may choose to regard some of their activities as robbery or, at best, a great treasure hunt (Hopkirk 1980), these men and their contemporaries believed they had rescued the glories of past civilization from oblivion and eventual extinction. Moral and political estimates of their work may have changed, but the scholarly benefits of their investigations are beyond calculation. In fact, a fair percentage of the objects in this exhibition were acquired during expeditions by Stein (Pls. 55–77) and von Le Coq (Pls. 46–50). The study and publication of the texts and artistic monuments these men discovered have continued in Centers for Central Asian Studies in many countries, in particular, France, Germany, Great Britain, Japan, the Soviet Union, and China.

The research on Esoteric Buddhist art and philosophy of the western Trans-Himalaya has relied on these Central Asian documents and on mediaeval Buddhist scriptures preserved in monasteries throughout Asia (Strickmann 1977). In the western Trans-Himalaya, texts were discovered, edited, and analyzed as result of the early field work by Csoma de Körös, S. Chandra Das, and Francke (Ruegg 1978) in the nineteenth century. This work was followed by the pioneering studies of Giuseppe Tucci, and, more recently, David Snellgrove, while F. W. Thomas and Richardson (see bibliography) provided an historical framework for mediaeval Tibetan studies. Tucci's contribution to the study of historical northwest India is equally important and continues through the researches in Pakistan and Afghanistan of the institute he founded in Rome (ISMEO). The study of the art and culture of the western Trans-Himalaya has expanded rapidly in recent decades.

There were other kinds of scientific expeditions to both Central Asia and the Himalayas. Some of these expeditions, such as by Troll (Austrian) Pls. 116, 117, 118; Koelz (American) Pl. 108; and Shelton (actually an American missionary) Pls. 132–135, also brought back art and ethnographic collections. In contrast to the Indo-Tibetan images bought in the emporia of the West, these objects are accompanied by documentation which allows us to place them within their geographical and, frequently, historical contexts. These objects, when combined with Tucci's well studied collections (Pls., 100, 101, 120, 121, 123) and the extant monuments provide the chronological framework for our study of the art of the western Himalayas.

THE THEME

The central theme of this study is the development of a distinctive regional style of Esoteric Buddhist art in the western Himalayas. As our purpose is to clarify the specific cultural, historical and economic factors which affected the development of this art, the equally important and contemporaneous Buddhist arts of Nepal and northeast India are not discussed here. In this context, "esoteric" refers to a form of Buddhism based on a group of texts called *tantras* and characterized by mystical, often "secret" practices transmitted directly from master to pupil. This form of Buddhism is sometimes called Mantrayāna (the Path of Spells) or, more frequently, Vajrayāna (*vajra,* meaning "diamond," symbolizes the indestructibility of Buddhist teaching and *yāna* means "the path"). Vajrayāna is the term used to describe the esoteric form of Buddhism practiced throughout the Himalayas and the Trans-Himalaya. As we shall see, art plays an important role in Esoteric Buddhist ritual and sacramental practice.

The term Tantrayāna (the path of the *tantras*) is sometimes used to distinguish the Esoteric Buddhism of Japan from the Vajrayāna or Mantrayāna of the Himalayas. Both forms of Esoteric Buddhism can be related to the earliest fully developed Esoteric Buddhist art which survives in the painted banners from the Central Asian Buddhist center at Dunhuang (Pls. 61,65–68).

Major settlements of this region were connected by a network of trade routes. The so-called "silk routes," the most important of these ancient trade roads, connected China to India and the Mediterranean world. The northern and southern branches of the silk route intersected in Chinese Central Asia (East Turkestan) where they joined the three main trade routes from northwest India. These latter routes traversed

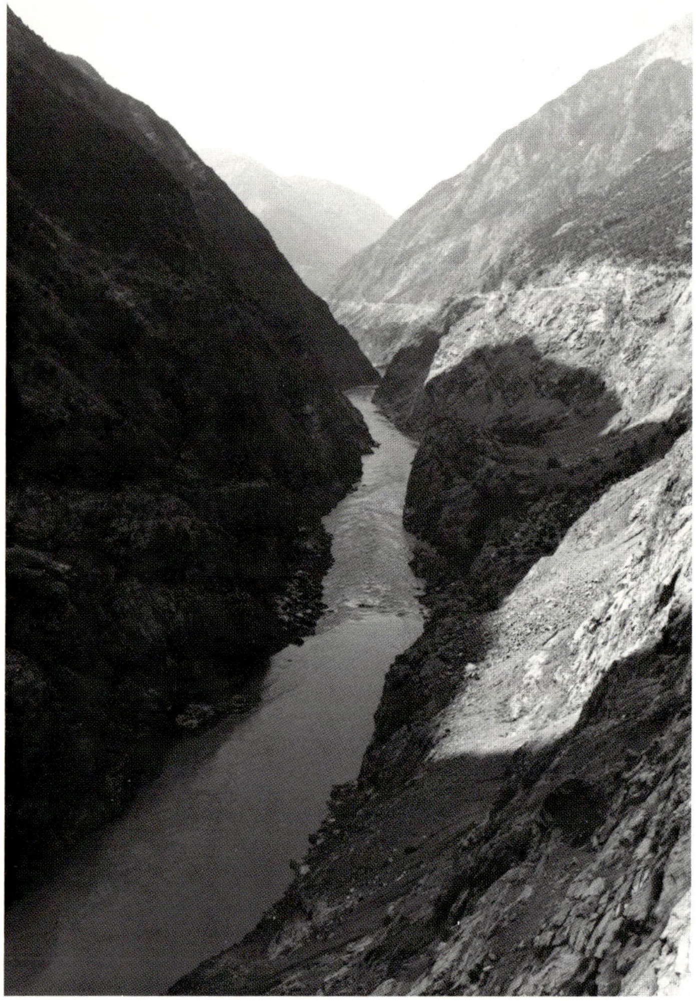

1. The Indus Valley between Kandai and Besham, Pakistan.

the Hindu Kush, the Pamirs, and the Karakoram (see Klimburg). The political and religious institutions that grew up along these trade routes facilitated contact among the diverse ethnic groups inhabiting the area. The Buddhist monasteries that lined the routes commissioned a vast amount of religious art and encouraged the development of distinctive artistic traditions. This monastic art reflected at different times the artistic traditions of the three great civilizations of the area: China, India, and Tibet. The similarity of patronage, function, and cultural heritage created a shared vocabulary of forms and styles which can be identified throughout the Vajrayāna monastic art of the Trans-Himalaya.

The monasteries clustered like economic nodes along the trade routes. Specialized commodities (such as horses, medicines, textiles, silks, wools, spices, precious stones, etc.) were exchanged in the nearby market places. Inside the monasteries, monks skilled in reading and writing taught literary languages and patronized religious arts. They thus enriched the cultural lives of the local inhabitants. Frequently their knowledge extended to the arts of magic, fortune-telling and medicine. Accordingly, they dispensed hospitality and catered to the spiritual and physical needs of merchants and missionaries bound on perilous journeys. In return, grateful merchants financed the monasteries facilitating the work of the monks.

This exhibition attempts to test the hypotheses that (1) a distinctive form of Vajrayāna art with definite stylistic and iconographic characteristics developed in the Trans-Himalaya between the seventh and thirteenth centuries A.D. and (2) that this art reflects the social and doctrinal evolution of Vajrayāna Buddhism in this region. In the course of this study we will chart the development of the art in several geographic regions, emphasizing the formative period of the art in the western Trans-Himalayas. The present status of the translation and study of contemporary Buddhist texts and historical documents allows us only to suggest the relationship between Buddhist art, doctrine, and society.

Until now, art historians have been concerned with the basic problems of chronology and attribution. The purpose of this study is to establish the larger cultural and historical contexts of the arts, considering questions of patronage and art production. The focus on the evolution of Esoteric Buddhist monastic art from the seventh to the thirteenth centuries A.D. allows us to identify the dynamic interaction of the different factors which characterized the trade route cultures.

The art historical evidence begins with the seventh century, a period that represents an historic watershed in the Trans-Himalayan region. In the last quarter of that century Tibetan armies advanced north into Central Asia and, in the following century, they moved west into India and Pakistan. By the eighth century, Tibet had emerged as one of the most important political forces in the Trans-Himalayan region. At the same time, Muslim armies were beginning their permanent conquest of present-day Afghanistan and parts of Soviet Central Asia. The Chinese Tang Dynasty, the most powerful in Asia, was constantly forced to defend its territory in Central Asia. The threat of Tibetan and, to a

2. Standing Buddha, rock engraving above Shyok River, opposite Khapalu, Baltistan. Graphically enhanced image.

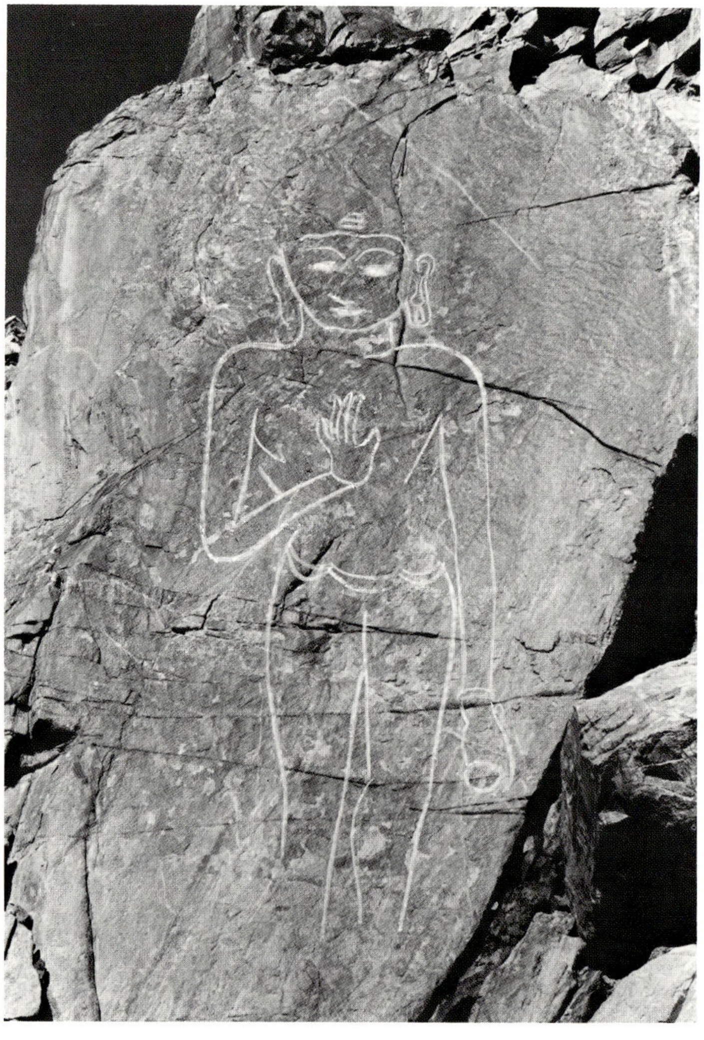

lesser degree, Arab expansion, motivated an alliance between the Tang Chinese and the Karkoṭa Dynasty, which, at that time ruled most of historical northwest India from Kashmir. The cultural interaction resulting from this alliance is reflected in the art of eighth-century northwest India.

This was a particularly creative period for the development of tantric Buddhist literature, especially the *tantras* of the *yoga-tantra* class (see Snellgrove). The earliest Esoteric Buddhist art was made during this period and appears, to a degree, to be based on the *yoga-tantras*. In addition, the earliest Tibetan Buddhist art (Buddhist art made either for or by Tibetans) can be identified, by virtue of Tibetan inscriptions and a distinctive style, among the eighth-century paintings recovered from the Central Asian Buddhist complex at Dunhuang by Sir Aurel Stein.

In the seventh century, Tibetan artists began to copy and adapt iconographic forms imported from Kashmir and Central Asia, and the tenth and eleventh century art of the western Himalayas (such as that at Ta-pho) still reflects its Kashmiri and Central Asian origins. By the mid-eleventh century these diverse influences had been integrated into a distinctive Vajrayāna monastic art. Under the patronage of the kings of Western Tibet, secular iconographic themes increased in the eleventh to thirteenth centuries.

In the following centuries, Tibetan religious orders expanded and allied themselves with the great aristocratic families. In time, these orders came, in effect, to rule over regional states. In the thirteenth century the Tibetan canon, consisting of the Kanjur and Tanjur (canonical works and commentaries), was closed. From this period onward many other literary works on sacred and secular subjects were produced. The art production of the monasteries continued to reflect earlier traditions, though by the fourteenth century the diverse artistic traditions had been somewhat systematized by the different Tibetan sects and figural representations had become more uniform. The various styles did, however, retain some regional characteristics.

The development of Vajrayāna Buddhist art was affected by the rise of the Mongols in the thirteenth century. Their conquest of Central Asia and considerable portions of the adjacent countries brought major changes in the political and cultural life of the Trans-Himalaya. Indeed, the conversion of the Mongol khans to Tibetan Buddhism significantly affected the form and direction of Buddhist institutions in the western Trans-Himalaya. These changes can be identified in the art produced between the fourteenth and sixteenth centuries in western Tibet. These events, however, are outside the time frame of this study and will not be treated here.

Art and ideology in Vajrayāna are strongly linked since art constitutes an essential component of the spiritual practices of Esoteric Buddhism. We attempt to demonstrate this interrelation through a discussion of the geographical, historical, and doctrinal contexts of the art. In addition, consideration of the process of cultural transformation assists us in understanding how Buddhism, as it spread along the trade routes, adapted to different sociocultural needs and circumstances. For example, Klimburg discusses the geographic and ethnic setting and the role geography played in determining the location of the trade routes. Snellgrove discusses the process of cultural transformation in terms of changes in Buddhist ideology and institutions between the seventh and thirteenth centuries in the western Trans-Himalaya. In broader historical contexts, Staal and Strickmann discuss the processes of cultural adaptation. Staal deals with the notion of religion in the Himalayas. According to his thesis, labels such as "Hindu" and "Buddhist" are misleading and fail to characterize the cultural unity of the Himalayan region. Strickmann discusses the Chinese response to, and transformation of, Indian philosophical systems. We thus gain an understanding of the nature of Chinese Buddhism during this period of cultural exchange between Buddhist institutions in Chinese Central Asia and the western Himalayas.

In order to understand both the genesis and development of Vajrayāna monastic art in the Trans-Himalaya, tenth to thirteenth centuries, as well as the function of the art in its ritual context, the art has been divided into four sections.

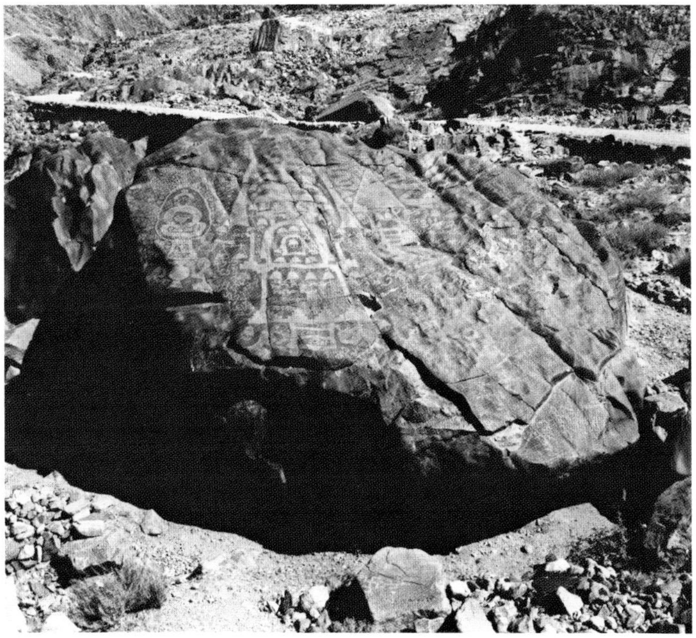

3. *Stūpas*, rock engravings near Chilas, Indus Valley, Gilgit Agency.

a. *The Early Phase: Northwest India: Seventh to Tenth Century*. This region, consisting of Kashmir–Jammuin India, north Pakistan, and east Afghanistan, is topped by the Karakoram mountain range and traversed by a few heavily traveled routes between India and Central Asia. These routes are still marked by numerous Buddhist engravings and rock engravings (Figs. 2, 3, 4, 5, 6a). Local traditions, including shamanism and Hinduism, contributed to the formation of Esoteric Buddhist concepts. The memory of these sources survives in the legend of Padmasaṃbhava (Pls. 100,123), the magician-saint who is said to have imported Buddhism from Uḍḍiyāna (the modern Swat Valley in Pakistan[1]) to Tibet in the eighth century. Examples of iconographic schemes, both Buddhist and Hindu, survive in bronze and stone sculptures. In this section, we shall discuss the arts produced under Śāhī (Pls. 10,22) and Kārkoṭa (Pls. 26,28) patronage, and demonstrate their impact on the later Esoteric Buddhist art of the Trans-Himalaya.

b. *Reflections from Along the Silk Route: Seventh to Tenth Centuries*. In the cosmopolitan oasis towns and trade centers of Central Asia one could find adherents of most of the great religions of the world—Zoroastrians, Manicheans, Nestorian Christians, Buddhists and, from the eighth century on, Muslims. The art reflects the extraordinary cultural diversity of the population and shows the influences of India, China, Iran, and the Mediterranean. It is not surprising, therefore, that the Tibetan conquest of the rich Central Asian cities along the silk routes, such as Khotan, Kucha, and Dunhuang, brought cultural and material wealth to Tibet.

Buddhist art first appeared in Central Asia about the second century A.D. Initially this art derived its inspiration from the Buddhist art of northern India, but later the influence of Chinese artistic traditions became progressively more important. Mahāyāna ("The Great Vehicle," as the second historical phase of Buddhism is called) teachings were important in Central Asian monasteries from an early date, and proto-tantric themes appear as early as the seventh century in the art of Khotan and Kucha, where Hindu themes were also known. A few examples of paintings (Pl. 50) and objects in bronze (Pl. 53), wood (Pl. 54), and clay (Pls. 51,52) from various sites in Central Asia reemphasize the importance of the relationship between the Buddhist art of northwest India and Central Asia. But our concern is to identify evidence for the early phase of Tantric Buddhist art in the western Himalayas. From this period no painted devotional images survive in India. Therefore, the walled-up library at Dunhuang preserved the

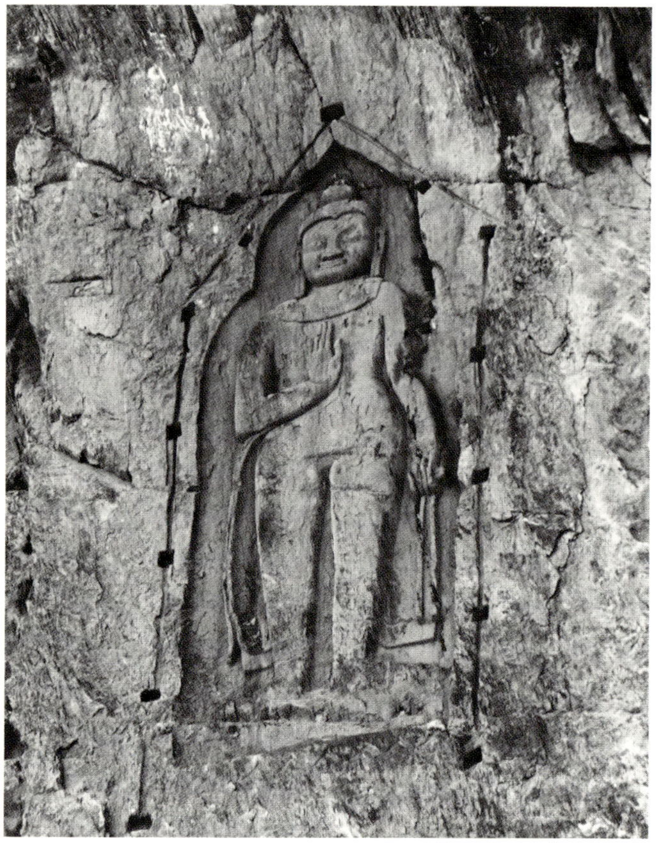

4. Standing Buddha, rock sculpture at Naupur near Gilgit.

most important testimony of this art during the seventh to tenth centuries. These Dunhuang paintings have been divided into "Himalayan" (Pls. 62, 68) and "Chinese" groups (Pls. 60, 70). As we shall see, at least three variants of the so-called Himalayan style can be identified. Apparently the earliest of these, produced during the Tibetan occupation of Dunhuang (786–848 A.D.) includes the first paintings that can be identified (by inscription) as having been made for or by Tibetans (Pl. 58). Furthermore, a large body of Dunhuang material contains tantric themes important for the subsequent monastic art of the western Himalayas. Iconographic examples from this "Himalayan" group include *maṇḍalas* of Avalokiteśvara (Pl. 61), and the five Jinas (Pl. 68), and images of fierce deities (Pl. 65), guardian deities (Pl. 59), and others. These objects represent styles, compositional themes, and gods found in the later art of the western Himalayas.

Central Asian art of the so-called "Chinese" type is not discussed here, but this subject has recently been treated in a number of publications (e.g., Nicolas-Vandier 1967). This exhibition does, however, present an initial inquiry into the impact of Central Asian art on the art of historical northwest India and the western Trans-Himalaya. China received Buddhism from India via Central Asia (Pls. 56,57) and subsequently Buddhist ideas returned to northern India and Tibet expressed in Central Asian forms. Several Dunhuang masterpieces allow us to illustrate this point (Pl. 61).

The art from Karakhoto, the most recent and farthest east of the Central Asian sites discussed here, also demonstrates the influence of both Chinese and Tibetan (Pl. 77) stylistic and iconographic parallels with the art of the western Trans-Himalayas (Figs. 47–50). The similarities in the painted banners from Karakhoto and the eleventh- and twelfth-century wall paintings from Alchi monastery in Ladakh are particularly striking. Works from both sites may have been commissioned by the same monastic order (Pls. 109,112). It is clear from this evidence that parallel themes emerged in the east and the west, and that an international style can be traced from the earliest period (e.g., eighth century in Afghanistan and Swat) to the most recent (twelfth-century Karakhoto).

c. *Monastic Buddhist Art of the Western Trans-Himalaya: Seventh to Seventeenth Centuries.* This region, as defined above, comprises the mountain zone stretching from the Pamirs to Mount Kailāsa in west Tibet and adjacent valleys in Himachal Pradesh to the south of the Great Himalayan Range. The central area, Ladakh (with Nubra and Zangskar), became a focus of interregional communications when, in the eighth to ninth centuries, as a result of political changes, travel between Central Asia and India shifted from the Pamirs to the trade routes traversing the eastern Karakoram passes (Yi-Liang 1944–45:309).

Monasteries of particular importance for the history of Vajrayāna were established in the new communication corridors linking India, Tibet, and Chinese Central Asia. Each of these areas nurtured Esoteric Buddhist art.

From the tenth and eleventh centuries the kings of Western Tibet subsidized scholar-monks, such as Rinchen Zangpo (958–1055 A.D.), who traveled to Kashmir and other parts of northern India in search of teachers, texts, artists, and art. During this period, Tibetan monasteries were built to house this living cultural heritage. The best remaining examples are the monasteries of Ta-pho in Spiti Valley (Himachal Pradesh), and Alchi in Ladakh, whose brilliantly colored frescos reflect the lost school of Kashmiri painting. However, surviving Kashmiri sculpture of the eighth to eleventh centuries, when compared with later (eleventh- to thirteenth-century) clay sculptures from western Trans-Himalayan monasteries, allows us to understand how the production of sacred art was transmitted, from master to student, across the mountains into Central Asia and back to Ladakh and west Tibet. In the same manner, artistic influences entered the Trans-Himalaya from other regions, particularly Nepal. Artists moved between the different Himalayan centers carrying their regional stylistic traditions with them.

After the fifteenth century a mature Tibetan art emerges. A few selected examples of Tibetan art from other regions demonstrate the integration of iconographic themes which, according to tradition, originated in northwest India or Central Asia. These iconographic themes include representations of the goddess Vajrayoginī (Pls. 112,114,128), who is said to have come from Uḍḍiyana (Swat); the magician-saint Padmasaṃbhava (the Lotus Born) (Pl. 123); and Kālacakra (the Wheel of Time) (Pl. 126). Traditionally, this meditational system is said to be of northern origin, and some claim it came from the mythical kingdom of Shambhala (Pl. 127), usually placed in Central Asia or specifically identified as Khotan.

5. Seated Buddha rock sculpture at Shakorai in Swat Valley ca. 7th–8th century. In style and technique this relief carving may be compared to 7th–8th century Tang sculpture in Central Asia.

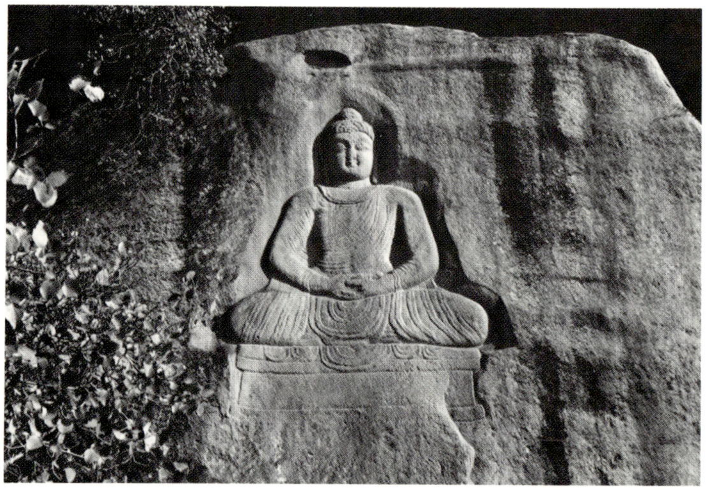

d. *Epilogue: Vajrayāna Ritual and Art, A Contemporary Example.* In order to understand the function of devotional art and liturgical implements in Vajrayāna ritual, the exhibition concludes with a reconstruction of a complete Vajrayoginī altar. The altar is the focus of daily Buddhist ritual and is found in both homes and monasteries. In some traditions, the *Vajrayoginī Sādhana* is the first rite performed by the new initiate to Vajrayāna (Esoteric) Buddhism. The altar—its history, symbolism, and liturgy—is explained by Chögyam Trungpa, Rinpoche, an incarnate lama of the Kagyud sect of Tibet. He also demonstrates how these same themes are retained today in daily Buddhist practice—even in America. These practices are the living reality of the historical themes explored in this exhibition.

This project is, in short, an attempt to show that by analyzing changes in the form and content of the art, as well as changes in the institutions that commissioned this art, one can understand the processes of cultural transformation which culminated in the establishment of a characteristic type of Himalayan Buddhist institution. In this study, art is seen as one component of a socioeconomic system which can be subjected to a comparative analysis. This perspective guides the analysis presented in the art historical sections. As our methods of analysis become more refined and our understanding of the production, distribution, and use of art works grows, we should be able to analyze the interregional exchange system more precisely. An understanding of this fundamental economic process should lead to a better understanding of the regional cultural traditions, their interaction, and their contribution to the evolution of Vajrayāna Buddhist art.

In summation, the underlying hypothesis of this study and exhibition is that a distinctive Esoteric Buddhist art evolved in the monastic centers located along the cultural corridors—or trade routes—through the western Himalayas.

FUTURE TASKS

Once the initial hypothesis is accepted, one can ask other questions: for example, in what way did the ethnically and linguistically diverse groups of this region come to share a common Buddhist culture at this time? I believe that this phenomenon can best be understood through an analysis of the interregional trade which linked this area with the international Eurasian trade network. Trade, however, is not considered the only cause of regional cultural change, but rather is seen as that aspect of the economic system which is most susceptible to analysis, given the available information and the nature of the questions raised.

Well before our period (the seventh through the thirteenth centuries), the impact of long distance trade had already reduced local self-sufficiency and encouraged the growth of urbanism and related institutions. Each trade center functioned as one link in the exchange system, and the resulting regional interdependence was a consequence of the interlocking nature of the trade network. A proper understanding of these patterns of interaction and the parallel process of cultural transformation could be gained through an inquiry which should include:

(1) A description and analysis of the network of exchange, including an identification of the trade centers, the materials exchanged, and the organization of the network (Earle and Ericson 1977: 89,127–139); and
(2) A definition of links between types of interaction within this network, and the correlation of changes within these centers and their attendant institutions with other changes occurring in the society at large.

The aim of such a model would be to allow us to understand how changes in Buddhist institutions, ideology, art, and patronage were linked to interregional and international interactions along the exchange network.

The description and analysis of an exchange network as long and complex as the trade network between Central Asia and the western Himalayas are arduous tasks. For example, many previous scholars thought that they could describe the overland trade routes between India and China and name the important settlements along these routes. In fact, as we shall see in the next chapter, political and strategic factors were as critical as geographical and climatic considerations in determining which routes were traveled. Discussion of the trade network must therefore be carefully defined within specific historical contexts. This is particularly crucial since the character of some settlements (or economic nodes) changed over time, in some cases as a result of changing ecology. Thus, for example, the importance of the routes which crossed the Karakoram and traversed Ladakh have been neglected in previous art historical research, which has concentrated on the better known routes via Afghanistan, although the importance of these latter, more renowned routes began to decline in the eighth century when traffic was rerouted over the Karakoram and the western Himalayas. It was as a result of this new trade network that the monasteries of the western Trans-Himalaya came into existence and flourished.

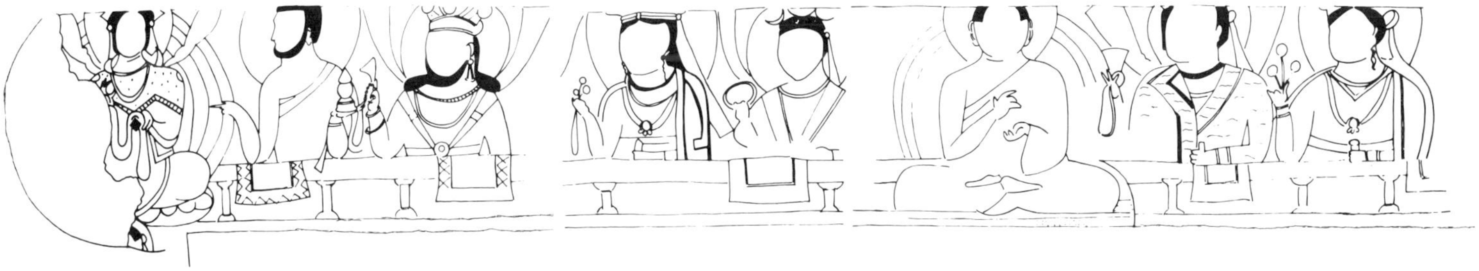

Ill. 1 38 meter Buddha, Pāñcavarsikam Bāmiyān.

Notes

1. The location of Uḍḍiyāna is of considerable interest to students of Buddhism. "The Tibetan authorities are of the opinion that the Tantric Buddhism originated from Uḍḍiyāna. The location of Uḍḍiyāna thus is important for the history of the Buddhist Tantric Literature" (Bhattacharyya 1958 reprint 1968:16). Bhattacharyya also believes that "Uḍḍiyāna has to be located in the Eastern and Assam area" *(ibid.)*. From this he concludes that the worship of certain deities, because they are associated in their liturgy with Uḍḍiyāna, also originated in the east. There is no question of the importance of northeast India, specifically Bengal and Assam, for the history of Tantric Buddhism. Nevertheless, most scholars today believe that Uḍḍiyāna was probably located in the area of modern Swat, Pakistan, rather than in northeast India.

II

The Setting:

The Western Trans-Himalayan Crossroads

Maximilian Klimburg

Cold snow joins to masses of ice,
Icy wind cracks open the earth,
An ocean of snow like a whitewashed terrace,
The rivers gnaw through high cliffs. . . .
How shall I cross over the Pamirs?
(Huichao, adapted from Fuchs 1938:454).

The huge mountain masses at the northwest of the Indian subcontinent, where the ranges of the western Himalaya, Karakoram, Hindu Kush, Kunlun, and Alai meet, with the Pamirs or "Roof of the World" in the center, have both attracted and deterred men through the millennia. They terrified the Chinese Buddhist pilgrims of the first millennium A.D., impressed Marco Polo in the thirteenth century, and fascinated European explorers and scholars more recently. For some, the main interest was in the source of the Oxus, the "great parent stream of humanity", "descending from the hidden 'Roof of the World' " (Curzon 1896:1). For others, the fascination was with the Pamirs' location "in the center" of the Asian continent, making them appear as "the most interesting part of the globe" (Paquier 1876:1). The contemporary viewpoint is less emphatic yet similar in view of the fact that both geographically and culturally, the three subcontinents of South, West, and Central Asia all meet in the Pamirs. Accordingly, this high mountainous region may be considered Asia's most prominent meeting place or frontier area, depending on one's perspective, deserving its haughty Persian epithet *bām-i-dunyā*, or "Roof of the World", as told by local Kirghiz to Wood in 1838 (Wood 1872:217).

Admittedly, the three Asian "worlds" of this larger regional nexus around the Pamirs are culturally less distinct now than they were in ancient times, due to drastic changes in the ethnic composition and the unifying impact of Islam. Clearly distinguishable is the South Asian sector which is best defined as historical northwest India, now divided between modern northwest India, north Pakistan, and east Afghanistan. The delineation of the West Asian and Central Asian frontiers, however, is very complex because their ancient cultures overlapped in the region to the north of the Hindu Kush which, from the geographical perspective, defines part of their eastern and southern limits respectively. From the historical viewpoint, the West Asian cultural sphere once included Iranian-dominated areas north of the Hindu Kush (such as Bactria, Transoxiana, Sogdiana, and Ferghāna). Iranian mediaeval traditions have denominated this eastern Iranian frontier region in Central or Inner Asia as "Turan" to distinguish it from Iran proper. Central Asia also includes this region, especially since successive migrations of Turco-Mongol peoples have changed its ethnic character. Nowadays it is identified as West Turkestan (including Afghan Turkestan), Soviet Central Asia plus north Afghanistan, or western Central Asia. The region of Xinjiang and its Tarim Basin, which is Central Asia proper in the present context, is also known as East Turkestan, Chinese Central Asia, or part of eastern Central Asia.

Avoiding the forbidding mountain zone in the center of the region, the main contacts between these three Asian "worlds" took place in Afghanistan to the west of the "Roof of the World." Thus, for millennia the main traffic lanes between Gandhāra (in northwest Pakistan) and Kashgar (in the western Tarim Basin of Chinese Central Asia), circumventing the Pamirs, described a wide curve touching Bamiyan to the west. The more direct connections through the high mountainous center were probably taken only by small and more venturesome groups of travelers and migrating peoples. However, from the eighth century A.D. onwards, as a result of the socio-political disturbances caused by the advancing Muslim armies, the major routes of communications between Central Asia and India were pushed into the Pamirs and even further to the east.

Through the ages, the main contacts between the Indian subcontinent and Central Asia consisted of migrations of predominantly nomadic peoples from the northwest to the southeast.[1] However, with the establishment of urban cultures in the West Asian and Central Asian areas of the region, long-distance trade communications intensified which stimulated the export of Indian goods and ideas towards the north. From the first to second centuries A.D. onwards, this expansion of trade was accompanied by the spread of Buddhism to the north along the same routes of communication. Merchants became increasingly important cultural agents whose ventures contributed to a thorough cultural change in vast portions of Asia: after assisting in the distribution of Greco-Roman ideas and concepts through trade connections with the Mediterranean, they participated in the propagation of Buddhism through trade with South Asia.

TRADE PATTERNS AND THE SILK ROUTES

A testimony to the importance of international trade for the region is the famous "Begram hoard," discovered by French archaeologists in Kāpiśa north of Kabul (Hackin 1939). Dating from the second to fourth centuries A.D., this hoard contained imported luxury goods from India (ivories), the Mediterranean (glassware, bronzes, and molds), and China (lacquerware), and thus demonstrates the luxury needs of a fastidious clientèle that presumably also encouraged the transcontinental silk trade.

Trade in this region, as in many other parts of the world, developed partially in response to the basic exchange needs of sedentary and nomadic communities, and partially as a result of increasing needs for raw materials and goods only found or produced in certain areas. Trade generated important economic and political interdependencies which, in many cases, became institutionalized. This happened in Central Asia, for example, with the practice of tribute paid by nomadic rulers to the Chinese court in exchange for political favors and access to Chinese markets and goods. Trade also stimulated urbanization and encouraged the emergence of an influential class of merchants and entrepreneurs who employed specialized craftsmen and service trades. In due course, the traditional providers of religious services developed powerful institutions staffed by priests and monks who benefitted from the increased need of both the local population and traveling tradesmen for spiritual and social solace.

Thus, as time passed, many communities or areas along the trade routes became famous for specific products and mineral resources, and also for religious, particularly Buddhist, institutions and festivals which generated pilgrimage parallel to trade. For example, Kucha was known for gold, copper, iron, lead, ammoniac and other minerals, fine felts, carpets, skins of fallow deer, perfumes, salt, etc., and also for extensive Buddhist cave monasteries and the Pāñchavarṣika Pariṣād, the quinquennial Buddhist state ceremony (Klimburg-Salter 1981b). Khotan was famed for jade, carpets, silken fabrics, and also for numerous wealthy Buddhist monasteries, Buddhist retreat centers in the nearby mountains, and a festival with car processions. Karashahr had a famous "Silver Mountain" where "the silver is dug which supplies the Western countries with their silver currency" (Beal 1911:36). Samarkand, "the resort of merchants from all over the world" (*Hudūd al'Ālam* 1937:113), was noted for its paper, cotton fabric, and hemp cords; while Bukhara produced fine carpets. Ferghāna was renowned for metal ore and products, for arms and chain mail, and for powerful horses. Balkh was noted for citrons and sugar cane, and for its large Buddhist and Mazdaist centers; Badakhshan, for lapis-lazuli, rubies and garnets; Bāmiyān, for its gigantic Buddhist cult figures and the Pāñchavarṣika ceremony (Klimburg-Salter, in press); and Tibet, for musk and valuable furs of ermine, black fox, etc. Historical northwest India was especially known for Buddhist sacred places and institutions of higher learning as well as sacred or ritual objects, but the region also produced some gold and silver and a large variety of precious textiles, gems, ivories, perfumes, spices, etc.—articles which are still exported by India today.

In addition, an astounding array of merchandise from faraway places found its way into and through the three Asian subcontinents. China exported silk, porcelain, lacquers, furs, cinnamon, vermilion, etc., and it received Mediterranean products like gold and silver, linen and woolen fabrics, coral, and glass. Indian articles were traded through Central Asia to China, and in part also to the Mediterranean. In short, the trade emporia of Central Asia, such as Kucha, Khotan, Kashgar, Samarkand, and Balkh, must have been stocked with local and imported products of widely differing value and nature. Presumably most prom-

Map 2 Historical Northwest India

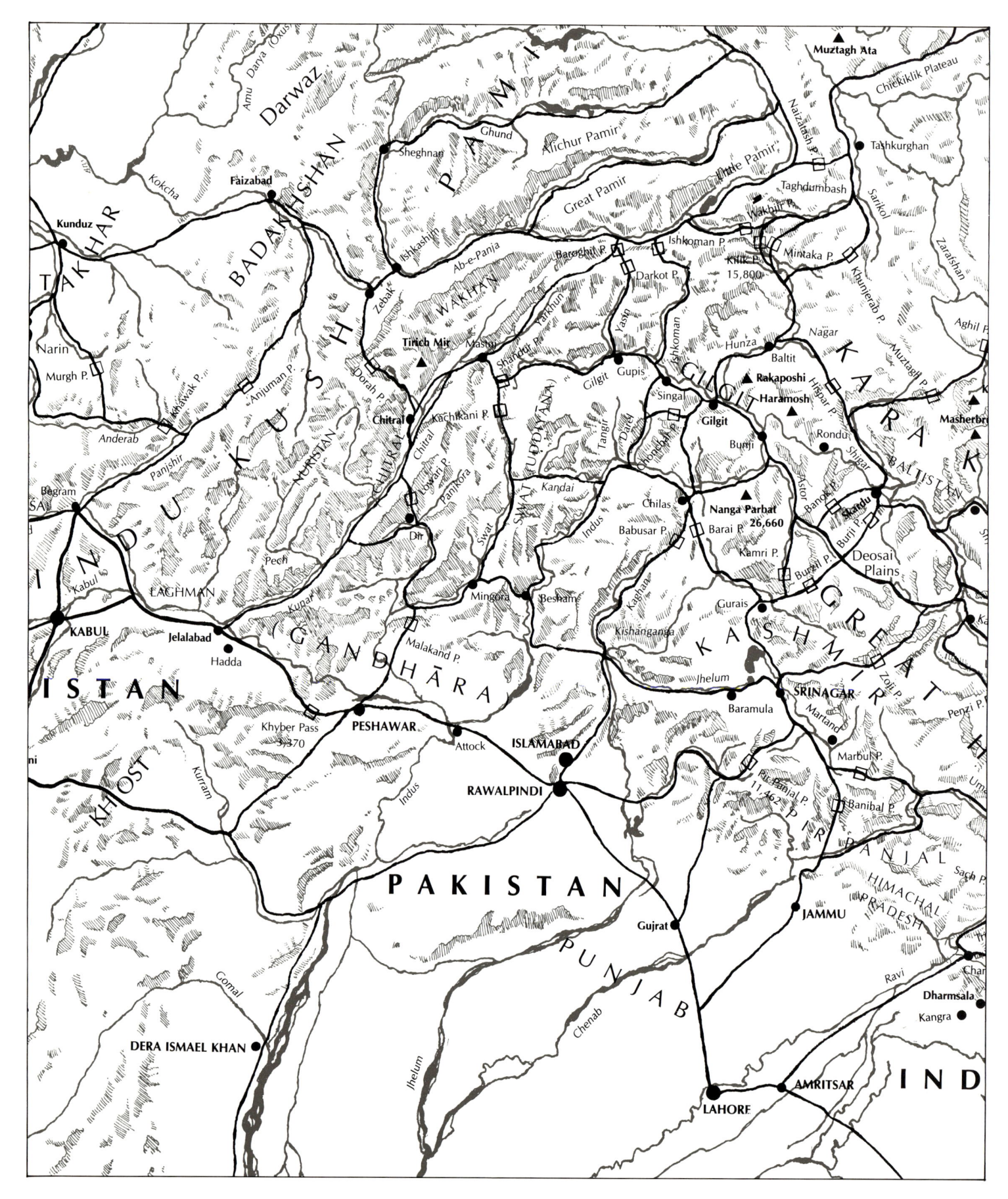

inent among these articles was silk, which was traded in both raw and finished form. In the Mediterranean world the demand for silk was so high at times that the purchase of this luxury item became a considerable drain on Roman gold resources.

Due to the assumed importance of silk, the main east-west trans-Asian trade routes have become known as "silk routes" or "silk roads" (a term coined by the nineteenth-century scholar Baron Ferdinand von Richthofen). Their total length (from China to the Mediterranean harbors) may well have been above 9,000 miles, and the transportation of items from one end to the other may have taken as long as one year. From the last centuries B.C. onwards a long line of caravanserais and trade emporia developed into important relay stations which profited through the levy of taxes. These taxes added to the drastic price increases of the items already caused by the costs of transport and frequent losses due to natural disasters and robbery. The looming danger of losing life and merchandise to robbers was verified by the famous Chinese pilgrim Xuanzang in 629, at the beginning of his long journey to India. While spending the night close to Karashahr in the northern Tarim Basin, a number of foreign merchants, who had left the camp earlier "for coveting an early sale of their merchandise," were murdered by robbers a short distance away. Xuanzang and his companions "found their dead bodies there, but all their riches gone; they passed on, deeply affected with the sight" (Beal 1911:36 ff.). Some two months later, when traveling from Kucha to Aksu, the pilgrim "encountered about 2000 Turkish robbers on horseback; they were in the act of dividing among themselves the booty they had got from a caravan" (ibid.: 40 ff.). Despite these considerable risks, the lure of huge profits continued to urge men to undertake long, dangerous expeditions. Crucially important was the trader's skill in reducing the risk by possessing intimate knowledge of the areas, practicing prudent diversification, and outmaneuvering slower competitors.

Iranian traders from Sogdiana appear to have been the most experienced and efficient entrepreneurs, and they secured a high income especially to their native towns in western Central Asia. The Chinese annals of the early Tang period describe how the shrewd and daring Sogdians "excel in commerce and like the profit; from his twentieth year onwards, a man leaves for neighboring kingdoms; wherever one can make a profit they have gone" (Chavannes 1903b:134). The Sogdians developed their own "Samarkand script" which they used not only for commercial transactions, but also for religious and scientific treatises and translations. Sogdian rock inscriptions of the period discovered in distant countries, such as Mongolia, the Indus Valley of north Pakistan (Jettmar 1980b:175), and Ladakh (Müller 1925), document the far-reaching expeditions of Sogdian entrepreneurs. In due course, a strong Sogdian merchant class emerged in competition with the local aristocracy, whose martial and courtly arts are reminiscent of the knightly culture of medieval Europe.

The silk routes can be most easily traced in the Tarim Basin of Chinese Central Asia, where traffic was forced into northern and southern routes in order to circumvent the deadly sandy wastes of the Taklamakan. Starting from the Chinese terminus, Luoyang, the trade caravans moved to Dunhuang and then proceeded by either of the two main roads. Apparently, the more important one was the northern route, which led via Turfan and Karashahr, or Loulan (in the Lobnor area) and Karashahr or Shorchuq, to the prominent trade center of Kucha, and continued via Aksu to Kashgar at the western end of the basin. From Aksu a secondary route, taken in 629 by Xuanzang, crossed the Tian Shan Range, led through their wooded, grassy northern foothills around the Issyk-kul Lake (a favorite summer campground for great nomadic rulers who were often important sponsors of trade), and continued onwards to the trade emporia of western Central Asia. The southern route passed through Miran, Cherchen, Khotan and Yarkand (where tracks branched off towards the Karakoram or Pamir passes on the way to India or Bactria), and then rejoined the northern route at Kashgar (see Maps 1 and 3).

The main silk road then ascended the Alai Mountains, which separate Chinese Central Asia from what is now Soviet Central Asia, by running alongside the Kashgar River, and crossed the Trans-Alai Range via the low Taun Marun Pass (11,200 feet) into the grassy Alai or Kizil-su Valley which leads down to the Oxus River (the modern Amu Darya) and onwards to Bactria. This valley "seems as if intended by nature to serve as a very convenient channel for traffic from east to west," and probably constituted "the channel through which passed in classical times the most important of the trade links between the Far East and the Mediterranean regions."[2] Another branch turned north after the Taun Marun and traversed the Alai Mountains by way of the Terek Pass (12,700 feet) into the Gulsha Valley which leads to the Yaxartes River (the modern Syr Darya) and onwards to the trade centers of Ferghāna and Sogdiana. Once past these regions, travelers did not stick to any particular routes, and varied their itineraries according to prevailing conditions. As a rule, they reached the Mediterranean by passing through Merv, northern Persia, and Syria, where Antioch essentially constituted the western terminus of the silk route. All trade with points further west went by sea.

Probably the most important among the leading trade emporia and communication centers were Kashgar and Balkh. Kashgar was situated approximately in the middle of the silk routes and linked the branches of the main east-west roads to the routes leading across the Pamirs to India or to Badakhshan and Bactria. According to Chinese sources, Kashgar was the largest and most populous principality of both the Tarim Basin and Sogdiana/Bactria. In the seventh century the town boasted several hundred Buddhist monasteries with 10,000 followers—more than twice the number in Khotan and Kucha (Beal 1884:II,307).

Balkh, the ancient capital of Bactria, was another important junction on the silk route, for it was there that travelers took the main road to northwest India. This trail proceeded via Samangan to the mountain valley of Bāmiyān (famous for the Buddhist monastery with gigantic rock Buddha images), crossed the major mountain ranges to the west of the Hindu Kush via the easy Shibar Pass (10,778 feet), continued through Kāpiśa and Laghman in eastern Afghanistan, and finally led over the low Khyber Pass (3,370 feet) into Gandhāra where trade emporia were stocked with Indian merchandise. A less important route, probably crossing the Hindu Kush Range at the difficult Khawak Pass (11,650 feet), connected Gandhāra with the silk route from Balkh via the Alai to Kashgar and with the paths leading through Badakhshan over the Pamirs directly into the southwestern part of the Tarim Basin.

The routes that crossed the inhospitable Pamirs were naturally much shorter than the main roads which circumvented them. Although most travelers were probably reluctant to expose themselves to the hardships of a prolonged high mountain journey, there was still considerable traffic on these trails. Most wayfarers probably just wanted to shorten the huge distances, but some may have selected the routes over the Pamirs for religious motives. Hidden among the mountains at the southwest of the Tarim Basin were religious centers of ascetics. Otherwise this remote area attracted only venturesome merchants and travelers pressed for time, or, by way of exception, armed forces.

THE SNOWY AND THE ONION MOUNTAINS

In Chinese sources the huge mountain masses at Asia's foremost meeting place are called the Xue Shan or "Snowy Mountains" and the Congling or "Onion Mountains". The first term appears to have been applied to the whole length of the long, "sky-high" mountain chains ranging from the Hindu Kush in Afghanistan to the Great Himalaya in Nepal. The ranges to the west of the Tarim Basin, connecting the Tian Shan in the north with the Snowy Mountains in the south and peaking at the eastern rim of the Pamirs, were known as the Onion Mountains. Their two dominant summits, the Muztagh Ata (24,757 feet), towering over the main access route from the north into the Pamirs, and the even higher Kungur (25,325 feet) descend gradually into Badakhshan and Tajikistan to the west. In between lie the high plains or plateaus locally called *pāmīrs*. Marco Polo claimed that these bleak and gloomy plateaus fringed with glacier-covered mountains and dotted with green patches of grassland were "the best pasturage of the world; for a lean beast grows fat here in ten days. . . . There are great quantities of wild sheep of huge size . . ." (Polo 1980:80)—the famous *ovis poli* or "Marco

Polo" sheep. Looking at the Pamirs from high on the Muztagh Ata, Sir M.A. Stein noted that "this seemingly endless succession of valleys and ranges were perhaps best calculated to impress me with a sense of the vastness of the 'Roof of the World.' " Turning south, Stein saw glittering "white pinnacles of bolder shape far away on the horizon, and in them I thought I could recognize the mountain-giants that guard the approach to the Indus Valley" (Stein 1904:95).

These "mountain-giants" in the "world of soaring peaks, glaciers, and deep gorges" (Ibid.: 73) are part of the longest and highest mountain range on earth, the Hindu Kush-Karakoram-Himalaya—the great "Snowy Mountains." Some of the giants, like the magnificent Nanga Parbat (26,600 feet), which rises abruptly some 24,000 feet above the Indus Valley, dominate adjacent inhabited valleys. Others lie hidden, unnoticed, and unnamed. In fact, the world's second highest peak, the K 2 (28,250 feet) of the Karakoram Range, was unknown until its "discovery" in 1856 by the surveyor T. G. Montgomerie who gave the giant its now famous geodetic mark. Deep valleys, often from 10 to 30 miles in length, intersect the mountains and often have "an embouchure so narrow that it is difficult to find a pathway beside the torrent which issues between overhanging rocks" (Biddulph 1880:1).

This magnificent but hostile mountain world is geologically the result of the relentless pressure of continental shelves which compressed, crushed, and pushed up the earth's crust so that a veritable "wasp waist" in Asia's central mountain barriers was ultimately formed. At one point, indeed, the distance between Gandhāra in historical northwest India (in present Pakistan) and Yarkand in Central Asia amounts only to some 700 miles. However, communication in and through this area was always severely obstructed by the problems of high altitude, harsh climatic conditions, and natural obstacles until, in 1979, the modern "Karakoram Highway" (along the Indus, Gilgit, and Hunza rivers into China) was opened.

This vast mountain region holds a huge water reserve, in the form of ice and snow, which runs off in three different directions. The southern portions are drained by the extensive Indus system which ends in the Arabian Sea. To the west and northwest, the streams flow into the Oxus system and out to the Aral Sea. In the northeast, part of the precipitation travels down the Kashgar (or Tarim) River to the lakes and marshes of Lopnor, while another part seeps away into the irrigated fields and desert sands of the southern Tarim Basin.

The Indus River system is by far the most important and extensive. From its source near Mount Kailāsa in west Tibet, the Indus flows half of its 1,900 mile-long course between and through high mountain ranges until it reaches the lowlands of Pakistan. Important tributary streams of the Indus in its upper course are the Shyok of Ladakh and Baltistan; the Gilgit whose feeders Yasin, Ishkoman, and Hunza drain the southern flanks of the Pamirs; and the Kabul which collects the water from the southern valleys of the Hindu Kush, particularly from the Chitral and the Swat valleys. Probably the most important among the ancient trails from the Pamirs down into Gandhāra followed the Chitral Valley.

As for the smaller Oxus (or Amu Darya) River system, only the uppermost portion is of interest here. Its two main headstreams originate in the Great and Little Pamir in the Wakhan of northeast Afghanistan, while the important Ghund affluent further down drains the Alichur Pamir and the Sheghnan Valley of Tajikistan (USSR). These *pāmīrs* served as "highways" in ancient times. Further down the Kokcha, which provided the main access route to the Pamirs from the west, drains most of Badakhshan in northeast Afghanistan and joins the Oxus from the southeast. Finally, the Waksh feeds into the Oxus from the northeast. In the upper regions where this river is known as the Kizil-su, it flows through the *pāmīr*-like Alai Valley which, situated between the Alai Range to the north and the Trans-Alai to the south, provides an easy track ascending the Taun Marun Pass on the way to Kashgar. This trail was probably one of the most important east-west connections.

The small Tarim system is fed mainly by the Kashgar River, the Zarafshan (or Yarkand), and the Khotan, most of which only periodically flow through the Taklamakan Desert. The southwestern feeder of the Zarafshan drains the Taghdumbash Pamir and flows past the small town of Tashkurghan, the chief settlement of the mountain area known as Sarikol. The Sarikol Valley provides the easiest access route from the Tarim Basin into the Pamirs.

All these rivers are serious obstacles to travel, but the difficulties encountered vary with the seasons. In winter, when icy winds whip through the mountains and fodder is scarce, the water level is low, streams are frozen, and travelers cross rivers and pass through gorges with relative ease. In summer many of the streams, swollen with water from melting snow, become impassable torrents, forcing travelers to bypass troublesome gorges and undertake dangerous river crossings. Thus travelers are often confronted with equally unattractive alternatives.

THE CLIMATE

Generally, the comparative dryness of the mountain weather provides favorable travel conditions. The Indian monsoon reaches only the southern mountains as far west as the eastern Hindu Kush. Consequently, the zone from Nuristan in east Afghanistan, Chitral, Swat, and Hazara in north Pakistan to Kashmir, Chamba, and Kangra (and farther to the east) in north India once was, and partially still is, heavily wooded. Conifers (Himalayan cedar and various pine trees) grow in the higher regions, and broad-leaved trees (holly oaks, poplars, maples, etc.) cover the lower slopes. Above 10,000 feet, alpine forests (consisting of white birch, juniper, rhododendrons, etc.) give way to alpine meadows which provide excellent pastures for livestock. However, considerable snowfall closes the local mountain passes for several months each winter.

North of this temperate zone there is a marked change in climate, characterized by a sharp decrease in precipitation and frequent strong winds. The exposure of the huge, high mountain masses to solar radiation in summer and the lack of it in winter leads to extreme variations in temperature, strong air currents, and characteristic seasonal weather patterns. In winter and spring, a western air stream brings low pressure systems across the Iranian plateau, leading to moderate precipitation. In summer, a reversal in the circulatory pattern moves warm air and the monsoon far into the north of the Indian subcontinent, but the shadow effect of the southernmost mountain ranges removes most of the air's humidity. This warm air stream does, however, affect the temperature in the highlands (cf. Raza et al. 1978:61).

The vegetation patterns change accordingly. The forested areas give way to lands sparsely covered with xerophytic shrubs. Trees grow only when planted and protected by local settlers, and firewood is scarce. Differences in the vegetation found in the valleys and higher mountain zones are minimal, and involve mainly differences in the types of shrubs and grasses produced by variations in the level of humidity. Most of the passes remain open in winter, but the prevailing arctic cold and frequent winds once took a heavy toll of lives.

The arid region of the low Tarim Basin (4,000-5,000 feet), with its hot summers and cold winters, presents an expanse of scrubby, drought-resistant weeds and shrubs interrupted by vast reaches of sand dunes and pebble flats. The annual precipitation is less than 5 inches, and in winter the strong western and northwestern winds blast rolling clouds of dust out of the denuded grounds and carry them over long distances to the east, creating Asia's largest "dust bowl." Fortunately, the high mountain ranges around the basin catch enough precipitation to permit irrigation of arable land in the densely populated oases at the rim of the basin and encourage the growth of forests, meadows, and steppe grasses at the middle altitudes.

THE "WESTERN BARBARIANS" AND THE "GOLD RACE"

The vast mountain area and the surrounding foothills and plains have historically been inhabited by an ethnically and linguistically diverse population. Unfortunately, our historical resources are meager. Among available sources only the Chinese annals of the Han, Sui and Tang dynasties, Chinese pilgrims' reports (see below), and Tibetan manuscripts from Dunhuang provide some substantial data. Textual documentation improves after the arrival of Islam, but the first comprehensive exploration was undertaken by nineteenth century researchers (such as Elphinstone 1815). The extensive movement, overlapping,

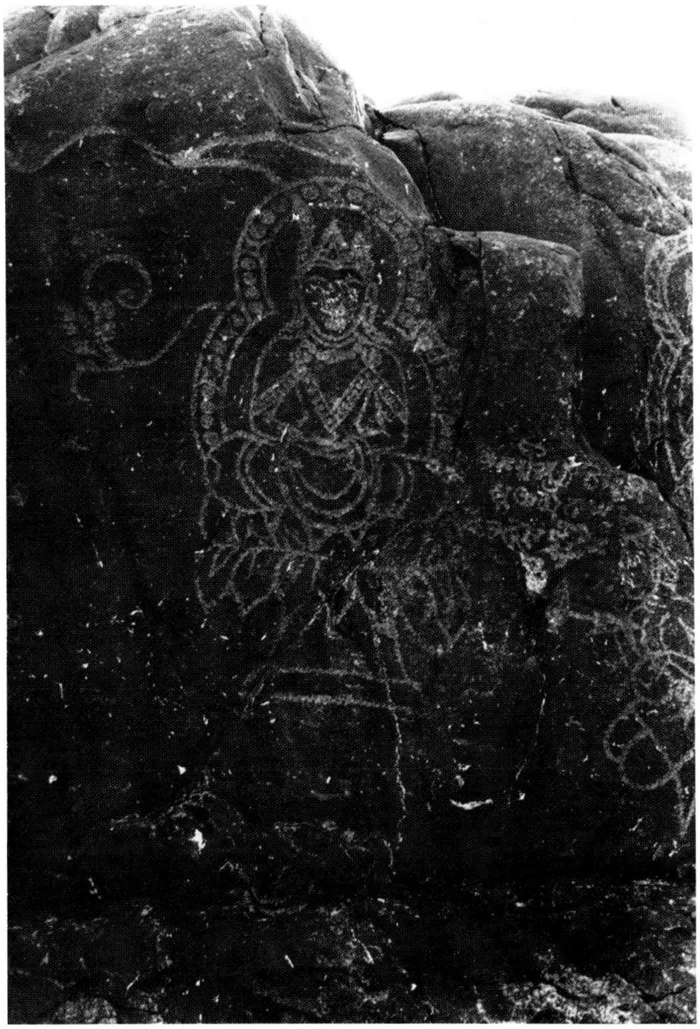

6. Jewelled Buddha, rock engraving near Chilas, Indus Valley, Gilgit Agency.

and mingling of peoples and their cultures through the millennia can thus only be assessed in very general, often hypothetical terms.

The routes from Central Asia over the Hindu Kush passes into historical northwest India first became well-trodden paths after the Indo-Aryan invasion of the subcontinent in the second millennium B.C. Numerous peoples have moved along these trails without leaving any traces except for their names appearing in Chinese and Western sources. The events of the first millennium A.D. are described (to a very limited extent) by the Chinese. They report that the Yuezhi (Yüeh-chih; Iranians?) were followed by the Hephthalites (Iranians or Turks? Cf. Enoki 1959 and Göbl 1967) who in turn were subdued or driven away by the Tujue (T'u-chüeh; Turks) in the sixth century. Consequently, the local population was subject time after time to ethnically and culturally different tribal rulers. But the Chinese sources tell us little about the indigenous inhabitants whom they mostly call Hu or "Western Barbarians" regardless of ethnic or cultural differences. They may have been mainly Iranian peoples, but nothing definite is known about them. Xuanzang disparagingly described the Hu as "rough and violent" (Beal 1884:II,292), "coarse and despicable in appearance," endowed with "little humanity and justice" (I,135), and "mostly false and deceitful" (II, 306). However, he speaks with respect of some urbanized Hu, such as the "honest people" of Kucha (I,19); refers to the "knowledge of politeness and justice" and "the behaviour full of urbanity" in Khotan (II, 309); and notes that "located in the middle of the Hu people" live the "brave and energetic" men of Samarkand (Sogdiana) who are also "skilfull in the arts and trades beyond those of other countries" (I,32).

This mention of the Sogdians corresponds to the contemporary Chinese view of the world to the west of them as the country of "the lord of treasures" where "the people have no politeness or justice. . . . They dwell in walled towns and are eager in profiting by trade" (I,14).

The view must have derived in part from the large quantities of gold shipped from west to east. Most of the precious metal came from the Mediterranean, but some may well have come from the famous golden hoards inside the western Trans-Himalayan mountains. Herodotus recorded the famous tale of "gold-digging ants," that lived in the sandy deserts of that mountain district and were "smaller than dogs, but larger than foxes," "exceedingly swift," and dangerous to Indian gold prospectors.[3]

The traditional practice of mining and panning for gold in the upper Indus Valley also inspired the fable of Suvarnagotra or the "Golden Race," living in the "Western Land of Women" mentioned in Indian and Tibetan texts. Xuanzang heard it while traveling in North India, and noted that "a superior sort of gold" (I,199) came from the homeland of this mysterious race. Some have identified this mythical kingdom of women with the similarly mysterious nation of Zhang-zhung on the high Changthang plateau of north Tibet, and there are, in fact, gold fields in the latter area. According to some Tibetan traditions, Zhang-zhung was a stronghold of Bon, the pre-Buddhist religion of Tibet (see Snellgrove and Richardson 1968:99 ff.).

We know that gold was found in the upper Indus Valley and traded by the people whose modern descendants, the Dards, inhabit a great portion of north Pakistan. Known to Ptolemy, Strabo, and Pliny as Derdai, Darada, or Dardae—and to Pliny as the possessors of significant gold resources: *fertilissimi sunt auri Dardae* ("the country of the Dards produces much gold") (Lib. vi., c.19)—the ancient Dards may have dominated the region as far east as Ladakh. Pressed deeper into the mountains by newcomers, they probably pushed their northern neighbors, the Burushos (whose ancient homeland, generally identified as the Bru-zha of Tibetan texts, is thought to have been located in the Gilgit area), into the northernmost valleys of Pakistan, Hunza and Nagar.

Unfortunately, our knowledge of these and other local tribes mentioned in ancient sources is sparse. Several tribes are mentioned, such as the Sattagydai, Aparytai, and the Assakenoi who fought against Alexander the Great in Swat, but they have disappeared without leaving any substantial traces. The Iranian equestrian nomads—the Saca, Tokhari, Asiani, and others—who subdued vast territories in Central Asia and formed the basis of the huge Kuṣāṇa Empire of the early centuries A.D., have also vanished from the ethnic scene. Only their memory lives on in some geographical names, such as in the modern Seistan (south Afghanistan), derived from Sacastene, and in the medieval Tokharistan, denoting the region east of Bactria (north Afghanistan).

Currently, the pre-Islamic ethnohistory of the region is a matter of great controversy. We can state with certainty only that Central Asia and much of historical northwest India were dominated by various tribes of Iranian origin until the gradual advance of Turkic tribes (gaining momentum during the latter part of the first millennium A.D.) thoroughly changed the ethnic picture of Central Asia. Presently Uzbeks, Turkmans, Kirghiz, Kazakhs, Uigurs, Mongols, etc., dominate most of the region. Central Asia itself is now known as Turkestan and is divided into a West Turkestan in the USSR and an East Turkestan in west China.

Similarly, little is known of the religious cultures the traders and pilgrims encountered on their way through the mountains between the Indian subcontinent and Central Asia. We can only assume that, independent of the Buddhist communities in the surrounding foothills, traditional animist and shamanist belief systems of widely varying types continued to exist at many locations within the mountains. Surprisingly enough, some of these nonliterate or "primitive" cultures survived until very recently (and, in one small district, are still present today), despite being surrounded by antagonistic practitioners of Islam. The most remarkable instance of survival existed in northeast Afghanistan, where the famous "Kafirs of the Hindu Kush" kept their "savage" and "prim-

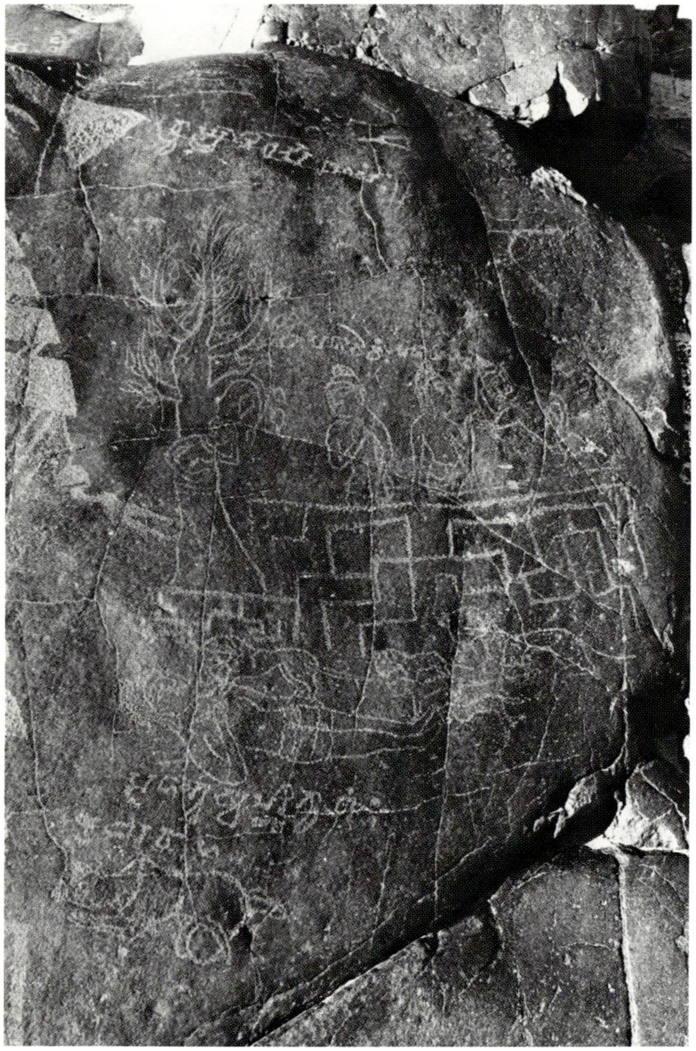

6a. Rock engravings of Tiger Jātaka near Chilas, Indus Valley.

itive" culture alive until the end of the last century. The culturally related Kalash Kafirs of Pakistan, living in several small communities in southern Chitral, have escaped Islamization up to the present, although at the cost of substantial erosion of religious and cultural integrity.[4]

The survival of such apparently ancient tribal religions allows us to reach some understanding of the cultural traits of the people living in the mountainous region of historical northwest India in the first millennium A.D. These traits probably included many of the features encountered with the "Kafirs of the Hindu Kush," such as animist polytheism, mountain worship, shamanism, magic, a goat and horse cult, a warrior cult and head-hunting, feasts of merit within the framework of rigidly defined social structures, extensive male-female polarity symbolism and concepts of pollution, sacrificial wine drinking, etc. Some of the features were of the "megalithic" kind, as is the worship of dominant rock formations, the use of sacred stones as cult objects, the erection of stone or wooden slabs around circular meeting and cult places, the heaping of stones as a reward for merit, etc. The remarkably elaborate Kafir arts and the extensive rock engravings discovered recently in the Indus Valley also suggest considerable artistic activity through the ages (Klimburg 1981 and Jettmar 1980b).

The surviving traits of magic may have originated in traditions related to those of two regions renowned in antiquity for their occult forces: the Swat Valley (ancient Uḍḍiyāna) and the Gilgit area (called Bruzha in ancient Tibetan texts). Uḍḍiyāna is believed to have been a center of magic and the occult even before the tales spread (early in the first millennium A.D.?) of miracles performed by Buddha in the valley (see Tucci 1977b: 68 ff.). Local Buddhist monks adopted some (of the earlier?) magic practices to the annoyance of Xuanzang who thought that their "art of using charms was detrimental to any form of higher learning" (Beal 1884:I, 120). Padmasaṃbhava, the great master of enchantments and supernatural events, is believed to have been born there in a miraculous way. Even now people fear the *ḍākinī* witches who were formerly believed to make up the powerful retinue of important local gods.

In Gilgit (Bru-zha) some of the features of Tibetan pre-Buddhist religion (later referred to as Bon), especially those relating to its systematization under Iranian and Buddhist influences, may have developed. Some early forms of Tibetan Buddhism, associated with the name of Padmasaṃbhava, may also have originated in the same area, and their mutual influence seems likely (see Hoffmann 1961:57ff.).

A third area, located in the mountains to the southwest of the Tarim Basin, was famed as a retreat for wandering Buddhist monks and almsmen. Xuanzang described these religious men who lived in caves, surrounded by "lofty defiles and peaks piled up one on the other," and sought "the *samādhi* of 'extinction of mind.' " Once they had entered that state of mind, their bodies started to wither away, but their hair continued to grow, "so that Shamans from time to time go to shave them" (Beal 1884: II,308), until the holy men finally reached *nirvāṇa*.

Traditionally, the mountain world attracted men seeking particular spiritual powers and enlightenment. This is still true today, and it is interesting to note that the inhabitants of valleys deep within the mountains adhere to the more mystical tenets of the Ismaeliyya sect which is very strong in Hunza and Yasin.

Since Islam has become the dominant religion in the area, Buddhism is practiced only in a few comparatively small areas in the east and southeast, such as Ladakh and Zangskar, while Hinduism is found in Himachal Pradesh and, in a minority position, in Kashmir. Nonetheless, ethnographic surveys taken since the last century show that many ancient indigenous traditions still existed very recently. The total picture, therefore, shows a striking combination of diverse and archaic features, which is not surprising in such inaccessible mountain areas.

THE PRESENT POPULATION

Linguistic studies best reveal the great amount of ethnic diversity. South of the great mountain divide, and in some areas to the north of it, the present population consists of peoples speaking Indo-Iranian languages. Some of them have preserved distinctive archaic features, as in particular the Kafir or Nuristani languages which are considered an early offshoot of the Indo-Aryan branch. The main Iranian languages are Persian, spoken by the Tajiks who also inhabit territories to the north of the Hindu Kush and the Pamirs, and Pashtu, spoken by the Pashtuns or Pathans who constitute one of the largest ethnic groups in Pakistan and Afghanistan. Indo-Aryan languages are represented by the Dardic group which consists mainly of Kashmiri, Kalasha, Khowar, and Torwali; the Shina spoken in the Gilgit Agency and beyond; the Bashkarik of Chitral and Swat; and the Pashai of east Afghanistan, which is spoken in the area south of the homeland of the former Kafirs and present Nuristanis (see Morgenstierne 1973). The only non-Indo-Iranian dialect of the area is the Burushashki, a language difficult to classify, and spoken in Hunza, Nagar, and Yasin in the Gilgit Agency.

North of the mountain divide, Turkic languages prevail. They are spoken by relative latecomers: Uzbeks, Kirghiz, and groups of Uighur origin. To the northeast, on the western uplands of the Tibetan plateau, Tibetan dialects are spoken.

All these ethnically and linguistically diverse groups had to adapt their modes of production and living to the local environment, and there has been little change in lifestyle through the ages. One of the few exceptions is the recent introduction of chemical fertilizer and some cash crop farming.

The local economies are normally based on both farming and animal husbandry, but the uplands have such limited agricultural potential that full-scale pastoralizing without any complementary farming was once widespread in the Pamirs and vast areas of the Tibetan plateau. The labor needed for farming is considerable, since terracing and artificial irrigation are generally required. Altitude also affects the farmers' chance of success. In lower altitudes the land can bear two crops a year, but at high altitudes a single crop hardly matures during the short, cool summers. Furthermore, in areas with a sufficient supply of wood, animal droppings can be used as fertilizer instead of fuel. Large quantities of maize, wheat, barley, millet, rice, beans, peas, etc., can thus be produced, stored, and exchanged in the lowlands, and also, to some extent, in the wooded valleys of the southern mountains. By contrast, in the highlands only moderate quantities of barley, the staple crop, are harvested. Accordingly, the need for supplementary products from animal husbandry tends to increase with altitude.

In the densely populated wooded valleys of the temperate zone, both farming and animal husbandry are carried out intensively. Animal husbandry has developed forms of transhumance that resemble Alpine dairy farming in Europe. Each spring large herds of goats, sheep, and cattle are driven up to the high mountain pastures. During the warm months large quantities of butter, cheese and/or curds are carried down to the village at given intervals. In the fall the herds are driven back to their stables down in the valley, and during the winter the animals' fodder comes from evergreen oak trees. Most of the herding and dairy farming is done by male family members and hired shepherds, and the work is organized either by individual livestock owners or by dairy cooperatives set up each spring for this purpose. Such systems, presently found in Nuristan, Chitral, Swat, and elsewhere were once instrumental in the production of sufficient surplus for feasts of merit.

Further to the north, outside the forested areas, a more generally encountered form of transhumance is prevalent. This consists of the seasonal migration of most of the village population and their livestock. During the summer, additional farming is carried out in mountain camps. While the herds are feeding in the alpine mountain pastures, another group of villagers works in the main fields.

Fully developed forms of migratory pastoralism are present in the Pamirs, the Kunlun, and the Tibetan highlands. Kirghiz and Tibetan nomads raise large herds of sheep, goats, and yaks by constantly moving the animals to new pastures, but exposure and malnutrition in the arctic winter take a heavy toll among the animals. The sedentary population keeps small herds close to the villages.

Most important for the economy of the uplands are the yak and the goat. The yak is a heavy ox-like animal covered with a thick, fleecy coat of long, silky hair. In addition to serving as a beast of burden, the yak provides herdsmen with rich milk and excellent meat. The hair is used to make tent coverings, ropes, and fine, strong cloth. The tails, if not attached to poles erected at tombs, are exported in great numbers to be made into fly-whisks. More recently, the fleece of the upland goats became a highly prized export item in connection with the famous Kashmir shawl industry, established in the seventeenth century.

The foothills and steppe-like plains to the northwest of the great mountain divide favor extensive livestock herding by both nomadic and sedentary stockbreeders. Best known among the fat-tail sheep commonly raised in this area are the karakul which provide the popular "Persian lambskin." The excellent horses bred in the region had such a repute in antiquity that the Chinese sent armed expeditions to acquire the "celestial horses" of Ferghāna and Tokharistan.

The heavy, two-humped Bactrian camels, presently widespread in Northwest China and Mongolia, once provided the chief means of transport through Central Asia's mountains, steppes, and deserts. Long trains of these animals, walking in single file and heavily laden with merchandise, were once a common sight in the vast expanses of the Asian continent.

Naturally, the material culture of the different ethnic groups was influenced by the availability of materials and fabrics. The ample supply of wood in the temperate climate zone is reflected in the elaborate wooden architecture, furniture, utensils, and art objects—all richly carved with floral and geometric ornaments which probably replaced formerly depicted religious and social status symbols. Most noteworthy is the traditional architecture with its use of scaffold and latticelike frames filled with stones and dirt, and its frequent employment of a "lantern roof" in the center of the ceiling.[5] The monumental and exquisitely decorated mosques, frequent victims of present modernization trends, may be considered indicative of the dominant appearance and careful execution of the former village temples (some of which have survived among the Kalash Kafirs). Outstanding "art provinces" with characteristic features are Nuristan, Swat, and Kashmir.

Farther north in the mountains the building materials are mainly stone and earth, and houses are often half-buried in the ground so that the earth will provide insulation against the winter cold. Here craftsmen mainly work with materials supplied by animal husbandry, and woolen products predominate. Among the tent-dwelling nomads the Kirghiz are noted for their skills in the textile crafts.

As the mountains descend into the foothills and plains to the north, the material culture gradually becomes enriched with sophisticated urban features and rich and varied supplies of agricultural and horticultural products. In view of the wealth and glamour of many Central Asian towns, ancient travelers must have felt awe, relief and gratitude when, after spending weeks in the icy, bleak mountains or desolate deserts, exposed to many dangers and tribulations, and unable to get adequate supplies and accommodation from local settlers, they finally arrived in a bustling town like Kucha or Khotan in the Tarim Basin. It seems likely that religious donations were often made as an expression of that gratitude.

In the past precious metals and stones mined in the mountains certainly added to the glamour of surrounding urban cultures. Today the situation is somewhat different. Of the once famous lapis-lazuli and rubies of Badakhshan, only the lapis is still mined. The formerly important silver mines in the Panjshir Valley (north of Kabul) are abandoned, and the fame of abundant gold finds in and around the Indus Valley is lost on the few gold washers who still search the sands of the Indus and some of its affluents with meager results. In ancient times the use of such precious materials within the mountain area was presumably modest, and mainly restricted to the wealthier Buddhist institutions and royal courts. In nonliterate societies such material may have had little objective material value, but its significance was probably great. The "Kafirs of the Hindu Kush," for example, prided themselves on their eye-catching silver jewelry and large silver cups used for wine-drinking at appropriate feasts (Klimburg 1981:164, fig. 47, 48).

Among the games played in the region, the western Trans-Himalaya favors *polo,* the originally Iranian "hockey on horseback," which once was played in the mountain valleys from Chitral to Ladakh. On the Pamirs and on the northern side of the mountains, the originally Turco-Mongolian *buzkashī* or "rugby on horseback," played with a goat or sheep carcass, is the chief recreation. Both these games are or were often sponsored by ruling or wealthy families as part of their perpetual struggle for local power.

"KINGDOMS" OF THE MOUNTAINS

The preserved reports by Chinese diplomats, pilgrims, and military men would be more informative, if the authors had been more careful in their general descriptions, orientations and transliteration of unknown or little-known local names and terms. The later accounts by Islamic geographers suffer from the disregard of the short vowels in the Arabic script, and this has resulted in mutilated renderings of many names. Indian sources are more attentive to religious didacticism and speculation than to pertinent information, and thus are of little value in historiography. Consequently, many of the small "kingdoms" in Badakhshan, the Hindu Kush, and the Pamirs mentioned by the Chinese dynasty annals and the pilgrims Faxian, Songyun, Xuanzang, Huichao, and Wukong cannot be localized with reasonable certainty. There were, for instance, the two kingdoms of Bohe, and those of Bolihe and Boluluo. While one Bohe can be identified with Balkh and Boluluo with ancient Bolor, the second Bohe and Bolihe, possibly two versions of one name, can only be located somewhere in eastern Badakshan or Wakhan.Such problems have produced a good deal of confusion; for example, it was once suggested that the Chinese pilgrim Faxian crossed from the Tarim Basin into India via the eastern Karakoram, Ladakh and Kashmir, while at present he is thought to have taken the easier Pamir route. Problems of this nature come up all the time and cause considerable difference of opinion.

Chinese sources do, however, convey the impression that the whole mountain region, with the possible exception of the rather deserted uplands of Ladakh and west Tibet, was ruled by a great number of kings or petty chieftains. Before the impact of the Chinese-Tibetan power struggle in the seventh and eighth century A.D., many of these states were probably independent. Those located on the periphery paid allegiance to Kashmir or to the shifting centers of power in the west or northwest. Succeeding dynasties—Kuṣāṇa, Hephthalites, Western Turks, Hindu Śāhī, and Islamicized Turks (the Ghaznavids)—brought both prosperity and destruction, promoted and opposed Buddhism, both courted and opposed the Chinese, and generally favored trade because of the profits. The center of the mountainous region, dominated by the comparatively large state of Bolor, probably escaped most of the turbulence until Tibet emerged in the late seventh century. The ensuing armed conflicts, first between Bolor and Tibet, and later between China and Tibet on Bolorian territory, shed some light on the otherwise dark scene inside the mountains.

The sudden advance of Tibetan troops into Chinese Central Asia in the late seventh century led to a large-scale conflict with Tang China in which Chinese troops soon gained the upper hand. A few decades later the Tibetans moved into Bolor, apparently in order to gain access to Xinjiang through the back door in the Pamirs. At the same time the Arab armies invaded Bactria and Sogdiana, and entered into an anti-Chinese alliance with Tibet. The Chinese retaliated by supporting Kashmir, which also felt threatened by the unexpected emergence of a military power on the deserted uplands to the east, and by embarking upon one of the riskiest undertakings in military history. In 747 a Chinese force ascended the inhospitable Pamirs and conquered the local Tibetan stronghold in the Wakhan at Lianyun near Sarhad, a settlement later known as Dar-i-Tubbat or "Gate of Tibet."[6] The Chinese then pushed down into the Gilgit area, referred to as "Little Bolor" in Chinese sources. This name was given to the Gilgit area after Great Bolor, or Baltistan, fell to the Tibetans in or around 722 A.D. Leaving occupation forces behind, Chinese troops then speedily reascended the Pamirs, returned to the Tarim Basin, and thereby terminated the whole expedition after only six or seven months. The effect of this brilliant military maneuver was such that "Fu-lin (Syria), the Ta-shih (i.e. the Tāzi or Arabs), and seventy-two kingdoms of diverse barbarian peoples were all seized with fear and made their submission" (the *Tangshu,* quoted from Stein 1921c:68).

A few years later, in 753, the Chinese advanced even farther and unsuccessfully attempted to conquer Great Bolor, or Baltistan, probably by taking the track through the Astor Valley.[7] However, the decisive Arab defeat of the Chinese in the Talas Valley in 751 soon prompted the Chinese to relinquish their hold on Little Bolor, and the Chinese episode in present-day north Pakistan thus came to an early end.

Contemporary accounts of these events reveal the names of several kings of both Great and Little Bolor, but provide few other points of historical relevance (see Jettmar 1977 and 1980a). Buddhist rock sculptures, art objects, and manuscripts (including the famous Gilgit manuscripts) found in this area testify to the presence of Buddhism, as did Xuanzang who reported the existence of 100 Buddhist monasteries "with something like a thousand priests, who show no great zeal for learning, and are careless in their moral conduct" (Beal 1884:I,135).

The presence of Buddhism was probably due in part to the trade caravan traffic and in part to the local wealth of gold and silver. Substantial wealth from these two sources of income may have made possible the building of a colossal wooden statue of the Buddha Maitreya, reported especially by the pilgrim Faxian (Beal 1884:I,xxix), which presumably once drew much attention to the small Darel Valley located to the west of Chilas (Indus Valley).

TRADERS, PILGRIMS, AND MISSIONARIES

The extensiveness of the network of ancient routes used by traders and pilgrims becomes apparent if the countless rock engravings and several large Buddhist rock images are seen in relation to each other and the topographical conditions. Recently Karl Jettmar, following first discoveries made by Stein (Stein 1944), found a great multitude of rock engravings of images and short texts, located close to Chilas and some other places further up and down the Indus Valley, and in the Hunza Valley (Jettmar 1980b). Many of them are Buddhist, and there is even a representation of the Tigress Jataka, the famous story of the Bodhisattva's sacrifice to a starving tigress (Figs. 3, 6, 6a). According to Xuanzang, this scene had taken place somewhere in the area (Beal 1884:I, 146). Striking is the concentration of the petroglyphs at locations where probably once rope bridges or ferries crossed the Indus (modern bridges exist at three of the four main sites).

More engravings were found at many other locations, such as at Hatun in the Gilgit Valley (Stein 1944: 6 ff.), close to the Darkot Pass (see ftn. 6), in the Satpura Valley south of Skardu (de Filippi 1923:65), close to Khapalu (Fig. 2), and elsewhere. There are also the monumental Buddhist rock sculptures in the Swat Valley (see Tucci 1958; Fig. 5), at Naupur close to Gilgit (Fig. 4), in the Satpura Valley (see Francke 1907), and in Ladakh and Zangskar (see Francke 1914b:I).

Only substantial income from trade would have induced the local communities to take responsibility for the construction and upkeep of bridges, ferries, and galleries inside gorges, and for the creation of inspiring Buddhist monuments. However, there are no records of the trade pattern and volume. Most probably silk constituted the most important merchandise moving south, while among the Indian export items Buddhist paraphernalia—from simple amulets to precious sacred writings, sculptures, and even relics—probably dominated in terms of value.

Except for traders, mostly Buddhist pilgrims and missionaries set out for these long and difficult journeys through intimidating gorges and over extremely high passes. But of the numerous pilgrims from East Asia who visited India via Central Asia (see Bagchi 1950), only four Chinese and one Korean have left us substantial reports. The names of these pilgrims are Faxian, Songyun, Xuanzang, the Korean Huichao, and Wukong. Their accounts are generally very short, with the exception of Xuanzang's.

Faxian, the first of the five men, left China in 399, apparently took one of the Pamir routes into Yasin or uppermost Chitral, continued via Darel and the Indus Valley into Swat (the ancient Uḍḍiyāna), and then traveled all over northern India until he returned by sea to China in 414 (Beal 1884, Legge 1886, and Giles 1923).

Songyun left China in 518 as head of an official Buddhist mission "to obtain Buddhist books in the West." He followed roughly the same route to Uchang (Uḍḍiyāna), also visited Gandhāra, stayed two years in the area, and returned to China via an unknown route in 522 (Beal 1884 and Chavannes 1903a).

Xuanzang, who left by far the most important report, the famous *Xiyu Ji* or "Record of the Western World," started his long journey in 629. After leaving the Tarim Basin north of Kucha, he passed through Ferghāna, Sogdiana, Bactria, Bāmiyān, Kāpiśa, and Laghman to Gandhāra and Uḍḍiyāna, visited Kashmir, toured northern India, and finally returned to China in 645 via the Hindu Kush, Badakhshan, the Pamirs, and the southern route in the Tarim Basin. From Khotan he sent his famous apology to the Chinese emperor Taizong for having undertaken his journey without the emperor's permission, stating the need to dare and sacrifice for the sake of "searching out the true learning, without any thought of personal safety." In that letter he described how he had traversed "vast plains of shifting sand," scaled "precipitous mountain-crags clad with snow," and passed "through the scarped passes of the iron gates" and "along by the tumultuous waves of the hot sea" (Beal 1911:209). The apology was duly accepted, and Xuanzang even received great honors upon his arrival (Beal 1884 and 1911; Watters 1904–05).

Huichao, the Korean, left China ca. 723 and traveled by sea to India where he stayed until ca. 726. His return journey led him through Bāmiyān to Badakhshan. He crossed over the Pamirs, took the northern Tarim route and reached Kucha in December, 727. His travel account appears to be somewhat poorly written, reflecting perhaps his imperfect command of Chinese (Fuchs 1938).

Wukong, a lay member of an official mission to Kāpiśa, set out in 751. Apparently he took one of the Pamir routes via Chitral into Laghman, and then continued eastwards via Uḍḍiyāna to Gandhara, where the eastern capital of Kipin or Kāpiśa was located. There Wukong converted to Buddhism. Subsequently he studied for several years in Kashmir, visited holy places in northern India, and in 790 returned to China via Badakhshan and the west-east tracks over the Pamirs. Unfortunately, his travel account is particularly short (Lévi and Chavannes 1895).

From India came numerous scholars who were needed in both Central Asia and China for the translation and interpretation of Buddhist texts. In the period between the fourth and seventh centuries A.D., most scholars probably started their hazardous trip from the Hīnayāna institutions of higher learning in Kashmir (which had a great reputation at least since the famous Buddhist council, organized by the great Kuṣāṇa Emperor Kaniṣka, was held there in the second century A.D.). Among these learned missionaries, Kumarajīva stands out. Born to Indian immigrants in Kucha and trained in Kashmir, he was taken prisoner by the Chinese (who held him in high esteem) in 383 after his return to Kucha.

After the eighth century, traveling through Central Asia to India became increasingly risky. There were political troubles within China, and Chinese armed conflicts with the Arabs and Tibetans turned out unfavorably; the Uighurs, Turkic people, took advantage of the power vacuum in the Tarim Basin, and China lost control of Central Asia and its vital overland routes. As Chinese power declined and Muslim armies steadily advanced towards the mountains, the Pamir routes lost much of their importance. Much of the remaining traffic between the Tarim Basin and India gradually shifted to the Karakoram routes further east.

PASSES, RIVERS, AND THE "HANGING PASSAGES"

It appears that the routes over the Pamirs provided the safest and quickest way across the stupendous mountain barriers between Central Asia and India. From the geomorphological viewpoint, the region these routes cross is, in fact, a "weak spot" in the subcontinent's natural northern defense system. At one point, the otherwise formidable mountain barrier is reduced to a single ridge, separating the headwaters of the Sarikol Stream (to the north) and those of the Hunza River (to the south), and it is easily crossed via the Kilik and Mintaka passes (15,800 and 15,430 feet). However, further down the road the wayfarer encounters ravines and canyons which enclose unfordable streams. Travel along the uppermost part of the Hunza River is virtually impossible without the help of laboriously constructed wooden galleries which are secured by wooden pegs driven into fissures of the rock. Pack animals could not use these fragile "bridges" and had to be led either along the river bed or across the mountain shoulder above the gorge. It can thus be assumed that major caravans avoided the Hunza Valley and took the Ishkoman Pass (14,060 feet) or Baroghil Pass (12,500 feet) farther west. This entailed, however, a longer journey during which men and animals were more exposed to the harsh climate of the Pamirs.

Chinese reports convey a vivid picture of the travelers' feelings

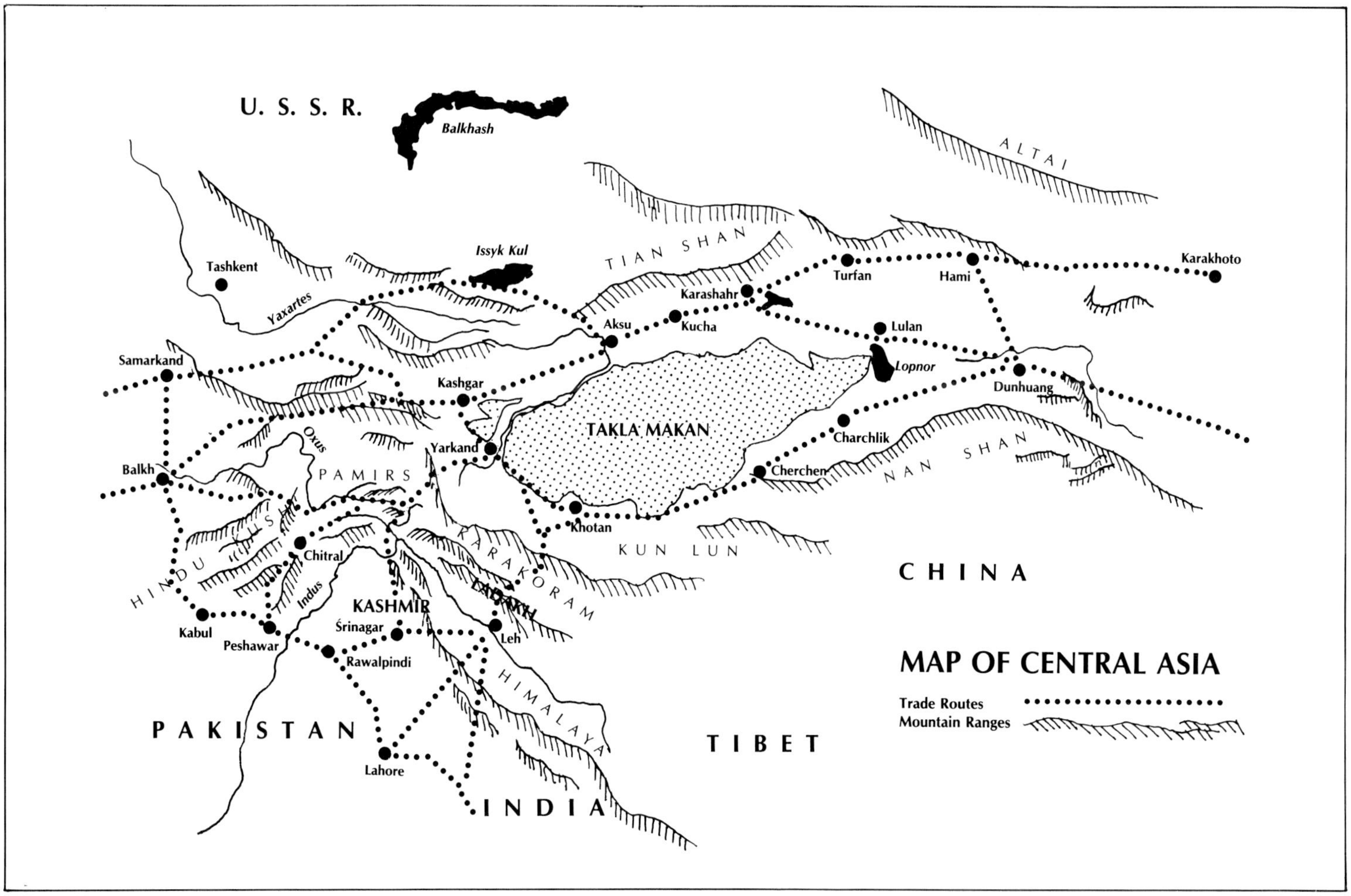

Map 3 Central Asia

when crossing these mountains. Faxian complains of "poison dragons who . . . spit poison, winds, rain, snow, drifting sand and gravel stones . . ." (Beal 1884:I,xxix). Songyun was unnerved by the altitude of the mountains, and remarked, after having reached the highest poin', "it seems just as though one was poised in mid-air. . . . Men say that this is the middle point of heaven and earth" (I,xc).

The hardships suffered on the high passes and uplands of the Pamirs were surpassed by those encountered on the routes to the north and south. The high Chickiklik plateau, over which the regular caravan route led from the Pamirs via Sarikol (Tashkurghan) to Kashgar or Yarkand, was particularly ill-famed. In his description of this spot Xuanzang noted that "even at the time of great heat the wind and the snow continue. Scarcely have travellers entered this region when they find themselves surrounded by vapour from the snow" (II,303). He also related an alarming tale about a company of ten thousand men and several thousand camels that once perished in a snowstorm on that plateau.

However, nothing seemed to frighten travellers as much as steep ravines. Again and again wayfarers described traversing the galleries (called "hanging passages" by the Chinese) along a steep scarp above the Indus River, probably at a point downstream of Sazin, between Darel and the Ghorband affluent which leads to Swat:[8] "The path is about one foot wide. The travelers walk step by step clasping each other" (Petech 1950:16). In his description the pilgrim Faxian said, "The mountain side is simply a stone wall standing up 10,000 feet. Looking down, the sight is confused, and on going forward, there is no sure foothold. . . . In old days men bored through the rocks to make a way and spread out side ladders; of which there are seven hundred in all to pass" (Beal 1884:I,xxx).

The commonly used bridges made of ropes of twisted twigs are mentioned only by Faxian. According to Biddulph, such a bridge "sways about with every gust, making it very unpleasant to cross in a high wind. . . . Where there is much traffic, these bridges are renewed yearly; but where little used, they are left for two or three years without repair, and become very dangerous" (Biddulph 1880:2). In spite of their untrustworthy appearance, these bridges were remarkably strong, and experienced men did not hesitate to carry heavy loads across.

The process of fording streams and crossing rivers by raft or boat is understandably also risky. Apparently the travelers were particularly afraid of "poisonous dragons and evil spirits" dwelling in the rivers and of sudden dangerous storms which would endanger the men "carrying with them the rare gems of India, or celebrated flowers" (Beal 1884:I,x). Xuanzang, in fact, lost "fifty manuscript copies of sutras, and the flower seeds of various sorts" while crossing the Indus on the return journey. He forded the river safely mounted on an elephant, but the boat with the precious load "was almost swallowed up" by a sudden storm (Beal 1911:192).

In addition to natural perils, there was the ever-present danger of robbery. Xuanzang himself fell victim to robbers on his way down from the Pamirs into the Tarim Basin. Huichao even accused the kings of Sheghnan in the Pamirs of frequently sending "two to three hundred men to the valley of the Great Pamir to attack and uncheckedly plunder the wealthy Hu traders and the envoys" (Fuchs 1938:455).

All things considered, traveling through this high mountainous world did not recommend itself. While the lure of potential profit certainly has motivated even riskier undertakings, the problems of transporting men and merchandise across these routes were considerable.

THE ROUTES

Today's traveler is confronted by the same problems that faced travelers in ancient times: the viability of a trail for pack animals; the existence of bridges or ferries; the fordability of streams; and the local availability of pack animals, porters, and food. Formerly the question of security was also of crucial importance.

Merchants, pilgrims, and scholars had little in common except the desire to move fast and safely. Merchants often had to choose longer, easier routes for the sake of their heavily loaded pack animals. Pilgrims could take shorter, more difficult routes or visit sacred places irrespective of additional travel hardships. We can thus assume that some roads were principally used by trade caravans, while others were favored by pilgrims, missionaries, or other travelers. All the different approach routes from the south probably joined at several places for passing over the inhospitable and deserted Pamirs. Most of them descended through the Taghdumbash Pamir and the upper Sarikol Valley—"a great natural thoroughfare over the 'Roof of the World' " (Stein 1904:64)—and over the Chickiklik Plateau into the Tarim Basin (see Map 2).

In attempting to trace the main routes from the south to the Pamirs, we must draw mainly on topographic evidence. This clearly shows that the road which leads through the Chitral-Yarkhun Valley to the Pamirs is reasonably convenient and safe for humans and pack animals throughout the year. Somewhat tellingly, Chitral is called "Little Kashgar" or simply "Kashgar" by neighboring Pashtuns and Nuristanis.

This track crossed the easy Baroghil Pass (12,500 feet) into the uppermost valley of the Oxus River (the modern Amu Darya, locally called Ab-e-Panja). From there the route either led east over the Wakhjir Pass (16,200 feet) into the Taghdumbash Pamir, or northeast through the Little Pamir and over the Naizatash Pass (14,920 feet) into the Sarikol Valley (see Stein 1932). The route probably taken in ca. 643 A.D. by Xuanzang, who had entered the Oxus Valley farther down, passed through the Great Pamir to the north and then joined the track running from the Little Pamir to the Naizatash Pass (Stein 1921b:I,72–80).

A secondary track left Chitral towards the northwest, crossed over the Dorah Pass (14,940 feet) into the Sanglich Valley of east Badakhshan, and met (in Zebak) an important track from Bactria and Kunduz, which was probably taken by Xuanzang and Marco Polo. The trail then passed over another mountain range and reached Ishkashim at the Oxus. From there one could travel upstream to the Great, Little, or Taghdumbash Pamir; downstream to Sheghnan, and from there up the Ghund Valley to the Alichur Pamir. This track then crossed over some smaller passes towards valleys leading to Kashgar.

Travellers on alternative direct routes from historical northwest India to Central Asia via the Pamirs encountered formidable problems in following and traversing the Indus Valley and in passing over the westernmost ranges of the Great Himalaya. One of these routes started in Swat, wound through the Ghorband Valley to the Indus River, and then traveled upstream (Fig. 1), past the "hanging passages."[8] to Darel which, reportedly, was once the political center of Uḍḍiyāna, and also prided itself on a gigantic statue of Maitreya. From there a track passed over the mountain range south of Gilgit to Singal on the Gilgit River, and then most probably ascended the Ishkoman Valley and Ishkoman Pass, also known as Karambar Pass (14,060 feet), for crossing the Pamirs. Another road went over the Chonchar Pass (ca. 14,000 feet), reached the Gilgit River just above Gilgit at Naupur, and then possibly proceeded via Hunza to the Pamirs (see below).

Another important set of tracks started in Kashmir, crossed the Great Himalaya, by-passing its enormous western "corner stone," the Nanga Parbat (26,660 feet), to the west or to the east. The western route traversed the Kishanganga Valley, took the Barai Pass (14,250 feet) into the Indus Valley, crossed the Indus at Thalpan near Chilas, passed over the mountains north of Gilgit and reached the Gilgit River at Naupur, where a large image of Buddha carved in rock (Fig. 4) may have served as a "welcome" sign to the pilgrims from the north. The route probably then continued upstream to Singal where it joined the track coming from the Darel Valley. The eastern route traversed either the Kamri Pass (13,500 feet) or the Burzil Pass, also known as Dorikun Pass (13,284 feet), into the Astor Valley. It reached the Indus south of Bunji, probably followed the Gilgit River upwards, and joined the tracks from Chilas and Darel.

Many wayfarers may have avoided the alternative route over the Pamirs through the Hunza Valley in view of serious local problems. The local population had a long-standing reputation for banditry, and communications in that area were further impeded by rocky canyons where passage was made possible only by the extensive construction of galleries. If travellers did choose the Hunza route—and the numerous rock inscriptions and images at Haldeikish provide ample evidence

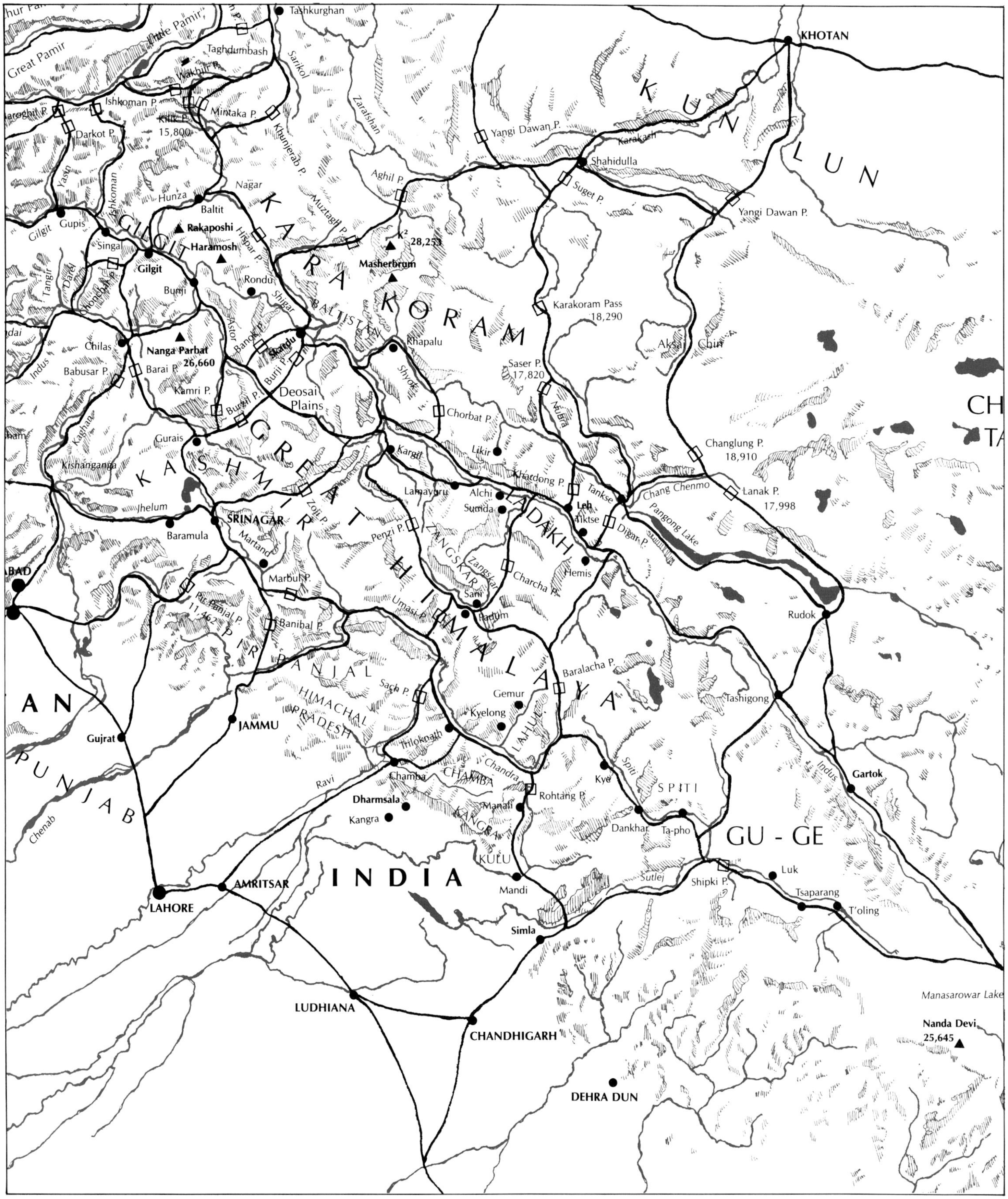

Map 4 The Western Trans-Himalaya

that they did (Jettmar 1980b:162 ff.)—the Taghdumbash Pamir could easily be reached over the gentle Kilik Pass (15,800 feet) or Mintaka Pass (15,430 feet). At these passes Central Asia and the Indian subcontinent literally meet "face to face."

The Pamirs thus constituted a very significant crossroads, and travel conditions on the Pamir trails were better than those on the routes that led over the Hindu Kush passes to the southwest and the Karakoram passes to the southeast. Except for the extreme cold, the strong winds, the danger of snowstorms, and the thinness of the air, these broad, stony 12,000- to 14,000-foot-high plains and the gentle mountain crossings around them constituted the easiest stretch of the long routes through the mountains.

The east-west connections inside the mountains to the south of the Hindu Kush-Pamirs-Karakoram divide focused on Uḍḍiyāna and Kashmir, two religious centers that differed widely in their Buddhist concepts and in their physical and social accessibility. There must have been considerable interaction between the two valleys in view of their religious roles and relative proximity. Tracks connecting Uḍḍiyāna with Kashmir probably ran through the Ghorband Valley to the Indus and then over the low mountains of present Hazara to the Jhelam River where the formidable Baramula Gorge cuts through the Pir Panjal Range. This gorge constituted the most important gate into the mountain-enclosed Kashmir Valley until the creation of Pakistan led to its closure.

Travellers from Chitral to Kashmir normally, unless hindered by political events, took the route over the easy Shandur Pass (12,250 feet) into the Gilgit Valley and followed the tracks connecting the Pamirs with Kashmir via the Astor Valley. The same route was followed by the British in 1888 when they advanced from Kashmir to secure the allegiance of the "Princely State of Chitral."

Gilgit and Baltistan, which apparently formed the state of Bolor (divided in the eighth century into Little Bolor and Great Bolor), were badly connected. The linking Indus Valley posed such difficulties that travelers probably took the route through the Astor Valley to the south, or via Nagar and the Hispar Glacier to the north. The track through the Astor Valley crossed the Banok (15,500 feet) or other nearby passes, and reached the Indus at Katsura (see ftn. 7). The alternative route via Hunza, Nagar, and the Hispar Glacier to the Shigar Valley in Baltistan was probably of local importance only.

The heavily traveled Astor Valley also served as a conduit for communications between Gilgit and Ladakh and as a path for the westward advance of the Tibetan armies in the eighth century. Ascending from the Astor Valley, the route crossed the inhospitable Deosai Plains or "Devil's Plains" (12,000-13,000 feet)—swampy uplands without any vegetation, but "swarming with mosquitos and marmots" (Gazetteer 1890:1068)—and then descended via Purig into the Indus Valley in Ladakh.

Intersecting with this road was a trail that ran from Skardu, the capital of Baltistan, across the Burji Pass (15,486 feet), or through the Satpura Valley, to the Deosai Plains, and further via Gurais into Kashmir. Buddhist rock carvings and engravings in the Satpura Valley close to Skardu may have signaled the start of this route to pilgrims from the north who may have crossed the great mountain divide via the Pamirs, Hunza, and the Hispar Glacier, or more directly over the forbidding Muztagh Pass (19,020 feet) inside the main Karakoram Range.

From about the eighth century on, the Chinese-Tibetan conflict, Arab advances, and the decline of Chinese power made the Pamir routes increasingly unsafe.[9] A part of the decreasing traffic was gradually diverted to routes east of the central Karakoram, but these pathways were never as important as the Pamir routes in the cultural and economic life of the region and the subcontinents beyond. While the overall decline of trade along the old "Silk Routes" reduced the general volume of traffic, the emergence of significant political and religious centers in Ladakh (with Nubra and Zangskar), and west Tibet generated specific Trans-Karakoram communications between the Tarim Basin and north India through those areas. The northwest Indian foothills were reached from Ladakh either via the Zoji Pass (11,300 feet) and Kashmir, or viat the Baralacha Pass (16,060 feet), Lahul, and the Kulu Valley in Himachal Pradesh. An eastern branch of the latter road led through the Spiti Valley to T'oling in west Tibet, located on the upper course of the Sutlej River (see Map 4).

People traveling along the eastern Karakoram routes generally chose the track leading over the Karakoram Pass (18,694 feet). From recent sources we know that the journey from Leh to Yarkand took some 28 days and necessitated crossing numerous passes—4 of them higher than 17,500 feet—constantly fording and refording streams and rivers, and spending some two weeks in uninhabited areas where supplies of grass were scarce or nonexistent. Camels can be used across the northern passes, including the Karakoram Pass, while only horses, or preferably yaks, can master the steeper and partially ice-covered southern passes. The Karakoram Pass itself is easy, but extreme cold and the lack of oxygen due to its high altitude severely stress men and particularly pack animals, as proven by an "almost unbelievable number of horse-skeletons which blaze the way for more than a day's march on either side. Where the death-harvest had been most rich, they could be counted a hundred to the quarter mile. Legs ridiculously in the air, heads absurdly ducked between legs, backs broken, backs curved, necks defiantly lurched upward, rampant, bodies half set up on haunches, every possible fantastic position was seen, as resultants of three forces—rigor mortis, gravitation, and vulture" (Crosby 1905:113). Similarly feared is the lower, but glacier-covered Saser Pass (17,820 feet), which connects the uppermost Nubra and Shyok valleys. A great number of weakened pack horses there regularly fell and had to be left behind, watched "by ravens, huge black birds that haunt the vicinity of the trade route. When a dying animal is abandoned by a caravan, these dismal birds of prey hover round it, pluck out its eyes before it has even died, and feast on its entrails." Many of the horse carcasses could be seen mummified "in strange attitudes, as though galloping, their heads thrown backward" (Roerich 1931:41). Merchandise left behind was marked with the owner's name and usually collected on the trip back.

Another route, rarely traveled in recent centuries, even though considered comparatively easy and feasible for camel transport, bypasses the Karakoram to the east. From the north, this Chang Chenmo route, as it was called by British explorers, leaves the Karakoram route at Shahidulla, ascends the Karakash Valley through the Kunlun Mountains, and leads across the high Aksai Chin Plain and the Chang Tang Pass (18,910 feet) into the Chang Chenmo Valley east of Ladakh. From there Leh could be reached via Tankse and the Digar Pass, or Gartok and T'oling in west Tibet via the Pangong Lake.[10] The route also connected with north India, leading by way of the same lake and Tashigong into Spiti and then continuing via Lahul and Kulu or via Simla towards the Indian plains. This road system may have been important during Tibet's rule over Chinese Turkestan, and during the existence of the powerful Gu-ge state in west Tibet. More recently, as it is known, the long stretches of snowfields and stony wastelands, the harsh climatic conditions and severe supply problems in vast uninhabited areas made traders prefer the Karakoram route, in spite of its numerous high passes from one deep valley to another and the limited feasibility of camel transport.

Despite such dismal aspects of traveling and trading over the Karakoram, at least in recent centuries considerable amounts of wool, furs, hides, textiles, tea, etc. were transported over this road by caravans mostly staffed by men from Yarkand. Much of this trade was doubtlessly generated by the sudden demand for wool, especially goat fleece from the Tibetan highlands and Central Asia, when Kashmir developed its famous shawl industry in the seventeenth century. Until the nineteen forties Leh was an important trade center, with caravans meeting from all directions—as in particular from Yarkand or Khotan in the north and Kashmir in the west.

THE VALLEY OF KASHMIR—INDIA'S PROSCENIUM OF THE WESTERN HIMALAYA

Kashmir's almost ideal location—embedded in high protective mountains which guard the valley from storms and invasions—its famous arts and crafts, and its institutions of higher Buddhist learning have attracted both merchants and religious men as well as fatigued travelers in need of recreation, regardless of their origin and profession. This peaceful, lake-filled country abounding with fruits and flowers was "a resting place for adventurous traders who seek the distant markets of Yarkand and Central Asia" (Lawrence 1895:12) and a haven for pilgrims and scholars like Xuanzang and Wukong, who both spent about two years there. Not by coincidence, three of Aurel Stein's four expeditions into Central Asia departed from Kashmir (in 1900, 1913, and 1930), taking the British-built "Gilgit Transport Road" through the Astor valley (in 1900 and 1930) or the alternative route via Chilas to Yasin (in 1913), and then crossing the Pamirs into the Tarim Basin.

It was not easy to reach this attractive staging, resting, and receiving area. Travellers had to either pass over the Pir Panjal Range, crossing the Banihal Pass (9,200 feet) on the way from Jammu (this route corresponds to the modern Indian road) or the Pir Panjal Pass (11,462 feet, preferred by the Moghul emperors) on the way from Gujrat; or they had to ascend the Jhelum Valley through the Baramula Gorge, the "Western Gate of the Kingdom" (Stein 1904:3), through which the Jhelum River passes with "extraordinary fury . . . on account, as the natives affirm, of its angry feelings at being obliged to quit the peaceful plains of Kashmir" (Vigne 1842:II, 163). Furthermore, the valley seems to have disliked the intrusion of too many foreigners—including merchants. It was feared that visitors would upset the delicate ethnic and economic balance and weaken the jealously guarded defense system. In the eleventh century Al-Bīrūnī noted that the Kashmiris "are particularly anxious about the natural strength of their country, and therefore take always much care to keep a strong hold upon the entrances and roads leading into it. In consequence it is very difficult to have any commerce with them. In former times they used to allow one or two foreigners to enter their country, particularly Jews, but at present they do not allow any Hindu whom they do not know personally to enter, much less other people" (XVIII,101). Admittedly, at that time there was particular reason for concern since the Muslim armies had already advanced far into north India.

Kashmir's political and cultural achievements added to the regional pride which appeared quite reasonable to Xuanzang: "As the country is protected by a dragon, it has always assumed superiority among the neighboring people" (Beal 1884:I, 148). In the eighth century, under King Lalitaditya-Muktapida, Kashmir even was one of the great powers of Asia. More specifically, according to the pilgrim, the valley had such high standards of Buddhist learning that its priests "could not be compared" with those of other nations, "so different were they from the ordinary class" (Beal 1911:71).

These Buddhist priests and their art and culture had a lasting influence on the surrounding areas, particularly throughout the western Trans-Himalaya, traversed by travellers and traders on their way to and from Central Asia, and destined to become a stronghold of Vajrayāna Buddhism in the tenth to the thirteenth centuries. However, in addition to direct influences, some of Kashmir's religious and artistic ideas are also likely to have traveled by way of the Tarim Basin into the western Trans-Himalaya. Carried to Central Asia over the Pamir passes, and enriched by the emerging spiritualism in the trade centers along the silk routes, they may well have recrossed the mountains, possibly by way of the Karakoram or Chang Chenmo route, into western and central Tibet, adding there to the philosophical diversity: "Although numerous religious writings come from Rgya (India), from Li (Central Asia), from Za-hor, from Kaśmīr and other countries, had been translated . . ., it was difficult to learn the Law, as sometimes the interpretations did not agree" (*Annals of Ladakh,* quoted from Naudou 1981:99). In time, Tibet integrated the diverse viewpoints resulting from cross-cultural contacts, a corollary to military conquests and long-distance trade.

Notes

---

1. A noteworthy exception to the perpetual north-south direction of the migration across the Hindu Kush is the newly excavated evidence for a south-north movement of some people native to the Indus culture of the late third millennium B.C. See H.-P. Francfort and M.-H.Pottier, "Sondage préliminaire sur l'établissement protohistorique harappéen et post-harappéen de Shortugai, Afghanistan du N.E." *Arts Asiatiques 34* (1978): 29–86.
2. Stein 1932:20–23. There is no consensus with regard to the location of the famous "stone tower" on the route to China ascending the Komedoi mountains which "trend to the east" and "unite with Imaus," as stated by Ptolemy in his *Geography* (I.xiii:8). Some modern authors still place the stone tower close to Tashkurghan, the "Stone Hill" or "Stone Tower" in the Sarikol Valley (first proposed by Sir Henry Rawlinson), and consequently trace the main silk road of antiquity across the inhospitable Pamirs. Stein's thesis (which concurs with Baron Richthofen's earlier suggestion that the Alai route corresponds to that described by Ptolemy) that the stone tower stood close to the village of Darautkurghan at the lower end of the Alai Valley, is much more reasonable. In more recent times this area became a favorite summer grazing ground of Kirghiz nomads.
3. Herodotus' "gold-digging ants" (Lib.iii:102–105) and the Indian myth of the "gold race" and its "kingdom of women" in the "gold country" are discussed by Thomas 1935:151–178. Thomas and authors before him have suggested that the "ants" actually refer to marmots which are plentiful in the region, and that the gold race were the mythical descendants of female demons (*rakṣāsī*) and merchants they had caught searching for gold.
4. The "Kafirs of the Hindu Kush" became famous at the turn of the century as a result of G.S. Robertson's travelogue and study of the same title. Islamized by force in 1896, the Kafirs were given their new name Nuristanis (inhabiting Nūristān, the "Land of Light"). Based on research done from 1971–1976, the author is preparing an extensive study on the Kafir arts and social structure. See Karl Jettmar 1975, Klimburg 1975, 1976 and 1981, and David J. Katz, *Kafir to Afghan: Religious Conversion, Political Incorporation and Ethnicity in the Vaigal Valley, Nuristan.* Ph.D.diss., University of California, Los Angeles, 1982.

   The Kalash Kafirs in Chitral, numbering only about 1,500, thrive on tourism, but are increasingly hard-pressed by their Muslim neighbors. See Jean-Yves Loude, *Kalash. Les dernier "infidèles" de l'Hindu-Kush.* Paris, 1980.
5. "Lantern roof" is the term for a roofing device in wood architecture whereby successive tiers of beams or boards are placed diagonally across the corners of the square opening which becomes progressively smaller with each layer. Probably invented in historical northwest India, where it was popular until very recently, the lantern roof spread through Iran and Central Asia. It can also be found in imitative cave architecture, for example in Bāmiyān (carved) and Dunhuang (painted).
6. *Hudūd al-'Ālam* 1937:120. Petroglyphs at the entry to the Darkot Pass seem to document the presence of Tibetan Buddhists at the Pamirs in the eighth century A.D. See Stein 1928:I, 46f.
7. The Chinese reportedly defeated the Tibetans near the town of Hosalao (Chavannes 1904:88) which, according to Tucci, can be located at the present village of Katsura in the Indus Valley to the west of Skardu, the capital of Baltistan (Tucci 1977b:79). In fact, at Katsura the route from Gilgit via the Astor Valley and Banok Pass to Baltistan reaches the Indus. This Chinese advance through the Astor Valley would also explain the otherwise unintelligible comment by the pilgrim Wukong, who stayed in Kashmir from 759 to 763, about the two roads leading to Bolor in the north; one "is always closed, and it opens only for a moment when an Imperial Army gives us the honor to come" (Lévi and Chavannes 1895:356). This road could only have led through the strategically important Astor Valley, which was then occupied by the Tibetans. In an earlier interpretation Stein thought of "an allusion to one of the routes which cross the mountain-range of the Pir Pantsal" (Stein 1896:23)
8. The Gazetteer of Kashmir and Ladakh (1890:911) mentions a particularly difficult spot in the area in question: "At 2½ miles from Sumar there is a very awkward bit of road called Chambai Kara along a steep scarp over the Indus."
9. A travel document from the tenth century, the "Saka Itinerary," is unfortunately very short and only partially intelligible. It describes a route from China through the Indus Valley to Kashmir, possibly referring to the main mountain crossing via the Taghdumbash Pamir and the Hunza Valley. See H. W. Bailey 1936.
10. Each of the two recently built Chinese roads from west Tibet to Xinjiang follows portions of this route. Their passing through Indian territory precipitated the armed Sino-Indian conflict over Aksai Chin in 1962, and the ongoing border dispute. See Fisher et. al. 1963 and Woodman 1969.

III

The Himalayas and the Fall of Religion

Frits Staal

For A. D. M. and T. C.

He who made fast the tottering earth,
who made still the quaking mountains,
who measured out and extended the sky,
who propped up heaven—
He, my men, is Indra.
Ṛgveda 2.12.2
[Plate 60]

Here Indra is heard of,
among us he is praised today,
holding the Vajra bolt:
our friend, he who has gained
unique renown among men.
Ṛgveda 10.122.2

A fundamental tenet of the Christian religion is that the Fall of Man occurred in Paradise. One tenet of the present chapter is that the Fall of Religion occurred in the Himalayas. By this I mean that the idea of religion is essentially a Western concept, inspired by the three monotheistic religions of the West; and that this concept is not applicable to the phenomena we find in and around the Himalayas. The Fall of Religion implies that "religion" is not a general term, like "language" or "society," but a name-like expression, such as "Yoga," "Zen," or "the Aztec Calendar." The referential extent of such names is not universal, but is confined to a particular cultural area.

The conceptual shift reflected in the thesis that religion is not a general term throws much light on Asian traditions. It also helps to solve two famous problems of Indian and Central Asian history. In order to elucidate and demonstrate these various theses I shall proceed under four headings: (1) Three Difficult Routes and Two Unsolved Problems; (2) Vedic, Buddhist, and Tantric Glimpses of the Himalayas; (3) Linguistic and Religious Approaches to the Study of the Vedas, Buddhism, and Tantrism; and (4) Continuities across Conceptual Boundaries.

I. THREE DIFFICULT ROUTES AND TWO UNSOLVED PROBLEMS

During the last several millennia, routes between India and Central Asia have lain chiefly in three areas: the Hindu Kush, the Western Himalayas, and the Eastern Himalayas. (See Chapter II; Map 1.) These routes share a significant feature: they do not cross the central portion of the Himalayas, through Tibet, or through Nepal. There have been such contacts between north and south through this region, but they were few and are attested only at a much later date, when Buddhism had reached Tibet. It should be recalled that Buddhism reached China in the first century A.D., Korea in the fourth, Japan in the sixth, and Tibet only in the eighth; and that it reached Tibet first from China and Central Asia. Direct contacts between Tibet and India across the central Himalayas and Nepal are known only after the eighth century A.D. From the seventh century onwards Chinese pilgrims went to India by sea. This was not only due to the fact that Arabs and Tibetans controlled the overland routes, but also and more generally to the extraordinary difficulty that characterizes all these routes.

Modern information pertaining to the route across the Karakorum into Leh and Ladakh provides greater and more reliable detail than is found in the earlier sources discussed in Chapter II. Even at the beginning of the present century, between 20 percent and 40 percent of all pack animals died on the two-month trek between Yarkand and Leh. This stretch comprises eleven major passes, of which only two are lower than Mont Blanc. The Karakorum Pass itself is 18,290 feet high. In spite of the difficulties of the terrain, at the beginning of the nineteenth century, India used this route to export shawls, brocades, leather, sugar, spices, tobacco, hardware, cotton and chintz piece goods, tin, iron, indigo, and opium. During the same period, China and Central Asia used the same route to export tea, silk, gold and silver, precious stones, carpets, sulphur, dried fruits, ponies, and marijuana. All these goods passed through Leh, where the gross value of the trade at the end of the nineteenth century was about 1,500,000 Indian rupees.

Between Leh and the valley of Kashmir, the terrain is easier and the passes are generally less than 12,000 feet high. Tourists can now fly from Śrīnagar to Leh, and there is also a road that can be used by cars after the snow melts, around June. If a traveler wants to walk across in May, just before the road opens, he has to trudge through snow for about 20 kilometers, thus getting an inkling of what these crossings were like in the past. There is one passage in Sanskrit literature that describes in some detail a trek across passes about 12,000 feet high in the Kashmir region. It occurs in the twelfth-century historical chronicle *Rājataraṅgiṇī* by Kalhāṇa, and describes a trip made by Prince Bhoja, probably early in April, 1144 A.D.:

> In some places the sharp edges of the frozen stones hurt like the points of the fangs of death. In some, the clouds hid the daylight, and produced darkness as if they were the snares of the god of death. Somewhere the falling avalanches resembled by their masses herds of elephants. In some places, the prince's body was hit by the hissing spray of torrents, as if by arrows. Elsewhere his skin would burst open under the piercing wind. Elsewhere again, the dazzling reflection of glittering snow would destroy his vision. At a wide open space he would expect a deep fall, and a clear way at a narrow passage. Often he would think he was ascending when in fact he was gliding down. (*Rājataraṅgiṇī* VIII. 2710–2713, translation Aurel Stein, with minor modifications.)

Prince Bhoja made his journey in order to escape the intrigues of some of his relatives (Stein 1900:1,27). Throughout history, the passes have also been used for a variety of military pursuits. The Zoji La, for example, was crossed from east to west by Turkish and Tibetan invaders in the fourteenth century and by the Mughal general Mirzā Muḥammad Haidar in 1532 A.D. (Stein 1900:II, 408, 490). To visualize such campaigns, one should turn to a modern example, which provides more precision and detail than any of the early sources.

British policy with regard to the northern frontiers of India has generally been straightforward, especially during the nineteenth century: its basic strategy was to create buffers, and entrust the expensive and dangerous job of defense to reliable allies. By the Treaty of Amritsar of 1846, the British made the Dogra Rāja of Jammu, Ghulab Singh, into Mahārāja of Jammu and Kashmir. They thus added Kashmir to his territories, and demanded in exchange, in the words of Sir Francis Younghusband, "the paltry sum of three quarters of a million sterling" (quoted in Staal 1982c). Earlier, Ghulab Singh had acquired Ladakh. In 1834, he had sent his general, Zorawar Singh, on an ambitious campaign into Zangskar, Ladakh, and western Tibet. With an army that is said to have consisted of 10,000 well-trained men, Zorawar Singh crossed the Umasi La, a Himalayan pass of 17,400 feet between the Upper Chenab (which flows down to Kishtwar and Jammu) and the Trans-Himalayan Zangskar valley. After making his way through Zangskar, Zorawar Singh defeated a Ladakhi army in the neighborhood of modern Kargil.

Zorawar Singh was an indefatigable warrior, at first considerate, but later notorious for cutting off the hands and tongues of his chief captives. He tried to conquer Tibet and Central Asia for the Jammu Rāja, but was defeated and killed in 1841 in western Tibet, on a battlefield at an altitude of 15,000 feet, situated between Gartok and the Kailās Range. We have various scholarly accounts of what happened to Zorawar Singh and his officials. According to two contemporary Ladakhi historians, Zorawar's corpse was cut into pieces by the Tibetans, who also pulled out his hair and kept it for good fortune (S. S. Gergan and F. M. Hassnain, in Francke 1977:45). According to A. H. Francke, the missionary author of *A History of Western Tibet*, published in 1907, those of Zorawar Singh's officers who were captured alive were taken to Lhasa, where they were "treated variously, but on the whole kindly." Only one of them, Ghulam Khan, a Muslim who had vehemently opposed idol worship and had a reputation for breaking Buddhist images, was slowly tortured to death with hot irons (Francke 1977:159). According to Swami Pranavananda, a scholarly explorer of Mount Kailas and Lake Manasarovar, Zorawar Singh fought so gallantly that the Tibetans believed him to be a Tantric endowed with supernatural powers. His testicles and some of his flesh are still preserved in the Simbiling monastery at Taklakot, while one of his hands is in the adjacent Sakya monastery. His other remains are buried under a *chörten (stūpa)*, of which the Swami publishes a photograph (Pranavananda 1949:79 and fig. 64). Throughout his campaigns, Zorawar Singh plundered palaces, monasteries, and temples, and sent all booty to the Jammu Rāja. In all, he is said to have accumulated 170 ponyloads of gold, silver, silk, carpets, Tibetan tea, etc., not to mention 37,000 Indian rupees in gold and silver coins (Gergan and Hassnain, in Francke 1977:4). We can only speculate about how such armies fed themselves in areas where food is almost unobtainable.

So much for the flavor of these campaigns. Can we generalize from these facts, and obtain an answer to the question why people venture into uninhabitable regions, and in particular the Himalayan passes between India and China? The evidence presented above certainly suggests that no one would wish to engage in such expeditions unless it were for profit or power. Anyone who does it for other reasons must be exceptional, if not maniacal.

We are now in a better position to address ourselves to two of the most interesting and important unanswered questions in the history of India and Central Asia:

I. Why did the Vedic nomads enter India from Central Asia on several occasions before 1000 B.C.?
II. Why did Buddhism move from India to Central Asia from the first century A.D. onward?

That these are significant questions is not open to doubt: the first movement resulted in the Sanskritization of India, which lasted for the next three thousand years. The second resulted in the Indianization and Buddhicization of large parts of Asia, which lasted for the next two thousand years. Both results could hardly have been imagined, let alone predicted, by anyone familiar with the preceding events. So how should they be explained? Will the key terms still be power and profit?

Let us first consider some of the answers that have been proposed in the past.

I. The Vedic Migrations

Basham, in a work that is general but balanced and insightful, attributes the migrations of the seminomadic Indo-European barbarians to the west (Europe), east (China), and south (India) in the second millennium B.C. to the pressure of population, the dessication of pasture lands, or both (Basham 1954:29). The migrations were possible because these nomads rode horses and chariots (*ratha*) with spoked wheels (*cakra*). The *Vedas* refer to numerous battle scenes, with Indra as the chief warrior. "It still remains an open question," writes Kosambi (1970:78), "whether Indra is not a deified ancestral war leader who had actually led the Aryans in the field, or perhaps a succession of such active human chiefs." The *Ṛgveda* also emphasizes the search for pastures, and *Lebensraum* generally, and cattle raids, which continue to be referred to throughout the Vedic literature. Several opponents are mentioned in the *Ṛgveda*; among them, the Paṇis, who were wealthy cattle owners. Warriors fought not only with ordinary arms (enumerated in a Ṛgvedic hymn: 6.75), but with incantations, recitations, and chants (*śastra* means both "weapon" and a ritual recitation of the *mantras* of the *Ṛgveda*). In later Vedic literature the dangers of travel are attributed to wild tribes, thieves, bandits, and other evil people (Rau 1957:29–30).

The Vedic nomads who crossed the mountains must have come on several occasions and in small groups. That their numbers were small is indicated by the *Ṛgveda*, which consists for a large part of "family books." It is likely that they left no archaeological evidence; if a census had been taken around 1000 B.C., no Vedic Aryan might have been listed. What is miraculous is that they imposed their language on a sedentary population that had known a much more advanced level of civilization several centuries earlier—the Indus civilization. The survival of the *Vedas,* orally transmitted until the present day, cannot be explained without reference to the Sanskrit grammar composed in Sanskrit by Pāṇini in the fifth or fourth century B.C., for this work fixed and canonized the language that became the standard of civilization for the following millennia.

II. The Buddhist Migrations

Unlike the Vedic and Hindu traditions, Buddhism was a missionary creed. After obtaining enlightenment and meditating for another four to seven weeks, the Buddha proceeded to Banaras and delivered his first sermon, referred to as *dharmacakrapravartana*: the setting-into-motion (*pravartana*) of the wheel (*cakra*) of the law (*dharma*). Walking all over the middle Ganges region, he continued to preach and proselytize for the next forty-five years (probably from 531 to 486 B.C.). Having received such a powerful push, it is not surprising that the momentum persisted and the wheel of the doctrine continued to turn. What is astonishing is that it started to cross the Himalayas, where no wheeled traffic of any kind is possible. The Aryans, earlier, could not have ridden their horses or chariots across the Himalayan passes. It is likely that they took horses with them (losing many), and possible that they transported some light chariots, as they carried fire in earthenware pots.

Buddhism could move into Central Asia because it followed the existing trade routes. It provided fortified monasteries defended by martial monks (Figs. *7, 7 a*); protection against armies, bandits, and criminal tribes; and bank vaults where traders could keep their money and gain interest. It should be noted that the goods of Buddhism were not as different from earlier products of trade as our modern dichotomy between material and spiritual suggests. Just as the Vedic Indians carried *mantras* that were as effective in warfare as actual arms, Buddhism promised the acquisition of special powers that had always been in demand on both sides of the Himalayas. Such powers are not merely "spiritual" and do not originate solely in the realm of the mind. Both (Hindu) *yoga* and Buddhist *abhidharma* sources specify that such powers (*siddhi; ṛddhi; abhijñā*) can be obtained by discipline, meditation, *mantras*, or drugs (described as "divine herbs": *divyauṣadhi*).

Power and profit may still be operative categories when it comes to explaining the Vedic and Buddhist migrations, but these terms should not be exclusively interpreted in a materialistic or commercial sense. It is here that our nineteenth-century parallels are to some extent misleading. It is equally misleading, however, to stress only the linguistic and religious dimensions of these migrations. This is a topic to which I shall return.

I have emphasized the similarities between the Vedic and Buddhist migrations which both turned the *cakra*. Such emphasis should not obscure certain differences. Buddhism was, at least in part, a princely reaction against the power of brahmins and a general reaction against Vedic ritualism. Such reactions also occur in Vedic literature itself, especially in the *Upaniṣads*. The strongest reaction against Buddhism came from the heart of orthodox, or rather *orthoprax* ("of right action") Hinduism: the philosophy of the Mīmāṃsā, which was the only system that made a real attempt to preserve the Vedic heritage. According to the Mīmāṃsā, the *dharma* is laid down by the Vedas. It is transmitted by word of mouth, like the Vedas themselves, from father to son and from teacher to pupil. At the beginning of this transmission there are no perfect, omniscient, or omnipotent gods or sages; the Vedas refer to gods and sages, but they merely participate in the work of manifestation and transmission. It is only the Vedas that are eternal, and of nonhuman origin (*apauruṣeya*).

It is obvious that the Vedas in the perspective of Mīmāṃsā are different from the Vedas as modern historians have reconstructed them. It is also obvious that, from the perspective of the Mīmāṃsā, the Buddha appeared as a renegade and a pretender: someone who claimed to know the *dharma* without having received it from a teacher (that is, without proper transmission) and who claimed to be able to set in motion a wheel that had been immutably fixed in the Vedas from the beginning of time. It is not surprising, therefore, that some of the most acid exchanges between Hindus and Buddhists took place in the later works of Buddhist and Mīmāṃsā philosophers. In those works the chief metaphysical difference between the Hindu and Buddhist traditions also comes to the fore: the Hindu emphasis on the existence of the soul or self as an everlasting substance and the Buddhist denial of the existence of any such substance.

These are momentous differences, indeed; yet they pertain almost exclusively to the lofty levels of philosophical and metaphysical speculation. Moreover, even on the level of technical philosophy, there are so many different Hindu and Buddhist schools that it is easy to find internal differences *within* each tradition that are larger than differences *between* the traditions. When it comes to the ordinary level

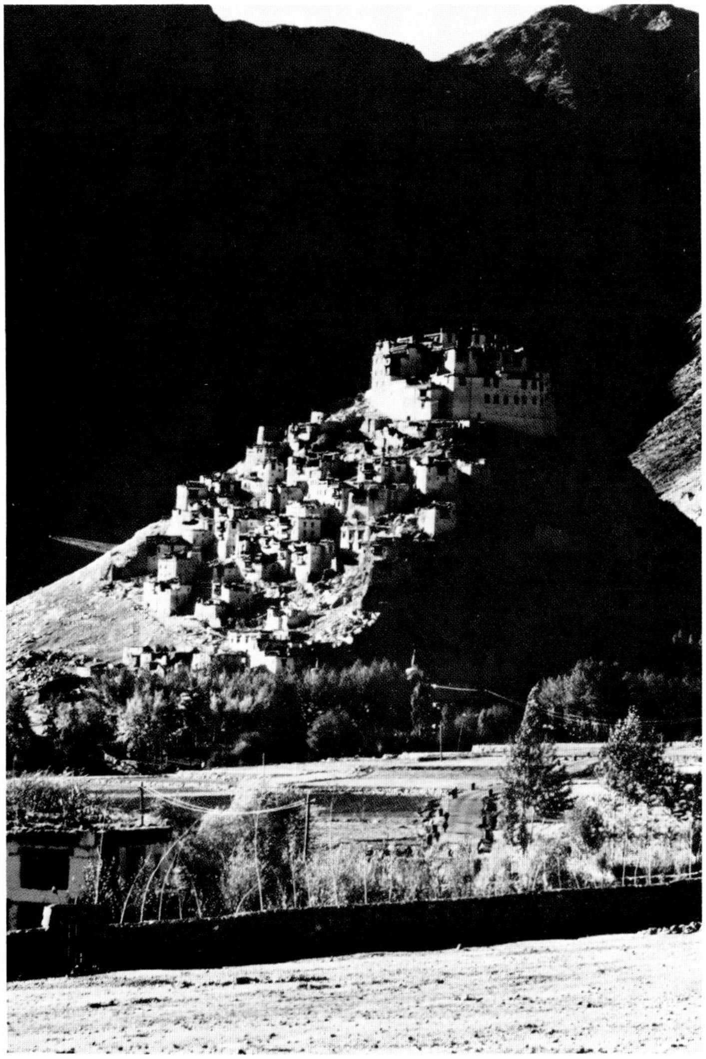

7a. Chemre Monastery, Ladakh. **(See Fig. 7 Color Plate)**

of daily life, it becomes more difficult to distinguish between Hindu and Buddhist ideas and practices. In later times their convergence becomes increasingly apparent and many differences appear merely terminological. Many differences are only due, as we shall see, to the difference of the *labels* "Hindu" and "Buddhist." For the follower of any of these traditions, the issue is not such labels, but where he received his teachings and through what kind of *immediate* transmission (*paramparā*). The teachings may originate from his natural surroundings (i.e., family, community, or village) or from a teacher (*guruparamparā*). Such immediate transmission is the only identifiable feature of what we tend to call "religious affiliation." However, many such transmissions taken together may not constitute a meaningful unit. The term "religious affiliation" is therefore a misnomer. It reflects labels that are attached primarily by outsiders.

If the differences between Hindu and Buddhist are not always distinct, it should not be surprising to learn that the same holds true of the differences between Hindu and Vedic. In spite of deep differences in their historical and geographical context, there are continuities as well as discontinuities between them. As we shall see, the main gap occurs between the *Ṛgveda*, on the one hand, and the later Vedas, with their Hindu ramifications, on the other. However, there is not an unbridgeable gap between Buddhism on the one side and the Vedic and Hindu traditions on the other. In fact, I have stressed similarities between Vedic and Buddhist traditions, that do not pertain to Hinduism. An important difference between Vedic and Buddhist traditions on the one hand, and Hindu traditions on the other, is that the former were on the move, especially in the beginning, while Hinduism, in spite of its numerous transformations, has remained a sedentary tradition, by and large. This difference is related to the aggressive characteristics of the Vedic and Buddhist traditions. The Vedic Indians were originally seminomadic pastoralists and fighters. The Buddhists, followers of the son of a chieftain belonging to the warrior caste, were equally aggressive in their proselytization, even if they stressed nonviolence and "compassion." Hence the emphasis, in both cases, on *cakra*. Of course, this picture is a generalization; but it should usefully complement the commonly drawn contrast between Vedic/Hindu on the one hand, and Buddhist on the other, which is also a generalization.

We have not yet satisfactorily explained why Vedic Central Asians and Buddhist Indians crossed the Himalayas; but we have come closer to such an explanation. I shall develop this line of thought by considering some direct references to the Himalayas that we encounter in these traditions, and also in Tantrism.

2. VEDIC, BUDDHIST, AND TANTRIC GLIMPSES OF THE HIMALAYAS

I. The Vedas

The Sanskrit term *himālaya,* "abode of snow," is common in later Sanskrit literature but does not occur in Vedic Sanskrit. In the Vedas, these mountains are referred to as "the snowy (mountains)," *himavantaḥ*, an expression which denotes the Hindu Kush as well as the (western) Himalayas. *Ṛgveda* 10.121.4 addresses the unknown god who, by his power, owns these snowy regions; 10.44.8 mentions earthquakes and moving mountains. There are numerous references to snow, hail, mist, and fog. Trees are described as "mountain-hair" (*Ṛgveda* 5.41.11). *Ṛgveda* 10.82.7 refers metaphorically to mists when ridiculing the ritualists and reciters of meaningless *mantras*: "enveloped in mists and stammering, taking life, the reciters wander" (see Staal 1982a:I,547).

There are numerous references in the *Ṛgveda* to the riches of the mountains, especially treasures, cows, horses, and Soma. The Vala myth refers to a demon or people who penned up cows in mountain caves, from where they were released by Indra. These cows have a secret name: "dawn." Dawn is similarly released from the mountains. Cows were rescued from the wealthy Paṇis, and Indra sent his bitch, Saramā, to threaten them (*Ṛgveda* 10.108). Before the fight, the Paṇis lived in the east; afterwards, they lived in the west (cf. Schmidt 1968:190). This may refer to dawn and dusk, but could also indicate that the Vedic Indians went from west to east as they continued to do throughout the Vedic period. Mountains were both to the west (*pratyañc*, behind) and to the east (*prāñc*, in front). In the later Vedic literature, mountains are to the north and the south (see Mylius 1972:372),* which refers to the Himalaya and Vindhya ranges, respectively.

The Paṇis were cattle owners and, possibly, landlords. They were warned, threatened, and attacked, not with ordinary weapons, but with incantations, recitations, and powerful language. The name Pāṇini is most probably derived from Paṇi, and it is likely that the great grammarian was a descendant of these Paṇis who lost their cows through the power of language. If language was the main cause for the loss of ancestral property, it was the chief weapon of the enemy, and therefore certainly worthy of analysis. Pāṇini himself was fully Sanskritized, of course, and it is unlikely that he preserved the language of his forefathers or, indeed, that he knew any language other than Sanskrit.

Wild animals live in the mountains, as does the Soma plant: both are called *giriṣṭha*, "mountain dwelling." The best Soma came from Mount Mūjavat (later: Muñjavat), probably a mountain in the Munjan area of Badakshan (northeast Afghanistan), where an Iranian language, Munji, is still spoken. (There is also a township called Shahr-i-Munjan.) The gambler of *Ṛgveda* 10.34.1 complains that dice keep him awake and excited, "like Soma from Mount Mūjavat." The strongest or "most inebriating" (*madintama*) Soma came from Ārjīkīya. The name probably refers to a river, since it occurs in a verse of the "Hymn of Rivers," *Ṛgveda* 10.75. Hillebrandt (1891–1902; English translation 1980:179) suggested that this river was in Kashmir, which is unlikely; Aurel Stein (1917), who identified the other river names occurring in the same verse, could not identify it. The new *Historical Atlas of South Asia*, published by the University of Chicago, places it in Afghanistan, which is most probably correct.

In the *Ṛgveda*, mountains are contrasted with plains (*samajya*), and also with deserts (*dhanvan*). There is no mention of the Kailasa mountain. Mount Mahāmeru is mentioned for the first time in the *Taittirīya-Āraṇyaka*, and seems to be located in some northern region, probably beyond the Pamirs. Morgenstierne (1931:443) mentions a mountain in Chitral still referred to as Mīr or Mēr, which could be the original Mount Meru, although it could also be called after a mythical original.[1]

Pāṇini and other grammarians provide much detailed information on the mountains. Pāṇini himself was born in Śalātura, a few miles north of the confluence of the Indus and Kabul rivers, then in a distant corner of the Achaemenid Empire. The word lists attached to his grammar enumerate various terms for paths and roads. These include *ajapatha* "goat track," which according to the later *Bṛhatkathā* is so narrow that two people from opposite directions cannot pass; and *śankupatha* "spike track," which indicates that spikes or nails (*śanku*) are driven into the mountains. The latter constitutes one of the earliest references to mountaineering (cf. Agrawala 1953:242–243). The term *uttarapatha* denotes a "northern route," but it is not clear where this was located. Pāṇini mentions goods or articles that were procured (*āhṛta*) along that route. One rule of his grammar (4.2.142) describes *kanthā* as a word often used as the second member of a compound indicating a place name; such a compound receives the adjectival ending *-īya*, which then induces *vṛddhi* vowel changes in the first member. This word occurs in similar forms in Khotanese and other Middle Iranian languages, and is still found in Samar*kand*, Tash*kent*, Yar*kand*, Chim*kand*, Kho*qand*, Panj*kand*, etc. (Agrawala 1953:68).

In later Sanskrit literature, the Himalayas recede into the background and references to them become more mythological. Even in the epics, mountains such as Kailāsa and Meru, sometimes identified with each other, are merely referred to as "king of mountains," or "crown of the earth." An attractive description occurs in the *Mahābhārata* (1.15.5–8; translated by Van Buitenen 1973:72):

> There is an all-surpassing mountain that blazes like a pile of fire and casts forth the splendor of the sun with its golden glowing peaks—Mount Meru! It is the many-splendored ornament of gold that is cherished by gods and gandharvas, immeasurable and unattainable by those of little merit of Law. Awesome beasts of prey range over it, divine herbs illuminate it, and the great mountain raises aloft to cover with its heights the vault of heaven. To others inaccessible even in their imaginings, it abounds in rivers and trees and resounds with the most beautiful flocks of many-feathered birds.

One detail is of interest. The expression of the original, *divyauṣadhividīpitam* "illumined" or "shining brightly" (*vidīpita*) with divine herbs, which commonly occurs in this kind of literature, is difficult to interpret literally unless it is taken to refer to the aura of hallucinogenic plants. In his ethnographic tales about Don Juan, Castaneda also describes peyote plants as shining in the night. The shine is visible only to the initiated, or those who have already ingested a fair amount of drugs. The "divine herbs" are the *divyauṣadhi* mentioned before that may cause supernatural powers.

II. Buddhism

The first Indian Buddhists went to China around the middle of the first century A.D. They came from Kashmir, which was then one of the chief centers of Buddhist learning and the location of the fourth council, held approximately during the same period under the auspices of King Kaniṣka. These early Buddhists probably went via Gilgit, to which the Chinese returned several times, and which they occupied during the eighth century (see Chapter II.) At that time the route via Gilgit, the gateway to India, was unsafe because of Tibetan military invasions and raids. The Chinese emperor, Xuanzang (Hsüan Tsang) (713–755 A.D.), therefore sent an army of 4,000 men under the prefect of Kashgar to assist the local king or chief, and protect, i.e., occupy, Gilgit (Stein 1907, reprint 1975:4–7, referring to Chavannes 1903). According to legend, the Indian Buddhist emperor Aśoka established Buddhist colonies in Khotan much earlier, in the third century B.C.; though this is possible, it is not supported by any evidence. It is, however, clear that Buddhist traffic between India and Central Asia increased gradually from the first century A.D.

Specific information about the route has been provided by Chinese pilgrims who later traveled in the opposite direction. Faxian (Fa-hsien) (around 400 A.D.) describes a large mountain range he encountered before entering India, the Bolor-Tagh, probably also on the Gilgit road:

> On these mountains there is snow summer and winter alike. There are also venomous dragons, which, if provoked, spit forth poisonous winds, rain, snow, sand, and stones. Of those who encounter these dangers not one in ten thousand escapes. The people of that part are called Men of the Snow Mountains. (Translated by Giles 1923:9).

Faxian also describes his descent to the Indus River. Seven hundred steps had been cut into the rocks, and several ladders were placed alongside these steps. The river itself was spanned by a suspension bridge.

Xuanzang, who journeyed in the western and southern regions for sixteen years (629–645 A.D.), traveled via Balkh and entered the Bāmiyān region of Afghanistan, about which his biographer Hwui Li writes:

> It is situated in the middle of the Snowy Mountains [i.e., the Hindu Kush]. The muddy roads and dangers of the passes and tracks are double those of the frozen desert [described before]. The pelting hail and snowstorms go on perpetually intermingled; then, the winding and crooked passes that are met with; then, in the level parts, the mud stretching for several *changs*. . . . (Translated by Beal 1911:52).

Should we still assume that the first Buddhists went to China, and the Chinese pilgrims visited India, for "power and profit"? The answers are obviously less straightforward. People joined the Buddhist order for a variety of reasons. Nāgasena, for example, told King Milinda:

> Some join the order so that sorrow may perish and no further sorrow may arise . . . others for other reasons: some have left the world in terror at the tyranny of kings; some have joined to be safe from being robbed; some harassed by debts, and some perhaps to gain a livelihood. . . . (Quoted in Kane 1962:V.II, 1023).

As for Xuanzang himself, his biographer tells us what he said:

> Alas! if it were not that I had determined to seek the incomparable Law for the sake of all that lives, much rather would I have pleaded that this body of mine, left by my parents, should have gone on its journey. . . . [i.e., if not for the *dharma*, he would rather have died than journey through all these dangerous regions] (Beal 1911:52).

Should we then add religious fervor and fanaticism to power and profit as possible motives for these journeys? The dichotomy is to some extent artificial, and of our own making. The *dharma* is sought because it provides power and profit, albeit not only to the traveler, and not only of the kind we regard as material; however, neither is there justification to assume that it is only the kind we regard as "religious." In some cases, Chinese pilgrims sought material profit in the more common sense. In the seventh century, Ming-yüan went to Ceylon, where he stole the tooth of the Buddha, the most precious relic in Ceylon. He could not keep it (Ch'en 1964:239).

III. Tantrism

In Tantrism, too, the Himalayas are portrayed in mythological terms, as in other Hindu traditions; but there are also more specific references to Himalayan regions. A typical mythological description, inspired by classical Sanskrit literature, occurs in the description of Mount Kailāsa at the beginning of the *Mahānirvāṇa-tantra*:

> The enchanting summit of the Lord of Mountains, resplendent with all its various jewels, clad with many a tree and many a creeper, melodious with the song of many a bird, scented with the fragrance of all the season's flowers, most beautiful, fanned by soft, cool, and perfumed breezes, shadowed by the still shade of stately trees; where cool groves resound with the sweet-voiced songs of troops of celestial nymphs, and in the forest depths flocks of cuckoos, maddened with passion song; where spring ever abides. . . . (Translated by Arthur Avalon [Sir John Woodroffe] 1927:1–2).

Since the real Mount Kailāsa is more than 22,000 feet high, this description is totally romantic. Barring its idealistic overtones, it could only apply to Himalayan foothills. However, its romantic excesses do not seem to be mere products of the imagination. The expression *nānāratnopaśobhita*, "resplendent with various gems," like the shining herbs mentioned before, is reminiscent of hallucinogenic experience (see Huxley 1963:100–101).* Actual gems are not displayed on the surface of mountains; they are hidden inside.

Hindu Tantrism also has real affiliations with Himalayan regions: the most important centers of the Tantra are situated in Swat, Gandhāra, and Kashmir, in the northwest; and in Assam and Bengal, in the northeast. Since there is no early mention of affiliations with the central Himalayas, this distribution appears to be related to the northwestern and northeastern routes across the Himalayas; this, in turn, suggests that there were connections with regions beyond the Himalayas. This is supported by the well-known Tantric references to *cīna* and *cīnācara*, the "Chinese way" or "custom." This expression need not designate China itself, but could apply to any region north of the Himalayan range. After the eighth century, when Tantrism began to come to the fore, direct connections between India and Tibet were also established. This helps to explain the simultaneous flowering of Indian and Tibetan, Hindu and Buddhist forms of Tantrism. It is significant that no one knows whether the Tantra was originally Hindu or Buddhist, Indian or non-Indian.

We are entitled to conclude from these scattered references that contacts between India and Central Asia across the Himalayas are attested in the Vedic, Buddhist, and Tantric traditions. Such contacts are more mythological in the case of (other) Hindu traditions. We know from political history about many other large movements across these mountain ranges. Around 100 B.C., for example, the Yüeh-chih, a group of Central Asian nomads, reached the Hindu Kush and settled on both sides of the Oxus. Under their pressure, the Scythians moved further west into what is now Afghanistan. Around the same time, the northern Śakas, who also came from Central Asia, crossed the Pamirs and the Hindu Kush, adopted Sanskrit, and became Indianized. By contrast, the Kuṣāṇas, who founded an empire which incorporated (during the first centuries A.D.) large parts of northern India and Central Asia, did not become fully Indianized.

The migrations of Buddhism into Central Asia and China resulted not only in Buddhicization, but in what may be referred to as Indianization: they included many features of Indian civilization that are not Buddhist or are not exclusively Buddhist (for example, *mantras*, meditation, fire ceremonies, martial arts, certain philosophical concepts, medical theories, cosmological views, etc.).[2] The situation is not entirely dissimilar to what we find in the contemporary West: many self-styled converts to Hinduism or Buddhism do not realize that the features that attract them in these so-labelled traditions are not exclusive to either tradition, but belong to both, and are in fact features of Indian civilization.

3. LINGUISTIC AND RELIGIOUS APPROACHES TO THE STUDY OF THE VEDAS, BUDDHISM, AND TANTRISM

The following remarks pertain not only to the study of the Vedas, Buddhism, and Tantrism, but also to the study of Hinduism; and, in fact, they apply to all or most of the traditional Asian "-isms" that Western scholars and other outsiders have given a name. All these are topics considered in classical Oriental studies, which developed in the West in the wake of Protestantism and the study of the Bible. Many Orientalists have therefore assumed, as a matter not requiring any proof, that the traditions which constitute the object of their investigation are "religions" based on a holy book regarded as the infallible source of religious authority. This holy book deserves careful, that is, philological, study, which emphasizes the importance of language for the study of religion, just as early Oriental studies in the West emphasized Hebrew as the language needed to study the Bible. The methods used in these early studies appeared to have universal validity because they also proved appropriate to the second area of study, where they were applied; the study of the Quran, Arabic, and Islam. However, they were much less relevant when applied to traditions that did not have a holy book. In these cases, the role of language was quite different either because the transmissions were oral; because the emphasis was on ritual and other activities rather than on carefully worded doctrines; or because both oral transmission and ritual were emphasized. The Vedic, Hindu, and Tantric traditions have these characteristics, as does Buddhism to a large extent. All these traditions began, accordingly, to be systematically misinterpreted.

These considerations apply to the traditions of India and China in general, but here another development has obscured the issues and hindered understanding. China was the favorite of the Enlightenment, or the Age of Reason (the eighteenth century); it was, for example, a source of fascination to Leibniz. Since then, the Chinese have been pictured as reasonable, practical, businesslike, and materialistic. India, on the other hand, was the favorite of the Romantic Period (the nineteenth century), as evinced, for example, in its idolization by Schopenhauer. The Indians have accordingly been portrayed as universally devoted to religion and mysticism, and interested only in the next world. All these notions were projected upon the sources, which were therefore largely misinterpreted.

It is obvious that these alleged characteristics of the Chinese and Indians may be justified to some extent; however, their uncritical and wholesale acceptance and the ensuing exaggerations have led to serious distortions. The contrasts between India and China have never been as absolute as foreign scholars have made them appear; conversely, the similarities are much more significant than has generally been noted. Many examples could be adduced to illustrate this. The same features which in China would be looked upon as symptoms of gross superstition, for example, tend in India to be interpreted as expressions of deep religiosity.

The result of all these confusions, misrepresentations, and projections is that the phenomena we are dealing with here have been approached by scholars from a perspective that overemphasizes language and religion. These two categories themselves are, of course, quite different in character and scope. Language is an "objective" category: human beings have languages and express themselves through them. Religion, on the other hand, is a "subjective" category. Although the term "religion" occurs in the dictionaries of Western languages, it does not necessarily have a universal, or even a wide, application. It is a useful concept when dealing with the Western monotheistic systems, because it originated in this context. Its applicability elsewhere is precisely the problem we are considering.

The Vedas constitute a good example of the distortions to which the use of the concept of religion has led. "The Vedas" are obviously not a religion; they are oral traditions concerned with history, social structure, myths, legends, beliefs, ritual, and other things and activities. That a religion cannot easily be extracted from this mixture is illustrated by the ambiguity and obscurity of the term "Vedism," and by the absence of boundaries that could demarcate it. For example, where does "Vedism" end and "Hinduism" begin? Is there another "-ism" in between, "Brahmanism" perhaps, a term met with in some of the older literature? Do Hindus who accept Vedic authority or perform Vedic rites belong to two religions at the same time—Vedism and Hinduism? (Staal 1980)

The study of the Vedas has long suffered from extraneous perspectives imposed from the outside: the linguistic perspective, which stresses the Indo-European background, and the religious perspective, which stresses the Hindu sequel. I shall briefly examine how these two concepts, language and religion, have been used in the study of the Vedas, Buddhism, and Tantrism, and discuss the extent to which their use in these contexts has been helpful.

I. The Vedas

A. The Linguistic Approach The Vedas appealed to European scholars primarily because they offered very early texts in one of the oldest languages of the Indo-European family: Vedic Sanskrit. Subsequently, the picture has become a little more complex. It is generally assumed that the original home of the Indo-European language family must have been somewhere between Europe and India, but probably closer to Europe: in southern Russia, for example. The reason for this assumption is that there are languages now spoken in Europe that belong to many branches of this family; they are well differentiated from each other even though they are situated in closely adjacent areas. The evolution of the Indo-European languages, moreover, should not simply be pictured as the branching of a tree: there need not have been one single trunk, since it is likely that there were Indo-European dialects from the beginning, or from a very early period.

There are two main subdivisions of the Indo-European language family: one in the west and one in the east. The western group incorporates not only most of the languages of Europe, but also includes Hittite, spoken in Anatolia from around 1700 to 1200 B.C., and two forms of Tocharian, both spoken in Chinese Turkestan (Sinkiang) between the sixth and the tenth century A.D. These two languages constitute the furthest eastern extension of the western branch of Indo-European, and their existence, though attested relatively late, suggests that these languages originated further to the east than is generally assumed.

The eastern subdivision of Indo-European is Indo-Iranian, presumably spoken in the Oxus Valley during the second and early first millennium B.C. The Tocharian languages must have moved east much earlier, for they are more closely related to the western group (e.g., Balto-Slavonic) than to any of the Indo-Iranian languages. The Indo-Iranians themselves moved south into eastern Iran, presumably in the period between 1700 and 1400 B.C.; and went west from there to western Iran, and east to India. In India, the *Ṛgveda* was subsequently composed, after an interval of perhaps two hundred years. There are no clear references to this migration in the *Ṛgveda* itself. The Iranian languages fall into three groups: Old Iranian (comprising Avestan and Old Persian), Middle Iranian (e.g., Khotanese and Sogdian, both found in Central Asia), and New Iranian (e.g., Persian). The Indian languages include Sanskrit, various Middle Indic languages, and modern languages such as Hindi, Panjabi, and Bengali.

This linguistic diversity and these patterns of relationship demonstrate that there have been numerous movements across the western Himalayas (including the Hindu Kush) in prehistoric times. The Indo-Iranians moved south to begin with, but the Middle Iranian languages show that migrations between Iran and Central Asia continued to take place in later times. This positive evidence for early contacts shows that the exchanges we are studying in the present context have a much longer history than is generally realized.

There are also certain negative conclusions that have to be drawn. Linguistic relatedness, in particular, does not demonstrate cultural relatedness. I shall illustrate this with two examples. The first is the Vedic *soma* and the Iranian *haoma*. The two terms are obviously related from a linguistic point of view. The description of the plant in the Indian and Iranian sources, however, is very different. Recently this has led to two recent theories about its original identity, one by Gordon Wasson and another by David Flattery. According to Wasson (1968),* the original *soma* was a mushroom, the fly-agaric (*Amanita muscaria*). According to Flattery (1982),* the original *haoma* was the wild rue (*Peganum harmala*). The arguments adduced by both scholars are not only different, but their sources are different: Wasson uses primarily Indian sources, Flattery, primarily Iranian. Since the original descriptions are not the same, the linguistic relatedness of the terms does not prove anything, and the two plants may very well have been different from the beginning.

My second example is the term *iṣṭakā*, which does not occur in the *Ṛgveda*, but plays an important role in the *Yajurveda* (presumably composed about two centuries later than the *Ṛgveda*) where it denotes a kiln-fired brick, made of clay. Such bricks are used in the construction of the fire altar of the Agnicayana, with which many texts of the Yajurveda are concerned. Since the Vedic nomads did not carry bricks around, the techniques for firing bricks were presumably inherited from the earlier sedentary cultures of the Indus Civilization, which were characterized by large constructions made precisely from such kiln-fired bricks. Whatever the etymology of the term *iṣṭakā*, it seems likely, therefore, that it denotes an object of pre-Vedic origin. However, this conclusion is puzzling because Old Iranian also has a term for brick which is related to the Vedic term: *ištya*. Though it seems that the term was inherited from the common Indo-Iranian mother language, its reference could not have been inherited. Since the two terms have the same meaning, one may be a later borrowing; or there may be a more complex explanation. Whatever it is, these facts demonstrate that linguistic relatedness may not prove anything about anything else.

The study of languages is of course indispensable for the understanding of anything composed or written in these languages; moreover, linguistic relatedness is of linguistic interest. Beyond that, linguistic relatedness is relatively unimportant, and potentially misleading.

B. The Religious Approach While the linguistic and philological approaches to the study of the Vedas may be misleading, the religious approach creates problems that are entirely artificial and of our own making. I referred already to the indefinite character of the term "Vedism," and the pseudo-problems it engenders when it is used to name the earliest Indian "religion." It is not clear what is so "religious" about the Vedas in any case. There is as much reason to look upon them as religious "books" (which they are not in any event, being oral recitations), as to regard them as classics of economics, history, ritual, or poetry. It is true that in later Hinduism the Vedas are often regarded as a sacred "revelation" (*śruti*). However, the Vedas themselves do not make or imply such a claim. Moreover, there is a paradox surrounding the Vedas to which Louis Renou has referred (especially Renou 1960): there exists a considerable gap between the *Ṛgveda* and all later Indian developments. Though the *Ṛgveda* is often invoked, it is rarely known, and the attention paid to it is purely ritual. Even if the forms of these compositions are carefully transmitted, their meaning is generally lost since there existed at no time a tradition that preserved the meaning together with the forms. The Vedas have gained enormous prestige in later India, but the service paid to them is lip service.

In order to illustrate some of these statements, I shall discuss one example in some detail: the case of the so-called Hindu systems of Indian philosophy. These six systems are often referred to as *vaidika*, "Vedic," to emphasize that they preserve the Vedic heritage as distinct from the Buddhist or Jaina philosophical systems, which reject the Vedas and are accordingly called *avaidika*. A closer look at these systems, however, will soon dispel the justification for these labels. Let us begin with the famous Vedānta system, often regarded as incorporating the end and goal (*anta*) of the Vedas. Actually, the Vedānta itself uses the term "vedānta" to refer to the latest Vedic, and sometimes post-Vedic, texts of the *Upaniṣads*. There is indeed a continuity between some of these *Upaniṣads* and the later philosophy of the Vedānta. But the *Upaniṣads* themselves are very different from the large majority of the Vedic texts, although they do in some sense "belong" to the Vedas. There is an enormous gap not only between the *Ṛgveda* and the *Upaniṣads*, but between most of the Vedic corpus and the *Upaniṣads*. The affiliation of the Vedānta to the Veda is therefore rather *recherché*.

The second system, that of the *Mīmāṃsā*, accepts the authority of the Vedas in a serious and literal manner, and regards the Vedas as eternal and of nonhuman origin (*apauruṣeya*). This system does not confine its attention to one portion of the Vedic heritage, but accepts it in its totality. Whatever its particular slant and interpretation, there is plenty of reason, therefore, to regard the Mīmāṃsā as Vedic.

The situation is very different with regard to the remaining four philosophical systems: Yoga, Sāṃkhya, Vaiśeṣika, and Nyāya. These systems refer to the Vedas very rarely or not at all. They are not reminiscent of the Vedas, and do not in fact accept their authority. The Nyāya system accepts *śabda*, "language" or "verbal authority" as one of the means of valid knowledge. This may be interpreted as referring to the Vedas, but in the Nyāya system itself, it is primarily used to denote the statements of an expert in some field of knowledge (*āptavacana*). We are therefore led to the surprising conclusion that of the six so-called "Vedic" systems of Indian philosophy, the Vedas play no part in four, are important in the remaining two, but are taken seriously only in one. The Vedas are therefore very different from the holy books associated with the three monotheistic religions of the West. This was appreciated and correctly evaluated in Islam, for the Quran refers only to Christians and Jews along with Muslims as *ahl al-kitāb*, "people of the book." Hindus, on the other hand, are included in the large category called *mushrikūn*, "polytheists."

II. Buddhism

A. The Linguistic Approach The study of Buddhism requires knowledge of so many different languages that its practitioners are relatively few. The chief Buddhist languages are Sanskrit, Pāli, Chinese, Korean, Japanese, Tibetan, and Mongolian. Unlike the languages of the Indo-European family, the last five of these languages are not related to one another. There exists a large literature of translations, especially from Sanskrit into Chinese and Tibetan. Something is known of the methods and techniques used by the translators, who were often Central Asians (see, e.g., Demiéville 1952 and van Gulik 1956). The lack of linguistic relatedness has not prevented the production of numerous reliable translations, including fixed vocabularies for the translation of technical terms. There are also bad translations, however, and some have been ludicrously inadequate. Amusing examples have been given by Brough, who studied a late (tenth to thirteenth century A.D.) translation into Chinese of a difficult Sanskrit text: the *Jātakamālā*, "Garland of

Former Birth Stories (of the Buddha)," by Āryaśūra (Brough 1964). The two Chinese translators, says Brough, "did persevere in the sad labour of forcing what little sense they could from the difficult Sanskrit." Their blunders were numerous. They believed, for example, that the Sanskrit numeral "ten" (which is *daśa*) was *darśa*. The word *darśa* happens to be a form of the stem of the Sanskrit verb "to see" or "to appear," which is exceedingly common. Whenever the Sanskrit text had expression like *dadarśa*, "he saw," *darśana*, "sight," etc., the translators brought in the "ten good courses of action" (*daśa kuśalāni*). "The word *kuśala*, indeed, did not appear at these places," writes Brough (1964:49), "but why strain at a gnat?"

The Chinese and the Indians had very different ideas about what constitutes a language (Staal: 1979a). The Vedic compositions were always transmitted orally, and were not written down until the Middle Ages. The Indians borrowed systems of writing only relatively late, and confined their use to commercial and administrative contexts, especially in the beginning; nothing important, and certainly nothing sacred (or secret, such as the *Upaniṣads*), was ever written down. The Chinese, on the other hand, were obsessed by writing, and developed their system of characters from a very early period. In this system each character denotes principally a unit of meaning; however, other characters may be used to further identify these meaningful characters, and to indicate features of sound. Since there were numerous mutually unintelligible dialects in the Chinese empire, learning a new dialect meant learning to pronounce characters in a new way. Applying these ideas to the study of Indian scripts seemed ludicrously simple: the "characters" are few, easy to write, and they correspond with pronunciation in a simple and straightforward manner. Having mastered these features of language, the Chinese assumed that they knew "the Indian language," for what else could there be to know? They were baffled only when they found that they did not in fact understand it.

A curious circumstance supported the original assumption of the Chinese, namely, that learning a language meant learning the pronunciation of a script. Buddhism introduced into China numerous *dhāraṇī*, magical spells, such as: *kirikiri vajrabhūr bandha hūṃ phaṭ* (a *mantra*, found as far east as Japan, which accompanies the gesture of the blue lotus). The Chinese were eager to receive such sacred noises not only because they sounded mysterious and therefore full of meaning, resembled the magical formulas of popular Taoism, and were suitable for recitation and meditation, but also because they conformed precisely to the Chinese idea of language. For as soon as one knows how to derive the pronunciation of a *mantra* from the way it is written, one knows all there is to know about it. The rest is speculation, and arbitrary at that. Arbitrary interpretations of *mantras* are not confined to later Buddhism. They go back at least as far as the *Upaniṣads*.

We can only imagine how mysterious Buddhism must have appeared to the Chinese—it was a tradition, moreover, that encouraged people to shave their heads and give up that most sacrosanct of all Chinese institutions: the family. Of course, here the road was again paved, at least to some extent, by popular Taoism.

B. The Religious Approach These considerations lead more or less naturally to a discussion of the status of Buddhism as a possible religion. I have so far abstained from attempting to define religion, although I have claimed that the term is applicable to the three monotheistic "religions" of the West, where it originated, and questioned its applicability to the Asian traditions we are considering. The reasons for the absence of a definition are clear: definitions can be given only at the successful completion of an investigation. The so-called religious phenomena we are dealing with have a conceptual status that is still largely unclear. A great deal of analysis and conceptual clarification has to be engaged in before a serious investigation can be said to have begun. During these preliminary investigations, we are led by intuitions, which are tested in the course of the work and may ultimately lead to adequate definitions. "Instinct, intuition, or insight is what first leads to the beliefs which subsequent reason confirms or confutes" (Russell 1953:19).

For the time being, it appears that Buddhism has some of the characteristics of a religion. First of all, with certain exceptions to which I shall return, and unlike the Vedic and Tantric traditions, Buddhism is relatively clearly demarcated. We can say, in most cases, who is a Buddhist and who is not. Moreover, Buddhism has a historical founder, the Buddha, and is in this respect similar to Christianity and Islam, though not to Judaism. At the same time, there are also considerable differences. There is no sacred book. The Western effort to raise the *Dhammapada* to such a status is ridiculous, and merely reflects a Western perspective. Like the *Bhagavad Gītā*, which has been assigned a similarly artificial role in Hinduism, the *Dhammapada* is one of many canonical writings, one that has been popular at certain times and in some regions. The same applies to the enormous literature of Buddhism, canonical or noncanonical, with which scholars are familiar: the value attached to these sources is uneven and variable. This is true of all so-called Hindu and Buddhist "sacred writings," including the Vedas and Tantras: they were recited, studied, followed, or invoked only by some people, at some times, and in some places.

The chief difference between Buddhism and the Western monotheistic religions is, of course, that Buddhism is atheistic and does not accept the immortality of the soul—in fact, does not believe in a soul at all. In this respect, it is similar to the Hindu system of the Mīmāṃsā, which is the most "Vedic" of the Indian systems of philosophy. When the concept of religion is defined, a decision will have been made whether a religion may be atheistic, in which case Buddhism may be a religion.

The relations between Hinduism and Buddhism are particularly fluid. Indian history provides many examples of Hindus becoming Buddhists, of Hindu temples turning into Buddhist temples, and *vice versa*. In these transformations, there are preferred alliances. For example, the reclining Buddha called *parinirvāṇa* tends to turn his head ninety degrees and be transformed into Viṣṇu lying on the serpent who is called *anantaśayana*. A contemporary example of such a transformation can be witnessed at the monastery of Spituk near Leh. This Buddhist shrine to the ferocious Mahākāla is in the process of being turned into a Hindu shrine to the equally fierce goddess Mahākālī by soldier-devotees from the Indian army encamped nearby, who have introduced prayer flags sporting the *mantra OṂ*, vermillion powder for the application of *kuṃkuma* to one's forehead, electricity to dispel the mystery-generating gloom, and last but not least water tanks, towels, and soap, emphasizing Hindu notions of purity.

III. Tantrism

A. The Linguistic Approach Languages needed for the study of Tantrism are Sanskrit, Tibetan, Apabhraṃśa (a Middle Indic language), Old Bengali, and Bengali. Since Tantric traditions are fluid, generally popular, and often esoteric, the so-called sources are admirably characterized by a favorite invective of philologists: they are corrupt. This refers not only to the state of the language, but often includes the style of the texts. Snellgrove (1959a:I,10) writes about the *Hevajra-tantra:* "The style is often crude and disjointed, and the whole work shows no logical construction." In his second volume he adds: "The language need not be graced by the term Buddhist Sanskrit. It is just bad Sanskrit" (Snellgrove 1959a:II, xi).

One style of language is characteristic of the *tantras*: the so-called *sandhābhāṣā* or "twilight language." This has also been interpreted as "intentional language," sometimes misinterpreted as *sandhyābhāṣā* which is of course unhelpful since all language is intentional. The correct interpretation of *sandhā* is "esoteric meaning." The simplest translation of *sandhābhāṣā* is, therefore, "secret language." In practice, this means that the language of the tantras should not be taken literally, but interpreted symbolically. Since it is not always clear where symbolism begins, the intent of many passages remains controversial.

B. The Religious Approach I have already mentioned that Tantrism is Buddhist as well as Hindu. It is not clear in which tradition the Tantras originated if, in fact, they originated in a single tradition, and had a single origin. There are very close connections between Tantrism and Yoga, an ancient complex of ideas, practices, and techniques found in both Hinduism and Buddhism. Further connections can and have been traced with the *Atharva-veda*, medicine, and magic in India, and with Taoism in China. It is certainly not easy to make Tantrism fit comfortably into the Procrustean bed of religion.

P.V. Kane (1962:II,1076) quotes a typical tantric verse:

> *antaḥ kaulaṃ bahiḥ śaivaṃ lokācāre tu vaidikam*
> *sāram ādāya tiṣṭhet tu nārikelaphalaṃ yathā*

"Inside a Tantric, outside a Śaivite, in worldly practice Vedic, let him live grasping the essence like a coconut." As Kane notes, the coconut is hard outside, liquid inside, and soft in between. In other versions of these lines, "Vedic" is replaced by "Vaiṣṇavite." Scholars, naturally, are baffled by such expressions as, for example, S. Gupta (1979:121): "There is a tendency among present-day Tantrics not to establish their exclusive identity, but take over other religious traditions which approximate their own." Actually, nothing about this phenomenon is confined to the present day. Moreover, who are we to ask for "exclusive identity"—census officials or police officers? Insistence on labeling in conformity with outside expectations may be called the "visiting card syndrome."

This syndrome is of course not confined to Tantrism, Buddhism, and Hinduism. A good example occurs in the otherwise excellent book by Ivan Morris on the Heian Period (1964:105–106), where a passage from *The Tale of Genji* is analyzed with labels in the following manner:

> Ukifune's visit to a Buddhist temple . . . is prevented by a defilement (Shintoism) and by a bad dream (superstition). Again, in order to prepare for the visit, Ukifune's ladies have purified themselves according to Buddhist practice by abstaining from meat and fish, and also have rendered themselves ritually clean by lustration and other Shintoist ritual; yet all their efforts become nugatory because of a taboo. Niou's excuse for spending the day at Uji is that he is on a retreat (Buddhist), while he keeps Ukifune with him on the pretext of Taboo (Shintoist).

The conclusion that may be drawn from all these facts and considerations is that neither language nor religion are natural and helpful categories of thought in the study and understanding of the Vedas, Buddhism, and Tantrism. Language is, of course, a necessary tool required to study and understand linguistic manifestations of the three traditions. Religion, on the other hand, has caused the issues to be obscured. Language and religion are categories that divide into separate groups entities that are clearly similar and closely related, and group together things that have nothing to do with each other. In an attempt at conceptual clarification, the use of such categories, therefore, evinces bad logic. That linguistic relatedness has nothing to do with historical relations follows immediately from two facts: first, the language of the Vedas is related to other Indo-European languages that have been vehicles for the expression of very different ideas and institutions; and second, the languages of Buddhism, though unrelated to one another, have all been used to express the same or similar ideas and doctrines. While this putting together of what does not belong together, and this pulling apart of what does belong together, are obvious in the case of language, they are less obvious in the case of religion. This topic therefore deserves more specific treatment.

4. CONTINUITIES ACROSS CONCEPTUAL BOUNDARIES

I shall now discuss seven examples in order to show that Vedic, Buddhist, and Tantric ideas and practices are closely related, or merge into each other, and also have close relationships with other Asian traditions. This discussion will not only demonstrate that these labels cannot be used to name religions, but also that there is not much justification for attaching any such labels.

I. Perforated Stones

In the Vedic ritual of the fire altar (*agnicayana*), certain "naturally perforated stones" (*svayamātṛṇṇa*) are used. They are put in the center of the first, third, and fifth layer of the bird-shaped altar of the *Agnicayana* by the chief priest, the *Adhvaryu*, who on each of these occasions—and only on these occasions—is assisted by a mysterious personage called the Ignorant Brahmin. I have argued elsewhere (Staal 1982a:I,139–166; 1982b:42–53) that the Vedic Indians imported the notion of these naturally perforated stones from Central Asia. Similar stones were found there by Aurel Stein; the Tibetans value them; and in various shamanistic practices in northern Asia use is also made of similarly perforated pebbles. The Chinese have long been interested in perforated stones, which they regard as miniature representations of rocks with caves, and in particular of the World Mountain. Such stones are placed in miniature gardens that exhibit the same correspondences between microcosm and macrocosm. The mountains are regarded as the abodes of spirits, presided over by a great deity who can be approached through caves and tunnels. At the same time, these stones are models of the celestial palaces of the gods. Their holes correspond to the stars.

Often such pebbles are found in river beds. In the Hindu cult of Viṣṇu, there is a similar stone, the *śālagrāma*, originally found in or near the river bed of the Gandak River in Nepal. It should be naturally perforated. Even the rosary beads of the *rudrākṣa*, so favored by Śaiva ascetics, are preferred when they are naturally, rather than artificially, pierced for the introduction of the thread (Ghurye 1953:92). So we have here a whole complex of practices and beliefs that makes its appearance in China and India, on both sides of the Himalayas, and is incorporated into a variety of traditions—Vedic, Hindu, Buddhist, Taoist, and Shaman. The multiplicity of these labels does not disguise the fact that we are dealing with ancient traditions that have many ramifications, and nothing to do with the "great" religions.

II. Breathing and Recitation

Breathing techniques are generally associated with Yoga, and rightly so. However, they also occur in the later Vedic literature, where the precise nature and meaning of five breaths (*prāṇa*, *apāna*, *vyāna*, *samāna* and *udāna*) continues to be a subject of controversy. Breath enables the *yajamāna* or patron of the ritual to recite the Vedic hymns; it therefore gives him direct access to the Vedas. In some rites breath is sacrificed, and all important rites are preceded by *prāṇāyāma*, which is an exercise of breath control. Breathing is also regarded as silent recitation; it is related to recitals described as *anirukta*, "unenunciated," and *upāṃśu*, "inaudible." Some rites are performed "in silence" (*tuṣṇīm*); they are accompanied by breathing only, or by recitations that are executed mentally (*manasā*) and that are therefore tantamount to meditations. In all Vedic recitation, breath control plays an important role. In the ritual of the chanters, for example, *aniruktagāna*, "unenunciated chant," is a protracted chant of "*o*" with the same structure and melody as the underlying *mantra*, which is represented mentally. The recitations of the *Ṛgveda* that are called *śastra*, "weapon," to which I referred before, are also rendered in accordance with special rules that prescribe where breathing should take place (always in the middle, and never at the end of the *mantra*), and where long "*o*" and other vowel recitations are to be inserted. It is in these contexts that we must look for the origin of the *mantra OṂ*.

In Yoga, we meet with *prāṇāyāma* as a regular part of the traditional techniques. The term *prāṇāyāma*, however, also refers to the natural process of breathing that is going on in the body in waking states as well as in sleep. Breath or *prāṇa* is a vibratory activity (*spanda-śakti*) basic to all forms of life. Speculation on this topic has been endless, and often reflects theories of traditional Indian medicine, which postulate the existence of channels in the body through which breath and breaths are flowing. I shall return to some of these theories in a later example (V: Sexual Techniques). For the present it is sufficient to note that these breath-related theories and exercises that are basic to the Yoga and to Indian medicine occur, with certain variations, in many forms of Hinduism, Buddhism, and Tantrism. In the Tantra, for example, the five breaths mentioned above are related to the mystic syllables *aiṃ*, *hrīṃ*, *srīṃ*, etc.

Breathing and reciting are similar in some contexts and complementary in others. Like breathing techniques, *mantra* recitation occurs in most Indian traditions. Gonda (1963) has demonstrated that the notion of *mantra* has remained fundamentally the same throughout its long development. In a recent unpublished paper, Wheelock described how in both Vedic and Tantric usages, *mantras* are primarily connected with ritual activity. The Tantric monosyllabic *bīja* or "seed" *mantras* carry one "beyond the boundaries of language" (Wheelock),* and in both the Tantric and Vedic rituals there is emphasis on meaningless *mantras* and on silent *mantras*. All *mantras* of this type point back to "the source of language" (cf. Padoux 1963:296). I have argued elsewhere (Staal 1980) that *mantras* preserve or remanifest a prelinguistic stage of development, during which man or his ancestors used sound in a purely syntactic or ritual manner. Later, language developed as meaningful communication. In essence, *mantras* are ritual, and therefore meaningless (Staal 1979b).

Similarities between Tantrism and Taoism have often been noted. They are not confined to the realm of *mantras*, but pertain to *prāṇāyāma* and to the sexual techniques I shall discuss below. In China respiratory techniques are also ancient. They are mentioned in an inscription on twelve pieces of jade probably dating from the sixth century B.C. (Needham 1956:II, 143–144). In China, these techniques are similarly connected with traditional medicine, or what has been called "ancient pneumatic physiology." Needham, who briefly discusses them, provides an explanation for some of the results of these techniques which is equally applicable to the Yoga: "There can be little doubt that the subjective effects which the Taoists experienced, and which they believed were so good for them, were due largely to anoxaemia, since they experienced asphyxic symptoms, buzzing in the ears, vertigo and sweating" (Needham, 1956:II, 143–144). The similarities in some of these developments are so close that there must have been historical connections between India and China in this domain. Scholars do not agree on whether the origins should be sought in India, China, or Central Asia. Connections between breath and wind (wind being the breath of a cosmic man: *Ṛgveda* 10.90.13) are certainly Indo-Iranian, and are also found in Shamanism.

A final word about the development of the theory of recitation in Buddhism. The earliest Buddhist position with regard to recitation was ambiguous: the sonorous recitation of the Vedas by brahmins was resented, but at the same time there is a tradition according to which the Buddha liked a young monk because of the beauty of his voice, and asked him to chant in his cell at night. Later, monks were not permitted to repeat aloud the syllables that were recited first by the master of ceremonies; they had to reproduce them mentally (Lamotte 1976:IV,1868). This resembles, as we have seen, the Vedic and Tantric traditions. A different attitude seems to prevail with reference to the *dhāraṇī* or magical spells, which resemble the *bīja mantras* of Tantrism. Lamotte has translated a Yogācāra text which makes a distinction between *artha-dhāraṇī*, "meaningful *dhāraṇī*," and *mantra-dhāraṇī*. The former have a meaning that is not yet formulated, or even expressed mentally. The latter are extremely effective: they are used by the Bodhisattva to alleviate the afflictions of all beings (Lamotte 1976:IV,1857–1858; the term *īti*, "affliction," which is used here, generally refers to diseases, thus underlining the Buddha's effectiveness as a medicine man). The difference between *samādhi*, "concentration," and *dhāraṇī* is that the former is always associated with thinking, whereas the latter can be associated with it or dissociated from it. In the final analysis, the situation is, therefore, extremely similar to what we find in the Vedas and in Tantrism.

III. Dīkṣā or Consecration

I shall translate the Sanskrit term *dīkṣā* as "consecration," though it is sometimes translated as "initiation." The English word "initiation" is better reserved for the translation of such terms as *upanayana* or *upasampadā*: the first denotes the ceremony during which boys become "twice-born," i.e., actual members of the high caste into which they were born; the second denotes the ceremony in which a person joins the Buddhist order and becomes a monk or nun. Many similarities exist between these two ceremonies. The term *dīkṣā*, on the other hand, refers to consecration ceremonies in which a person prepares himself for a specific position, task, or status. This occurs in Vedic and Hindu contexts; in Tantrism its function is, in fact, closer to that of an initiation. However, here I am interested not so much in functions (which vary with the circumstances), as in specific ritual features (which are often invariant).

In Vedic ritual, the *dīkṣā* ceremony occurs at the beginning of each of the larger *śrauta* rituals (see e.g., Staal 1982a:I,317–333). The ritual patron or *yajamāna* is partially shaved, his nails are pared, he bathes, changes dress, butter is put on parts of his body, and he is struck with blades of *darbha* grass. His wife undergoes similar rites. This is followed by an offering of clarified butter placed into the fire. In the Agnicayana, the *ukhā* pot, a large clay vessel, is brought and fire is supposed to originate in it. The *yajamāna* sits down on an antelope skin, a rope (*mekhalā*) made of hemp is tied around him, and a long piece of cloth is wound around his head into a kind of turban that looks as if it has horns at four corners. Next he is given a staff, and is tied with a string to the *ukhā* pot; a breastplate is fastened to his neck with another string and a band of antelope skin is put around him. After three "Viṣṇu" steps and numerous recitations, the band is removed. The turban is removed during the next ceremony. At the end of the *dīkṣā* itself, the *yajamāna* is addressed by a senior member of the community.

In Tantrism, the *dīkṣā* ceremony begins with the consecration of the ground (which in the Vedic ritual had been done earlier) and with the placing of vessels in which *aṅkura* shoots are put (see Hoens 1979:80–84; these same shoots are utilized in other Vedic rites, but not in the *dīkṣā*). The teacher should bathe, keep silent, purify himself, and then worship an image of the deity. The pupil should sip water, perform, mentally an "application" (*nyāsa*) on different parts of his body, and brush his teeth. The teacher and pupil pass the night together on *darbha* grass. The next day begins with an offering of clarified butter into the fire. The teacher looks at his pupil "with a divine look" (*divyacakṣuṣā*) and touches different parts of his body. The pupil is blindfolded and throws flowers toward a jar. Then the teacher, by means of meditation and *mantras*, mentally destroys the pupil and restores him. He applies different *mantras* to the pupil's body. From that moment on, the pupil dedicates his body, his wealth, and his whole life to the teacher. He feeds him and pays him a sacrificial fee (as is done in the Vedic ritual on a later occasion). (For Vajrayāna consecration ceremonies, see Chapters V and VII.)

In another form of Tantric *dīkṣā*, called *nirvāṇa-dīkṣā*, threads that represent fetters or forms of bondage are tied to different parts of the pupil's body. Subsequently, these threads are cut and thrown into the fire. In a variant of this rite, a string is wound around the pupil's body twenty-five times and then cut and burnt. In this way the pupil is said to have died and be reborn.

I shall not comment in detail upon the similarities and dissimilarities between these various forms of *dīkṣā*. It seems obvious that we are dealing with closely related ceremonies about which we happen to be informed in detail with respect to two stages of their complex and probably continuous development: the Vedic and the Tantric. As for intermediate or otherwise related forms (both Hindu and Buddhist), let me only mention that in the *upanayana* ceremony we also find similar purification rituals, a girdle, an antelope skin, and the famous "sacred thread." Omitting such parallels, we possess two snapshots made at an interval of more than a thousand years. We can only guess at what a complete film of this ritual development would be like.

IV. Fire Rituals

Agni ("fire") is the basic substance and deity in all Vedic rituals. We have already seen how fire ceremonies and oblations into the fire are incorporated into the consecration ceremonies, and how the perforated pebbles of our first example are inserted into a fire altar. The Vedic fire ceremonies continue in the *homa* rites of medieval Hinduism and are incorporated into Tantrism. They were also transferred with surprisingly little change to Buddhism, where they flourished in Vajrayāna Buddhism, and in the Japanese Shingon and Tendai sects, as well as among the Yamabushi, or mountain-dwelling ascetics. The Japanese term for the *homa* rite is nothing but the Japanization of the Sanskrit term as *goma*.

To study the forms and interconnections of all these various related fire rituals would require major investigation such as cannot be undertaken here. The basic features are described in various sources, but in the present context it may be sufficient to refer to a publication on the Vedic ritual of the fire altar: Staal 1982a. The first volume of this book contains a detailed description of the Vedic ritual; the second volume includes several contributions on related forms, such as chapters on Agni offerings in Java and Bali (by C. Hooykaas),* on Tibetan *homa* rites (by Tadeusz Skorupski), and on *homa* in East Asia (by Michel Strickmann). The Tibetan and Japanese fire ceremonies are still very much alive. They clearly derive from Indian Buddhist forms which no longer exist.

Strickmann refers in the introduction to his chapter to many related fire ceremonies: for example, the Śaivite traditions of Tamilnadu and Kashmir and the practices of the Hindu-Buddhist Vajrācāryas of the Kathmandu Valley of whom Snellgrove has written: "Their one need is to know how to perform the rites, of which the *homa*-sacrifice is the most important." Strickmann regards all the contemporary instances of *homa* as a Tantric metamorphosis of the Vedic ritual. There are, in fact, countless continuities and discontinuities. The emphasis on fire-sticks (sticks of firewood), which are put on the fire to the accompaniment of *mantras,* is found in all Vedic, Hindu, Tantric, and Buddhist fire ceremonies. However, in China there appears an incense burner which has no counterpart in India. In these later Buddhist traditions, the three basic fires of the Vedic ritual, the "domestic fire" (*gārhapatya*), the "offering fire" (*āhavanīya*), and the "southern fire" (*dakṣiṇa*), are identified respectively with three classes of persons deserving honor and attention: wives, children, and domestic servants; parents; and brahmins and ascetics. A new development in Buddhism is a fire-meditation, in which the adept visualizes himself as completely consumed by fire so that he perceives that he is entirely without self. Side by side with such spiritual developments, the fire rituals persisted. The recited *mantras* continue to refer to Agni, and are sometimes distinguishable from the Vedic only by their pronunciation. Most of the ritual implements are direct counterparts of their Vedic predecessors. In many offerings, for example, two ladles are used: clarified butter is scooped by the smaller ladle from its vessel, poured from the smaller ladle into the bigger, and the oblation is then made from the bigger ladle. (See Fig. 8.) In all these examples there is evidence of the gradual transformation of ancient ceremonies that have nothing to do with the labels "Vedic," "Hindu," "Buddhist," or "Tantric". Those who insist that the term "religion" be employed might find it simpler to refer to a single Fire Religion with a long and varied history on both sides of the Himalayas.

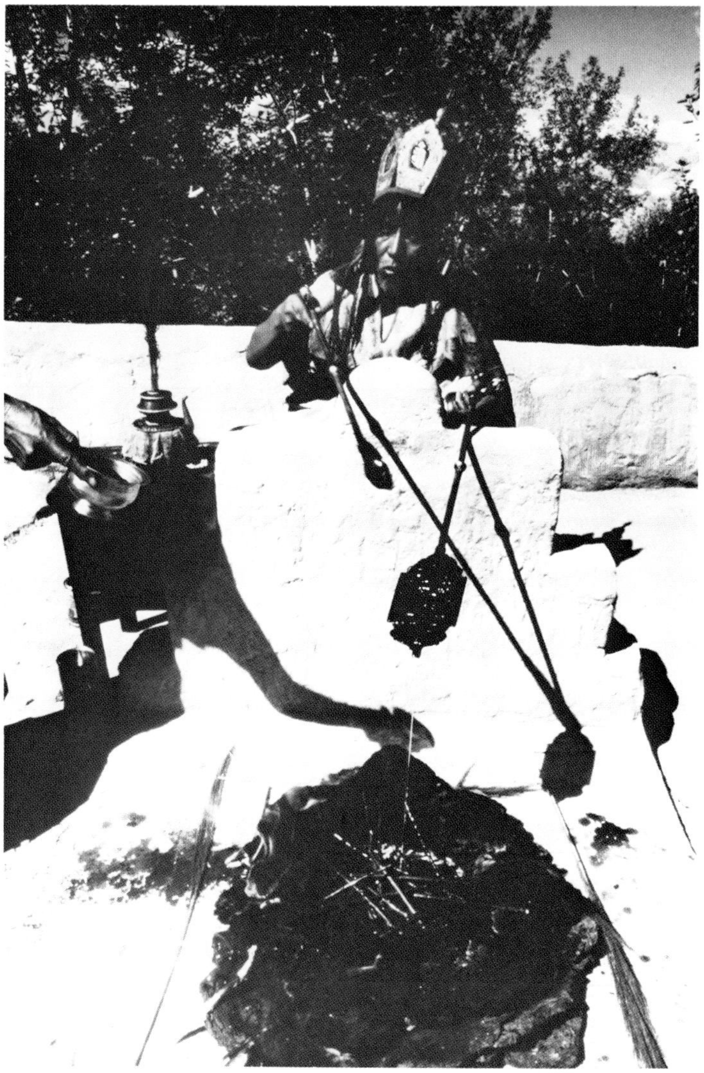

8. Fire Ceremony, Zangskar.

V. Sexual Techniques

One of the basic notions of Kuṇḍalinī Yoga (or "Yoga adorned with earrings"), adopted and adapted in the Tantra, is a mysterious power called *kuṇḍalinī* that ascends through the body via a path characterized by equally mysterious centers, each called *cakra*. This term, which we have met several times, suggests that this ascent is akin to the movements of the Vedic nomads and of Buddhism across the Himalayas. The *cakra* centers are not found in traditional Indian medicine, but they are combined in generally unclear ways with theories about the spine and other "channels" in the body adopted in this system of medicine. The *kuṇḍalinī* is described as a "fine fibre like a lightning flash" (Dasgupta 1932:II,356). It is not clear whether it is actually a physical nerve or some kind of nervous or other energy. Its descriptions vary, as do descriptions of the *cakras*.

The lowest *cakra* is sometimes described as a cave located at the foot of a cosmic mountain. In nonmetaphorical terms, it is located between the anus and the genital organs. In the Hindu Tantra, this *cakra* is regarded as the lowest of seven, located respectively at the base of the penis (only male anatomy is taken into account), near the navel, in the heart, between the eyebrows, and at the top of the head (or slightly above it). In the Buddhist Tantra, always slightly more puritanical, we generally find only the four highest of these *cakras;* but there are variations, as I mentioned. The *cakra* at the top of the head, represented by a thousand-petaled lotus, is referred to by Buddhists as *uṣṇīṣa* after the protuberance on the top of the Buddha's head that is also visible in sculpture (Pl. 82). It is also assimilated to Mount Meru, or Kailāsa, as the case may be; it should not surprise us that these *cakras* take us again across the Himalayas.

In the *Śiva-saṃhitā* there is a passage (1.196) translated as follows by Jean Varenne (and from his French by Derek Coltman):

> *At the top of the body, above the head,*
> *there is the lotus with a thousand petals,*
> *shining like the light of heaven:*
> *it is the giver of liberation.*
> *Its secret name is Kailāsa,*
> *the mountain where Śiva dwells.*
> *He who knows this secret place*
> *is freed from* saṃsāra *[transmigration].*

Varenne (1976:175) has correctly brought out the associations implicit in this verse: "It is significant that the name Kailāsa should be given to this 'place outside the body' . . . For Śiva's paradise is a region of delight where the supreme being joys eternally in his union with his *śakti*: the final liberation is thus presented as being a sort of perpetual wedding feast, an orgasm without end."

A contemporary Indian mystic provides a description that is not altogether different. Though it avoids any mention of sex, it is replete with animal references:

> There are five kinds of *samādhi*. First, he feels the Mahāvāyu (the great nerve current whose rising is felt in the spinal column) rise like an ant crawling up. Second, he feels It rise like fish swimming in the water. Third, he feels It rise like a snake wriggling along. Fourth, he feels It rise like a bird flying—flying from one branch to another. Fifth, he feels It rise like a monkey making a big jump; the Mahāvāyu reaches the head with one jump, as it were, and *samādhi* follows. (Sri Ramakrishna 1947:677; cf. 174.)

The notion that *kuṇḍalinī* is related to orgasm is even supported by contemporary popular magazines. In *Cosmopolitan* (August, 1976), C. Dragonwagon published some answers he received to the question, "What is orgasm like?" An unnamed but perceptive nurse replied: "The sensation is very, very diffuse at first and then focuses, moving up the spine. The better the sex is, the higher the tingling goes, and (when everything is flowing perfectly) you somehow *leave* your body—disappear right out through the top of your head."

Books and articles on *yoga* are widely available these days, and it is not impossible that our nurse was familiar with such literature. Whether she was or not, connections between *kuṇḍalinī* and sex are undeniable. There is an ancient belief in Tantric Yoga that the seminal fluid can be made to ascend through the body, and reach the brain. Whether this notion is itself the origin of *kuṇḍalinī* is not clear. At any rate, when semen reaches the head, wonderful powers are said to result. However, for this to happen, semen must not be spilt elsewhere, and therefore, the basic concern in the Tantra, Hindu as well as Buddhist, is its retention. One method for achieving this aim is by exerting pressure, prior to ejaculation, on the urethra at the lowest *cakra*. This forces the seminal secretion into the bladder. According to the Yogins, however, it thus begins to make its way up to the brain.

This practice and the underlying theories are still very much alive. Swamī Muktananda (1974:98),* for example, writes: "the entire seminal fluid accumulated in the testicles starts flowing upwards towards the heart. Then it gets purified by the gastric fire and moves on into the brain, strengthening all the sensory nerves and greatly enhancing a yogi's power of memory and intelligence." Compared to these ideas, Freud's notion of sublimation is mere child's play.

The remarkable fact is that similar practices and theories were adopted by the Taoists. This is described by Needham (1956:II, 149,428), who also mentions that similar techniques have been used as a contraceptive device by Turks, Armenians, and Marquesan Islanders. What is interesting about the theory of the "nourishing of the brain" is that it is so patently false. For Indians and Chinese to share such an erroneous theory, there must be a historical explanation. Again, it is not obvious whether the source lies in India, China, or Central Asia. Not surprisingly, Needham is inclined to accept a Chinese source; whereas Indologists, such as Filliozat (1969), prefer an Indian origin.

In India, these sexual techniques are especially associated with the northeast. It is possible, therefore, that the link with China was across the eastern Himalayas. This region is in any event implied when, in the seventh century, the *Tao Te Ching* was translated into Sanskrit for the benefit of a king of Assam (cf. Pelliot 1912). Unfortunately, this translation is lost.

VI. Dismemberment

We have seen that the corpse of General Zorawar Singh was cut into pieces, and also that the breath of a primeval person was believed to be the origin of wind. Actually, these facts are related. The hymn of the *Ṛgveda* (10.90) that refers to this primeval person describes how the entire universe originated from his dismemberment. In later Vedic literature, the same is said of Parjāpati: the world comes into being from his sacrifice. According to Mus (1935), this myth of dismemberment is not of Aryan origin. It is common in the religious ethnography of Southeast Asia and parts of the Pacific. It is related, on the one hand, to human sacrifice and, on the other, to the belief in relics. The deposition of relics of the Buddha within a *stūpa* or *chorten* is therefore not so different from the treatment given to parts of Zorawar Singh's body.

Macdonald (1975) has placed Mus' ideas in a wider perspective by providing more ethnographic evidence from south, southeast, east, and central Asia. At an Oxford conference in 1979, he reported on the practices and beliefs of Sherpas and Tamangs with reference to this "démembrement créateur." As is well known, the Parsis leave the bodies of their dead in the open air for vultures to dispose of. Some Tibetans dismember dead bodies and dispose of them in a similar manner. This has been filmed in Dolpo by Kawakita Jiro.

It is likely that these practices were once more widespread than they are at present. In the southwest Indian state of Kerala, for example, Nambudiri brahmins touch various parts of the dead body with a knife. The traditional explanation for this custom involves the most famous Nambudiri brahmin of the past, the philosopher Śaṅkara. Śaṅkara became a *saṃnyāsin* or wandering ascetic and was, accordingly, excommunicated by the orthoprax Nambudiri followers of the Mīmāṃsā. When his mother died, there was no one to help him carry her to the funeral pyre. Since he could not carry her himself (being a weakened ascetic, perhaps, or because his mother was too heavy), he dismembered the body. Of course, this legendary explanation is a rationalization; it is more likely that the Nambudiri custom reflects a widespread ancient practice.

The Parsi custom refutes Mus' belief that dismemberment is not of Aryan origin. Actually, it may be Central Asian. Some Siberian Shamans place a knife or an axe on a person's dead body (Chernetsov in Michael 1963:30).* Eliade refers to several cases of shamanistic initiation, where the body of the initiate is first symbolically dismembered and then put together again (1969:320–323). We have already considered the Tantric variety, and it is not impossible that the "application" rite (*nyāsa*), to which I referred in that context, is connected with this. In all these cases, the initiate is thought of as dying and being reborn. We find this illusion also in the famous Indian rope trick. The Buddha himself convinced his kinsmen of his miraculous attainments by a similar exhibition: he rose into the air, cut his body to pieces, let his limbs and head fall to the ground, and then joined them together again before the spectators' wondering eyes (*Buddhacarita* XIX, 12–13, quoted by Eliade 1969:321). Similar stories are found in China, Java, ancient Mexico, and medieval Europe. Not very long ago, a political murder in Vietnam was followed by a dismemberment of the corpse (Popkin 1979:55).[3]* So here is another ancient belief, found on all sides of the Himalayas.

VII Power Spots

"Power spot" is Castaneda's term for what in the phenomenology of religion is tamely referred to as "sacred space." I have already mentioned Mount Kailas and the Manasarovar Lake as places of pilgrimage that have attracted Hindus, Buddhists, and others. Mount Everest itself is similarly sacred to different people. The Kashmir region and northwest India in general became, in Lamotte's words (1970:III,xi), the second Holy Land of Buddhism (the first being Magadha).

Holy places are of universal interest, and pilgrimages are the precursors of our contemporary holiday trips. To visit Buddhist power spots was one of the motivations of the Chinese pilgrims. Even at present, Hindus and Buddhists who have no special interest in Christianity are often keen on visiting Lourdes. All such facts are well known and there would be no point in recalling them, if it were not for the opportunities they afford to observe that the greatest power spot on earth is undoubtedly the Himalayas themselves. To see them, no religion is needed; merely the right perspective. Mountaineers generally have it:

> It seemed as though our first view of the Himalaya was to be indefinitely postponed. Again the great cloud screen rose tall above the curve of the world. I was about to turn away disappointedly when a wild thought made me raise my head higher. They were there . . . an arctic continent of the heavens, far above the earth and its girdling clouds: divorced wholly from this planet. (W.H. Murray) W.H. Murray, quoted from Horbein 1968).

CONCLUSIONS

Any tourist, traveler, or mountaineer who crosses the Himalayan range from south to north is struck by dramatic changes when he reaches the other side, or even when he ascends to some of the higher regions still to the south of the summits and passes. The luxuriant vegetation of the foothills and southern slopes is gradually replaced by a few scattered shrubs and blades of grass; the humidity and intermittent monsoon rains give way to aridity and cold winds; instead of green, brown, and yellow hues, the traveler sees white, blue, and the reds of dawn or dusk reflected on rocks, ice, and snow; animals and humans have become rare, and present a very different appearance: the rigidity of the caste Hindus of Nepal and the fanaticism of the Muslims of the northwest is replaced by the cheerful smiles of Tibetan Buddhists. There is every reason, under such circumstances, for religious prejudice to harden.

Yet these are all appearances, and appearances deceive. At present, Hindus and Buddhists in these areas may look very different from each other. In reality, even a cursory inspection of past events demonstrates that the transitions between Hinduism and Buddhism have generally been fluid and uncertain. Most features of Tibetan Buddhism were originally Indian. Though Buddhism is closer to a Western religion than any of the other -isms we have discussed, it remains true that facts such as those assembled in the present chapter demonstrate that the notion of religion itself vanishes in the thin air of these mountains.

The myth of religion has not only been adhered to by scholars of religion. It has been perpetuated by textual scholars, for the simple reason that most texts are labeled. Anthropologists, on the other hand, aided only by their field work and unhampered by a knowledge of history, have long felt uncomfortable with the concept of religion as applied to China or India. In China, the myth has strengthened traditional prejudice: it was not, in any event, supposed to be a very religious country. In India, the traditional bias is that it is a land of religion; this has caused numerous problems, primarily of a conceptual nature. Instead of rejecting the concept of religion itself, Indian anthropologists have therefore introduced new notions, such as the Great Tradition and Little Traditions. If we look closely, we discover that the Great Tradition is made up of what resembles Christianity and the Little Traditions is made up of what deviates from it. Another concept, Sanskritization, was postulated as a process by which the Great Tradition allegedly spread to the Little Traditions and absorbed them. Actually, Sanskritization may not amount to more than social climbing (Bailey 1960:188).* I have submitted this concept to a critical examination elsewhere (Staal 1972a), and mention it here only because Sanskritization is a good example of a notion that becomes unnecessary as soon as one rejects the equally dispensable idea of a Great Tradition, which itself is superfluous because it is nothing but a reflection of the equally misleading parent notion of religion. All we witness is the collapse of a house of cards consisting of popular and scholarly clichés.

In China, it has often been felt that the concept of religion is inapplicable; in India, only Western prejudice has prevented a similar discovery. And yet, its inapplicability should be patent to anyone who merely looks. Here is another, and final example. With regard to two of India's greatest philosophers, Bhartṛhari and Gauḍapāda, there has been a long controversy as to whether they were Hindus or Buddhists. The absurdity of such a dispute should make us wonder how such questions can be meaningful at all. Can one even conceive of asking whether al-Ghazzālī or Thomas Aquinas were Christians or Muslims?

The inapplicability of the notion of religion is not confined to the region of the Himalayas, though it is particularly obvious there; it is inapplicable to most parts of Asia. We have already noted that in southern India, "Hindus" perform "Vedic" rites. Similarly, in the southeast of Asia, in Bali, we meet with "Buddhist Brahmins." In the northeast, the situation is not different. In contemporary Japan, it is not unusual to hear young engaged couples discuss whether their wedding ceremony will be Shinto, Buddhist, or Christian.

Earlier in this chapter we asked two questions: why the Vedic nomads entered India from Central Asia and why Buddhism moved in the opposite direction. These questions obligingly vanish into thin air as soon as we remove the labels. Such labels as we are enamored of affixing obscure the fact that the underlying reality of the last several millennia is best described as a continuous movement and exchange of people, goods, and ideas between India, Central Asia, and China, across the mountain ranges of the Himalayas.

*Specialized Bibliography

Bailey, F. G.
1960 *Tribe, caste, and nation.* Manchester.
Flattery, David S.
1982 *Harmal and the origins of the Indo-Iranian soma/haoma rituals.* Berkeley.
Hooykaas, C.
1982 "Agni offerings in Java and Bali." In *Agni: the Vedic ritual of the fire altar,* Frits Staal. Berkeley and Los Angeles.
Hornbein, Thomas F.
1968 *Everest: the west ridge.* London.
Huxley, Aldous
1963 *The doors of perception and heaven and hell.* New York.
Michael, Henry N., ed.
1963 *Studies in Siberian shamanism.* Toronto.
Muktananda Paramahansa, Swami
1974 *The play of consciousness (Chitshakti Vilas).* Shree Gurudev Siddha Yoga Ashram.
Mylius, Klaus
1972 "Das geographische Milieu der mittelvedischen Literatur." *Mitteilungen des Instituts für Orientforschung* 17:369–382.
Popkin, S. L.
1979 *The rational peasant: the political economy of rural society in Vietnam.* Berkeley.
Wasson, R. G.
1968 *Soma: divine mushroom of immortality.* New York.
Wheelock, W.
n.d. *The mantra in Vedic and Tantric ritual.* Unpublished manuscript.

Notes

1. In the same article, Morgenstierne discusses several explanations of the name Munjan, not linking it to Mūjavat.
2. I shall return to several of these topics. An interesting example is the belief in demons, studied by Filliozat, who writes: "Aussi Noël Péri avait-il bien raison d'écrire: 'Il semble que le bouddhisme et ses personnages, je ne dis pas ses idées ni ses doctrines, y soient (dans le tantrisme) simplement surajoutés à des croyances, à des pratiques d'une autre origine et qu'il n'a pu déraciner. Au fait, nombre de termes techniques et d'observances y décèlent l'influence persistante d'anciennes idées indous.' " Filliozat comments: "Il est seulement contestable dans ces phrases que le bouddhisme n'ait pas 'pu déraciner' ces croyances et ces pratiques, car il n'est pas du tout certain qu'il l'ait tenté. Ce sont là simplement les idées indiennes et le bouddhisme a renié le brahmanisme, non pas l'Inde" (Filliozat 1937:152–153).
3. I owe this reference to Ms. A. Spiro.

IV

India in the Chinese Looking-Glass

Michel Strickmann

ONE HALF OF EURASIA

India and China share Eastern Eurasia between them, not so much in terms of political entities, "blocks" or states, but in the more vast and inspiriting realm of social and cultural history. Even those cultural configurations originating west of the Indus, outside the Serindic subcontinent (like Islam) have been definitively marked by the Indian or Chinese societies which have played host to their eastward diaspora. Moreover, the interaction between India and China, now reduced to journalistic banality, was formerly intense and ravelled. Each acquired and retained elements of the other, and aspects of each have met and melded on neutral ground, in the vast expanses that stretch between them, Southeast Asia and Insulindia on the one hand, Central Asia and Tibet on the other. Here we will be occupied with reflections in and projections from the more easterly partners in this grand work of fusion and diffusion: the Chinese and the denizens of those Central Asian kingdoms that began to come within the Chinese sphere of influence from ca. 150 B.C. The chief object of our concern will be Buddhism, now in its death agonies, but in happier times an all-embracing set of interlocking systems that absorbed and mobilized vast tracts of Indian tradition, drilled them across Central Asia, and set them down in China, there to mingle with various other systems of local manufacture.

The stages of Chinese expansion and westward probing which ultimately led to the introduction of Buddhism began not long after China's consolidation under centralized rule (221 B.C.). The path of the first Buddhist missionaries is better known as the Silk Route, commerce thus nominally winning out over religion—but in fact, Buddhism and commerce were closely allied from the start. Yet neither was a factor in the great road's opening; it was a simple question of military expediency. The grazing-lands of the puissant Xiongnu, mounted nomads, marched with China's northwestern frontier. The establishment of the first Chinese empire provoked an answering consolidation of Xiongnu forces. Xiongnu raids were a constant threat to Chinese agricultural colonies in the border regions and, in addition to treating with the Xiongnu themselves, the rulers of China attempted to form alliances with peoples further west so as to establish bases in the Xiongnu's rear. The Xiongnu treaties were accompanied by shipments of Chinese luxury products calculated to appease their lust for conquest. It may be, too, that by exporting the paraphernalia of sinic gracious living, the Chinese hoped to corrupt the simple martial spirit of their formidable enemies (in ancient times, rival Chinese states had sent one another troupes of dancing girls and musicians with this intent). At all events, the first silk to leave China went as a bribe, a payoff. Thus it was hardly a nascent spirit of free enterprise (as some have innocently supposed) that first opened the Silk Route to the west, but rather a concerted policy of defense. In the view of the eminent historian of Han China, A.F.P. Hulsewé, there was but a single reason for the Chinese expansion into Central Asia in the second century B.C., which in time led to cultural and commercial contact with western and southern Asia: the desire to stop the Xiongnu invasions by depriving the enemy of their western bases (Hulsewé 1974:120). With Han garrisons eventually stationed at cities all along the route to Khotan and points west, the way was open for a more diversified civilian traffic in both directions. The fortunate recipients of silk and other civilised goods had meanwhile been able to exchange them with their own neighbours; thus, in time, Chinese silks reached Rome, and Chinese silk and mirrors have been found in a number of remote sites, including the frozen tombs of Pazaryk and elsewhere in Siberia (Rudenko 1970:304–306).*

SOME PRECOCIOUS CHINESE EXPLORERS

The Chinese were to figure as some of the world's greatest travellers, and their literature of exploration was suitably precocious. The Chinese literature of exploration was rooted in a long mythological tradition. The travels of the legendary Monarch Yu had been undertaken with a sound hydraulic goal, channeling off the waters of the primordial Deluge, laying out the fields, levelling the rough places, and generally making the world safe once more for Sinology. His exploits shaded in the map of China with rude tribes and surrounded it with formidable neighbours in demonic or theriomorphic guise. This is the picture we find in the *Book of Mountains and Seas* (*Shanhai jing*), which enshrines a classic sinocentric view of the world and its startling denizens. Small wonder that travel, under such conditions, should be hedged round with magical caveats, and shrouded in spiritual significance. The awesome catalogue of demons, monsters and marvels likely to be encountered has been drawn up by Kiang Chao-yuan (Jiang Shaoyuan), in a work revealingly titled *Travel in Ancient China Considered Principally under Its Magic and Religious Aspects* (1937). Only by a thorough knowledge of the precise nature and mode of dealing with the uncanny creatures he might meet could the traveller hope to survive. And defense was only part of the stock of needful lore; who, without special instruction, would know that many of the demonic apparitions were in fact edible, and might usefully supplement his rations? The water monster *wangxiang* for example, resembles a small child with flaming red eyes, large ears, and long talons—sufficiently off-putting, one would suppose—yet you have only to strangle it with a rope and it becomes susceptible of boiling, and is moreover a most beneficent, luck-bringing viand (Kiang 1937:72–73). Ingestion (rather than expulsion) as a means of dealing with otherwise troublous phantoms has always recommended itself to the economical and food-obsessed Chinese; it was still being counselled in a booklet published in Peking in the sixties (*Bupa guidi gushi; Ne pas avoir peur des fantômes*).

Expeditions were sent forth to find the Eastern Isles of the Immortals; wave-subduing Chinese generals postured and curvetted their dragon-steeds on the strands of Southeast Asia; but perhaps the most haunted voyage of all was that undertaken, in legend, by King Mu of Zhou. Mu, Son of Heaven, travelled to the West—to the mysterious domain of the Mother Queen of the West, Xiwang Mu, who dwelt in her splendid palace amid the peach orchards, ringed with tigers and other heraldic beasts, on Mt. Kunlun—the point, in the Northwest, where heaven and earth met: the Gate of Heaven (Mu's tale is translated in Mathieu 1978).* There are echoes of this voyage to a western paradise throughout later Chinese literature, especially in Taoist writings, but it is likely that even the Western Paradise of Amitābha was, in China, touched by Kunlun's eery sunset glow. The Son of Heaven's long and arduous journey to the west was also a journey heavenwards. It partook of the nature of a pilgrimage, and the allegorical potential of the narrative was not lost upon subsequent generations of readers and travellers (Loewe 1979). The common mediaeval Chinese name for India, Tianzhu ("celestial bamboo"), reflects the same positive otherworldly aspect of the distant west.

All this may seem sufficiently remote from the workaday world of Buddhist missionary activity, but there is no doubt that much of this phantasmagoric aura continued to suffuse Central Asiatic travel, for Indians and Chinese alike, throughout the ten centuries of active Buddhist transmission eastwards; glimmerings of it might indeed still be caught until recently, even by such stalwart explorers as Sir Aurel Stein. The marvelous and the fantastic permeate the long series of accounts by Chinese pilgrims to the great sites of India, and are reflected, too, in the systematic précis of their narratives which were incorporated into Chinese works of history and geography (Petech 1950,1966). Without the records made by these Chinese monks, our knowledge of the history of mediaeval India and Central Asia would be utterly impoverished and inchoate. But it would seem that much of the appeal of their narratives for Chinese readers lay in a taste for exoticism, a thirst for marvels. The monkish travellers themselves were no less susceptible to the spell, and the physical perils with which their venture was fraught were often scarcely to be severed from the spiritual or demonic. They were all of a piece, the desert was animate, the Silk Route alive with phantoms, and protective spiritual power was no idle, abstruse notion. All this was taken up and further spun out in the countless accretions of story-telling that recalled the pilgrims' experience. The world's greatest novel of travel, the *Journey to the West* ("Monkey"), is in this sense faithful to the spirit of the mediaeval travellers, and through its incomparable verve and sway, the adventure of Central Asian pilgrimage and cultural encounter has become for all time integral to traditional Chinese theatre, story-telling, and religion (Dudbridge 1970).

The discovery of their western neighbours helped the Chinese towards the discovery of themselves. It was in taking stock of the alien nature of the "barbarians" that the touchstones of Chinese ethnic identity were installed and contours of self-defining idealism were modelled. First of all, there was a centralised rule, a focused imperium of which the divine authorisation was embodied in the person of the Monarch, the Son of Heaven. Concurrently with political focus came easy, reasonable communication. This in telling contrast to the slipshod diversity and heterogeneity of alien arrangements: for example, the "thirty-six tribes" of the Western Regions, that could only communicate via "multiple interpreters." These oft-encountered *topoi* of foreign relations serve to underscore the Chinese pride in their own centralised state and single, unifying language; more properly, in their *written* language, the standardisation of which had been a natural concomitant of the third century B.C. political unification. The Chinese politeia and the Chinese written language were the cardinal pieces in the whole ethnic edifice, and we shall see that if they are vital to an understanding of the Chinese view of themselves in relation to the outside world, they have also been essential in the elaboration of Chinese spiritual life, seen from within. The creation of a centralised empire manned by hyperliterate bureaucrats and scribes was a triumph indeed, and in a way China never got over it.

Thus began the long chronicles of exotic anthropology, born of the perceived distinctions between China's wall-, mountain-, and sea-girded inner world and the great, menacing outer waves of jabbering, fantastical barbarians. The hunters and herders were seen as a threat to settled Chinese agrarian civilisation, and this must serve as adequate justification for their cruel demonification—though every foreign group sufficiently temerarious to invade and rule China was quickly sinified and rendered nearly human. That the Chinese should term their civilisation the "Central Realm" (Zhongguo) was only the most obvious blazon of its distinctive identity; China the focus, all else mere periphery.

Yet there is considerable irony in this formulation. It works stark violence on both geography and ethnography. The Chinese may have seen themselves as radically separate and distinct from the encircling peoples, may indeed have thereby defined their own "centrality;" but they all too often chose, in their writings, to veil from view the countless aliens in their very midst. Even in 1982, the geopolitical entity designated "China" includes numerous groups not ethnically or culturally Chinese. The situation would have been even more striking in the first centuries A.D., when such non-Chinese groups could be found in many more regions of which the sinic ethos has since become indisputable. Virtually the only appearance of these peoples in the literature of Late Chinese Antiquity is in the form of laconic eruptions in the official chronicles of imperial prowess, when these surly indigenes collided with the inexorable Chinese advance. In the Middle Ages, their uncouth mores occasionally drew the wondering attention of Chinese administrators. Yet this disturbing alien presence did not disappear for centuries, and—despite the even harsher measures of a more recent regime— has still not quite disappeared. The Yao of Hunan, in Central China, were not thoroughly subdued until the twelfth century, and much of the Southwest was brought under effective Chinese control only very much later. The final pulverisation of Tibet (now also on the map of "China") and the numerous peoples of Sichuan and the Sino-Tibetan frontier is very recent history indeed. Wolfram Eberhard must be credited with having discerned the vital implications of this ethnic diversity within ancient and mediaeval "China"; he has tried to determine the precise contribution of each of the major ethnic groups to the conglomerate culture which we complacently term "Chinese" (Eberhard 1968).

In this internal wilderness country of the alien unknown, exploration and development followed the patterns of Central Asian cultural discovery. As in Central Asia, only the spiritually strong might safely venture into the alien heart of "China, " and once more, in history as well as legend, it is the self-sufficient Buddhist monk who emerges as the epitome of the intrepid pioneer. We find him blazing unknown tracts, conciliating and instructing the rude natives, discovering life-giving springs of water and founding monasteries that will, through a proper marshalling of labour and capital, open the forests and fens to cultivation, civilisation, sinification (Soymié 1961; Ch'en Yuan 1941). Other forms of spiritual discipline besides Buddhism might also serve: the once formidable Tao are tranquil now, refugees absorbed in their Taoist mysteries and proud of their Chinese system of writing, the fruits of assimilation and the means of a narrow escape from annihilation (Lemoine 1982).

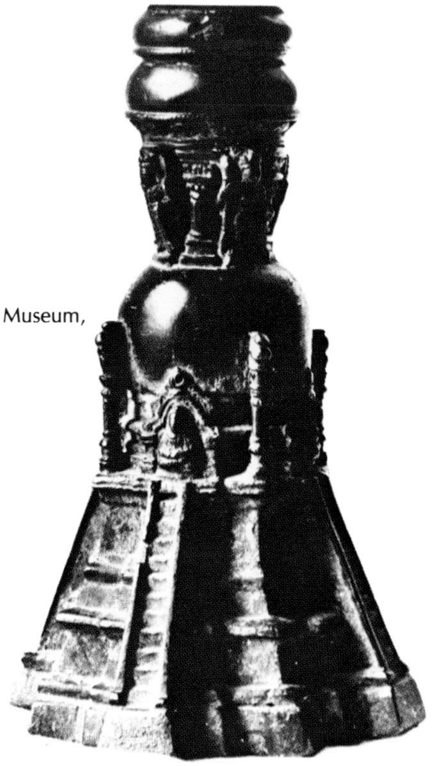

9. Reliquary *stūpa*, Peshawar Museum, Pakistan.

Thus in beginning with the balanced images of "India" and "China" we were yielding to the evocative power of a fiction: two fictions, really, for "India" is no less an ethno-political figment, a congeries of distinct cultures, not infrequently mutually hostile (Kosambi 1964:1–2). Perhaps our neat sense of things is simply the product of recent nationalism, journalistic convention, and modern cartography. For though our minds cling to an India where people wear white garments, eat with their hands, and revere the creative force of sound, and a China where people wear blue, eat with sticks and bow before the sacral character of writing, there is conceivably very much within these configurations that has not yet entered our books, much less our newspapers. And what then of the intervening societies, which we are accustomed to align with India or China in accordance with their mode of dress, eating habits, writing systems? It would not be difficult to pepper the reader with unsettling selections from the long roster of contradictions inherent in our received view of Asia. But we have already seen that we can destroy an Asian country without even having begun to understand its *present* state, let alone its past. Suffice it to remember that these ancient interlocking social conglomerates, the "Chinese" as well as the "Indian," were complex to a degree that few of us supposed specialists have the capacity to render. What is simple, too simple, are the official pronouncements of the dominant groups. But the emperors of China were not, as a class, distinguished ethnologists or social historians; still less were most of the chroniclers who crouched and cringed before the throne. And we shall find that the non-Chinese were not alone in suffering from the distortions or malign neglect of official authors.

ENIGMAS OF CHINESE RELIGION

The figure of the solitary Buddhist monk setting off into the unsubdued wilderness naturally grips our attention. In Chinese, religious conversion is styled "transformation" (*hua*). What was the role of religion in this great Babel of peoples? If the overlooming monoliths of race, language, and state were heaved aside, should we in fact find that religion offers a master key to understanding, a straightaway through the maze of ethnic profusion? Such has not been the view of historians of China writing in English. It is regularly implied that religion, for the Chinese, was at best a distinctly marginal phenomenon, at worst a form of low-class self-indulgence. Most puzzling of all, we are presented at the very outset with another basic problem of definition, regarding not only the nature of religious identity in traditional China, but the very identities of the several religions themselves. The historian's dilemmas are compounded when he turns to the anthropological literature. There he discovers that a reigning question concerns plurality or singularity: are there many religions in China (or, Chinese religions), or simply one runaway phenomenon, "Chinese religion," with a multiplicity of aspects? Sino-anthropologists perhaps too easily divorce themselves and their work from a long, well-documented history which they are unable to plumb in the original classical Chinese; yet their perception of a large number of beliefs and practices fully shared by the bulk of the population in Taiwan and Hong Kong, whatever their nominal sectarian affiliations, is accurate enough; the problem becomes even more intriguing when one realises that a comparable state of affairs goes back at least 1500 years, to the fifth century.

What, then, *are* China's religions? So far we have taken notice of Buddhism, an import, and Taoism, a native creation. The oft-mentioned "Confucianism" is, in my opinion, best seen as something else, not strictly comparable—more a Paideia, a system of culture and its graduated inculcation, rather than a faith professed by a guild of ritual technicians claiming otherworldly authority. The paradigm later styled "Confucian" was simply a broad base of Sinic letters, a fundamental view of cosmos and society which we might better term "common Chinese," for it was also fully shared by Taoist priests and Chinese Buddhist monks. Indeed, in mediaeval times, Taoist abbeys and Buddhist monasteries often sheltered academies providing training in this common Chinese literary culture, full assimilation of which, whatever one's regional or even ethnic origins, certified a man as civilised: respectably Chinese. The embarrassment of modern scholars who retain the old Chinese rubric of the "Three Teachings" is apparent when they have to deal with the cult of the dead ("ancestor worship"), and sacred sciences such as divination and geomancy. It is customary to vacillate, assigning these wayward phenomena now to one of the great Three, now to another. But in fact they belong to none of them exclusively, and are freely used, when needed, by all. This might also serve to describe the attitude of most Chinese to Buddhist and Taoist institutions, and for the mediaeval period, as well as the modern, a functional rather than sectarian approach to the question of religious identity might best serve for the great majority of the population.

The poverty of the "Three Religions" formula becomes increasingly apparent with each shuffle through the dossier of evidence. Where, for example, is Islam, which has counted an enormous Chinese following (and presumably exacted a more exclusive allegiance from its adherents than either Buddhism or Taoism)? But most glaring of all is the omission, from many accounts of one strand of Chinese spiritual life that can be traced back well beyond the formation of Taoism and the introduction of Buddhism, and which is still highly visible today in surviving traditional societies on the periphery of China. Spirit-possession, ecstatic religion, or shamanism has attracted the attention of philologists and literary historians working with pre-Han texts, as well as anthropologists doing field work in Taiwan, Hong Kong, and the Chinese communities of Southeast Asia. In China as elsewhere, the descent and embodiment of the gods has always offered the most direct means of access to knowledge of the invisible world; the most immediate response to disease or disaster has been consultation of a medium or oracle, often through the exorcists (local, nonhierarchised priests) who control them. Properly ordained Taoist priests and Buddhist monks have always made it clear that the gods whom the people thus honour through their mediums and through costly animal sacrifice are in reality not supreme or disinterested beings at all, but rather mere spirits of the dead, keen on prolonging their dubious posthumous survival with offerings made by the deluded populace. Far from being able to aid those who call upon them, they are themselves the source of sickness, material ruin, delirium and death. Yet despite the eloquent denunciations of the officially recognised spiritual hierarchies, an attitude which neatly coincided with the overarching State's distaste for all unofficial "degenerate cults," the mighty ecstatic substrate endured as what R.A. Stein has called "the nameless religion." If we know it chiefly from literary texts committed to writing near the beginnings of our documentation and from field work carried out today, apparently at the tradition's end, we should not imagine that the evidence has been exhausted. The literature of mediaeval China reveals that spirit-possession and exorcism held centre stage in mediaeval Chinese life, and many of the aims and techniques of ecstatic religion were taken up, in sublimated form, into Buddhism and Taoism. On the whole, the Chinese evidence seems strongly to support the analysis put forward by I.M. Lewis in 1971, who relates the various forms of possession-cults to the two dominant classes of spirits, the morally-binding shades of departed ancestors and the amoral, spontaneous cults of peripheral beings. Lewis also makes an excellent case for bringing together spirit-possession and trance-mediumship with the phenomenon of shamanism, which it has become more usual to treat as an exotic complex unto itself. Here too, Chinese texts and practice might lend compelling support to his thesis. Yet few scholars have acknowledged the strength and persistence of the Chinese ecstatic tradition, and this is ironic, for even as it long predates the organised, officially-sponsored "higher" religions, Buddhism and Taoism, so it seems very likely that it has already outlasted them in China; the dependence of these elaborate and cultivated institutions upon the State, though it made their fortunes in the Middle Ages, has ultimately resulted in their near-disappearance. As the curtain now falls upon traditional religion in China, the spiritual mantle of Buddhism and Taoism will henceforth presumably revert to those impulses of direct experience and ecstatic realisation out of which the great religions themselves once long ago emerged.

RELIGION IN AN EMPIRE

If we turn then to China in quest of that land's particular contribution to religion, we will first of all find it in the imperial ideology and the tentacular, centralised State. There is a remarkable parallel in historical development at either end of Asia. The conditions of Late Antiquity are strikingly similar in both contexts—the decline and reappraisal of classical culture in an age of invasions; and a plurality of exotic religions, eventually ceding to a single, universal religion in close alliance with the State—such are the circumstances both of the declining Roman Empire in the West, and the failing Han Empire and ensuing Three Kingdoms and early period of disunion in the East. The differences, of course, are equally obvious. The most remarkable is the apparent prolongation in East Asia of the Late Antique circumstance of a number of religions tolerated, if not actively sponsored, by the central government. Though there were brief periods of particular proscription, though one or another of the organised religions might run into a squall of intense disfavour (most usually for political rather than doctrinal reasons), and though the socioeconomic strength of Buddhism made it clearly paramount, the essential balance of religious pluralism was effectively maintained for nearly two millenia. The State was greater than the sum of its parts, and transcended religious particularism. The imperial cult came to draw freely upon the messianic ideologies of both Buddhism and Taoism, but as effective Pontifex Maximus, the Monarch sat enthroned above all ordinary spirtual lineages. He was the worthy companion of Taoist celestials and the Buddhas, and ideally united all faiths and suffrages in his sacrosanct person.

To this special state of affairs religion in China owed much of its prosperity as well as its special character; to it, we too owe nearly all our resources for discovering more about Chinese religion. For today, perhaps the most conspicuous monuments to the intimate alliance between organised religion and the State in China are the enormous, officially-sanctioned collections of Buddhist and Taoist literature. In India, individual schools had assembled what they believed to be the authentic word of the Buddha, together with commentaries and amplifications set down by their own patriarchs. But the idea of a totally inclusive collection comprising not only the entire corpus of the Buddha's pronouncements but the writing of every available Buddhist author, as well, seems to be a uniquely Chinese conception (duely imitated by the Koreans, Tibetans, and Japanese). With the resources and patronage of the State, the Chinese Buddhist community had the means of realising this ambitious undertaking.

An obsessive official concern with the written word had already determined Chinese excellence in bibliographic classification and the collection and preservation of documents. These skills met their greatest challenge in the unending flood of Buddhist literature with which mediaeval China was deluged. But classification of the numerous translations of Indian originals was hardly a sufficient response to the impact of Buddhism on Chinese society. An original Chinese Buddhist literature began, which soon rivalled the translations; moreover, when Indian Buddhism declined and new Indian texts no longer reached China for translation, Chinese Buddhist literature continued to flourish, in a genre it had made peculiarly its own. The official concern with record-keeping was manifested early on among Chinese Buddhist scholars, though (as in the parallel tradition of secular chronography) it might be sounder to term it hagiography rather than historiography. In bringing the prosaic devices of Chinese chroniclers to bear upon a Buddhist subject-matter, however, the Chinese were making a distinctive contribution to Buddhist literature as a whole. The Chinese example had enormous influence upon the Tibetans, and though the great chronicles of Buddhism by Bu-ston, Tāranātha, the Fifth Dalai Lama, and dPa'o gtsug-lag 'phreng-ba are ironically far better known in the West (Vostrikov 1970), it should not be forgotten that Tibetan historiography shared the heritage of the great Chinese Buddhist universal histories of the Song and Yuan.

No less influential than chronography or hagiography was the Chinese contribution to Buddhist scriptural literature. This statement may occasion surprise—we are accustomed to envisage the sacred traffic as being all one way. It is undeniable that Indian *sūtras*, as well as the copious literature of tales (*jātaka, avadāna*) had an incalculable influence upon Chinese literature and art. The inexhaustible Indian "Ocean of Story, " long recognised from its westward influence into all the literatures of the Near East and Europe, was equally available to East Asia. Moreover, it reached China, for the most part, in a rather more pristine form: whole Indian works of literature were brought there intact, over the Silk Route, for translation. Though "Bodhisat" may still be dimly visible through the Iranian and Syriac permutations that brought the mediaeval West the *avadāna* of Barlaam and "Joasaph," much of the Chinese tale-literature came, if not straight from Sanskrit originals, at least from the languages of complacently Buddhist Central Asiatic kingdoms.

The vast body of Indian parables and exempla worked like fresh genetic stock on mediaeval Chinese literature: both on written literature and oral narrative. Literary form as well as content was affected: it has often been remarked how the scriptural convention of intermingled prose and verse inspired the Chinese *chantefable* (*bianwen*), which has been seen as anticipating the later full-scale novel. But perhaps the most potent effect of all was exerted by the idea of the sacred book itself. For Mahāyāna Buddhism was bodied forth in works which insisted upon their own supramundane status, works which cried out incessantly for recitation, copying, diffusion and respect and which guaranteed their obedient votaries all manner of protection and rewards (Schopen 1975). Their setting was awesomely otherworldly, their players mighty and numerous beyond belief, their scenario often miraculous and uncanny: a cosmodrama. And their substance was quite literally a revelation—the word of the Buddha himself. It is fitting that the books in which this eternal message was embodied should themselves become objects of extreme veneration.

THE IMPACT OF INDIAN FORMS

The effect of these imported sacred books upon Chinese literature and art was utter and definitive. It can be gauged, obviously, by the rapid proliferation of manuscript copies of the Chinese translations of such works, which demanded and were given all the respect due the Indian originals. The multiplicity of scripture-copies found at Dunhuang, especially the thousands of transcripts of the *Lotus Sūtra*, attest the ready acceptance with which the literature's claims were met. It even appears that the art of printing developed, in the first instance, in response to the requirement for innumerable copies and/or repetitions, most forcibly advanced in one class of revealed scriptures, the *dhāraṇī-sūtras*, or books of spells, since Buddhist *dhāraṇīs* are the oldest examples of printing to survive. But there are other indications of the effect of Mahāyāna literature upon China, which are perhaps all the more telling for being somewhat off the beaten track. The Taoist religion had come into being during the second century A.D. in studied opposition to the frenzied cults of the profane; it seems to have taken for its earliest sacred book the *Laozi* or *Book of the Way and Its Power*, a third-century B.C. work which had already been subjected to a variety of interpretations, political as well as mystical. A practical literature of rulebooks and manuals for the conduct of ritual and meditation also arose. But it was clearly the example of the Buddhist sacred book that inspired the great Taoist scriptures that came to be written from the fourth century on. In the earliest and most brilliant instances, the cosmic setting and the alternation of prose and verse, the most immediately striking formal features of the *sūtra* genre, have been employed to frame contents still essentially Taoist: astral rites and meditations. But soon more of the substance of Buddhist *sūtras* was incorporated in their Taoist counterpart, including many of the same parables and key phrases embodying points of doctrine. Mediaeval Taoist authors, the cream of the sacerdotal community, represent a consciously nativistic reaction to Buddhist literary exuberance and social success. In this respect (like the Bön-po priesthood in later Tibet) they provide, in spite of themselves, testimony all the more convincing because unconscious, to Buddhism's inexorable advance. The standards of religious professionalism exemplified by the Buddhist monastic community eventually became obligatory upon all religious practitioners conspicuous in the public eye. We therefore see upper-class Taoists adopting, for example, celibacy and vegetarianism, but sedulously discovering and elaborating reasons for this new code of conduct drawn from China's own native repertory of symbols (Strickmann 1978b).* Taoism had begun its history as an organised religion in opposition to local ecstatic cults of the deified spirits of the dead. This conscious dichotomy persisted throughout the Middle Ages, and is still found today. Yet Taoists were not above putting Buddhism firmly in its place, above all as a religion chiefly concerned with *death* (in contrast to Taoism's obsession with eternal Life), and also, as a doctrine not really meant for Chinese consumption at all. For if Laozi's early career seemed to have terminated mysteriously when he disappeared through the Pass that led to the Western Regions, it was revealed to the Taoists that he had in fact proceeded to India. There he transformed himself, first into Queen Māyā, then into an embryo in her womb, and by means of this twofold docetic effort enabled himself to be born as Gautama, the destined Buddha. Laozi would thus have to be added to the roster of Western travellers—some centuries before the Silk Route opened at all. And the religion which this master of metamorphosis taught his benighted Indian votaries was in fact a debased form of Taoism. Indeed, according to one account, he devised the institution of celibate monks and nuns as a means of sterilising and so eliminating the troublesome barbarians entirely! (Zürcher 1959:288–320).

This Taoist fantasy, first attested in the third century A.D., is perhaps the earliest theory of China's influence on Indian religion, bravely advanced in the face of the overwhelming evidence of the eastward movement of books, institutions, and specialists. It has found a curious latter-day echo in the notion that Chinese, and more particularly Taoist, sexual practices may have been a leaven in the fermentation of Indian Tantric ritual (R.H. van Gulik 1961:356).* The timeless quality of most Indian religious documents renders difficult any clear proof of imports from East Asia. Yet in attempting to trace the originality of Chinese Buddhism, we may also discover evidence of its influence, if not on India, then at least on certain non-Chinese communities of Central Asia. The chief concern of even those Buddhist scholars specialising in China has hitherto been with canonical (or better: normative) Indian Buddhism. The study of Chinese Buddhism has consequently fastened on Chinese conceptions—or misconceptions—of normative Buddhist thought. To discover and appreciate the true originality of Chinese Buddhism, we must for the moment abandon this conventional perspective and we must also avoid the opposite extreme of Taoist sinocentricity. It is on the intervening terrain that our evidence is to be found, in a largely neglected tract, between Buddhism and Taoism, occupied by the Chinese Buddhist "apocrypha."

ORIGINAL CHINESE SŪTRAS

It is paradoxical that while the potent effect of the Mahāyāna scriptures has long been noted, the creation of an original Chinese Buddhist scriptural literature has seemed a fact barely worthy of comment. The term "apocryphal *sūtras*" already says it all, and it comes as no surprise to find that these Chinese scriptural creations have been taxed as "forgeries" and "fakes." The Sino-Japanese vocabulary of bibliographic abuse is equally damning: such works are "doubtful," "dubious," "false," and "fabrications." It seems significant that the compilation of critical classified bibliographies of Chinese Buddhist literature began under an emperor who prided himself upon the orthodoxy of his Buddhist faith, Liang Wudi (502–549). The basic criterion of scriptural authenticity was simply the existence of a foreign original, from which the Chinese version had been translated. Since we are not obliged to credit every Mahāyāna *sūtra* with being the authentic word of the historical Buddha, we may wonder how a scripture composed in fifth-century China can possibly be less "authentic" than one written at the same time in Kashmır? Both are at an equal remove from the ideas of the historical Buddha. Yet each is potentially valid and valuable in its own right, with regard to the Buddhism of its time. The more closely we study Chinese Buddhism, the more obvious becomes the State's obsession with control. The copying and distribution of Buddhist literature was a highly meritorious act, to be sure, and there is no doubt that each successive dynasty that sponsored the collection and transcription of a Buddhist Canon counted on thereby accruing otherworldly merit that would guarantee the stability of the realm, the longevity of the reigning house, and the empire's general immunity from pestilence and natural calamities. But it is no less clear that the periodic calling-in and editorial scrutiny of religious literature was used as a check on potential dissidence and unauthorised spiritual pretensions. Thus the guarantee that a scripture *was* foreign in origin not only made it *ipso facto* of a piece with the foreign religion (and hence less likely to contain matter that might prove seditious in a Chinese context); since nearly all translations were done under official supervision, it also assured the authorities that the text had, as it were, already been properly filtered for Chinese consumption.

Thus it is natural that the greatest number and variety of original Chinese *sūtras* should have been produced during periods of relatively slack central control: the fifth century, and the second half of the sixth. Not surprisingly, these periods were also the chief epochs of Taoist scriptural production, since both classes of work shared all their essential formal features. Both were sacred texts claiming otherworldly authority (for the "India" of the Mahāyāna *sūtras* was no mere mortal realm, but rather a never-never land of celestial marvels). Both were written by Chinese authors, directly in Chinese, for a Chinese readership—and no doubt much of their popularity was due to the relative fluency of their language, for Chinese Buddhist translationese is decidedly an acquired taste. Nearly all Taoist scriptures and a substantial proportion of the Buddhist scriptures composed in China are written in excellent classical Chinese. Even this positive feature has sometimes told against them, given the common bias in favour of Indian Buddhism. Some Chinese pseudepigrapha are so brilliantly written that their Indian origin was long maintained even in the face of overwhelming evidence to the contrary. Here the most celebrated cases involve *śāstras* and commentaries, rather than sūtras. *The Awakening of Faith in the Mahāyāna* (*Dasheng qixinlun*)is the best-known example (Demiéville 1973:XXXIII). Though composed in China in the second half of the sixth century, it simply seemed too good to be Chinese. Conversely, it is interesting to note that a few translations were so well done that, lacking Sanskrit manuscripts or Tibetan translations (in which it has been customary to place more confidence than the often far earlier Chinese versions) scholars for some time suspected them of crypto-sinicity. In this class falls the great commentary on the *Large Sūtra of Perfect Wisdom* (*Mahāprajñāpāramitāsūtropadeśa; Dazhidu lun*), whose claims to "authenticity" had to await Lamotte's convincing demonstration of Kashmıri authorship (Lamotte 1970:VIII-XLIV).

Far more significant than the readable style of the "unofficial" *sūtras*, of course, is their contents, since Chinese authors naturally wrote on topics of the most intense interest to a potential Chinese readership. These original Chinese works sometimes give us glimpses of that eldritch will-o'-the-wisp, the otherwise unrecorded oral tradition. A good example is the celebrated *Sūtra of the Wise Man and the Fool* (*Xianyu jing*). Typically, this fascinating collection of tales is better known from a later and incomplete Tibetan translation based on the Chinese original. A sixth-century Chinese Buddhist author has recorded the circumstances of its compilation. Not long before the middle of the fifth century, eight Chinese monks from Gansu had travelled west in search of sacred texts. They reached Khotan at the time of the *pañcavarśaka* ceremonies, held every five years. This was the occasion for one of those enormous Buddhist festivals for which Central Asia was renowned; the custom was implanted in China during the same century. The most distinguished clerics from all the great monasteries of the region were present for the prolonged festivities; the most accomplished preachers embroidered on their favourite parables. The Chinese monks recognised their opportunity and gathered whatever material they could. Their collection was apparently first put together in sequential form at Turfan on their way back to China, in 445, and though the text was subjected to further editing, it is probable that our *Book of the Wise Man and the Fool* still embodies a portion of the Buddhist lore recounted in Khotan on that memorable occasion. Though much of the work's contents are not known from Indian sources, it is remarkable that one of the tales was discovered in a fragment in the Kuchean language; the Chinese book clearly represents a stock of traditions once current in Central Asia (Lévi 1925).

Or we may take the example of an Indian rite, the *abhiṣeka*, or royal consecration. This was to become the crucial ceremony marking the disciple's initiation into the mysteries of Tantric Buddhism; it is perhaps best known in the West by its Tibetan equivalent, *dbang*. Even as the son of a king was enabled to come into his royal inheritance through consecration, so the Buddhist *abhiṣeka* marked the spiritual coming of age of the Buddha's lineal heir. By the eighth century, the rite was found throughout the area of Tantric Buddhist diffusion. Consecration was already listed among the ultimate attributes of the Bodhisattva in the *Avataṃsaka sūtra*, translated into Chinese at the beginning of the fifth century. But the Indian work gave no indication that the rite of consecration was already being practised within the Buddhist community. Our earliest description of the rite is found in a *sūtra* composed in China, near Nanjing, in 457, and appropriately named *The Book of Consecration* (*Guanding jing*, T 1331). Thus in the absence of prior textual evidence, the Chinese work offers a unique reflection of contemporary Buddhist practice (Strickmann 1978c).*

The authors of original Chinese *sūtras* clearly did much towards the acclimatisation of Indian beliefs and practices in a Chinese milieu, and a considerable amount of valuable information from Central Asia as well as India has been preserved in texts of this large and varied category. But one of the chief aims of such authors was the elevation of traditional *Chinese* beliefs and practices into the framework of Buddhism; they sought and found the Buddha's authorisation for many of the customs without which Chinese spiritual life, even in Buddhist vestments, could never have been viewed as complete—components which Buddhism had to assimilate if it was to survive and prosper at all levels of Chinese society.

It is in this glib scriptural context that we find the Buddha's seal of approval being set upon various Chinese forms of divination, healing practices, mortuary customs, and reverence for parents and ancestors. In the same class of original scriptures we find the most explicit directives for Buddhist rituals in the service of the State: protective rites against internal and external enemies, and rites for bringing needed rain to the fields of the empire. Wondrous to relate, those original Chinese *sūtras* most useful for the State's purposes managed to weather the periodic government scrutinies and, like the defensive rites, survive in successive official Buddhist Canons. Other works, no less wholly Chinese but of less obvious utility to bureaucrats, were plucked out and proscribed, and were it not for the discovery of a cache of some 30,000 mediaeval manuscripts at Dunhuang, Gansu, at the beginning of this century, many of them would have remained only names of works stigmatised as "doubtful," "false," or "fabricated" in the *index expurgatorius* of the hypercritical official bibliographer. In the unofficial scriptures, then, we find all shades of opinion represented, from the ascetic to the self-indulgent, in all styles of scriptural syntax, from the most sedulously indianizing to the Taoist-in-spite-of-itself. We might well wonder how widely some of these works were diffused and what segments of the population they reached. Statistics on these points do not come readily to hand. But it is noteworthy that many of the original Chinese *sūtras*, like the Taoist scriptures which they in so many ways resembled, are known to have been composed in the Lower Yangtse region. There, in an area embracing the vicinity of modern Nanjing and extending southwards into northern Zhejiang, was the font of much new spiritual literature from the fourth through sixth centuries, the formative period of Chinese religious life. Thence new scriptures percolated northwards into regions of China then under alien rule, and so the presence of such works in the distant repository at Dunhuang, at the gateway to the West, is a most significant indication of their broad diffusion. But most intriguing of all, the progress of many of these Chinese scriptures did not stop at Dunhuang. A number have been identified in translation, in several languages of Central Asia, including Sogdian and Khotanese (MacKenzie 1976; Utz 1978; Emmerick 1979). It has been suggested that many of the still perplexing fragments of Central Asian Buddhist literature which have not yet been identified, and which appear to correspond to nothing known from Indian Buddhist writings, may quite probably represent translations from original Chinese scriptures. This is bound to become a fruitful line of inquiry, as more scholars recognise the importance of the Chinese creations. There are already scattered indications of how elaborate the chain of transmission and transformation might become, as in the case of the *sūtra* in the Tibetan Buddhist Canon (Otani no. 1028), on the cult of the Big Dipper (Ursa Major), which was translated from an Uighur text, itself a translation of a Chinese Buddhist *sūtra* which had been adapted from an original Taoist scripture (which in turn represented a systematisation of widespread common Chinese belief). In reconstructing the lost Buddhism of the peoples of Central Asia, a series of vital links in the chain of Serindian cultural transmission, we must recognise the influence of Chinese Buddhist enclaves upon the environing Sogdian, Kuchean, Uighur, and Khotanese communities. Among lay members of the western outposts of Chinese Buddhism, it would appear that original Chinese scriptures were accorded primacy in much the same way that they often were by lay devotees within China proper. It was natural that their Central Asian neighbours should take many of their Buddhist sacred texts from this proximate source—a source doubtless seen as representing *in partibus* the wealth and power of China itself. Small wonder, then, that Manichaeism arrived in China at the end of the seventh century already draped respectably in the garments of Chinese Buddhism (Haloun and Henning 1952). Where surviving documents have given us the means, we can frequently detect elements of a characteristically Chinese Buddhism making their way westwards, in the company of Chinese commerce and Chinese military might.

MOTIVES AND MEANS OF BUDDHIST EXPANSION

The "Buddhist Conquest of China" and the lesser-known Chinese impact on Buddhism itself are long-term historical phenomena, most vital phases of their history extending over more than a millenium. Various spiritual and literary explanations for this gigantic movement in the life of East Asia have been advanced in western writings. But it is perhaps not entirely likely that China began its involvement with Buddhism in response to an overpowering craving for the interminable subtle verbiage of the *Sūtra of Perfect Wisdom*, or that Buddhism owed its warm welcome in China to the eager quest of Chinese authors for Significant Form. Philologists tend naturally to batten on texts, particularly scriptural texts, their right and natural fodder, to the exclusion of contexts and institutions. And the study of Buddhism has so far been more the purview of the philologist than the historian. Part of this is due precisely to Chinese bibliographic acumen; the scriptures, statutes, commentaries, and hagiographies of Buddhism were long ago neatly relegated to the great Canons, and this deft pre-packaging has served virtually as a *cordon sanitaire* around what is, after all, a vast body of primary sources for Chinese social, cultural and economic history. It is to the serious historians who have worked directly with Buddhist texts that we owe many of the most cogent observations that have so far been made on the origins, growth and spread of the Buddhist community. A succinct account of early mediaeval Indian conditions has been given by D.D. Kosambi. The primitive poverty enjoined upon *bhikṣus* ("beggars") by the Buddha soon gave way; within a century of the Buddha's death, monks had begun to accept and even solicit donations in cash. In time, "the accumulated monastic wealth often provided some of the capital so badly needed by early merchants and caravaneers in the Indian hinterland" (Kosambi 1965:182). Monasteries came, *inter alia*, to serve as banks, fulfilling an essential economic function closely allied with the spread of trade. Kosambi takes as an example the early monastic foundations at Kārle (Western India). He notes the opulent style of the surviving sculpture and the voluptuousness of its worldly themes: "hardly what one would expect in an assembly place for monks, but precisely what rich merchants would have liked" (Kosambi 1965:183). The donors' names are inscribed upon the pillars; prominent among them are the names of merchants and bankers, high officials, physicians; the local merchants' union is there, together with records of entire villages donated by the king and his governor. Craftsmen's guilds are also inscribed among the donors, as are numerous still more humble individuals. This complex of cave-monasteries was situated in the uncultivated outlands, not in a major centre of habitation. But its locus was strategic, for it lay hard by a much-travelled road leading from the seacoast to the inland plateau. The nominal requirement of ascetic isolation was thus cleverly combined with proximity to a major route of commerce.

Kosambi also points out that a monastery like Kārle will itself have been a considerable consumer of goods, all of which had to be brought from afar: "cloth for the monks, incense and costly perfumes for the service, metal images, metal lamps in large numbers" (1965:185). Beyond their function as banks and repositories of supplies, monasteries also served as way-stations for the caravans; pilgrim-routes and trade-routes were thus superimposed. In view of these early developments in Indian Buddhism, it is hardly surprising that the religion spread and flourished along the arteries of trade. Kosambi's reconstruction helps us towards a clearer view of the probable activities of the great monasteries of the Central Asian city-states. But it is the remarkable Chinese documents recovered from Dunhuang that bring the glow of homely realism to the picture. Here were found original manuscripts documenting the daily life of mediaeval Chinese monasteries and lay organisations: monastic accounts, contracts, lists of offerings, official monks' certificates, circulars to the members of laymen's groups, and census rolls. The full range of this unique corpus has been surveyed in a brilliant work by Jacques Gernet on the economic aspects of mediaeval Chinese Buddhism—a masterpiece of historical scholarship still insufficiently recognised in the English-speaking world (Gernet 1956). Gernet traces a vivid tableau of Buddhism's socioeconomic impact on China from the fifth through tenth centuries. Members of the *saṅgha* enjoyed special status, exempt from taxes and corvée labour. They accumulated wealth through offerings and trade, sponsored monastic agricultural colonies and founded the institution of monastic serfs, activities which eventually resulted in the dispossessing, by the monks, of vast number of peasants. Huge sums were realised from monastic monopolies on water mills and oil presses, and of course, from interest on loans to merchants as well as peasants.

Most striking of all, perhaps, are the offerings made by the laity—offerings remarkable not only for their number and diversity, but also for the enthusiastic spirit of emulation that seems to pervade this pious phenomenon. In an atmosphere of lavish ceremony, a lively competition in sacrifices was mounted, and the luxurious appointments of the great monasteries bespoke the eagerness of members of the self-respecting classes to outdo one another in conspicuous and merit-accruing generosity. This process, too, began in the fifth century. Beyond the obvious social distinction that redounded to the donor, some of the otherworldly motivation behind such lavish gifts emerges only too blatantly in this extract from a *sūtra* composed in mid-fifth century China. Regarding the efficacity of offerings made on behalf of a deceased relative who had, during his lifetime, occasionally wavered in his commitment to Buddhism, the Buddha declared:

> Of the felicity cultivated for that person, he will receive one part in seven. Why is this so? Because during his lifetime he did not have faith in the Tao and its merit. Therefore he is made to obtain only one seventh of the merit of those felicitous acts. But if all the appurtenances with which the deceased enhanced his person—his halls, mansions, chambers, his gardens, groves, and ponds—are bestowed upon the Three Treasures, this will produce the very greatest felicity and the most powerful merit. By that means he can be drawn forth from the miseries of the hells and will directly obtain deliverance from the affliction of sorrow and suffering. He will attain lasting liberation and will be reborn in one of the pure lands of the Buddhas in the ten directions. (T. 1331, ch.11.)

In such cases of doubt, only a total donation would guarantee total beatitude. Indeed, if a single formula were sought to explain the phenomenal success of Buddhism in mediaeval China, we might suggest that Buddhism did so well precisely because it offered the Chinese unlimited means of turning material wealth into spiritual felicity.

The special grace accorded merchants in the Buddhist dispensation was naturally mirrored in scripture and legend. The Central Asian caravans enjoyed the protection of particular divine guardians (Bareau 1959). It is significant that it was two merchants, Trapuśa and Bhallika, who were said to have been the first persons to make offerings to the Buddha immediately after his enlightenment. They gave him parched grain and honey from their travelling provisions and received some of the Buddha's hair in return. Their memory has consequently been hallowed throughout the Buddhist diaspora. In Balkh (northernmost Afghanistan) Xuanzang heard of the two *stūpas* northwest of the city which the merchants had built over the relics. Far to the south, in Ceylon, a similar tale is told. Whilst in Burma, the building of the great Shwe Dagon pagoda of Rangoon is also linked with the inspiring tale (Lévi 1929). In return for making the initial offerings to the Buddha and thereby founding the fecund rite of offering, Trapuśa and Bhallika were chosen to inaugurate the potent cult of relics—itself vastly productive of prestige and wealth. To this well-balanced construct of legends and rites, the Chinese made a characteristic contribution. The monkish catalogues list a "fabricated" scripture passing under the name of *The Sūtra of Trapuśa and Bhallika* (or, in jejune Chinese contraction, *Tiwei jing*). This fifth-century work was prudently expunged from the Buddhist Canon; like so many good things, it has only been restored to us through the finds at Dunhuang. It is clear from the text that the merchant-saints were being invoked to sponsor a scripture directed to Chinese laymen, themselves perhaps merchants. This is made clear by the emphasis on the Three Refuges and the Five Precepts, the most elementary undertakings of lay Buddhism. But the good Trapuśa and Bhallika might have shuddered to learn the nature of the book on which their blessing was invoked, for as we read further in the text we discover that much of its matter has been lifted directly from a Taoist work on the internal spirit-personnel that run the body (*The Inner Book of Laozi, Laozi zhongjing*). Such is the teaching which the Buddha is alleged to have bestowed upon his first disciples; such is the message they are supposed to have borne away with them, to China (Makita 1976; Strickmann 1978c).* Once again, the Chinese contribution to Buddhist lore and practice reveals a truly admirable inventiveness.

THERAPEUTIC RITUALS

Quite beyond their mercantile and savings-and-loan activities, religious institutions were supposed to provide aid and comfort to the faithful—particularly after having so rudely awakened them to their full eschatological peril (Strickmann 1978d).* There is copious testimony to Buddhist professional activity in the treatment of disease. The Buddha himself was of course the Great Physician, his prime medicine the universal solvent of Insight. In theory at least, physical health was a function of spiritual health (Demiéville 1937). The monastic rule had consequently exhibited the clearest logic in restricting the range of medicaments which holy men might use to those effluvia produced by their own bodies. Communities of saintly monks maintained ample stockpiles of this panacea, which (according to a fifth-century Chinese author) they enticingly styled "broth of the yellow dragon" (May 1967). The egesta of high lamas still figure as an esteemed medicine among pious Tibetans today. But as usual this was only one side of monastic practice, the aspect of self-consciously strict *vinaya* observance. The creation of a specific patron of healing techniques, the Master of Pharmaka (Bhaiṣajyaguru, Yaoshi) suggests the growing importance of therapy as well as its cultic associations. This Buddha was seen as having an especially close bond with China, for his paradise was situated in the East (Birnbaum 1979). He was frequently depicted as bearing a myrobalan in his right hand, and under the informal aegis of this benign figure Buddhist monks played a capital role in the infusion of the already abundant Chinese pharmacopeia with Indian, Iranian, and Central Asian materia medica. Huc and Gabet provide us with a colourful description of Buddhist medical practice a century and a half ago—but surely these practices go back many centuries, and helped consolidate the position of monasteries in local communities. The dispensary at the monastery of sKu-'bum (Kumbum) attracted purchasers from hundreds of miles around to buy the monks' botanic simples at exorbitant prices, inflated because the herbs grew on the holy mountain that gave birth to Tsong-kha-pa. Each summer, young monks betook themselves from the monastery to nearby Chogortang, where they would botanise daily, carrying osier baskets, and fortify themselves with leathern bagfulls of tsampa gruel and pots of buttered tea. Instead of herbs, roots, and fungi, the lowest grade of monk would gather argols (i.e. dung), which were divided into four separate grades depending on the species of animal, and used for everything from fuel to medicine. (Huc and Gabet 1928:II, 108–110.)

The therapeutic aspect of Buddhism, in the medical as well as the spiritual sense of the word, lent powerful support to capital formation in promoting the religion's eastwards diffusion (Filliozat 1934). But for the special circumstances attendant upon the end of Buddhism, which was also to be the end of the world, material means alone of dealing with disease were not adequate. It was necessary to channel the full resources of the spirit-realm against the demonic menace, and this could best be done through ritual. Indian scriptures offered potent *mantras* towards this end, each to be recited under the proper ritual conditions, and each embodying the concentrated force of a particular Buddha, Bodhisattva, or a benevolent guardian deity. Moreover, by mobilising the hitherto despised forces of ecstatic religion (a licit proceeding when faced with acute danger), Indian monks created powerful rituals of exorcism through spirit-possession (*āveśa*). Properly harnessed and yoked to a Buddhist ritual vehicle, spirit-possession was an important method of prophecy as well as therapy, and under the aegis of Buddhist masters it became highly popular, even fashionable, at the Tang court (as well as among the aristocracy of Heian Japan).

Once more, however, Chinese monkish authors were not content to restrict their demon-quelling to imported methods. They too responded to the challenge of their apocalyptic times by creating appropriately Chinese exorcisms for a wider Buddhist following. Only quotation at length could give the flavour of these original Chinese *sūtras*. The formula, though, was to drape colourful Indian trappings over a framework of tested Taoist healing ritual. Written talismans, burnt and given to the patient in charmed water, and pressed on the sufferer's body, and graven seals of apotropaic datewood, were favourite media of demon-dispelling among the Taoists, and thus were duly assimilated into Chinese Tantric Buddhist rites (Strickmann 1978c).*

Ritual, then, was central in this apocalyptic age. Somewhat mechanical and contrived-seeming, perhaps, when compared with the instantaneous enlightenment (swift as thought!) among the Buddha's direct disciples, it was nonetheless the right and proper path to salvation under the Counterfeit Law. And no complex of rituals was given greater attention than the rites for the salvation of the dead. The rise of individualism, the cult of personality, the glimmerings of "personal religion," for which twentieth-century scholars are forever scanning the horizons of the Chinese past, appears to be a mirage. Henri Maspero claimed to detect its emergence at the fall of the Han, in the birth of Taoism. Others now see it coming forth in the Song, or under the Ming. Chances are that all the reports are false; the visionaries have been guided by the shimmer of hagiography, rather than the darker bulk of more substantial historical documents. There is no doubt that the extended family was and remained the fundamental cornerstone of Chinese society, and that it was the primary focus of the great majority of rituals. The emphasis of ritual was therefore a collective rather than an "individual" or "personal" one. Families expanded along a patrilineage whose members, living and dead, were in some sense virtually consubstantial, living descendants curiously incarnating their deceased ancestors. The weal and woe of living and dead communicants was intimately linked by a chain of mutual causality and collective responsibility. Hence the care taken with the siting of graves, hence the dread punishment of extermination of the culprit's family to the ninth degree of kinship. The decisive nature of the choice of the monk's life is underscored, in Chinese, by its being termed "leaving the family" (*chujia*). Yet the all-embracing grip of the family system is equally well shown in the organisation of monastic life itself, for the ordinee has only left his family to join a still greater lineage, the fictive family of masters and disciples which allies its members as "children of the Buddha." It is not surprising, then, that the greatest concern of the Chinese under the Buddho-Taoist dispensation was the salvation of their dead, which not only sanctified the family's past but also guaranteed its beatific future. Chinese Buddhist monks and Taoist priests quickly perceived and responded to the demand. From the fifth century on, they elaborated wonderfully complex funeral and memorial rituals, Buddhist and Taoist versions both keeping step in an admirable spirit of social service. Mortuary rites were a substantial source of income for religious foundations in the Middle Ages; nowadays Buddhism in particular subsists mainly on revenues from memorial services, and in consequence is cynically referred to as "mortuary Buddhism" in Japan. Mediaeval Chinese would have found the cynicism misplaced. As the fifth-century *Consecration Sūtra* puts it, "The case of the dead person is like that of one who has broken the Law in the world of the living; in his heart he thinks longingly of his family, and looks to them for forceful assistance in escaping from his peril. Acquiring merit on behalf of the deceased is like bestowing provisions on travellers: it always has a good result" (T 1331, ch. 11). The dead are indeed travellers into a realm more fearful even than the Western Regions, because dominated by Law. Every family should therefore amply provide for its own pilgrims into the Infinite, and both Buddhism and Taoism early equipped themselves to mediate in that function.

DUNHUANG

Thus after a long and circuitous journey, sounding once again the themes of travel and the protocols of the frontier, we come at length to Dunhuang. Here the full range of Chinese symbols was marshalled on the imperial frontier, and the settled Chinese agrarian population might behold the stately procession of polyglot merchants and pilgrims from the countries of the West. Yet it was some time before Dunhuang became the comprehensive focus of cultures that we are accustomed to visualise under the Tang, when natives of India, Iran, Tibet, and the kingdoms of Central Asia met and mingled there, and chants rose up to the Buddha, Mani, Lord Lao the Most High, and Christ.

It was the decisive defeat of the Xiongnu and their expulsion to the north, in 119 B.C., which made possible the Chinese settlement of the long and fertile Gansu corridor. From that point on, China was in direct contact with Central Asia (Hulsewé and Loewe 1979:41). There followed a series of military campaigns against Central Asian cities which refused to provide facilities for Chinese garrisons, including distant Ferghāna (104–102 B.C.), and the Han were soon manipulating the internal politics of the Wusun people in a manner that would do credit to our own intelligence operations. Sometime during this period, a Chinese *agent provocateur* was credited with a plot that resulted in the murder of the king of Jibin, a name traditionally taken as standing for Kashmir. As the ground was steadily softened up by such all too familiar tactics, the heroic exploits of Han expeditionary forces came to be supplanted, from ca. 65 B.C. on, by the founding of stable agricultural colonies of veterans in Central Asia, by way of maintaining a lasting Chinese presence (Hulsewé and Loewe 1979:50). Dunhuang had been founded sometime shortly before 91 B.C.; it marks the limit of cultivable land, at the western end of the great Gansu corridor, and hence truly represents a Chinese *finis terrarum*. It was from this outer rim, shielded by the strongly fortified portals of the Yumen guan and the Yang guan, that Chinese expeditions set out for Central Asia.

If, as Hulsewé has shown, the Chinese government was the principal interested party in the silk trade, making use of its most celebrated commodity in its burgeoning international relations, there is nevertheless notice in Chinese sources from the first century B.C. on of foreign merchants arriving at the frontier posts. By the first century A.D., there were traders from the Western Regions at Luoyang, the Eastern Han capital, and another reference reveals that by 120 A.D. there was a constant traffic of foreign merchants at Dunhuang "from the most opulent Western Regions," who repeatedly attempted to win over the Chinese commandant with gifts of slaves, horses, gold, silver, incense, and carpets (Hulsewé 1974:133). In the course of this intense commercial activity Buddhism had already made its entrance on the Chinese scene, and monasteries were established at Dunhuang. From Dunhuang came one of the greatest of the early translators and expounders of scripture, Dharmarākṣa (Fa-hu), who in 286 completed the first integral translation of the *Lotus Sūtra*. And at some time in the 350's or 360's, work was begun on the first cave-sanctuaries in the long cliffside, southeast of the city, that (owing to the pious work thus begun and long continued) eventually came to be known as the Caves of the Thousand Buddhas.

It is this cave-complex that leaps to the mind's eye with the mention of Dunhuang. After the Great Wall, perhaps, and the city of Beijing, it has become one of China's best-known archaeological sites. This is due in great part to its pioneer explorer, Sir Aurel Stein, whose circumstantial narratives of Central Asian discovery reopened the Silk Route to twentieth-century scholarship. His massive works record an odyssey of travel and discovery no less stirring and informative than the journal of his patron saint, the seventh-century Chinese pilgrim-monk Yuanzang. The paintings found at Dunhuang, and the manuscripts brought out by Stein, Pelliot, and a succession of Russian, Japanese, and Chinese scholars, have revolutionised our knowledge of mediaeval China and its relations with the peoples of Central Asia.

Apart from having preserved a remarkable hoard of treasures, the caves exert their own fascination. Here we find the East Asian expression of the cavern-sanctuary, already well-attested in early Buddhist India. The first council was reportedly held in a great grotto (latterly reconstructed, in Rangoon, as the headquarters of the Burmese *saṅgha*!); after the council's conclusion, Mahākāśyapa, most responsible of the Buddha's disciples, retired into a cave, there to await the coming of Maitreya (Lamotte 1958:227). More tangibly, we have already mentioned the cave-monasteries at Kārle, in Western India. Thence we may follow the trade-route to the northeast, through the Buddhist cave-complexes of Elūrā and Ājantā, renowned for their opulent murals and sculpture. The ascetic's barren retreat became the focus of intense patronage; ravishing art was the outcome. Yet once again, the Chinese monuments are no mere replicas of Indian originals. The mountain- and cavern-shrines of China already had their own highly-evolved traditions, and yield to none in spectacular setting and iconic riches. Architecturally, they invite comparison with the rock-hewn churches of Cappadocia and Ethiopia, whilst much of their deeply ingrained symbolism is uncannily realised in the Mayan cavern-cults of Yucatan (Mercer 1896).*

Superimposing their own interpretation on prior chthonian worship, the Taoists termed their sacred grottoes "cavern-heavens" (*dongtian*) and visualised them as celestial paradises, secreted deep within sacred mountains. Into their dark declivities illuminati would descend in quest of sacred knowledge. Heaven the Taoists envisioned as "the vault of space" (*kongdong*), whilst an inch-square recess of the brain, a focal point in meditation, was called the "Cavern-chamber" (*dongfang*). The entire three-tiered speleology was peopled by supramundane beings—heaven, earth, and brain all conceal sacred caverns. The Western Mother Queen's dwelling on Mt. Kunlun was a "stone chamber" (*shishi*), glossed as a habitable cave; significantly, the same term occurs in Han official texts, denoting a vault for written records of particular value. The Taoist Canon was itself divided into three "caverns," and mediaeval adepts were instructed, when they perceived death's approach, to conceal their scriptures in a cliffside cave. There they would be safely shielded from the defiling gaze of the profane, until their discovery by the next destined initiate. It is a curious chance that the finder and guardian of the Dunhuang manuscripts, just before Aurel Stein arrived on the scene, should have been a Taoist priest.

Thus in mountain caverns paradise might be pictured, and sacred texts preserved. This is precisely what we find at Dunhuang's Caves of the Thousand Buddhas. The complex, with neighbouring cavern-sites, offers some 600 grottoes, many elaborately adorned, on which work proceeded for centuries. Here too, safely preserved for 900 years in a "stone chamber," was a great hoard of mediaeval manuscripts in Chinese and Central Asian languages: Sanskrit, Khotanese, Sogdian, Uighur, and the earliest known examples of Tibetan. The total, now dispersed to libraries throughout Europe and Asia, has been estimated at some 30,000 items. Both Chinese Buddhist and Taoist sources state that the mountains and their cavern-paradises will serve as sacrosanct places of refuge during the world's final apocalyptic convulsions. At that time the saints and the elect among the faithful will seek sanctuary at designated points within the earth. Meanwhile, by ritual means, through pilgrimage, they may anticipate this happy conclusion to the annals of mundane suffering. Their offerings could be brought to the stone coffers of holy mountains, where their pious donations subsidised depictions of paradise and its denizens, limned on cavern walls. There, too, they might undertake scripture-copying, most often in fulfilment of a vow. For this they would often have recourse to the services of a skilled professional scribe, since the rules for transcribing sacred texts were stringent: ritual purity, the finest paper, the clearest of formal calligraphy: cursive script was not tolerated, nor scribal errors condoned. Lasting till the end of time, such scripture-copies (like the paintings) were duly labelled with their donours' names and pious intentions. They would bear perpetual witness to the donation, and would provide eloquent testimony on behalf of the donours and their ancestors, first at the tribunals of the dead, ultimately before Maitreya's throne. Hope for eventual salvation in Maitreya's messianic kingdom became the determining motive of the great collective ritual assemblies for scripture-copying, and this is one of many aspects of mediaeval Chinese Buddhism that survive in Japan (Sekine 1968).

Japan also provides the closest analogies with the art of this vanished world of mediaeval Chinese craftsmanship and piety. The pantheon represented at Dunhuang is that rich Six Dynasties and Tang conglomerate that was to be transplanted and preserved in Japan, and a Japanese scholar, Matsumoto Eiichi, has written what remains, after forty-five years, the most comprehensive guide to its complexities (1937). In the first rank, of course, are the Buddhas: the Buddha of our own era, Śākyamuni (Pl. 55), and his canonical predecessors, as well as Maitreya (Pl. 14), still to come. Yet save perhaps for Maitreya, whose unmanifest potential made him a logical focus of eschatological yearning, the active cult of the Buddha during the Chinese Middle Ages was most particularly the cult of still another Buddha, Amitābha (Pl. 85), patron of the Western Paradise or Pureland into which a majority of the faithful aspired to be reborn. Depictions of his realm of bliss are frequent on scrolls and cavern walls. But though these great, static paradise-*mandalas* promised an enviable infinite serenity, for iconographic variety and exuberance the emphasis had long since shifted from the Buddhas to the Bodhisattvas, more directly accessible as saviours and guides. Paramount among them is Guanyin (Avalokiteśvara) (Pl. 61), whose numerous functions are reflected in a dazzling variety of forms: thousand-armed, eleven-headed (Pl. 122), wishing-jewel-bearing, noose-wielding, succouring the faithful reciters of his scripture (ch. 25 of the *Lotus*) from shipwreck, fire, robbers, demons and lustful thoughts.

More highly specialised was Dizang (Kṣitigarbha, "Earth-matrix"), the psychopomp, guide of the spirits of the dead through the labyrinthine courts of purgatory and out to the lands of the blessed. In socio-economic terms Dizang was the patron of burial societies as well as the mainstay of bereaved families, and it is significant that he came to be represented in the guise of a stalwart, trustworthy monk (Soymié 1966). A less well documented personage, Yinlu pusa ("The Bodhisattva who leads along the road") was, like Dizang, frequently figured on funeral banners, borne (perhaps as soul-supports) in the procession to the tomb. He too was venerated as a guide and protector in the dominant mortuary cult. Also often shown on banners was Bishamen (Vaiśrāvaṇa), patron of Khotan and world-guardian of the northern quarter, chief of the host of all the lesser, local godlings and spirits who submitted in good time to the Buddha's Law and were consequently entrusted with the protection of the faithful.

The paintings on silk, the paradise-*maṇḍalas* and mortuary banners, were mobile complements to the immobile mural paintings; they were discovered among the manuscripts, and their marked signs of wear suggest that they were retired to storage only after long and useful lives in ritual. The manuscripts themselves include a number of scrolls and booklets illustrated with paintings in colour, among them a codex depicting the courts of the Ten Kings of the underworld. The kings are shown as infernal magistrates, and the tortures and punishments applied to the dead are represented in the lively fashion that changed but little over a thousand years. Such paintings were still being produced in Formosa in the early years of this century, and important cognate material has been preserved, once again, in Japan (Ogawa 1973). However stereotyped these traditions may have become, in the earliest known examples of such sequences we are freed, for a time, from the overwhelming scholasticism of Sino-Japanese Buddhist art. Could we only realise it, we are also liberated from the tyranny of "fine" art: the "amateur" current which has been exalted by Western art historians (following their mandarin masters) into a Great Tradition of Chinese painting. As in the mediaeval West, the bulk of artistic production was not the work of decorous scholar-painters or long-nailed imperial academicians, but rather of well-trained professionals, working to order. To understand this art, a thorough knowledge of the abundant textual sources is essential. But Chinese art history has still not found its Panofsky, and the Warburg Institute is overshadowed, in East Asia, by a swarm of aesthetic "authenticators."

At Dunhuang, artistic activity flowed beyond the confines of the painted scrolls and into the margins of texts, in rapidly brushed sketches and doodles. But most interesting, for the history of art, are the ink drawings in black and white, the "monochrome paintings" (*bohua*), found among the manuscripts. Some represent leaves from craftsmen's notebooks, working drafts or cartoons—a type of material hitherto missing from the documentary evidence for mediaeval Chinese painting. It is clear, moreover, that a number of these drawings were intended for direct use in preparing murals. The drawing would be applied to the prepared surface of the wall and the outline of the design pricked with a pin; the sketch removed, the pin-pricks would be joined by brush-lines on the wall's surface. Or the inked contours of the sketch on paper would be cut out, and the resulting stencil applied to the wall and painted over. Thus in addition to being forceful examples of brushwork and design, the surviving ink drawings provide fascinating evidence for the way in which complex mural constructions were assembled (Jao et al. 1978:12). The presence of this considerable ensemble of graphic work at Dunhuang permits us to approach certain long-standing scholarly debates regarding the cave-decor in a spirit of optimism. For example, it has long been averred that the painting in the earlier caves betrays clear technical and stylistic affinities with Central Asian examples, notably the caves at Kizil, near Kucha, and this view still finds currency (Akiyama and Matsubara 1969:12). The Jātaka scenes in the sixth-century friezes at Dunhuang, with their abundance of faunal forms in severely geometrical landscapes, predictably evoked reminiscences of the Central Asian animal style. Against this interpretation it has been plausibly argued that these continuous narrative sequences represent a natural application to mural art of the technique of the Chinese illustrated scroll (Sullivan 1962:152).*

Testimony of a more prosaic nature is found in the colophons of murals and manuscripts alike, which give the names and titles of artists and artisans who realised the caverns' decor. There was a guild of painters at Dunhuang, whose members appear to have been responsible for the designs which the artisans executed *in situ*. Typically, it has been surmised that this body included Indians and Central Asians, but this must be regarded as unproven. On the contrary, the painters seem to have been Chinese members of a Chinese corporation, and though naturally indebted to Indian narrative and iconographic sources, the characteristically Chinese style of the paintings is beyond doubt. The outlandish elements, curiously garbed foreign potentates and highly stylised alien landscapes, reflect the perennial Chinese taste for exotica. From the earliest dated cave-paintings (520) down the centuries, the art of Dunhuang embodies technical and stylistic developments in the art of China.

This was only to be expected, in view of the city's close ties with China's metropolitan centres. From Dunhuang, the Chinese lap of the Silk Route led south and eastwards to the capital cities of Changan and Luoyang, and there is no doubt that their refined art and literature were familiar in the frontier town. But before the traveller reached the rugged defiles that gave access to the Chinese heartland, he was presented with an alternate route, veering sharply southwards into the western province of Sichuan (Shu). Dunhuang maintained a special relationship with Sichuan's major city, Yizhou (modern Chengdu). From 925 on, Western Sichuan was an independent kingdom, and the Dunhuang collections include a number of manuscripts copied there in the tenth century. Indeed, the whole class of scriptural texts with inset paintings appears to derive from the ateliers of Western Sichuan. The idiosyncratic poet- and painter-monk, Guanxiu (832-913), settled in Sichuan around 902; his fame and examples of his work soon reached Dunhuang (Jao et al. 1978:I, 16). The art of printing, too, seems to have begun in Western Sichuan, and it is doubtless there that the several incunabula found at Dunhuang originated.

Yet however much Dunhuang may have owed to the vigorous culture of Shu, the frontier city maintained a distinct identity of its own. Witness the proud eulogies of local worthies, the long lists of donours and patrons at its shrines and monasteries, and the minor epic of Zhang Yichao, the indigenous hero who delivered the city from Tibetan occupation (it had fallen in 787, after a siege of more than ten years) in 848 (Demiéville 1952:167–68,176–77). The copious documentation on Dunhuang's Buddhist devotees' societies vividly illustrates an institution that must have been a prime vehicle of social cohesion and local identity. Thus even if we must recognise the influx of metropolitan culture in the arts, we should not allow Dunhuang to resubmerge in the vast ocean of the Chinese State. Whether in tenth-century Dunhuang or twentieth-century Tainan, there is abundant evidence that the life of China has always lain with its multiplicity of local cultures, and that these cultures have been based upon temples and shrines, the spiritual Law—in fact, upon ritual. If there is merit in this view, it will be clear how effectively China has struck at the roots of its own culture by the systematic despoilment and destruction of temples throughout China and Tibet since 1966. We may sense how ill many historians have served the cause of Asian history by diverting attention from local cultures to the central government, that paperwork empire so reminiscent of our own, and by focusing "intellectual" and "religious" history on elite abstractions like "The Three Religions" or "Neo-confucianism." Regional wholeness is blazoned forth in the symbolic totality of the local pantheon, integrated within the ritual year—whether Dunhuang's thousand Buddhas, the 360 gods of the Kulu Valley in the Western Himalayas (G. Jettmar 1974: 15), or the traditional "hundred temples" of the old city of Tainan (Schipper 1977:651).*

Dunhuang represents a virtually inexhaustible fund of textual and artistic remains, the speculum of a complex local society. Continuing research on this mighty corpus, when integrated with the evidence of the printed tradition and the results of ongoing archaeology, should in time utterly transform our appreciation of mediaeval China. How sad, then, that so little work should have been done with these materials in the United States, and that until quite recently, Dunhuang studies were not even represented here in academic curricula. In 1980, a seminar in Dunhuang studies was inaugurated at the University of California, Berkeley; this year another begins, at Princeton. It is to be hoped, then, that the long period of neglect by American scholars is now over. An attempt has been made to present the essential bibliography of Dunhuang research in succinct handbook form (Strickmann 1980b).

If we were to seek a Western parallel to Dunhuang and its cultural riches, we might well choose Dura-Europos, another frontier city, near the Western terminus of the Silk Route. Like Dunhuang a confluence of trade and cultures—Persian, Parthian, Hellenistic, Hebraic, Roman—Dura's artistic remains testify in spectacular fashion to the presence there, too, of a plurality of religions: Mithraism, Judaism, Christianity, all duly moulded in accordance with the dominant Hellenistic cultural canons, and a close parallel to the way in which Chinese culture and style determined the form of southern and western Asian faiths on China's frontier. Just as the exuberance of Indian Buddhist sculpture and mural art was subdued and acclimatised within a Chinese matrix at Dunhuang, so were the diverse strands of Near Eastern inspiration moulded, at Dura, to the suave decor of the Grecian mode. Nor do the parallels stop there. Like Dunhuang, Dura was a garrison city; first Greeks, then Romans, held it against "barbarian" encroachments. Dura was destroyed in A.D. 256, and the site was afterwards deserted. Its abandonment virtually coincided with the end of Antiquity, and the Syrian sands have therefore preserved for us an urbane cameo of that vanished world and its diversity. Dunhuang's decline coincided with a mushrooming series of new alignments on the checkerboard of Central Asian peoples, leading in time to China's withdrawal from the cities of the Silk Route and the refocusing of Chinese geopolitical interest within a circuit closer to the imperial still point of a rapidly moving world. Not long after the Uighur and Tibetan threats had been contained came the steady Chinese retreat before a boisterous and varied company of Tanguts, Khitan, Jürchen, and finally, most dire of steppe-born perils, the Mongols. And the seeds of change were not all of alien devising. Tucked away among its thousands of manuscripts, Dunhuang preserved a number of the earliest known examples of printing. As much as any foreign political or military presence, printing was to revolutionise China's own culture, before wreaking more global changes. The sealed-off compartment adjoining Cave 17 appears to have originally been intended as an honourable repository for two imperially-commissioned manuscript sets of the Chinese Buddhist Canon, each presented to a great Dunhuang monastery during the Tang (Fujieda 1981). It seems safe to assume that their relegation to the storage-chamber sometime not long after the year 1000 was connected with the arrival at Dunhuang of the first printed Buddhist Canon, a project which had been started in Chengdu in 971. We can reasonably surmise that the installation of the great *Editio princeps* must have dictated the consignment of the sumptuous Tang manuscript canons to storage. The sealing away of the Dunhuang manuscripts thus epitomizes the progressive decline of the long Chinese manuscript tradition consequent on the rise of large-scale printing, a phenomenon that resulted in not only increased preservation and diffusion, but also much selectivity and loss. Thus the caverns and their hoard encapsulate an entire past age of traditional China, for with the decline of the manuscript tradition ended China's Middle Ages; printing and the Song Dynasty ushered in the beginning of modern times.

Michel Strickmann

Specialized Bibliography

Aziz, Barbara Nimri
1978 *Tibetan frontier families*. Durham.

Demiéville, Paul
1955 "Les apocryphes bouddhiques en Chine," *Annuaire du Collège de France*, reprinted in Demiéville, *Choix d'études bouddhiques*. Leiden 1973, pp. 153–157.

Dudbridge, Glen
1978 *The legend of Miao-shan*. London.

Guilk, Robert Hans van
1961 *Sexual life in ancient China*. Leiden.

Kabutogi, Shoko
1978 *Sutain Perio shūshū Tonkō Hokkekyō mokuroku*. Tokyo.

Magnin, Paul
1979 *La vie et l'oeuvre de Huisi* (515–517). Paris.

Makita, Tairyo
1976 *Gikyo Kenkyu*. Kyoto.

Mathieu, Remi
1978 *Le Mu Tianzi zhuan*. Paris.

Mercer, Henry C.
1896 *The hill-caves of Yucatan*. Philadelphia.

Rudenko, Sergei I.
1970 *Frozen tombs of Siberia: The Pazyryk burials of Iron-Age horsemen*. Berkeley. and London.

Schipper, Kristofer M.
1977 "Neighborhood cult associations in traditional Taiwan," in G. William Skinner, ed., *The city in traditional China*. Stanford.

Soymié, Michel
1966 "Notes d'iconographie chinoise: les acolytes de Ti-tsang (I)." *Arts Asiatiques*, 14:45–78.

Strickmann, Michel
1977 "The Mao Shan revelations; Taoism and the aristocracy," *T'oung Pao* 58:1–64.
1978a "The longest Taoist scripture," *History of Religions*, 17:331–54.
1978b "A Taoist confirmation of Liang Wu Ti's suppression of Taoism," *Journal of the American Oriental Society* 98:467–75.
1978c "The Consecration Sūtra, A Buddhist book of spells." Ms.
1978d "Buddhist eschatology and Chinese sovereignty," lecture at the University of British Columbia; ms.
1981 *Le Taoïsme du Mao Chan; chronique d'une révélation*. Paris.

Sullivan, Michael
1962 *The birth of landscape painting in China*. London and Berkeley.

V

Buddhism in North India and the Western Himalayas

Seventh to Thirteenth Centuries

David L. Snellgrove

In the course of its long history of some 2,500 years during which Buddhism has spread from the central Ganges Valley in India, first over the whole Indian subcontinent, and thence by land and sea to almost every country in Asia, local scholars in different places and at different times have analyzed its progress in diverse ways. During the first century B.C., while still limited to the Indian subcontinent (including Śrī Laṅkā), it was known as a doctrine and as a monastic rule which, having been promulgated by Śākyamuni Buddha, had already split into eighteen sects—all claiming to preserve the words of the Master in an authentic form. Comparisons of the various sets of scriptures that have survived to the present day suggest that a substantial core of oral teachings must certainly go back to an early period of formulation which can only have taken place within the decades immediately following the decease of Śākyamuni; this, according to calculations based upon the very much later Great Chronicle (*Mahāvaṃsa*) of Śrī Laṅkā, took place in 483 B.C.[1] Although this date has won a kind of conventional acceptance in popular books on Buddhism, it remains quite unreliable; but unfortunately, no better one can be suggested. No complete "life" of Śākyamuni was composed until several centuries after his decease; and despite his certain historical existence, his life story and the collections of stories of his supposed previous series of rebirths were composed almost entirely from legendary materials. The theory of reincarnation is fundamental to Buddhist doctrine, and thus it was assumed that Śākyamuni had won his way to final enlightenment as a result of his heroic striving throughout many previous lives when he was referred to not as Buddha, but as Bodhisattva (lit. "enlightenment being" with the sense of "would-be" Buddha). Moreover it was assumed that since world ages followed one another in cycles, there must have been Buddhas in the past and a future Buddha, eventually known as Maitreya, would follow him in this succession of World-Teachers. According to the earliest literary sources and archeological evidence, Buddhism presents itself not only as a philosophical doctrine and as a religious rule for monks and nuns, but also as a religious cult centering on Śākyamuni himself. The primary cult object was a type of funereal mound, corresponding exactly to the tumulus under which great men have been interred in many early civilizations, and of which the pyramids of Egypt are a particularly well-known type. The Sanskrit term for this is *stūpa*, meaning simply a pile (of earth and masonry). After Śākyamuni's death, eight shares of relics, the shovel used for dividing them, and the remains of the fire are said to have been divided between ten townships over which the first Buddhist *stūpas* were constructed. Shrines of this kind certainly existed in the third century B.C., for records show that the emperor Aśoka (who died 232 B.C. after a reign of thirty-six years) visited some of them and had others opened so that further shares of relics could be obtained for the many other *stūpas* he founded. By this time the *stūpa* was regarded as representing the ideal of Buddhahood as achieved by Śākyamuni when he passed into final *nirvāṇa*, while retaining to some extent its significance as a tomb. Similar monuments were constructed over the relics of his early disciples, and to this day the relics of revered Tibetan lamas are honored in precisely the same way. The cult of the *stūpa* as symbolizing the goal of all Buddhist striving underwent ever more detailed elaboration in the later periods (Figs. 10 and 11).

Like all great religions, Buddhism continued to develop and enrich its teachings, drawing upon those accumulations of Indian beliefs and theoretical constructions which lie likewise behind all the various forms in which Hindu religion has expressed itself. Thus by the first to second centuries A.D. we find that it embraced not only changed philosophical teachings, but also a much wider cult of other Buddhas and Bodhisattvas apart from Śākyamuni. The earlier philosophical views had been pluralistic, in keeping with the then contemporary theories of existence. Not only were the continuing cycles of existence (known as *saṃsāra*) regarded as distinct from the state of *nirvāṇa*, but both these planes of existence (often referred to as the "mundane" and the "supramundane") were analyzed as compositions of elemental particles, whether physical or mental. Over against these rather complicated theories there now developed a monistic interpretation of expe-

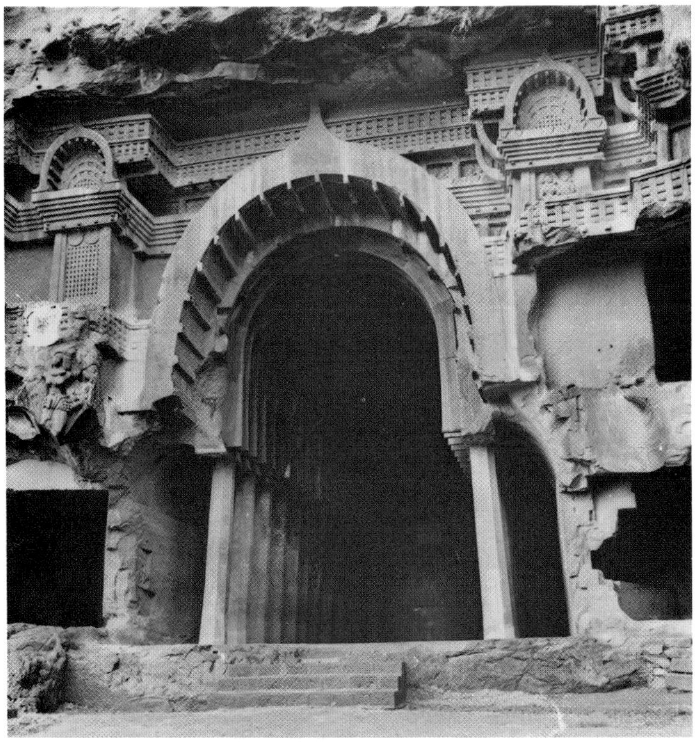

10. Cave temple (2nd century, B.C.) *stūpa*, Bhaja.

11. *Stūpa* cave temple, Bhaja.

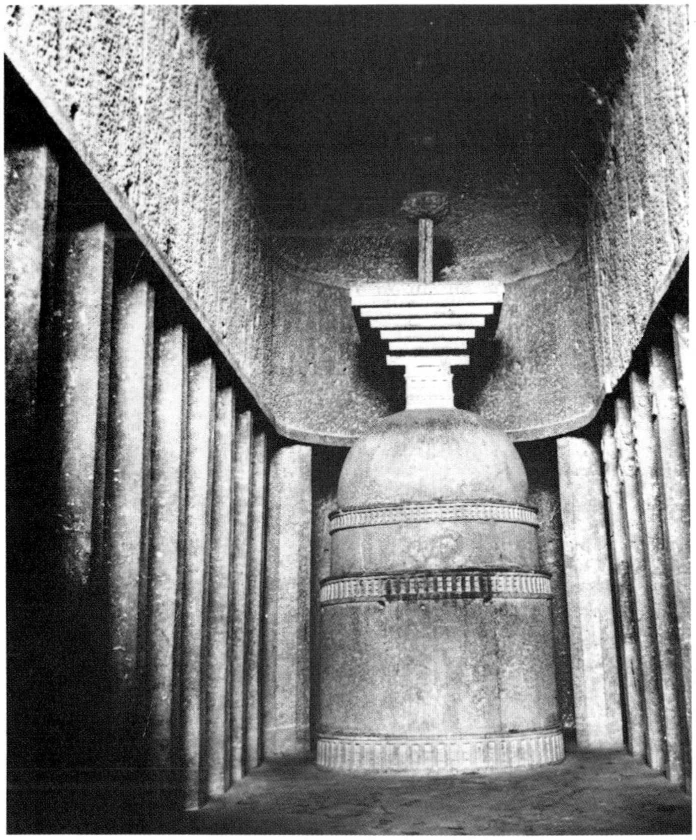

rience which argued that there was no essential difference between *saṃsāra* and *nirvāṇa* and that the apparent difference existed solely in a false point of view. So deep-seated, however, was this erroneous interpretation of reality, that exactly the same kind of moral discipline and meditational exercise continued to be taught; and thus the monastic structures remained largely unchanged. Monks holding the earlier and the later philosophical theories continued to live together within the same communities, and the codes of monastic discipline as preserved by the earlier sects continued to be respected. A synthesis was gradually developed whereby all the complicated categories of the earlier pluralistic system were reinterpreted in monistic terms. Looking back on these developments, which were complete in all respects by the seventh century, Indian Buddhist scholars who were at pains to attribute all these various teachings to Śākyamuni argued that he had taught the doctrine in three stages out of concern for the varying abilities of human beings. First, said the scholars, he had taught the theories that were preserved by his early disciples (known as *śrāvakas*, literally "hearers"); next, he taught the theory of the essential sameness of *saṃsāra* and *nirvāṇa*, both regarded as equally ungraspable by philosophical disquisition; finally he had taught the theory of "pure thought" according to which the earlier categories might still be used for pedagogic purposes, as means to an end where their essential relativity must be realized if enlightenment was to be won. These three phases, referred to as the three "turnings of the Wheel of the Doctrine," were all incorporated in the later versions of Śākyamuni's life story without any sense of historical anachronism. In order to inculcate the later theories, new teachings (modeled to some extent on the earlier ones) were gradually composed, and all were attributed in the first instance to Śākyamuni himself. The two later "turnings," known as the "Middle Course" (Mādhyamaka) and "Just Thought" (Cittamātra), were regarded as a superior way by their propounders, so they referred to themselves as followers of the Mahāyāna ("Great Way") and castigated the earlier sects as followers of an "Inferior Way" (Hīnayāna). Their teachings included not only the new philosophical interpretations, but also a more welcoming attitude to all those who sought perfection, layfolk quite as much as the monks. They argued in effect that since Śākyamuni had achieved Buddhahood as a result of a whole series of earlier lives, any other person of good will could undertake the same heroic course, if only he were prepared to make the personal sacrifices involved. This might take aeons, but ultimately Buddhahood was the one goal from which no living being need be excluded. Such universalist views were an inevitable corollary of the philosophical theory of the sameness of *saṃsāra* and *nirvāṇa*, experienced once all false views and conceptions had disappeared. It further followed that if other beings were on their way to Buddhahood, then some would already have reached the high state of divinity within one of the paradises associated with the plurality of Buddhas who were now assumed to exist in all the various directions of the universe. Thus a religious cult was devoted not only to the Buddha Śākyamuni, but to other Buddhas as well; notably, Amitābha ("Boundless Light") of the western quarter; Akṣobhya ("Imperturbable") of the east; and the various Bodhisattvas who came to be associated with them (Fig. 17) and with Śākyamuni himself, who continued to hold a central position. In this central position he was characterized as "Resplendent," and this epithet (Sanskrit: Vairocana) became yet another Buddha-name. In the earlier stages of this development, various other names appear, and it was only gradually that a few great names came to predominate. The leading Bodhisattvas were: Mañjuśrī or Mañjughoṣa ("Gentle Voice"), usually associated with Śākyamuni; Avalokiteśvara ("Lord of Compassionate Glance") (Fig. 21), associated with Amitābha; and Vajrapāṇi ("Thunderbolt-in-Hand"), associated with Akṣobhya. Not only was the cult of the great Hindu divinities, especially Śiva and Viṣṇu, paralleled by the corresponding Buddhist cult of the great Bodhisattvas, but many Hindu divinities were also adopted by Buddhists: benign ones were eventually made subject to Avalokiteśvara and fierce ones were subject to Vajrapāṇi.

By the seventh century, the volume of Buddhist scriptures had reached enormous proportions, and Buddhist monks had carried the Buddhist religion from northwest India across Central Asia to China, Korea, and Japan, and across the Indian Ocean from ports on the east coast to all the lands of Southeast Asia. Lay craftsmen often accompanied the monks, for even when local styles of architecture were used, painters, image-makers, and wood-carvers were required in order to reproduce paintings and images of Buddhist divinities in the correct conventional manner. Few Indian Buddhists traveled as far as China, for the route was long and several city-states, such as Khotan, Kucha, and Turfan, operated as intermediaries. The ancient land of Gandhāra, spanning what is now eastern Afghanistan and northern Pakistan, had known of Buddhism since the time of Aśoka; and by the first and second centuries A.D. the new religion became predominant after the conversion of recently arrived barbarian rulers, known to Indian tradition as the Kuṣāṇas (Fig. 13). This far northwestern part of the Indian subcontinent was already occupied by the descendants of previous invaders, Greeks, Scythians, and Parthians; and these people were mainly responsible for the considerable missionary endeavor which followed the Silk Route along both sides of the Taklamakan to China and beyond. East of Gandhāra was the Hindu kingdom of Kashmir where Buddhism also flourished, and whence, from the seventh century onward, it passed into western Tibet (Fig. 16).

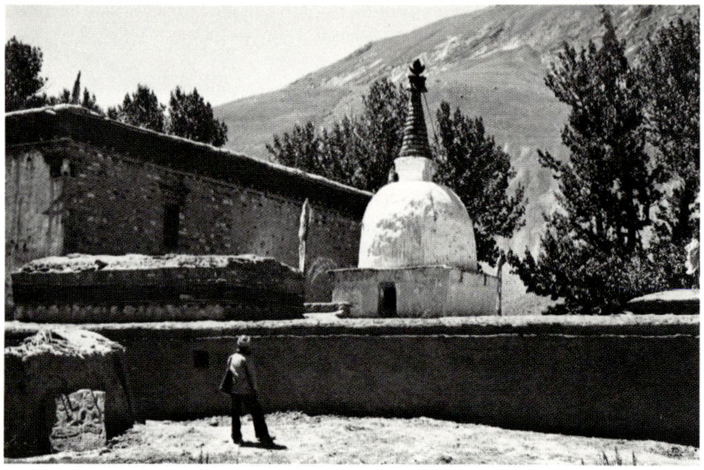

12. A freestanding *stūpa* traditionally identified with a *stūpa* built by the Kuṣāṇa Emperor Kaniṣka (1st–2nd centuries A.D.), but probably very much later, Sani.

The question may be asked what selection of Buddhist literature was employed in such considerable missionary ventures; one may answer that there was usually little real choice, for the texts and traditions that happened to be available in any particular area were simply passed on. Reference was made above to the existence of many early sects, conventionally numbered as eighteen, although there may have been many more. Of these the Sarvāstivādins and especially a branch sect, known as the Mūlasarvāstivādins, were strong in the northwest. It is not surprising, therefore, that it was the Monastic Rule (*vinaya*) of this particular sect which was transmitted both to China and Tibet, although other localized versions also reached China. By this time an agreed "canon" of Buddhist scriptures had long since been fixed by another important sect, the Theravādins, who were strong in southern India and had established a main stronghold in Śrī Laṅkā. But in northern India, where Buddhism continued to develop in the manner briefly described above and where so many later scriptures had to be accommodated, the fixing of a canon must have been a far more contentious proceeding. Some sects that adhered strictly to the earlier teachings certainly had canons of scriptures corresponding to the Theravādin one, but these are scantily known. It was generally agreed that Śākyamuni's teachings embraced the Monastic Rule (*vinaya*) and General Discourses (*sūtras*); but, to these some sects added a third part consisting of philosophical disquisition and doctrinal inventories known as "Further Doctrine" (*abhidharma*). Here was the cause of dispute which predated the Mahāyāna developments. These developments were based upon other compositions which purported to show the deficiencies of the earlier Discourses which, although attributed to Śākyamuni, had been added to and amended over the centuries in order to fit sectarian views. Thus voluminous works known as Mahāyāna *sūtras* began to appear in large numbers and, thanks to their popularity in the far northwest, they were rapidly passed through Central Asia to the Far East. As a radical rebuttal of the *abhidharma* literature which stated that "real elements," both physical and mental, were the basic substance of existence, there appeared the remarkable works known as "Perfection of Wisdom" (*prajñāpāramitā*) which teach the nonexistence of all such elements and the futility of such philosophical disquisition (Pls. 100 and 101). Existing in several recensions of varying lengths, this particular literature has provided the philosophical basis for the whole Mahāyāna. So it came about that the scriptures of the followers of the Mahāyāna consisted of the Monastic Rule (*vinaya*) available in their locality, the Perfection of Wisdom literature, and an ever-increasing number of Mahāyāna *sūtras*, replacing the *sūtras* of the "early disciples." These Mahāyāna *sūtras* were now all in Sanskrit, the classical language of India, which had prevailed over local dialects in which the earlier scriptures had been recorded since the first century A.D. All the later *sūtras* were written in Sanskrit, while the earlier works (notably the *vinaya* literature) which were still considered valid, were transcribed from dialect into Sanskrit. Only in Śrī Laṅkā has a complete canon survived; it is written in the mixed Indian dialect known as Pāli, and this is the important "Hīnayāna" canon of the Theravādin order. By contrast to Śrī Laṅkā where the Buddhist tradition was fixed at a comparatively early period, the fluidity of the religious situation in India and the continual appearance of scriptures for which canonical status was claimed, resulted in no Mahāyāna Sanskrit Buddhist canon ever receiving a fixed form. The Chinese and the Tibetans created canons of their own devising in due course, incorporating all the scriptures attributed to Śākyamuni and other Buddhas which they had managed to amass before Buddhism finally disappeared from northern India in the early thirteenth century. They also accumulated vast numbers of commentarial works by Indian Buddhist writers which were then arranged as a voluminous collection attached to the supposed canonical works. However, by the time they were engaged in this ambitious program, the works known as *tantras* had appeared, and so these too being treated as "Buddha-Word" were incorporated into the canons.

13. Image of Buddha preaching, identifiable as Buddha Vairocana—no later than 13th–14th centuries.

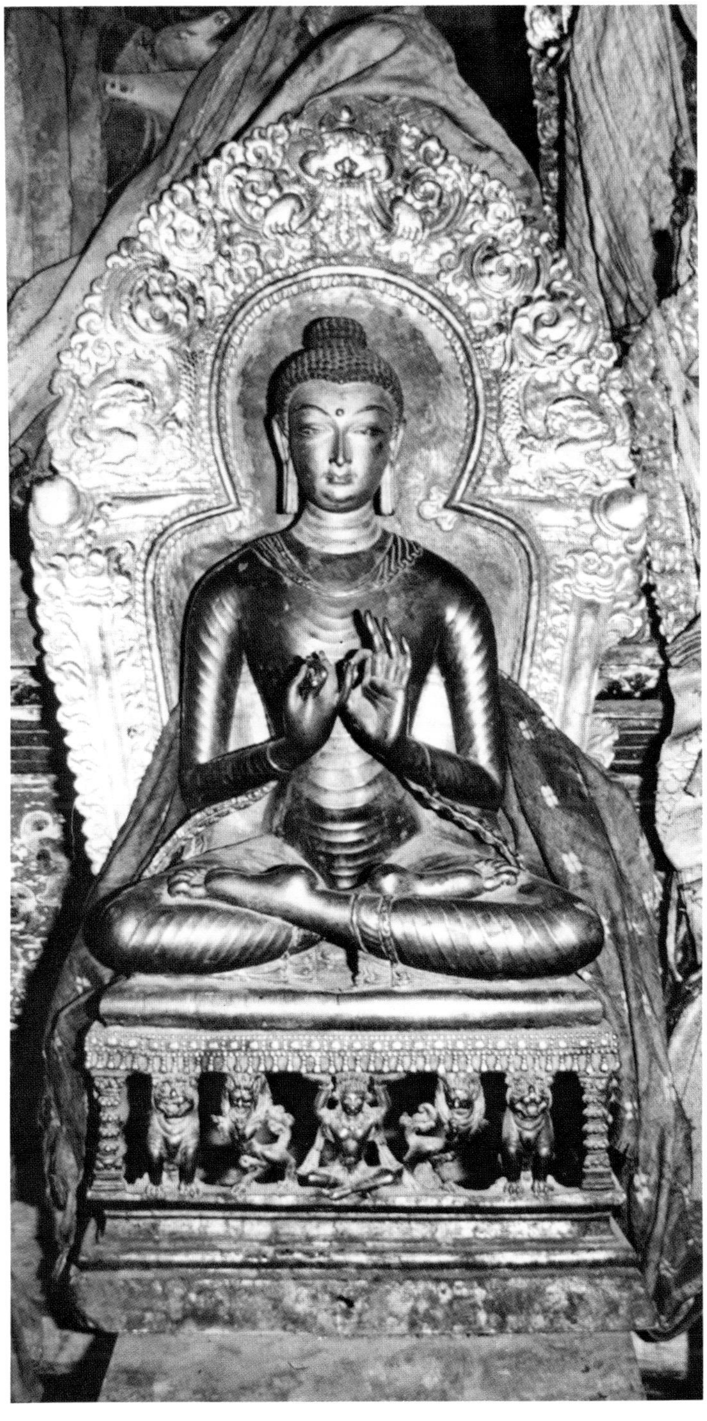

The promulgation of the *tantras* resulted in the gradual emergence of an entirely new phase of Indian Buddhism, known as the *Mantrayāna* ("Way of Spells") or *Vajrayāna* ("Adamantine Way"), which can be dated conventionally from the seventh century onwards, although some of the actual texts may have much earlier origins. One may note that its exponents did not evisage it as a separate "Way" (*yāna*), but rather as part of the whole Mahāyāna movement, in which they now distinguished two branches, that of the "Perfection of Wisdom" and that of "Spells." It was agreed that the final goal of Buddhahood remained the same, but whereas aeons of time were needed for a Bodhisattva to complete such a course according to the "Perfection of Wisdom" teachings, a resolute *yogin* by the practice of "Spells" could achieve enlightenment in the course of a single life-span. I am aware that the use of the term "spell" to translate *mantra* may displease some modern Western Buddhists, but there can be no doubt that its use is entirely suitable. The spell consists of a set of syllables, sometimes with no apparent meaning, the correct utterance of which should compel the presence of some other being, whether human or superhuman. Such is a *mantra*, and it is precisely with such an intention of coercion that the *mantra* was used. Much more is involved in tantric practices than the utterance of spells, but their use is so universal that it is not surprising that the term *mantra* has given its name to this whole latest phase of Buddhism. Modern Westerners often refer to this phase as "The Tantra," but there is little if any justification for the use of *tantra* in this general sense. Like *sūtra*, *tantra* means a text of a particular kind; and when used in a general sense, the plural is preferable. Thus a Tibetan may ask if one follows the way of the *sūtras* (long-term practice based on the "Perfection of Wisdom" teachings) or the way of the *tantras* (the quick path). Now although some *sūtras* contain some material that can be properly classed as tantric (in that spells to coerce certain divinities are taught) and although some early *tantras* are referred to as *sūtras* in their colophons, clear distinctions can be made between these two classes of literature.

A *sūtra* is generally philosophical and doctrinal in content. The Mahāyāna *sūtras* commend the career of a Bodhisattva, sometimes defining the various stages of his advance, and they preach interminably on the emptiness (*śūnyatā*) of all elements of existence and all theories based upon them—except where such theories serve as means to an end. It was recognized that a Bodhisattva must embark upon his long career in whatever situation he may find himself at the time of taking his vow. It is likely to be an auspicious situation, earned by his acts of virtue in previous lives, but he finds himself in the everyday world, where he is called upon to practice the perfections of liberality, morality, patience, meditation, and knowledge; but although he practices them, he must never think of them as absolutes. Thus while he gives generously, indeed recklessly, he knows that ultimately there is no giver, no gift and no receiver, and so on with all the other perfections. He worships Buddhas in their various paradises, but he must know that Buddhahood is essentially one. He prays to his favorite Buddha, Bodhisattva, or even a lesser being, asserting notionally their existence, but at the same time passing beyond to the ultimate reality that guarantees their apparent existence. If they did not exist conventionally he would have no means of apprehending that ultimate reality because all along the way of his progress, he needs mental supports.

A *tantra* may be generally defined as a ritual work centering on the cult of one's chosen divinity. Although it may be interspersed with doctrinal assertions, these are quite arbitrary and may even appear contradictory, for the object of the practicer is to coerce a particular divinity for a specific end. For this reason the divinity is usually described in the most detailed terms and he or she is regarded as real, more real than the person of the actual practicer, who transcends himself precisely by identifying himself with the divinity. In short, "one is oneself the Destroyer, the Creator, the King, the Lord" (*Hevajra-tantra* I.viii.47) and yet "nothing is mentally produced in the highest bliss, and no one produces it; there is no bodily form, neither object or subject" (*ibid.* I.x.33).

Taken as a whole, tantric literature comprehends the following subject-matter: descriptions of various divinities; lists of "spells" required for their invocation; descriptions of their sacred abodes (known technically as *maṇḍala* or mystic circle); details of ritual, involving consecration in the *maṇḍala* by means of which the pupil is identified with the divinity of his master's choice and is able to exercise the corresponding powers. These powers are generally classed as mundane or supramundane. Mundane powers include magical rites of all kinds, such as producing rain, increasing prosperity, subduing others to one's power, causing dissension among one's enemies, and even killing them. Supramundane powers include the gaining of enlightenment and the ability to assist living beings in the intermediate state between death and rebirth, so that they may at least be saved from evil states of reincarnation.

Later commentators grouped the vast number of *tantras* under four headings, translatable as "rites of magic" (*kriyā-tantra*), "rites of religious practice" (*caryā-tantra*), "rites of yoga" (*yoga-tantra*) and "rites of supreme yoga" (*anuttarayoga-tantra*). The *tantras* of the first three classes show definite direct connections with the Mahāyāna *sūtras*. some of which already contain chapters dealing with spells for the coercion of divinities; at the same time the Great Beings, Buddhas, and Bodhisattvas invoked in the early *tantras* are those who also appear in Mahāyāna *sūtras*. In the first two classes of *tantras*, there is usually a so-called "Three Family" arrangement of the divinities: those grouped under Śākyamuni (or Mañjuśrī) are known as the Buddha Family; those under Avalokiteśvara are known as the Lotus Family; and those under Vajrapāṇi are known as the Vajra Family. Pupils are accepted for consecration depending upon their aptitudes as interpreted according to this "Three Family" structure. The Buddha Family is envisaged as including *pratyekabuddhas* ("solitary Buddhas") and disciples who have taken monastic vows. The Lotus Family includes those, originally outside the Buddhist fold, who place their faith in benign divinities; while the Vajra Family includes those, also originally outside the Buddhist fold, who place their faith in fierce and horrific divinities. We have already noted how the Mahāyāna teachings urge layfolk as much as monks to embark upon the long and heroic career of a Bodhisattva. The *tantras* take this process of popularization a stage further in that they welcome those outside the Buddhist organization, permitting them to be Buddhists while continuing the cult of their own favorite divinities.

It must be emphasized that Buddhism was essentially an Indian religion, and that all the developments that it underwent on Indian soil were related to the life of India. India certainly possessed its great centers of learning, known to us today as archaeological sites, where Buddhist traditions were maintained and the inmates were set apart from Brahmanical learning. But were the layfolk in these areas Buddhist or Hindu? The craftsmen who built and decorated the temples and shrines were usually laymen, and they need not necessarily have been Buddhist laymen. Even if they were, they probably lived with their families in neighboring villages, where the cults of local divinities and maybe of the Great God Śiva (Pl. 24) and his bloodthirsty spouse were taken for granted. The monks never lived in isolation from their fellowmen, and it was inevitable that while preaching the Buddhist virtues they should accept the cult of other divinities besides their specifically Buddhist ones. The problem could be solved by the supposed conversion of these divinities to an expression of faith in the Buddha, his Religion and his Community. Thus an important *yoga-tantra*, "Symposium of Truth of all the Buddhas" (*Sarvatathāgata-tattva-saṃgraha*) contains an account (in part II, ch. 6) of how Vajrapāṇi reduced Śiva and all his company to subjection and formed them into a *maṇḍala* (ch.11). As Vajrapāṇi says: "I have received the *vajra* in my hands and have been consecrated as Vajrapāṇi (Thunderbolt-in-Hand) by all the Buddhas. I shall fix the places in the Great Maṇḍala of Victory over the Threefold World for these divinities who are extraneous to the Vajra Family, so that they will not be backsliders on the way to supreme and perfect enlightenment."

If the larger monasteries were open to these developments, how much more so were the many small religious centers, which doubtless also existed? The Mahāyāna made available to married laymen the possibility of practicing religion in all seriousness, and the general situation which developed in Tibet from the seventh century onwards is likely to have been typical of India also. We know from their biographies that when Tibetans went in search of teachers in India, they found them not only in monasteries but in hermitages and in otherwise ordinary households. Also typical of the Indian religious scene, then as now, are wandering *yogins*, free to seek religious teachers, wherever they will. Buddhist monks were not bound to their monasteries in the manner in which Christian monks have usually been bound, and they were free to wander and find teachers of their choice elsewhere. The pursuit of enlightenment was often regarded as an internal process, supported by solemn acts and words, leading to a conversion of thought. Despite its nobility, there is something unrealistic in the theory of the Bodhisattva who strives through innumerable rebirths in the pursuit of final enlightenment for his own salvation and that of all other living beings. Why, one asks, did the formulators of these Mahāyāna theories conceive of this vocation in these extravagant terms? Their primary model was Śākyamuni (Fig. 14) himself, who saw with his divine eye at the moment of his enlightenment his countless previous rebirths. This claim was made in his own words:

> Thus with mind concentrated, purified, cleansed, spotless, with the defilements gone, supple, dexterous, firm and impassible, I directed my mind to the knowledge of the remembrance of my former existences. I remembered many former existences, such as one birth, two births, three, four, five, ten, twenty, thirty, forty, fifty, a hundred, a thousand, a hundred thousand births; many cycles of dissolution of the universe, many cycles of its evolution, many of its dissolution and evolution; there I was of such and such a name, clan, colour, livelihood, such pleasure and pain did I suffer, and such was the end of my life. Passing away thence, I was born here. Thus do I remember my many former existences with their special modes and details. This was the first knowledge that I gained in the first watch of the night. Ignorance was dispelled, knowledge arose. Darkness was dispelled, light arose. So it is with him who abides vigilant, strenuous and resolute.[2]

Having thus achieved enlightenment, involving also knowledge of the previous lives of all other living beings and the knowledge of his own final release, Śākyamuni gradually gathered disciples around him,

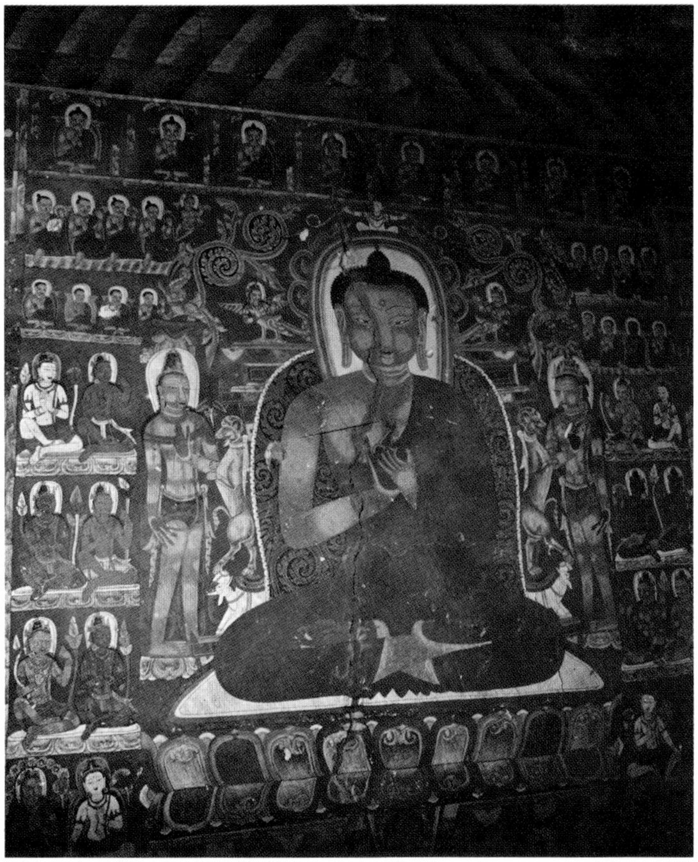

14. Śākyamuni Buddha wall painting, Lhakhang Soma, Alchi, 12th–13th centuries.

showing them the way to the state of *nirvāṇa* which he himself had realized. *Nirvāṇa* and enlightenment are then synonymous terms; many of Śākyamuni's early disciples attained *nirvāṇa* in that very same birth, and were subsequently referred to as *arhat* (worthy), a title which is also used for Śākyamuni himself. Thus according to the early schools, there was no difference between his state of enlightenment and that achieved by his disciples; but they were followers while he was the greatly revered teacher who had shown the way. The Mahāyāna theorists began to dispute this, arguing that *arhats* (Fig. 15) remained subject to various human frailties and thus their supposed state of *nirvāṇa* could not be the final *nirvāṇa* of a fully enlightened Buddha. In the "Perfection of Wisdom" literature Śākyamuni converses with Śariputra, one of his two most stalwart disciples, and contrasts the aspirations of a Buddha with those of a mere disciple: "What do you think, Śariputra, does it occur to any of the Disciples and Pratyekabuddhas that, after he has practised the six perfections, has brought beings to maturity, has purified the Buddha-field, has fully gained the ten powers of a Tathāgata, his four grounds of self-confidence, the four analytical knowledges and the eighteen special *dharmas* of a Buddha, after he has known full enlightenment, he will lead countless beings to *nirvāṇa*?," Śariputra says no, and the Lord continues:

> But such are the intentions of a Bodhisattva. A glow-worm or some other luminous animal does not think that its light could illuminate the Southern Continent or radiate over it. Just so the Disciples and Pratyekabuddhas do not think that they should, after winning full enlightenment, lead all beings to *Nirvāṇa*. But the sun, when it has risen, radiates its light over the whole Southern Continent. Just so a Bodhisattva, after he has accomplished the practices which lead to the full enlightenment of Buddhahood, leads countless beings to *Nirvāṇa*.[3]

Thus a distinction came to be drawn between the lower state of *nirvāṇa* of an *arhat* and the final *nirvāṇa* of a Buddha. There was some discussion of whether one might progress from the lower *nirvāṇa* to the higher, or whether one was so set in one's selfish conviction of a kind of personal *nirvāṇa* that there was no hope of progress without reentering cycles of human rebirths.

With such a daunting series of rebirths ahead, it is not surprising that some followers of the Mahāyāna sought ways to shorten the lengthy process, and the means they lighted upon are described in the *tantras*. It was a matter of experimenting with techniques of meditation; many of these had been long practiced in India, but had been regarded with some suspicion in the earlier stages of the doctrine. Buddhists never denied the existence of higher and lower beings of all kinds, but a Buddha was thought to have transcended them all. However in all worldly affairs, in which a monk might be properly engaged when dealing with faithful layfolk, serious account might well be taken of these beings. Magical powers, altruistically employed, were assumed to be the property of a Buddha and of an *arhat*, but the gods or demons who were coerced had no part in assisting one towards enlightenment. As observed above, the Mahāyāna, by contrast, accepts the existence

15. Wall painting, one of a set of sixteen Arhats, Sani Monastery, Zangskar, probably 17th century.

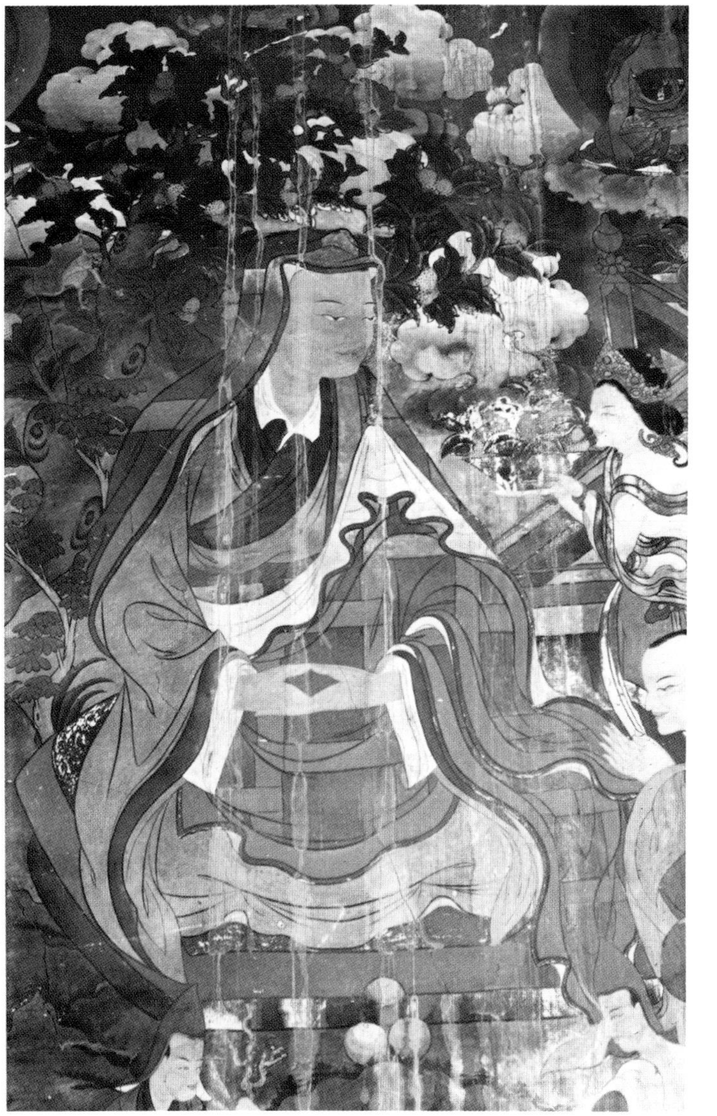

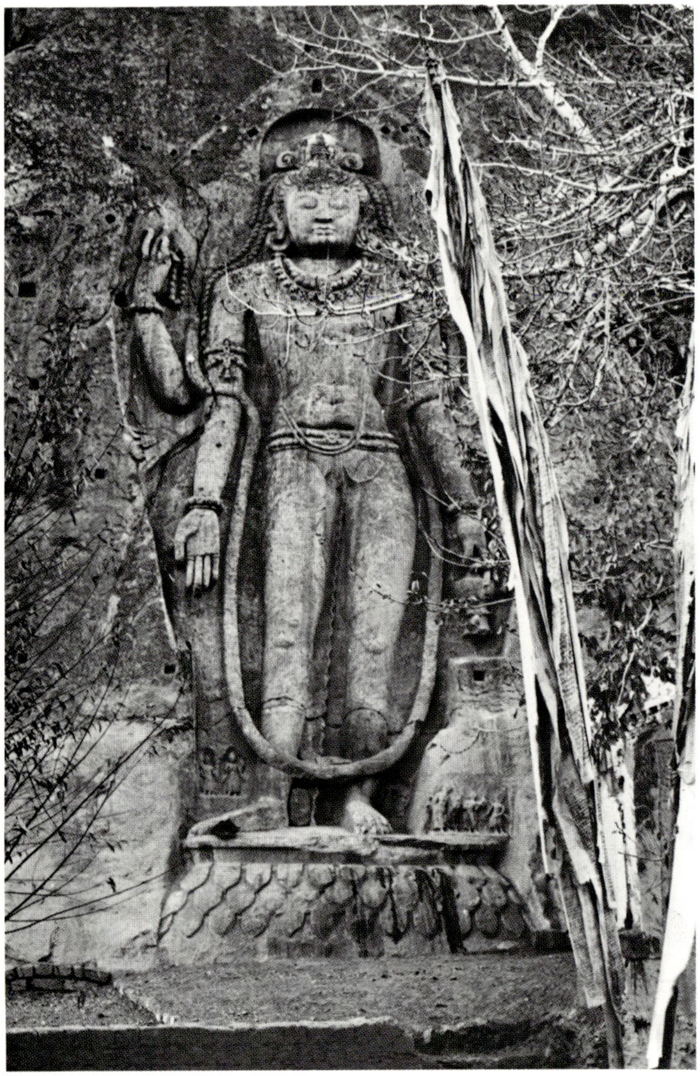

16. Rock carving of the Bodhisattva Maitreya, Mulbek Ladakh, 9th century.

of Great Beings, in the form of celestial Bodhisattvas, who can assist a believer towards his goal. As far as the practicer is concerned, they correspond to the many worshipful beings already accepted in Hindu religion, although they are naturally possessed of all wholesome Buddhist qualities. Once it was accepted that intense devotion to such a higher being assisted one on the path to enlightenment, the way was open for acceptance of the many practices referred to as tantric. The essence of tantric practice may be described as the visualization of a certain "chosen divinity," believed to be of the very essence of Buddhahood, and the deliberate identification of oneself with this divinity. Once this state of self-identification is realized, one achieves the state of enlightenment which the chosen divinity embodies. He is the means towards the wisdom that is then achieved. Wisdom is to be understood as the "Perfection of Wisdom," i.e., the sameness of all phenomena whether relating to *saṃsāra* or *nirvāṇa* and the emptiness or vanity of all concepts whatsoever of which the chief ones are the notion of a personal self and the notion of elemental particles of which the whole universe was said to consist according to the theories of the early Buddhist schools. But without the means, which are embodied in one's personal chosen divinity, recognized as both real and unreal at the same time, such a state would be unobtainable. (Pls. 16 and 17).

The *tantras* were arranged in classes because it was supposed that they operated at different levels. The "Rites of Magic" (*kriyā-tantras*) are usually concerned with successes of a mundane kind, such as tranquilizing evil influences, gaining worldly prosperity for oneself or others, subduing foes, and doing works of destruction. These are known as the "four rites," and Buddhist monks were often asked to perform them. (Pls. 18 and 19). The "Rites of Religious Practice" operate with similar objectives but raised to a higher level. For example, the rite of tranquilizing may be performed on behalf of a deceased individual in order to negate the effects of his evil actions in the past and assist him to a better state of rebirth. A whole *tantra* entitled "Elimination of Evil Rebirth" is devoted to this subject, as well as evocations of the Buddhas and many circles of lesser divinities, such as the *maṇḍala* of the Four Kings of the Directions, the *maṇḍala* of the Guardians of the Ten Directions, the *maṇḍala* of the Eight Great Planets or that of the Eight Great Snakes (*Nāga*). As might be expected, Vajrapāṇi presides over these groups of Indian divinities that have been subdued to the service of Buddhism. Since this particular *tantra* has the final intention of helping the practitioner achieve Buddhahood, it was liable to be classed with the next highest group, the *Yoga-tantras*, which are intended to enable the devotee to achieve this highest of objectives. These *tantras* are distinguished by far more elaborate circles of divinities, arranged according to a basic fivefold pattern corresponding to a center and points in the four main directions. In this way the *maṇḍala* was given a psychological significance lacking in the earlier conception of just three "families," those of the Buddha, the Lotus, and the Vajra. The "families" were therefore extended to five with the addition of those of the Gem and the Sword; and each was presided over by a Buddha of the corresponding cosmic direction with whom a set of four Bodhisattvas was associated. This *maṇḍala* was then completed with four Buddha-Goddesses placed in the intermediate directions, eight lesser goddesses symbolizing the workship that must be offered, and four guardian divinities placed at the four entrances to the *maṇḍala* (Fig. 23).

17. Wall painting, Bodhisattva Maitreya, Lhakhang Soma, Alchi, Ladakh, 12th–13th centuries.

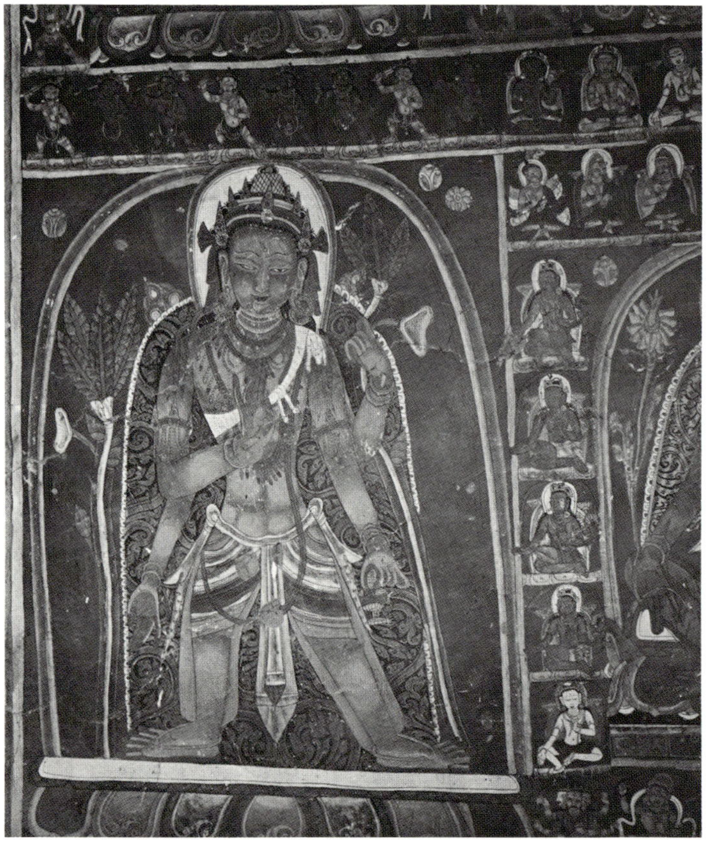

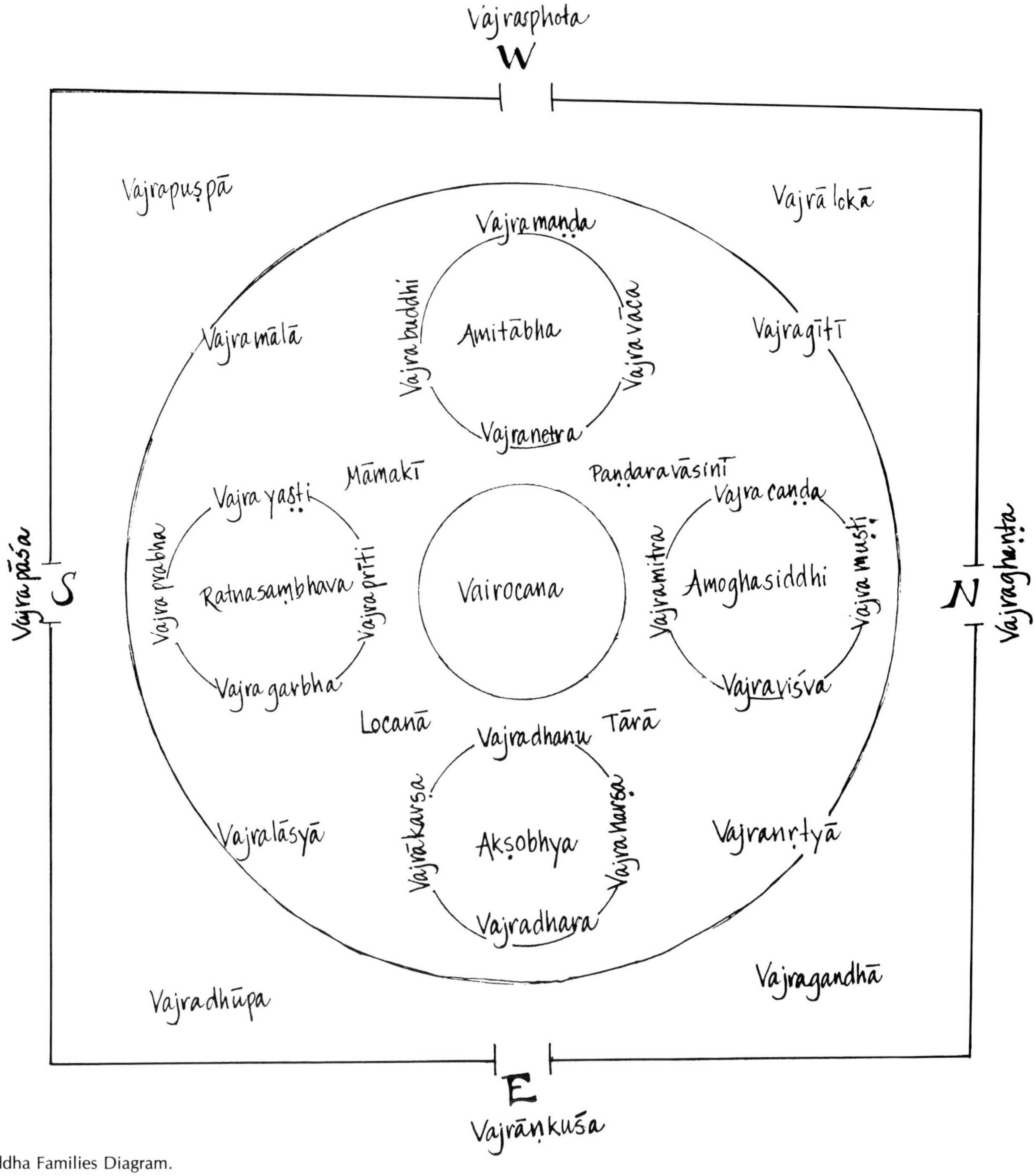

Ill. 2 — Five-Buddha Families Diagram.

This fivefold arrangement means that such a *maṇḍala* becomes the symbol of both *saṃsāra* and *nirvāṇa* (seen ultimately as nondifferentiated), as well as of the macrocosm (the universe) and the microcosm (the false idea of an individual person). In this arrangement, the corresponding elements are:

Direction	*Buddha*	*Saṃsāra*	*Nirvāṇa*	*Elements*	*Personality*
Center	Vairocana	Delusion	Wisdom of Pure Absolute	Space	Consciousness
East	Askṣobhya	Wrath	Mirrorlike Wisdom	Earth	Body
South	Ratnasaṃbhava	Malignity	Discriminating Wisdom	Water	Feelings
West	Amitābha	Passion	Wisdom of Sameness	Fire	Perceptions
North	Amoghasiddhi	Envy	Active Wisdom	Air	Impulses

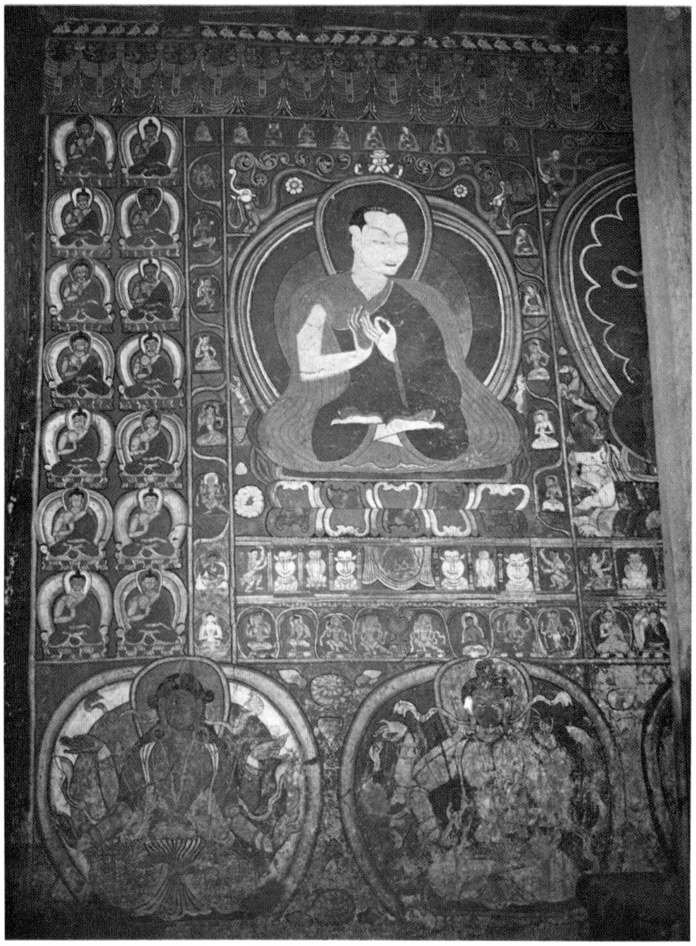

18. Portrait of Rin-chen bZang-po, the "Great Translator," in the Lotsawa'i Lhakhang (the Translator's Temple) at Alchi, probably 13th century.

One of these sets, that of the Five Elements of which the universe consists, is found in so many other early traditions that it requires no explanation. The five components of personality represent a very early Buddhist list of the factors into which the person is dissolved. The early schools, followed by all later phases in the history of Buddhism, accepted the dogma of "no self, no person, no being." The Five Evils into which *saṃsāra* is divided are an extension of the early set of Three Evils, Delusion, Wrath and Passion, which, according to the early Buddhist schools, lie at the root of the whole cycle of continual rebirths. The five aspects of Wisdom or Supreme Knowledge (*jñāna*) have been drawn from the terminology used in Mahāyāna works concerning the state of final enlightenment. The Wisdom of the Pure Absolute is self-explanatory; Mirrorlike Wisdom implies that the whole of *saṃsāra* is reflected in the mind of the Sage as objects are reflected in a mirror; Discriminating Wisdom means that he can direct his thought at will to any situation; the Wisdom of Sameness means that he is imbued with the knowledge of the ultimate sameness of *saṃsāra* and *nirvāṇa*; Active Wisdom means that he is ever active on behalf of living beings by his readiness to manifest himself in the form of teachers and guides in the various worlds, thus cutting off the Five Evils of *saṃsāra*.

Each of the Five Buddhas is the head of a separate Buddha-Family, although the central Buddha Vairocana (Resplendent) comprehends all the others. His family is simply known as Buddha or Tathāgata Family. His immediate entourage consists of four Buddha-Goddesses, who are identified as aspects of the Perfection of Wisdom (*Prajñāpār-amitā*—feminine in Sanskrit). They are identified either by the names on the diagram or simply by the names of the other four families; in the latter case they are known as Vajra-Being, Gem-Being, Dharma-Being and Action-Being. Locanā (meaning Buddha-Eye), Māmakī (meaning My Very Own), Pāṇḍaravāsinī (Possessing a White Garment) and Tārā (Saviouress) are the names of four attendant goddesses who appear rather haphazardly in an earlier *tantra* (the *Mañjuśrīmūlakalpa*) where the Three Family system prevails. Here they have been used as mere appellations to complete a fourfold set covering the four intermediate directions. Whoever deals with tantric materials must become accustomed to seemingly quite arbitrary lists of names.

The names of the Sixteen Great Bodhisattvas (Pls. 21 and 21a) assume a variety of forms, and while it may be of some interest to analyze the names given on the diagram, the reader must be aware that other sets also occur.[4] We may take each of the families in turn.

Akṣobhya (Pl. 10) (Imperturbable), head of the Vajra (Thunderbolt) Family has as his chief Bodhisattva, Vajradhara *alias* Vajrapāṇi (meaning Vajra-Holder and Vajra-in-Hand), also often referred to as Vajrasattva (Vajra-Being). In some tantric schools these three names are later distinguished iconographically, and Vajradhara and Vajrasattva become names for a sixth all-comprehending Buddha, of whom more will be said below. The other three Bodhisattva-names of Akṣobhya's set of four may be translated as Vajra-Coercion (*Vajrākarṣa*), Vajra-Bow (*Vajradhanu*) because he hits the mark, and Vajra-Joy (*Vajraharṣa*).

Ratnasambhava (Pl. 109) (Gem-Born), head of the Gem (*Ratna*) Family has as his chief Bodhisattva, Vajragarbha (Vajra-Embryo), who may also be referred to as Vajraratna (Vajra-Gem) or Ratnapāṇi (Gem-in-Hand). The other three are Vajra-Light (*Vajraprabha*), Vajra-Standard (*Vajrayaṣṭi*) and Vajra-Happiness (*Vajraprīti*).

Amitābha (Pl. 85) (Boundless Light) or Amitāyus (Boundless Life), both titles of the Buddha of the western quarter, is head of the Dharma or the Lotus Family. His chief Bodhisattva is Vajranetra (Vajra-Eye), also known as Avalokiteśvara (Lord of Compassionate Glance). The other three are Vajra-Knowledge (*Vajrabuddhi*) who is identified with Mañjuśrī, Vajra-Essence (*Vajramaṇḍa*) and Vajra-Speech (*Vajravāca*).

Amoghasiddhi (Infallible Success), head of the Action Family, has as chief Bodhisattva, Vajra-Universal (*Vajraviśva*); the others are Vajra-Friend (*Vajramitra*), Vajra-Wrathful (*Vajracaṇḍa*) and Vajra Handclasp (*Vajramuṣṭi*).

19. The ruins of Nyar-ma Monastery in Ladakh, which was founded by Rin-chen bZang-po about 1000 A.D., as related in his biography.

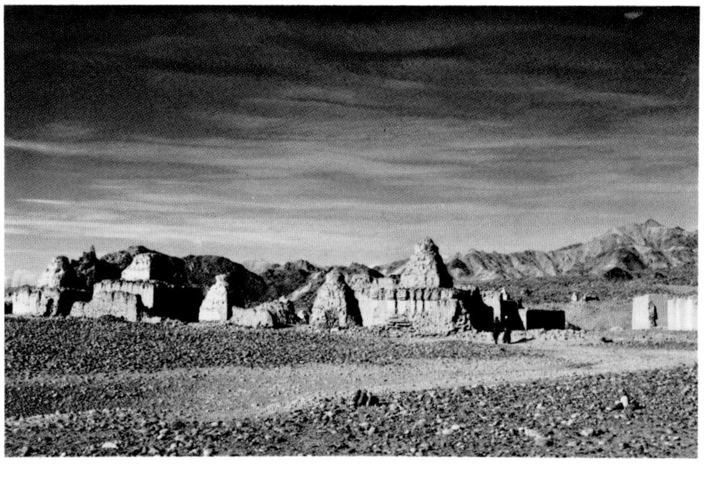

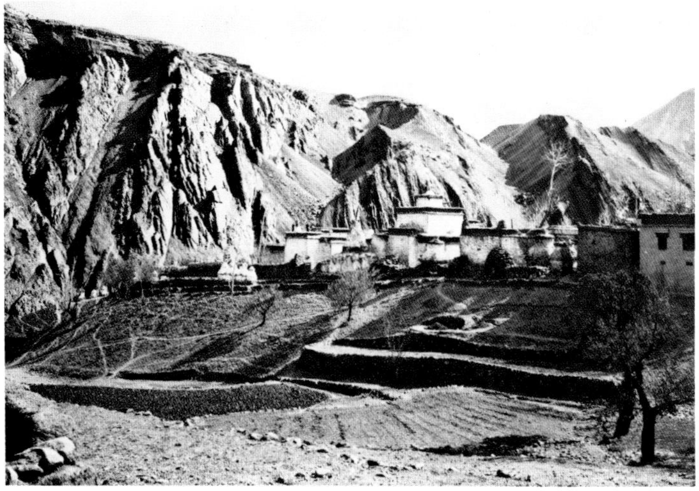

20. Alchi Monastery in Ladakh. This is nowadays popularly attributed to Rin-chen bZang-po, but inscriptions in the two main temples inform us that the founders were two wealthy prelates named Ts'ul-khrims-'öd and *sKal-ldan Śes-rab*. The latter studied at Nyar-ma, and thus the foundation of Alchi can probably be dated to the second half of the 11th century.

These are the main divinities in the third class of *tantras* known as Yoga-tantras. The principal divinity is Vairocana (Resplendent), who is also known as "Omniscient One" (Sanskrit: *Sarvavid*; Tibetan: *Kun-rig*) (Fig. 22). A variation in Buddha-names occurs in the *tantra* "Elimination of Evil Rebirths" which is also allocated to this group; here Akṣobhya (of the eastern direction) is represented by the "King who Eliminates Evil Rebirths" (*Sarvadurgatipariśodhanarāja*), Ratnasambhava (of the south) by Ratnaketu (Gem-Banner), Amitābha (of the west) by Śākyamuni, and Amoghasiddhi (of the north) by Vikasitakusuma (Flower Fully in Bloom). Such sets of five were made up from Buddha-names occurring in the Mahāyāna *sūtras* and the earlier *tantras*, and their formulation depended upon the predilections of teachers in different religious centers (Fig. 24). For example, also in the main *maṇḍala* of this same *tantra* the Sixteen Bodhisattvas may be arranged in one full circle around all five Buddhas, instead of being arranged in separate sets of four. The permutations are many, and it would be impossible to treat them all in a short account of this kind.

The eight goddesses of the offerings, arranged in two sets of four, are fortunately constant and appear thus in many different *maṇḍalas*. The first set includes Vajra-Gestures of Love (Vajra-lāsyā) and—omitting "Vajra" in all the other cases—Mālā (Garland), Gīti (Song), and Nṛtyā (Dance). The second set consists of Dhūpā (Incense), Puṣpā (Flower), Ālokā (Lamp), and Gandhā (Scent).

The four door-guardians are Vajra-Hook (Vajrāṅkuśa) in the east, Vajra-Noose (Vajrapāśa) in the south, Vajra-Fetter (Vajrasphoṭa) in the west, and Vajra-Possession (Vajrāveśa) or Vajra-Bell (Vajraghaṇṭa) in the north.

Maṇḍalas such as these might be marked out with colors on a specially prepared floor for the purposes of ritual, but they are far more frequently painted on temple walls for the purpose of general edification and private meditation; or far more rarely, they may be represented by life-size images arranged around a temple. A fine example of the latter arrangement can be seen in Ta-pho Monastery, founded in Spiti old western Tibet ca. 1000 by the great translator Rin-chen bzang-po (Fig. 18). An amazing collection of *maṇḍalas* of the *yoga-tantra* class may be seen at Alchi Monastery in Ladakh (Fig. 20), founded during the eleventh century. Related *maṇḍalas* of the same *yoga-tantra* class, centering on Vairocana (Fig. 13), have been found in the Tunhuang Caves, and by the ninth century these tantric traditions reached Japan as the main ingredient of the Shingon sect. Thus from the far northwest of India they passed right across Central Asia to the eastern limits of the Buddhist world.

One of the factors that distinguishes the *Yoga-tantras* from the two lower categories is the far greater significance attached to the term *Vajra*, which is prefixed to most names in the *maṇḍalas* just described. In the *Kriyā-* and *Caryā-tantras* there are only three Buddha-Families, those of the Buddha or Tathāgata, the Lotus, and the Vajra, arranged in this order of precedence. Thus it is taught that anyone who has received consecration in the highest family, the Buddha Family, is authorized to invoke divinities in the other two; whoever has received consecration in the Lotus Family may invoke divinities in this family and the Vajra Family; but whoever receives consecration in the Vajra Family is limited to this family only.

The Vajra Family seems to comprise in the first instance aggressive, originally non-Buddhist, divinities who have been subdued by the Bodhisattva, erstwhile Yakṣa Vajrapāṇi. This wielder of the thunderbolt first appears in Buddhist tradition as the personal guardian of Śākyamuni, and he is depicted in this role in many sculptures dating from the first century B.C. onwards. He is then referred to as a *yakṣa* (a local divinity and possibly tree-spirit) or even as the Lord of *Yakṣas*, and he is regarded as such throughout the early Mahāyāna period. Thus it is said that he protects not only Śākyamuni, but any Bodhisattva who is well advanced on the path towards enlightenment. He is thus

20a. Facade, Sum-tsek Chapel, Alchi.

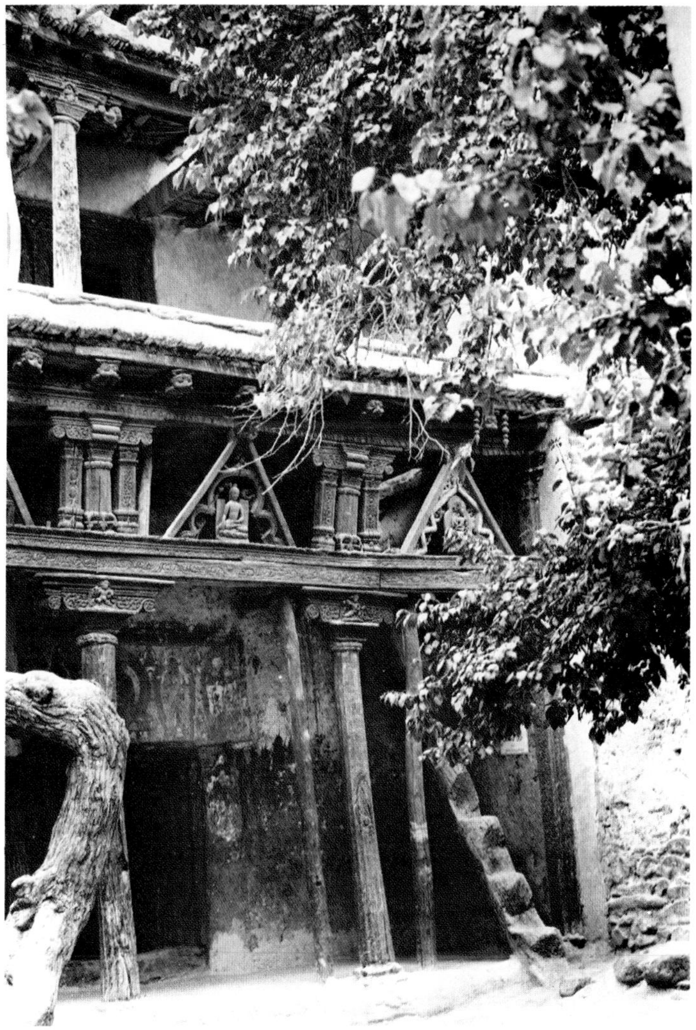

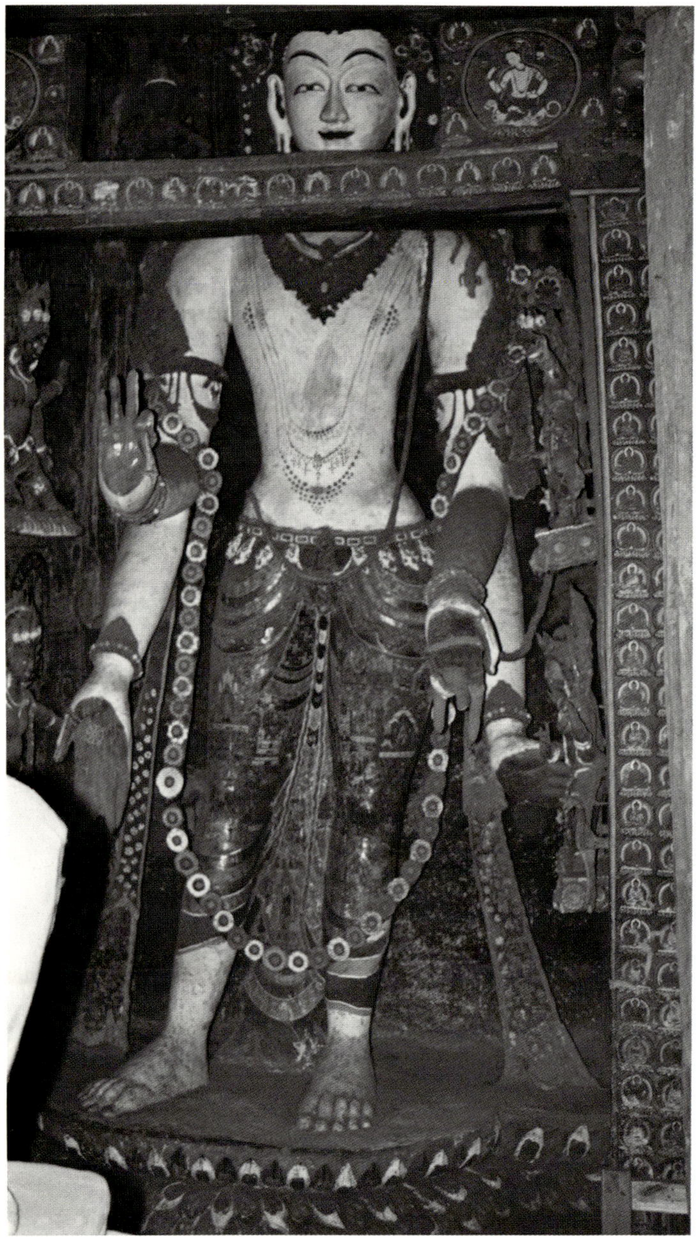

21. An image of human proportions of the Bodhisattva Avalokiteśvara in the Sum-tsek ("Three-tier") Temple at Alchi. His lower garment is painted with scenes of Buddhist shrines and worshippers, all of Indian inspiration, ca. 12th century.

a kind of "guardian angel" of a potentially ferocious kind, and the task of subduing subversive non-Buddhist divinities falls easily to his lot. In early *tantras* he is referred to as a Bodhisattva, although his *yakṣa* origins are still remembered, and his family is the lowest of the three. However in the *yoga-tantras*, the Five Families, now presided over by five cosmic Buddhas, are treated as all having the same effective worth. Thus a blindfolded pupil, led to the *maṇḍala* by his teacher, throws a flower or a toothpick onto the outspread *maṇḍala*, and depending on the section of the *maṇḍala* where this falls, his family association is decided. In this respect Vajrapāṇi (Pl. 92), who is chief Bodhisattva of the Vajra Family under the Buddha Akṣobhya, is on fully equal terms with leading Bodhisattvas of the other families. In fact he quickly assumes a preeminent position simply because all these *tantras* are concerned with powerful means of coercing higher beings, and he has a long tradition of being the most powerful influence for good. Thus his progress knows no limits. In the fourth and so-called highest class of *tantras*, the Tantras of Supreme Yoga (*Anuttarayoga-tantras*), his family (with Akṣobhya as its presiding Buddha) comes to the center, and Vairocana's family is moved to the eastern quarter. The actual name of Vajrapāṇi is retained as the name of the most powerful of Bodhisattvas; but under his alternative names of Vajradhara (Vajra-Holder) and Vajrasattva (Vajra-Being), which are often used in the *yoga-tantras*, he is regarded as a sixth absolutely supreme Buddha, of whom the set of Five Buddhas is his primary manifestation. The final triumph of Vajrapāṇi and the preeminence of his Vajra Family, explain why the whole phase of tantric Buddhism became known not just as the *Mantrayāna* (Way of Spells), as it was conceived during its earlier development, but as the *Vajrayāna* (Adamantine Way). (Pl. 24).

Just as all the Mahāyāna *sūtras* were attributed to the Buddha Śākyamuni, so too were the first three classes of *tantras*. The central Buddha was still Śākyamuni in the two lower classes, while in the *yoga-tantras* Vairocana is still thought of as a glorified form of Śākyamuni, whose actual name is sometimes used. However, it could scarcely be denied that these later teachings were of a very different kind from those propounded in the *sūtras*. The long career of the heroic Bodhisattvas was now replaced by a highly ritualized series of consecrations, leading to the final consecration into the very nature of Buddhahood. The process is, in fact, somewhat analogous to the elaborate ceremonial of the crowning of a British monarch or perhaps to the ordination of a Catholic priest. In all these cases, the ritual actions are held to have validity in their own right, but their effectiveness on the person concerned depends upon his preparedness and inward disposition. Thus the traditional account of Śākyamuni's achieving of enlightenment under the famous Bo tree at Bodhgayā was retold to

21a. An image of Maitreya in the Sum-tsek Temple, Alchi, Ladakh, ca. 12th century.

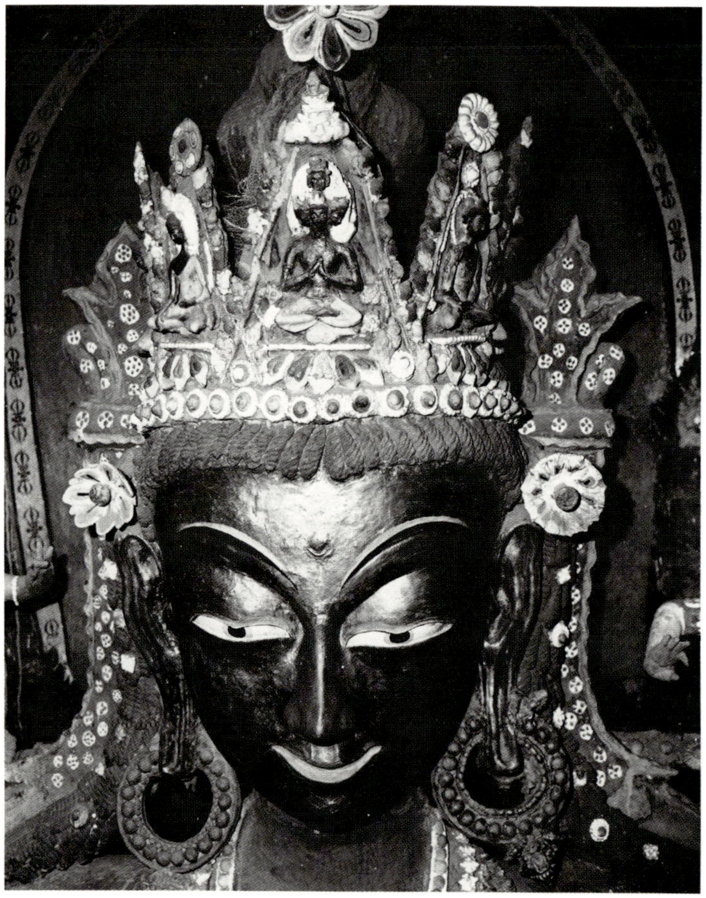

suit this new manner of reaching the final goal. While in earlier traditional accounts Śākyamuni's final progress towards Buddhahood is marked by four ever higher stages of "inner composure" (*samādhi*), now the process is interrupted by the Buddhas of the Ten Directions, who arouse him from the fourth stage of composure by snapping their fingers and saying, "You cannot become a perfected Buddha just by means of this inner composure." Then leaving his physical body by the banks of the Nairañjana River, they conducted his "mind-made body" (*manomayakāya*) to the Highest Heaven, where they bestowed upon him the preliminary consecrations, followed by the five stages of perfect enlightenment, as marked by five formulas of self-consecration. Thus he became the perfected Buddha with the name of Vairocana; and having taught the *yoga-tantras* on the summit of Mount Meru, he descended to the banks of the river, reassumed his physical body and thereafter the traditional account of his ministry follows this elaborated version. The consecrations he received from the Buddhas of the Ten Directions are precisely those bestowed upon the worthy disciple in the *maṇḍala* of the Vajra Sphere *(Vajradhātumaṇḍala)*

22. Maṇḍala of Vairocana in the Sum-tsek Temple, Alchi. It represents Vairocana (four-headed) in the centre with the Four Buddhas to the four main directions (east being downwards, signified by the blue Akṣobhya), the four Buddha-Goddesses in the squares of the intermediated directions, the eight goddesses of the offerings in the corners of the outer square and in line with these outside the circle, the Four Guardians by the gates, and the Sixteen Bodhisattvas, four on each side of the square, spaced between the four goddesses of the offerings (in the corners) and the Guardians, as already mentioned.

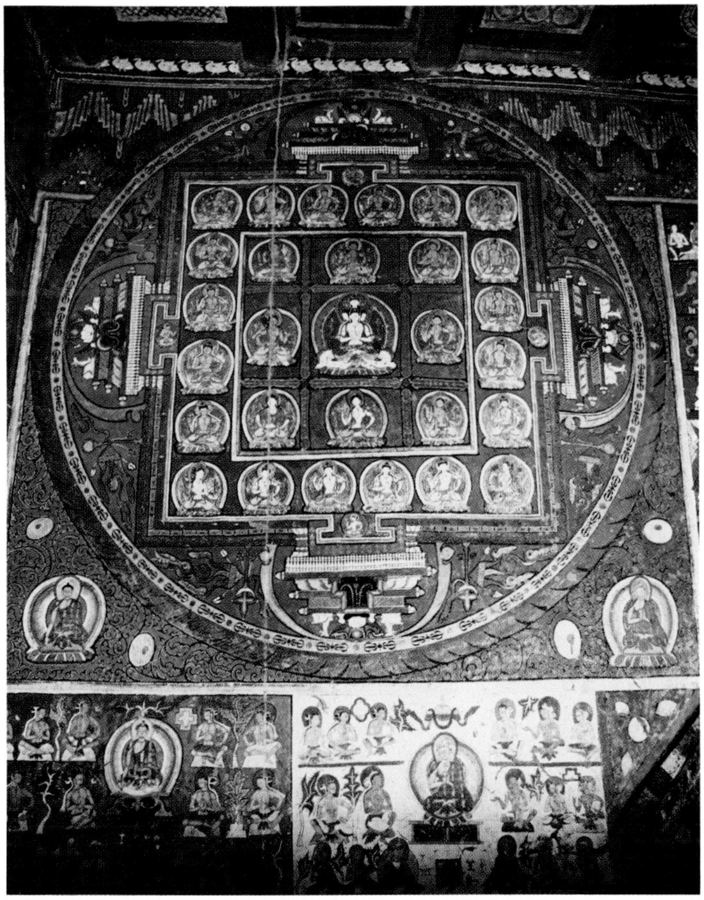

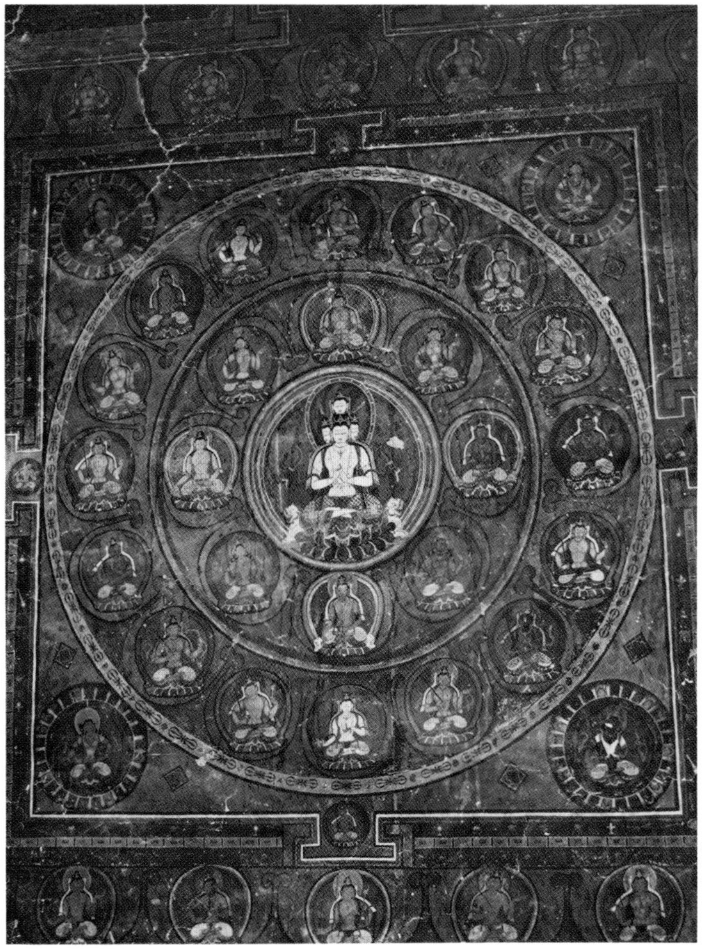

23. Wall painting of a Vairocana maṇḍala in the *'du-khang* at Alchi. Vairocana in the center, surrounded by the Four Buddhas and Four Buddha-Goddesses in the next circle, who in turn are surrounded by the Sixteen Bodhisattvas in the outer circle. Only four of the eight goddesses of the offerings are visible in the outer corners of this photograph. Ca. 12th century.

which is the primary one taught in the *yoga-tantra,* "Symposium of Truth" (STTS).

The preliminary consecrations are those bestowed with water, with a crown, with a *vajra*, with a bell, and finally with a name. As a set of five they bestow one by one the five aspects of Wisdom listed above.

The five formulas of self-consecration that result in the achievement of perfect Buddhahood are:

1. The Teacher, embodying himself the essence of Buddhahood, approaches the neophyte and says:
   "O son of good family, how will you realize the highest enlightenment, you who undergo all privations in your ignorance of the Truth of All the Buddhas?"
   The neophyte asks instruction and is told:
   "Proceed with this *mantra* properly recited, which clarifies and composes one's own thought and which succeeds spontaneously:
   OṂ CITTAPRATIVEDHAṂ KAROMI" (meaning OṂ I penetrate thought!).
2. The neophyte then says: "I beseech you, O Lord Buddhas. I see a form of lunar disk in my heart."
   The teacher replies, "This, O son, is Thought which is naturally translucent. As one regards it, so it becomes, just like stains (disappearing) on a white garment." Then in order to

produce the Thought of Enlightenment the neophyte is instructed to pronounce this *mantra:*
OṂ BODHICITTAM UTPĀDAYĀMI" (OṂ I produce the Thought of Enlightenment).

3. Having thus raised the Thought of Enlightenment, the neophyte says:
"That appearance of a lunar disk, I see it really as a lunar disk."
The Teacher says: "The essence of All Buddhas, Samantabhadra (Universal Good), the Rising of Thought has become manifest. Practice it well!"
Then in order to make the form of the *Vajra* firm in his heart on that lunar disk, he is given this *mantra:*
OṂ TIṢṬHA VAJRA (OṂ Stay *Vajra*).
4. The neophyte says: "O Lord Buddhas, I see a *vajra* on the lunar disk."
He is told: "Stabilize the Samantabhadra-Thought-Vajra of All Buddhas with this *mantra:*
OṂ VAJRĀTMAKO 'HAM" (OṂ I am the very essence of the Vajra!)
Then the Vajra-Element (*vajradhātu*) of the Body, Speech, and Mind of All Buddhas enters that *vajra* in his heart and he is consecrated with the *Vajra*-name of ———. Then he says: "O Lord Buddhas, I see myself as the Body of All Buddhas."
5. He is told: "O Great Being, conceive of yourself as the *Vajra* of Being, as the Buddha-Form which comprehends all wonderful appearances, using this *mantra* which succeeds spontaneously:
OṂ YATHĀ SARVATATHĀGATĀS TATHĀHAṂ" (OṂ as all Buddhas are, thus am I!)
Saying this, the one consecrated knows himself to be a Buddha, and bowing before All Buddhas, he says: "Consecrate me, O Lord Buddhas and stabilize this enlightenment." When he says this All Buddhas enter his *Vajra*-Being and all the divinities of the *maṇḍala* are manifest to him.

Such a form of initiation was available to laymen as well as to monks so long as they were acceptable to a qualified teacher (*guru*) of the requisite tradition. Having been initiated with the consecrations, the practicer was free to meditate upon the divinities of the *maṇḍala*, invoking them to his presence and absorbing them into his own being. With the proper disposition he was thus able to enter a state of enlightenment at will. Such consecration ceremonies were probably also performed on behalf of larger numbers of believers, who while not adequately prepared, might benefit from the merits of such a performance. One must also bear in mind that many Buddhist monastic ceremonies consist essentially of invoking just such a set of divinities, to whom symbolic offerings are made and to whom praises are intoned. They are called forth out of the Void, which is the Perfection of Wisdom, then identified with the performers, bestow their blessing for the benefit of all living creatures, finally requested to take their leave. Thus the *tantras* provide the substance of much monastic liturgy.

The *yoga-tantras* had followers in Central Asia, China and Japan from the eighth century onwards; and they still provide the basis of Japanese tantric Buddhism (Shingon) to this day. They were introduced into Western Tibet from the tenth century onwards as a major part of the so-called "second diffusion" of Buddhism in Tibet; the "first diffusion" took place in Central Tibet between the mid-seventh and mid-ninth centuries under the three "Religious Kings," Srong-btsan-sgam-po, Khri-srong-lde-btsan, and Ralpachen (Ral-pa-can). After the extinction of their dynasty in 842, some descendants made their way to Western Tibet and established three kingdoms in the area west of Mt. Kailās (Mt. Meru), which includes present-day Ladakh. These rulers did much to sponsor Buddhism, financing scholarly expeditions to northwest India and the central Ganges Valley (see Chapter VIc). This was the original home of Buddhism; and although the eastward advance of Islam had already caused its eclipse in western and central India, it was not until the early thirteenth century that Buddhism was finally effaced from the eastern tracts, known now as Bihar and Bengal. In Kāshmīr it also maintained a firm hold until the mid-fourteenth century, when a Muslim dynasty gained power.

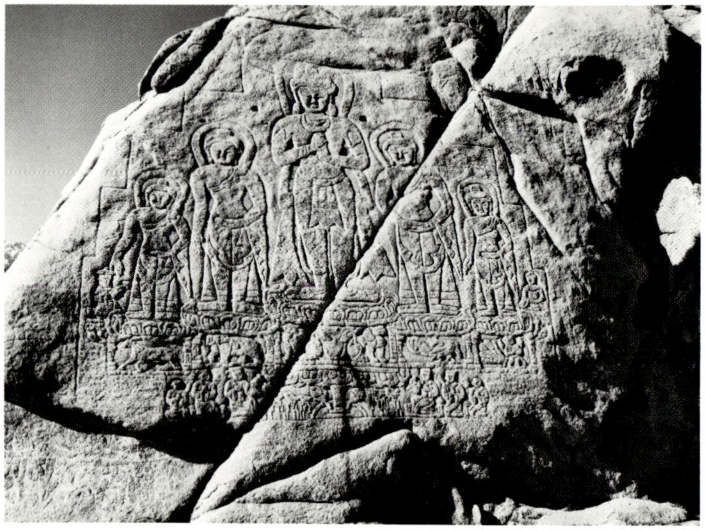

24. A rock carving of the Five Buddhas near Shey in Ladakh. It is undatable, but certainly belongs to the earlier period before the Tibetanization of this area, thus prior to the 10th century A.D.

In earlier Western accounts Tibetan Buddhism has often been referred to as degenerate and corrupt, and it is important to record that the royal sponsors in both Central and Western Tibet were interested in importing the religion in its more conventional Mahāyāna form. As has already been noted, this included the monastic rule (*vinaya*) common to all the earlier schools. That less acceptable practices claiming to be Buddhist were entering the country in the guise of Buddhism is proved by an edict issued by King Yeshe Ö, who reigned at Tsaparang in Western Tibet in the early eleventh century and who was also the chief sponsor of the Great Translator and importer of Indian Buddhist styles of painting and imagery from Kāshmīr, Rin-chen bzang-po (958–1055). The edict stated:

> You abbots, tantrists, living in the villages,
> Without having any relationship with these Three Ways
> (those of the Early Disciple, Solitary Buddha and Bodhisattva),
> Claim: 'We follow the Mahāyāna,'
> Entirely devoid of the conduct of the Mahāyāna,
> Claim to be a Mahāyānist.
> This is like a beggar saying that he is king . . .
> Village abbots, your tantrist way of practicing,
> Will shock if the people of other countries hear of it.
> These practices of you who say 'We are Buddhists,'
> Show less compassion than a demon of action.
> More avaricious for meat than a hawk or a wolf,
> More lusty than a mere donkey or ox,
> More greedy for beer than a beetle (?) in a rotten house,
> More indifferent to pure and impure than a dog or a pig.
> By offering excrement, urine, semen and blood to the pure divinities,
> Alas! you may be born in the mire of corpses.
> By denying the existence of the Dharma of the Tripiṭika,
> Alas! you may be born in hell.
> By way of retribution for killing living beings through 'the rite of deliverance,'
> Alas! you may be born as a demon of action.
> By way of retribution for indulging in lust through 'the sexual rite,'
> Alas! you may be born as a microbe in the womb.
> Worshipping the Three Jewels with flesh and urine,
> Ignorant about the significance of 'implicit' and therefore practicing it literally,
> You, Mahāyānist, may be born as a demon.
> What a strange Buddhist adhering to such practices!
> If these practices, like yours, bring about Buddhahood,

> Hunters, fishermen, butchers and prostitutes,
> All of these would certainly have attained Enlightenment by now.[5]

The main cause of these religious aberrations was the *tantras* of the fourth and supposedly highest class, known as "Supreme *yoga-tantras*." These works met with little favor in Central Asian and Far Eastern Buddhism, and their claim to be the highest form of tantric practice has certainly been disputed in Japan. Writing of the origins of Shingon in an introduction to his study of the *Mahāvairocana Sūtra* (of the *yoga-tantra* class), the eminent Professor R. Tajima states:

> Indian esoterism has had two sources: the monastery of Nālandā and that of Vikramaśīla, with the result that it has separated into two traditions. The first was a development of Mahāyānist thought; this was an orthodox esoterism based on the Vinaya (Monastic Rule). The second took shape along rather popular lines towards the end of the eighth century and quickly degenerated into 'esoterism of the left-hand' (Sadōmikkyo). This last has not inspired Japanese Shingon. . . . Merely considering the chronology, the (Buddhist) esoterism of Tibet was introduced into this country after the foundation of Chinese esoterism. As for its affiliation, we have historical proofs that it derived principally from the centre of Vikramaśīla. On the other hand, researches based on the Tibetan versions of the scriptures are precious for the texts themselves, but one observes that the strange esoterism of lamaïst religion is in fact rather remote from the teachings of the Buddha. One must never lose sight of the considerable gap between Chinese esoterism, which is the source of Japanese Shingon, and that of Tibet.[6]

This short passage, while helpful in making such a clear distinction between Tantric Buddhism in the Far East and in Tibet, makes an overall distinction between the two cultures, which has subsequently become true, but does not apply during the period we are considering, namely the seventh to the thirteenth centuries. During that period the *yoga-Tantras* had generally established themselves as a form of orthodox Buddhism as much in Tibet as in Central Asia, China, and Japan. Other *tantras* of the so-called "Supreme Yoga" class were meanwhile being translated into Chinese (and are still included in the Chinese Canon and the Japanese which is based upon it); as we note from the edict quoted above, responsible Tibetans were quite as disturbed by these teachings as were the Chinese and Japanese. By the end of the eighth century doubts had been raised about whether some *tantras*, especially those of the "Supreme Yoga" class, should be practiced literally. Finally, it was decided that such *tantras* should be translated into Tibetan only when royal permission was given.[7]

SUPREME YOGA-TANTRAS

We have already observed how throughout the 1,700 years or more that Buddhism flourished on Indian soil, ever later and more developed forms of doctrine have been superimposed upon all that went before. The latest formulation in any one period is usually made by the proponents of the latest theories, and it is not surprising that they should regard their particular teachings as the last word in excellence. This is surely the overall context in which one may regard the name "Supreme Yoga" as attached to a particular group of *tantras*; Chinese and Japanese Buddhists thus had some good reasons for treating them as suspect. In defense of the Tibetans one must recall that they were very much closer to the actual sources of Indian Buddhist practice in the seventh through thirteenth centuries, and that during this period they held their Indian teachers in high respect, regarding themselves as mere students of the new religion. It was only after the eclipse of Buddhism in India that the Tibetans found themselves as the full inheritors of the Indian Buddhist tradition, and there is no doubt that many distinguished Tibetan teachers could make spirited rejoinders to any suggestion that their form of tantric Buddhism is less orthodox than present-day Shingon. At the same time they might readily admit that some tantric teachings can have a completely wrong effect if practiced by those who have not been properly initiated into their use. Maybe such an admission already accepts in effect the contention of others that Buddhism has generally been available for open practice to all men and women of a good disposition, and any suggestion of "hidden teachings" is contrary to the whole ethos of Śākyamuni's doctrine. Why should there be scriptures which have to be interpreted in an "implicit" sense, if the practicer is not to be castigated for entirely falsifying the doctrine; accused of immorality and obscenity by those who reject these strange "scriptures" altogether; and even threatened with rebirth in one of the hells by his fellow-practicers, if he does not practice them as "implicitly" intended? The answer to this question is simply that these "scriptures" had been produced in certain circles which claimed to be Buddhist; they incorporated a certain amount of Buddhist philosophical theory; that their yogic practices claimed a degree of success, that Indians, whether Buddhists or Hindus by general affiliation, have always been tolerant of the strange ways of any man of religion (even if he is only self-declaredly so), and chiefly because there were already so many different styles of Buddhist practice in India with no central authority which might claim the right to proscribe any of them; that the tantric Buddhists who were responsible for the teachings of the "Supreme Yoga" class were no more or less acceptable than the many other groups. One significant factor so far as acceptance is concerned may distinguish them. Whereas all earlier "scriptures" for which "canonical status" was eventually claimed were presented in one way or another as the direct Word of the Buddha, the *tantras* of the "Supreme Yoga" class, while subsequently included in the Chinese and Tibetan canons, were not attributed to Śākyamuni in the same way that the yoga-tantras were. They are said to have been taught by Vajrapāṇi on the instruction of the Buddha.

This last group of *tantras* differs from all other Buddhist canonical works in that the central figure, although given the title "Lord" (*Bhavagān*) with all its accumulated Buddhist associations, is no Buddha manifestation known of throughout the Mahāyāna or in any of the other classes of *tantras*. He is known as Heruka (a title of Śiva in an horrific manifestation) or as Saṃvara (Pls. 34 and 111) (or Śambara, another name of Śiva); or as Cakrasaṃvara (which the Tibetans translated as *'Khor-lo sdompa*, the "Wheel-Vow," since *saṃvara* happens to mean "vow" in Sanskrit—although such is scarcely its origin in the present context); or as Bhairava (the Terrible) (Pl. 33), also a title of Śiva. Some leading names of a quasi-Buddhist nature were coined by the use of the all-important term *Vajra*, as in the compound name Vajrabhairava, now the main tutelary divinity of the Tibetan Yellow Hat order; and especially by the name, Hevajra, presumably formed from the salutation given to a neophyte at the consummation of his consecrations when he is addressed as 'He Vajra (meaning something like "Behold O Vajra!"). All these Great Beings are described in horrific forms and since their main characteristic is wrath, they are all identified with Akṣobhya's Family of Wrath which involved transferring Akṣobhya's family to the center of the *maṇḍala* and placing Vairocana to the east. This is largely a theoretical rearrangement, for most of these Great Beings have their own *maṇḍalas* consisting either of *yoginīs* (feminine companions of noncelibate *yogins*) or of emanations of themselves.

While the *tantras* of the three other classes were produced within thoroughly Buddhist circles and are available both to monks and to layfolk, the "Supreme Yoga" *tantras* clearly arose amidst groups of noncelibate *yogins*; and many of their practices, especially those involving sexual *yoga*, are quite unsuitable for monks. It is true that they were later accepted in monastic circles and reinterpreted accordingly in terms of their supposedly "implicit" meanings, whereby the whole process became one of mental visualization. Reinterpreted in this way, they had nothing to offer that was not already available according to the practice of the *yoga-tantras*.

Indian *yogins* are renowned for their power to control the natural processes of breathing, which can greatly assist in the experiencing of higher states of trance. This is as much a part of Hindu as of Buddhist yogic practice. It is thus not surprising that some groups of *yogins* experimented with the control of the natural force of sexual involvement. They discovered that the seminal fluid could be withdrawn at the very peak of enjoyment thus producing a psychological state, often referred to simply as "Great Bliss" (*mahāsukha*), which in relation to certain Buddhist philosophical theory, they defined as the final state of enlightenment. They were quite aware of the abuses to which such teachings might lead; hence their insistence on strict secrecy. It is only fair to regard the leaders of this movement as quite sincere in their intentions. However the circles in which they moved, as quite clearly described in some of these *tantras*, must have appeared to many outsiders as thoroughly objectionable. They deliberately flouted all Hindu and Buddhist conventions, partaking at their gatherings of sacramental offerings consisting of the flesh of man, cow, elephant, horse and dog, accompanied by alcoholic brews, of which a whole variety are listed in at least one such *tantra*. Victims might be killed by what was euphemistically referred to as an "act of deliverance," whereby they were given assurance of an improved state of rebirth. A special offering referred to as the "five elixirs" consisted of excrement, urine, semen, flesh and blood. Ritualized copulation also took place at such gatherings, which any outsider might quite reasonably regard as orgies.[8] Strangely enough, all these very un-Buddhist proceedings were accepted by those who did not belong to such circles and scholars gave them new interpretations more in keeping with conventional Buddhist ideas. Thus readiness to accept unclean and even revolting food could be interpreted as a quite proper indifference to the sightly and unsightly, the palatable and the unpalatable, such as all forms of asceticism seek to inculcate. Even slaying might be accepted when interpreted within the terms of the heroic conduct of a Bodhisattva, who might find it necessary to kill in order to save others; even if as a result of such an immoral act he should have to spend an appropriate length of time in one of the hells. The union of the sexes was quite easily interpreted in terms of the union of "Wisdom" and "Means," without which the realization of enlightenment according to later Mahāyāna theory would be unattainable. The Perfection of Wisdom, which transcends all conceptual notions and is thus characterized as the Void, could never be realized unless one made use of approved means; ideally, these are the practices recommended for a Bodhisattva which, while having no absolute validity in themselves, served, as it were, the purpose of a boat which, having transported one across the wild ocean of the *saṃsāra*, is abandoned on the further bank. Since the word wisdom (in Sanskrit as in Greek) is feminine, the female partner was identified conventionally as "wisdom" and Buddhist *tantras* normally refer to her precisely by the corresponding Sanskrit term, namely *prajñā*, while Hindu *tantras* use the term *śakti*, meaning "power." In fact the male and female roles are reversed according to Buddhist theory, which was presumably already fixed by the importance which the Perfection of Wisdom holds in the Mahāyāna, not only philosophically but also as the Great Goddess, Mother of All Buddhas.

It would seem that most of these *tantras* reached Tibet direct from eastern India through Nepal, but some of them must have had a limited following in northwestern India. One very important and altogether acceptable *tantra* of this class, the *Tantra* of the "Wheel of Time" (*Kalacakra*) (Pl. 126), probably originated in that general area. Another entitled "Secret Union" (*Guhyasamāja*) was already translated into Tibetan in the eighth century, and the translation was reworked by no less a scholar than the great Rinchen Zangpo (Rin-chen bzang-po) (Fig. 18). This *tantra* refers to magical rites of all kinds, enjoins the use of all the "objectionable" sacramental items listed above, but has none the less continued to be respectfully regarded by the most saintly of Tibetan lamas as containing a collection of the most excellent meditational practices. While Guhyasamāja is envisaged as embracing his female partner (in the manner known as *yab-yum*, "father-mother," in Tibetan), the features of both three-faced divinities are tranquil, and the implements they hold—the *Vajra* and Bell (symbolizing Means and Wisdom), a gem, a lotus, a wheel, and a sword—indicate that they comprise in their union all five Buddha-Families. While this *tantra* uses as its primary *maṇḍala* the Five Buddha arrangement, moving, as already noted, Akṣobhya to the center, a sixth supreme Buddha is also present. This figure, which can be identified as the all-comprehending Guhyasamāja couple, is also known as Great Vairocana (*Mahāvairocana*); thus suggesting, despite the slight disarrangement, an essential unity with the *Vajradhātumaṇḍala* of the *yoga-tantras*. The introduction of this sixth supreme Buddha in the *tantras* of the "Supreme Yoga" class may suggest a claim to an even higher goal of spiritual attainment, but this is not consistently argued. All that is claimed is a speedier, more effective means of attaining the one goal of universal enlightenment.

The two main routes through which Buddhism reached Tibet from India between the seventh and thirteenth centuries passed through either Nepal or northwest India, leading via Gyantse to Lhasa (established as the capital of central Tibet in the seventh century A.D.) on the one hand, and to Tsaparang, the capital of the western Tibetan kingdom of Gu-ge (established in the tenth century A.D.) on the other. The so-called first "diffusion" of the new religion centered on Lhasa, where several early temples dating back to the seventh and eighth centuries have been identified. It was not until the second part of the eighth century that the first Tibetan monastery, *Sam-ye*, was built southeast of Lhasa at the lower end of the Yarlung Valley. This region was the homeland of the line of kings of this period, some of whom took an active interest in Buddhism. The first monastery was a small affair with seven ordained monks under Indian tutelage. Buddhist influences from Central Asia and China also reached Tibet at this time, and the contentions which seem to have developed between various factions led to an official debate at Sam-ye (c. 792), sponsored by King Khri-srong-lde-btsan, where the Indian party arguing in favor of conventional Mahāyāna teachings is said to have prevailed. Any semblance of official protection of the Buddhist religion came to an end in 842 A.D. with the assassination of the last of this line of kings, who since his enthronement in 836 had been doing his best to oppose the new religion.

Buddhism continued to make progress in Tibet, but without any central controlling interest roving monks and *yogins* gained the initiative. Many of them may have been men of serious religious intentions, but others purveyed the kind of practices which King Yeshe Ö castigated less than two centuries later. Just as most people nowadays are more interested in technological innovations than in basic research in the natural sciences, most people of the past were more concerned with miraculous events and magical rites than with the practice of serious religion. One has but to read the biographies of renowned Tibetan lamas to realize how those who recorded their lives were often more interested in their hero's supernatural powers than in his supernatural knowledge. With the breakup of the old kingdom in central Tibet, the initiative for furthering organized Buddhism passed to the rulers of western Tibet. Their enthusiasm was soon matched by that of other aristocratic families in the central and eastern parts of the country, who with the regaining of their petty territories saw the advantage of supporting the new religion, if not from religious conviction, then certainly from their recognition of the cultural advancement it introduced. Just as the early Christian religious communities brought the advantages of what remained of Greco-Roman civilization to western Europe, so the newly established Buddhist monasteries brought the advantages of Indian and to some extent also Central Asian civilization (in which West Asian, northwest Indian, and Chinese influences were mingled). The art of writing was introduced together with Buddhism, and although some pre-Buddhist materials were recorded, the mainstream of Tibetan literature has remained thoroughly Buddhist.

Up to the thirteenth century monasteries remained small, consisting of maybe six or seven monks, occasionally more, with an abbot in charge, who was either appointed by a local ruler or was himself of noble family. It was not until the second half of the thirteenth century, when the Mongols gained control of Tibet and found it convenient to appoint an abbot of the monastery of Sakya (Sa-skya) as their representative for the whole country, that monasteries began to become wealthy and populous, serving the function even of local administrative center. In order to vie with the growing wealth and influence of Sakya (Sa-skya), other religious houses looked for powerful sponsors, usually among other groups of Mongols, who were seldom united for long. Monasteries that were successful in this "power game" soon transformed the outward appearance of Tibetan Buddhism, so that it became a powerful state religion, ordered by whoever happened to

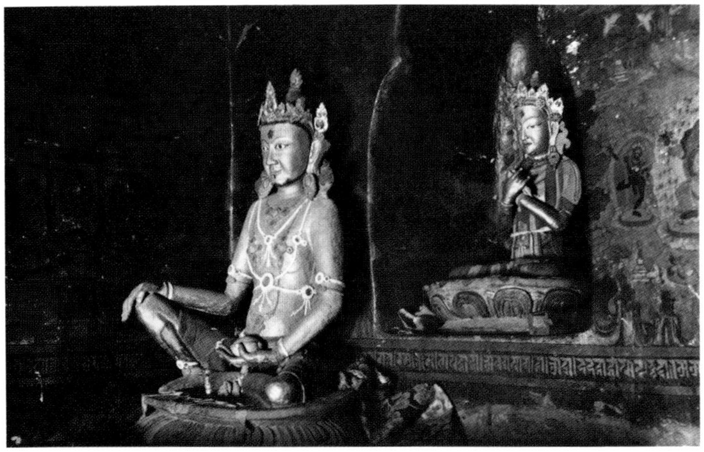

25. An image of the Great Yogin Nāropa with the Supreme Buddha Vajradhara (Holder of the Vajra) in the alcove behind him. Nāropa (956–1040) is believed to have spent some time in Kashmir and, according to local tradition in Zangskar, is also said to have meditated in this cave at Dzong-khul, near which the present monastery of Dzong-khul (Zangskar) was subsequently built.

be successful in any one period. Some of these powerful religious orders found it convenient to maintain a family relationship between those who exercised lay and religious authority, therefore both offices remained hereditary. Other smaller religious houses elected the religious authority by agreement between the elders of the community. But already in the twelfth century successors to the headship of some communities began to be discovered by applying the principle of reincarnation. Thus a child was sought for, who showed signs of being a reembodiment of the deceased lama. This strange system seems to have been adopted first by some of branches of the religious order known as Kagyud-pa (bka'-brgyud-pa, meaning "Transmitted Word"). Its lines of succession go back to the famous yogin Milarepa (Mi-la Ras-pa) and his teacher Marpa, and from there to the Indian tantric *yogins* Naropa and Tilopa. Among the Indian *yogins*, conventionally numbered as eighty-four, who were the chief promulgators of tantric traditions of the "Supreme Yoga" class from perhaps the eighth to the thirteenth centuries, such ideas of identifiable reincarnations of religious teachers certainly existed, and it was from them probably that the Tibetan religious sects originally connected with them derived the idea. It proved extremely popular; and was later adopted by other religious orders, among them the Yellow Hats, whose reincarnating grand lamas became, from 1642 onwards, the nominal and in the case of the fifth and thirteenth incarnations actual rulers of Tibet. But this takes us far in advance of the period with which we are concerned, and the later period is mentioned only in order to draw a proper contrast between Tibetan Buddhism as it developed modestly between the seventh and thirteenth centuries and far more grandiose and its overpowering expression which began to form as the first period came to an end and became fully effective from the seventeenth century onwards.

Monasteries were inevitably small in the earlier period for the straightforward reason that they were not yet wealthy enough to become large. Political power was in the hands of local lay rulers, styled kings or chieftains, and it was thanks to their beneficence that lands were made available for the building of a temple with a monk or two in charge or more ambitiously for a monastic community. We have the example of King Yeshe 'Ö (Ye-śes 'Od) of Gu-ge and his most successful religious protégé, Rin-chen bzang-po, upon whom he is said to have expended much, not only for his scholarly visits to India, but also to enable him to found religious communities on his return. The only actual monasteries founded by him which are known are Tholing near Tasparang, Ta-pho in Spiti, Nyar-ma in Ladakh, and perhaps Sumda in Zangskar (Map, 1). All are still standing today (although Nyar-ma is a ruin, Fig. 19), and their actual size can be seen. None of them can be expected to have housed more than twenty monks at the most, and probably less. Rin-chen bzang-po, thanks to the bounty of his royal benefactor, is said to have also founded 108 (a conventional number) temples also, but they would usually have had just one resident monk to look after them. Monasteries might also be founded by a wealthy individual and Alchi in Ladakh is an excellent example of this practice. An inscription there informs us that it was founded by a Religious Teacher named Kalden-Sherab (sKal-ldan śes-rab), who was a wealthy man of aristocratic family. There is no reason why he should have taken monastic vows himself. One is reminded in the Christian tradition of Saint Paulinus of Nola (353–431), who used his inherited wealth to establish his own monastery and finance other works of charity. Thus it is written of Kalden-Sherab (sKal-ldan śes-rab): "Free from avarice in his thoughts, he made gifts without distinction of persons. Remembering favors received, he did favors in return. In order to help living beings he constructed with difficulty the fort and the bridge. Disinterested acts of virtue and strict meditation he practised continually. . . . He built here in the Alchi valley this great monastery, his faith being the main factor and his wealth the secondary one."[9]

A very different figure would seem to be Marpa (1012–96) who must have been Kalden-Sherab's contemporary, although living in a different part of Tibet, where Buddhism was more easily imported from Nepal than from northwest India. He lived the life of a regular householder, plowing his own fields and quarreling with his neighbors. His religious interests seem to have depended on no one else for material support and having at his own cost visited Nāropa (Fig. 25) in eastern India in quest of tantric doctrines, he quite reasonably expected his students to make fair compensation to him for what he passed on to them. His disciple Milarepa (Mi-la Ras-pa) lived all his life as a strict ascetic, scarcely encouraging students. However, he had one determined follower, a certain Gampopa. Born of an aristocratic family, he began to turn his thoughts to religion, and having discovered Milarepa (Mi-la Ras-pa) and been accepted by him, he became effectively the mainspring for the whole later glorious expansion of the Kagyudpa Order. He founded with his own resources a monastery in Dvagspo in the south of Tibet and from his direct disciples derived in due course the six main suborders of the Kagyudpas. We mention here only one of them, P'agmo Dru (Phag-mo Gru) (1110–70), because he founded another monastery, gDan-sa-mthil, which subsequently became one of the greatest of the whole order. But in his own time, the monastery consisted of his own simple hut, surrounded by the even simpler huts of his few disciples. It was not until after his death that this place began to develop, thanks as was so often the case to the patronage of a local noble family, into the impressive establishment it still was in the mid-twentieth century. These grandiose developments began in the thirteenth century, when some of the leaders of the Kagyudpa suborders were trying to hold their own against the pretensions of the Sakyapas (Sa-skya-pas), who were receiving outside support from their Mongol overlords.

All such references to later developments serve to illustrate the great difference between nineteenth- and twentieth-century Tibetan Buddhism and the religion that was slowly gaining hold in Tibet between the seventh and thirteenth centuries. At that time, there was considerable dependence on outside assistance, and Tibet was by no means the closed land that it became during recent centuries. Contacts with India and Nepal were continual, and thither came not only religious teachers, but religious craftsmen who embellished the new religious buildings—painting according to the correct iconographic norms, carving woodwork, casting images, and thus guiding the Tibetans in all the arts of the new religion. Building styles generally remained traditionally Tibetan, for, as in other countries, these were largely dictated by the available materials and climatic conditions. However, it is said that bSam-yas, Tibet's first monastery, was laid out on the pattern of the great Indian monastery of Odantapuri (in modern Bihar); but as all traces of this have long since disappeared any comparison with Indian styles is difficult. This was a royal foundation, built at a time when Tibet was the center of a vast Central Asian empire, and so the account of craftsmen being brought from surrounding lands is very likely to be true. By the twentieth century it had inevitably undergone much rebuilding as with other great religious centers which have been in continual use over the centuries. The main temple of Lhasa, the Jokang (Jowo Khang, literally "House of the Lord"), named after a famous image said to have been brought by a royal wife, dates back to the seventh century; and it is still the center of Tibetan religion, although vastly different in outward appearance from the simple temple that it must once have been. The carvings on the doorways and lintels may well be original; they suggest early Central Asian associations. Temples on the Gyantse route as described by Professor Giuseppe Tucci[10] although founded in the thirteenth century continue to show similar influences, and it is clear that such cultural imports have continued to persist a very long time after the actual physical contacts came to an end. Certainly the main influences in Central Tibet came from Nepal and eventually from northern India, whether in imagery and painting or in doctrinal traditions. Thus we note that representations of the great divinities of the *tantras* of the "Supreme Yoga" class soon prevailed over the traditions of the "Yoga" class of *tantras*, which are so well preserved for us in western Tibet. This can only have been because this later class of *tantras* flourished especially in eastern India and Nepal from the tenth to the twelfth centuries; and we certainly know that they were cultivated by the Sakya (Sa-skya-pa) and the Kagyud-pa orders—albeit in their "purified" or "implicit" interpretations.

Chinese influences in painting and imagery began to penetrate Tibet as a result of the Mongol connection at a time when a Mongol dynasty ruled over China (1280–1368); but it was not until very much later, especially during the Manchu dynasty (1644–1911), that its effects were fully felt (Pl. 128).

The temples of old western Tibet, as preserved in a few monastic complexes, notably Tholing (now beyond our reach), Ta-pho, and Alchi, have been out of regular use for a long time. Thus they have not been subjected to the redecorations which in most other places have entirely obscured the earlier styles of painting and imagery. In Tibet the *tantras* of the "Supreme Yoga" have become more popular than those of the "Yoga" class, centering on the cult of Vairocana and the other four Buddhas of the directions. So far as personal meditational practice is concerned, this probably makes little difference, since much of the subject matter which outsiders (and this includes followers of Japanese tantric Buddhism, as we have already observed) find objectionable, has been interiorized and thus rendered purely symbolic. As far as the liturgies based on these *tantras* are concerned, there is inevitably a difference in content because completely different sets of divinities are invoked, be it Vajrabhairava, Heruka, Hevajra, or Padmasaṃbhava (Fig. 26) in one of his many manifestations. The last named is widely invoked by all orders of Tibetan Buddhism except the Yellow Hats, but they, too, in the present unhappy days of exile admit him to their altars. He is famed as the "Great Magician," the *yogin* of miraculous powers, who assisted in converting Tibet to Buddhism in the latter half of the eighth century by his power over the many local demons who opposed the new religion. In fact Tibet was converted by the enthusiasm, generosity, and self-sacrificing labors of thousands of Tibetans of all classes, who in this early period accomplished the seemingly superhuman task of transferring the vast heritage of Indian Buddhism in all its manifold doctrinal diversity together with all the cultural expressions required for its transfer from one country to another across some of the most difficult mountain routes in the world. Moreover the Nepal Valley, even Kāshmīr, and certainly the plains of northern India were most unsuitable climatically for Tibetans and many went there in quest of teaching and, struck down by fever, never returned. For the present writer the earlier period remains the more interesting one and certainly the more heroic.

David L. Snellgrove

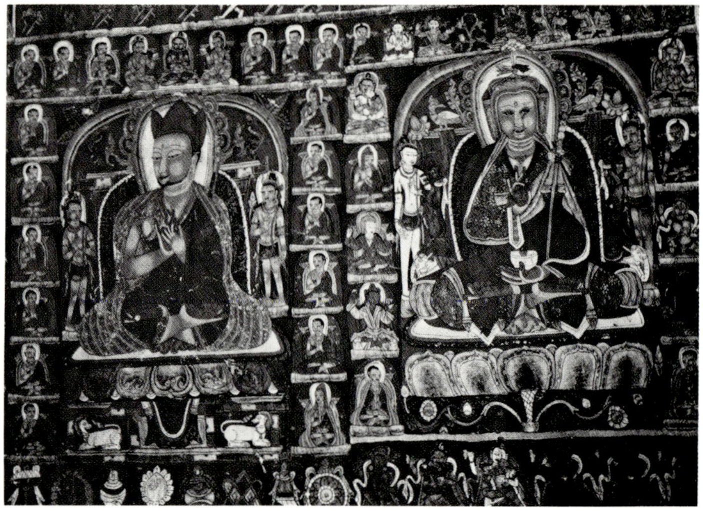

26. Mural of Atīśa who came to western Tibet in 1042 as a missionary from the famous Indian monastery of Vikramaśīla (in modern Bihar) and remained there until his death in 1054; and of Padmasaṃbhava, another great yogin who played an important part in central Tibet when Buddhism was being introduced there in the 8th century. This painting is in the Lhakhang Soma at Alchi, probably 13th century.

NOTES

1. Concerning the uncertainty of this date and its relationship with the reign of the Emperor Aśoka (second half of the third century B.C.), when the new religion can first be related to a clearly identifiable historical background, see Romila Thapar, *Aśoka and the Decline of the Mauryas*, Oxford University Press, London 1961, pp.13–14.
2. See E.J. Thomas, *Life of Buddha,* p.67.
3. Compare E.Conze, *The Large Sūtra of Perfect Wisdom,* pp. 58–59 and also our *Buddhist Texts through the Ages*, pp.119–128, where the same theme is illustrated by this and other extracts.
4. Lists of the several variations will be found in my introduction to the *Sarva-tathāgata-tattva-saṃgraha*, (facsimile edition), pp. 26–28.
5. I am grateful to Dr. Samten G. Karmay for this quotation, taken from his article, "The Ordinance of Lha bla-ma Ye-shes-'od" in *Tibetan Studies in honour of Hugh Richardson* (Oxford 1979), pp.150–162.
6. See R.Tajima, *Étude sur le Mahāvairocana-Sūtra*, Paris 1936, p. 7.
7. This information is given by the Tibetan historian Bu-ston (1290–1364). For the actual source see Samten G. Karmay, *op. cit.* p.159, note 27.
8. Those interested in these practices as still performed in India by a sect of Hindu yogins may refer to G.W. Briggs, *Gorakhnath and the Kanphata Yogis,* Calcutta 1938.
9. Snellgrove and Skorupski, *Cultural Heritage of Ladakh*, vol. I, p. 30.
10. See his *Indo-Tibetica*, vol. IV, part I, p.138 ff. (text), and part 3, fig. 50.

Section Two

Art and Ritual

VI

Esoteric Buddhist Art of the Western Himalayas

Deborah Klimburg-Salter

(a) The Early Phase: Northwest India – Seventh to Tenth Centuries

The "Abode of the Gods," the great Himalayan massive, stretches from Afghanistan in the west to Assam in the east, and separates the Indian subcontinent from the great inland steppes and deserts of China and the Soviet Union. It is the source of the great rivers of the subcontinent, the Indus, the Ganges, and the Brahmaputra. Along these rivers the earliest civilizations of India developed; throughout the millennia, these waterways have provided rich agricultural land, served as avenues of trade, and helped establish the economic foundations of the ancient civilizations of the subcontinent. These great rivers and mountains divide South and Central Asia into several regions, each of which has an identifiable cultural history.

From a relatively early period, the area stretching from Afghanistan to the Tarim Basin (including north Pakistan and Kashmir) has been distinguished by a common history and shared cultural characteristics. For most of the first millennium of our era, large portions of this region were economically interdependent, but the center of political power shifted a number of times. The Esoteric Buddhist art of this region will be discussed in three sections: the early phase, seventh to tenth centuries in 1) northwest India and 2) Central Asia, and the mature phase in the 3) western Trans-Himalayas where Vajrayāna art flourished in monasteries, some of which are still in use today.

Historical northwest India is defined here as including parts of eastern Afghanistan, all of northern Pakistan and in northwest India, the state of Kashmir-Jammu. Two events profoundly affected the development and character of Buddhism in northwest India: the conquests of Alexander the Great and the expansion of the Mauryan Dynasty. In the fourth century B.C., Alexander and his successors extended Hellenistic culture to historical northwest India. By the beginning of the third century B.C., the Mauryan Dynasty, whose capital was in northeastern India, extended its control as far as Afghanistan. Under the greatest of the Mauryan kings, Aśoka Piyadāsa, Buddhism spread throughout the realm.

By Aśoka's time, a settled agricultural society had evolved and the village had emerged as a basic unit of production. Trade gradually expanded and the merchant class expanded with it. Buddhist institutions also became prominent at this time, and they were the first Indian institutions for which the merchant class was a primary source of patronage (Kosambi 1970). This alliance between the Buddhists and mercantile institutions affected the nature of Buddhist monuments at that time and subsequent times in Indian history. Aśoka himself established numerous Buddhist institutions which played a critical role in the redistribution of wealth. In contrast to the rather exclusive system associated with the later Vedic religion, Buddhism as well as other religious movements espoused a more flexible social philosophy. This relative egalitarianism and its appeal to the expanding merchant class played important roles in the expansion of Buddhism.

Aśoka's propagation of Buddhism throughout his empire supplied the ideological justification for the large-scale sociopolitical reforms he introduced. The edicts that proclaimed these reforms (the Aśokan edicts) were engraved in stone, and some have been found as far west as Afghanistan. Among the ideas contained in the edicts was the concept of *ahiṃsa* advocated earlier by Jainism. This term can be translated as "nonviolence," but in this context it specifically meant "no killing." This ideology, selectively applied, allowed Aśoka to cease both the burdensome state sacrifices and military campaigns (Kosambi 1970). The socioeconomic impact permeated all levels of society. The reforms reflected changing attitudes which had developed in Indian society as it evolved to an agrarian economy and sedentary villages. From the beginning in India, these Buddhist ideas were part of broader changes in social philosophy (Kosambi 1970).

The importance of such reforms for the prosperity of an agrarian economy is demonstrated by a later historical parallel in the early fifteenth century. The king of Ladakh, Grags-'bum-lde (ca. 1410–1440), like Aśoka inspired by the ideology of Buddhism, promulgated an edict, the Mubhe edict (Francke 1906:75–76) against animal sacrifice. Just as in the third century B.C., these reforms were intended to prevent needless destruction of important economic resources (Fisher, Rose, Huttenbeck 1970:29).

The oldest surviving Buddhist art dates from the period of Aśoka's reign. The iconography (such as the lion, associated with Śākyamuni) tends to reflect an imperial as well as a Buddhist ideology. Aśoka is famous for constructing a large number of great *stūpas*, or reliquary mounds (such mounds were originally intended for royal burials). The *stūpas* attributed to Aśoka were called the Dhārmarājika *stūpas* and several are located in historical northwest India. These *stūpas*, symbolizing the body of the Buddha, became a focus of pilgrimage and worship; and great institutions, such as the monastery at Taxila, grew up around them. The construction and endowment of a *stūpa* may have been seen as an imperial obligation, for the Kuṣāṇa emperor Kāniṣka also built monumental *stūpas*. Subsequent generations built many more, and the remains of these structures can still be seen along the main routes connecting Afghanistan, Pakistan, northern India, and Central Asia (Fig. 12). In addition, a large number of reliquary *stūpas* were used as personal shrines (Pl. 1). These small shrines also contained symbolic relics in the form of small pieces of sacred material, such as portions of the *sūtras* (words of the Buddha).

BUDDHIST ART

All of the surviving early Buddhist art was associated with Buddhist monastic and pilgrimage sites. In this early art, there are no icons of the Buddha Śākyamuni. He is represented only by symbols such as the *stūpa*; and, thus, this phase of Buddhist art is known as aniconic. This period lasted about four hundred years, and at some time in the first century of the Kuṣāṇa period (the first to fourth centuries A.D.), the image of the Buddha first appeared. During this period there was an explosion in the production of Buddhist monuments and works of art. The Great or Imperial Kuṣāṇas ruled northwest India from capitals at Kāpiśa (near Kabul, Afghanistan) and at Mathura (near Delhi) from about the first to the mid-third centuries A.D. (Kuṣāṇa chronology is still not established). This dynasty was followed by the so-called little Kuṣāṇas (Kidara Kuṣāṇas) who ruled until the Hephthalite invasions in the mid-fifth century. The Kuṣāṇa rulers were responsible for instituting both a well-organized system of administration and the so-called "Pax Kuṣāṇa," which facilitated the lucrative silk route trade between China, the Mediterranean, and India. Under Kuṣāṇa patronage, both trade and Buddhism flourished; and monasteries, particularly those along the great trade routes, came to serve a complex of religious, educational, and financial purposes.

Two important developments which occurred during this period and had a great impact on the later arts of historical northwest India were the increased importance of Mahāyāna Buddhist institutions and the establishment of a dynastic cult centered on images of the Kuṣāṇa king.

At about the same time that the anthropomorphic image of the Buddha became current in northern India, images of deified kings were installed in Kuṣāṇa dynastic shrines (Rosenfield 1967:202; Kosambi: 1977:189). Both Buddhist and dynastic worship in India and Afghanistan were, therefore, focused on a cult image. This phenomenon seems related to the general climate of the time when "biographies" of Śākyamuni and anthropomorphic images of Hindu and Jain gods were produced in increasing numbers.

The style of the Buddha image from Shotorak and Paitava (near the Kuṣāṇa capital at Kāpiśa) suggests that dynastic arts affected the formal evolution of the Buddhist arts. I have elsewhere proposed that slight modifications in the style and iconography of the Buddha image were associated with a changing view of kingship in northern India. Unfortunately, because of insufficient historical evidence, it is not yet possible to define the relationship between Buddhist and dynastic institutions in the Kuṣāṇa period.

Royal patronage resulted in Buddhist institutions near the Kuṣāṇa capitals. Members of an affluent merchant class were also important patrons. In Kuṣāṇa art, these two groups of donors are represented in two different ways. One group is represented in a style which reflects their long tradition of Greco-Roman and Mediterranean-oriented culture. The other group is shown in Central Asian dress. It has been suggested that Buddhist narrative art can be seen in part as a statement of social identification, particularly among the merchant and urban middle classes (Taddei 1978a:96–101).

Changes in Buddhist iconography follow changes in doctrine,[1] and reflect changes in social organization and patronage; however, interpretation of the original iconographic meaning and doctrinal associations is severely limited by the fragmentary condition of the surviving images. These images were once part of larger configurations in specific architectural settings which are now mostly lost. It is difficult to understand the meaning of the images in their present isolated state. Recent research, however, has identified major philosophical and ideological tendencies which are reflected in both the form and content of later Kuṣāṇa art (Klimburg-Salter in press). This new ideology is clearly expressed in Kuṣāṇa dynastic arts. These visual symbols remained important in the art of northwest India through the early Islamic period (Pl. 59; Fig. 28) (Belenitsky 1968:213).

Toward the end of the period of the little Kuṣāṇas (ca. the third and fourth centuries A.D.) emphasis on narrative images declined and there was an increase in the number of iconic images accompanied by a tendency toward large-scale—even colossal—images, particularly of the Buddha. In the fourth and fifth century art of historical northwest India, the Buddha image is usually placed in the center of a triad or pentad. The Buddha is represented in hieratic scale, notably larger than other figures in the composition (Pl. 108).[2] In Esoteric Buddhist art, more figures were added to the pentad. Eventually, each of the Buddhas became associated with a family *(kūla)*. These deities are considered to be emanations of the principle deity and to partake of his essence. The various deities are commonly organized into a cosmic diagram known as a *maṇḍala* (Pls. 68, 126). In the *maṇḍala* all the deities are presented according to their place in the divine hierarchy. Early, *maṇḍala*-like compositions survive in the wall paintings of the Hindu Kush. No paintings of fully developed *maṇḍalas* survive in northwest India, but their iconography can be inferred from the painted *maṇḍalas* of the eighth to tenth century which have been found at Dunhuang.

The earliest known *maṇḍala*-like compositions survive in wall paintings found in the Hindu Kush. The single three-dimensional example is the eighth century bronze *stūpa* in the Peshawar Museum (Fig. 9). The next examples of this form are the ninth-century *maṇḍalas* from Dunhuang (Pl. 69).

Our understanding of the compositional devices used in the art of Afghanistan and Pakistan in the sixth through the tenth centuries is severely limited because only fragments of paintings from this period have been found outside the Hindu Kush. These fragments (from the Hephthalite and Turkic periods) have been excavated at Hada, Tepe Sardār, and Kandahār; but these have not yet been systematically studied (Tarzi 1976; Taddei 1978b).

From the middle of the fifth century A.D., for about one hundred years, the Hephthalites (nomadic invaders from Central Asia) ruled much of present-day Afghanistan, north Pakistan, and northwest India. Like the Kuṣāṇa before them, these peoples from the steppes were changed by acculturation, and their adaptation to urbanism involved adopting Buddhism. Until recently, it was believed that the main legacy of the Hephthalites was the destruction of Buddhist institutions. This was certainly true in some areas, particularly Pakistan. It is also true, however, that the late fifth and sixth centuries in eastern Afghanistan were characterized by an increase in Buddhist art production.

About 557 A.D., a confederation of Western Turkic peoples became the predominant military power in northern Central Asia and Afghanistan. Between the seventh and tenth centuries, groups identified by the dynastic title Śāhī were present in both eastern Afghanistan and northern Pakistan. We use the blanket term "Śāhī" (rulers) to refer to a group of rulers who used this title in inscriptions on coins and monuments; however, these rulers can be divided into at least two successive groups, known in contemporary literature as Turki Śāhīs and Hindu Śāhīs. In the eighth century, Kashmiri rulers included descendants of the Turki Śāhī in their administrative system. Clearly, the period between the sixth and eighth centuries was one of considerable political and cultural change in historical northwest India.

Recently, scholars have attempted to identify the distinctive cultural characteristics that emerged in Afghanistan and Pakistan during the period of Śāhī rule (Pl. 59) (Klimburg-Salter). This research has shown that both the Hephthalites and the Western Turks, like the Kuṣāṇas before them, inhabited the eastern Iranian cultural sphere which was then under considerable Indian influence. They shared a number of cultural traits, including multilingualism and Buddhism. It is, in fact, quite difficult to distinguish between the different cultural contributions of Hephthalite and Turkic rulers.

During the Śāhī period, both Buddhism and Hinduism were patronized in the area stretching from Afghanistan to Kashmir. In fact, the Korean pilgrim Huichao, who visited the area in 726–727 A.D., tells us that Buddhism had become the state religion in Gandhāra, Uḍḍiyāna, and Kāpiśa; and the kings, whom he identifies as Turkic, were aligned with the monastic hierarchy.[3]

According to Huichao, the king of Uḍḍiyāna performed the *pāñcavarṣika pariṣad* twice a year. In this ceremony, surplus wealth was redistributed to the Buddhist community *(saṅgha)* through the agency of the king. Previously, this ceremony was performed annually. It was held even less frequently when the Chinese pilgrim Faxian reported witnessing this ceremony in the mountains south of the Tarim Basin in the early fifth century.

The art and archaeology of eastern Afghanistan and Pakistan from the sixth to the ninth centuries offers the largest body of information pertaining to the Śāhī, and a critical and systematic analysis of this material should lead us to a better understanding of their society (Klimburg-Salter in press).

After some six centuries of more or less continuous artistic activity, the general art production in Buddhist monasteries decreased from the seventh century onwards. There is, however, evidence in northern Pakistan of a significant increase in the production of portable objects (both Hindu and Buddhist), such as sculptures in bronze and stone (Pl. 4), as well as an increase in Buddhist images carved or cut into the rocks along the Karakoram trade routes (Fig. 1-6). Many of these images show a varied and unusual iconography (Pl. 18), and the association between these themes and contemporary belief systems (including earlier schools and Mahāyāna) has scarcely been explored. Despite the abundance of extant objects and images, this late Buddhist culture of northern Pakistan is little understood. Similarly, we know little of the organization and social function of the local Buddhist monasteries.

The art of the sixth through the eighth centuries is, however, becoming better known as a result of Karl Jettmar's survey of rock engravings and inscriptions along the pilgrimage routes connecting Central Asia to India via the Indus Valley (Jettmar). The inscriptions associated with the carvings will provide an historical context for the art, while a comparative stylistic analysis of the rock carvings and the large number of bronze sculptures attributable to Swat and northern Pakistan, perhaps Gilgit (Pl. 10), may assist us in dating the more extensive Kashmiri sculptural remains (Pl. 28).

At present we are only able to distinguish two chronological groups in the Buddhist art of Pakistan: the so-called Gandhāran group (Pls. 1,2,3,5) (ca. first through fifth centuries A.D.), which takes its name from the geographic area; and the later Śāhī art ca. sixth through ninth centuries) (Pls. 6–8), named after the dynastic title, Śāhī. It is only in this latter group that we have evidence of Esoteric Buddhist iconographic themes (Pl. 20).

Evidence of these Esoteric themes is seen in the arts of Afghanistan and Pakistan, especially in the painting of the Hindu Kush. In Pakistan, these themes appear in portable stone sculptures and a few bronze images, e.g., a *stūpa* depicted as the *vajradhātu-maṇḍala* and decorated with images of the five Buddhas (Fig. 9), Hayagrīva (Pl. 20) and Vajradharma Lokeśvara (Pl. 19).

HINDU ART

In the same region, the practice of Hinduism had been increasing since the Gupta period (fourth through fifth centuries). The Hindu Paśupati and Kāpalikas sects were particularly important in Afghanistan and Pakistan. There was a growing interest in Hindu tantric sects. In the

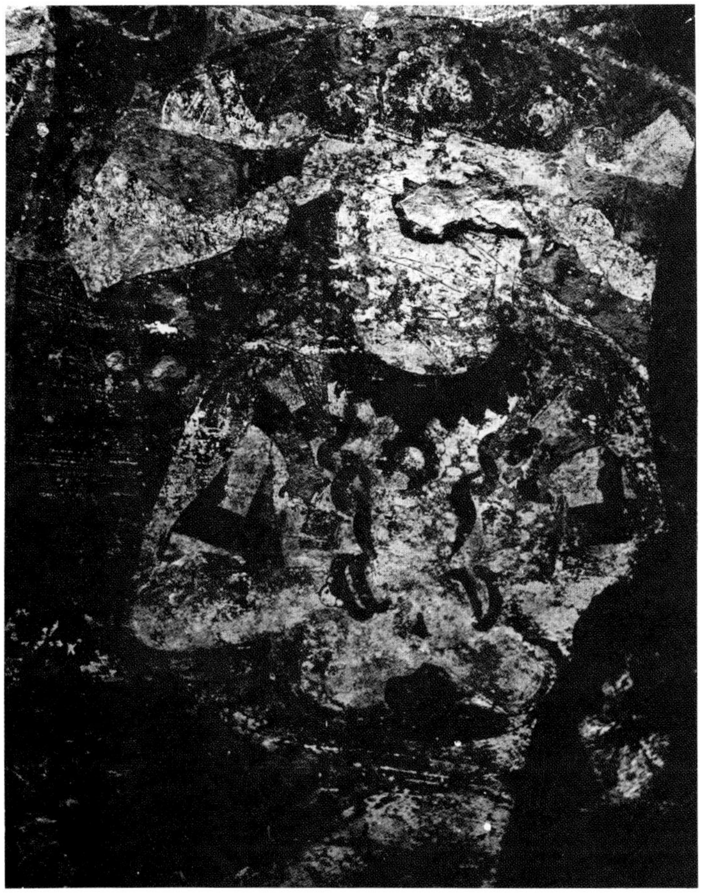

27. Maitreya, Cave "K", Bāmiyān, Afghanistan.

ninth century, Hinduism became the state religion under the Hindu Śāhīs ruling from Kabul.

Artistic evidence for the practice of Śaivism may date from the fourth and fifth centuries in Afghanistan and Central Asia. From the seventh century onwards a variety of Hindu cult images were worshipped in Central Asia and throughout northwest India. In the Kabul and Kāpiśa areas worship of Śiva (Pl. 22), Mahiṣāsuramardinī (Pl. 23), and the sun god, Sūrya (Pl. 21), was particularly important.

There is abundant evidence for the association between the Hindu kings of northwest India and sun worship. Several images of Sūrya, all in expensive materials and executed with impressive technique, have been found throughout the area. The earliest comes from Khair Khaneh (Kuwayama 1975; Bernard and Grenet 1981) where a temple to Sūrya was excavated many decades ago by French archaeologists (Hackin 1936). This site is located on a hill overlooking the road between Kabul and Kāpiśa (both Śāhī capitals) and further excavation might provide information about the cultic practices of these kings. It is worth noting that Kabul's New Year's celebration (which is called "Farmer's Day" in Afghanistan) continues to be celebrated on this same hill.

Although a great deal of Hindu sculpture dating from the seventh, eighth, and ninth centuries has been discovered in recent years (Pl. 24), only one Hindu shrine complex has been excavated with modern methods. This is the Japanese excavation of Tepe Sikandar in Kāpiśa (Kuwayama 1972). The archaeological evidence from this site together with the cult image of Umā-Maheśvara (other names for Śiva and his consort) and its inscription provide a relative chronological context for Hindu practices and art (Kuwayama 1974, 1976) within the period of the Turki Śāhī of Kāpiśa-Kabul. Thus, the ruling class appears to have patronized both Hindu and Buddhist cults (Pls. 2,22)

It has long been known that this pattern of coexistence characterized all of northern India. It has only recently been recognized that this occurred in Afghanistan as well. Recent archaeological evidence allows us to replace the earlier model of a succession of Buddhist, Hindu, and Muslim societies with a more complex and realistic picture. It is now believed that Buddhism and Hinduism coexisted through the early Islamic period, at least into the ninth century. According to Staal, one can understand why Hinduism and Buddhism have always been compatible if one does not define these systems according to the Western concept of religion. The syncretism which evolved in this environment is well known from literary sources and is reflected also in Tantric Buddhist iconography.

The archaeological finds from Tepe Sardār at Ghaznī in Afghanistan demonstrate the effect of Hindu practices on Buddhism. While excavating Chapel 23 workers found the statue of the Hindu goddess Durgā-Mahiṣāsuramardinī along with the figure of a bejeweled Buddha wearing the three-pointed jeweled cape current in the contemporaneous arts of Afghanistan and Pakistan (Pl. 9). Both images, the bejeweled Buddha and the Durgā-Mahiṣāsuramardinī, appear to have been eighth-century additions to the original Buddhist chapel (Taddei 1978b:47–57). Other marble images of Mahiṣāsuramardinī (Pl. 23) from Afghanistan testify to the importance of the deity in the Śāhī period. There are other images of the goddess from Kashmir (Pl. 42), but they may have been associated with Hindu rites.

What place in society was held by those who adhered to Hinduism? The significant amount of high quality marble sculpture (Pl. 24) suggests that the patrons were from the ruling class. The sudden appearance of Hindu cult images made only in costly materials would seem to suggest the migration of a new group who brought their Hindu practices with them. Might these people be associated with Göbl's "Alxon," who returned to Afghanistan from India about 600 A.D. (Göbl 1967:II,70)?

There was a steady increase in the popularity of Hinduism throughout northern India beginning in the Gupta period. To date, however, there is no substantial evidence for Hindu cult practices in Afghanistan prior to the sixth century; the one possible exception is the painting from Delvarzin Tepe in northern Afghanistan which may represent a syncretized form of Śiva worship (Kruglikova 1974). It is possible that these Hindus were a military class that lived under the rule of the Buddhist Turki Śāhī in Kāpiśa-Kabul in the seventh and eighth centuries, and came to power as the Hindu Śāhī in the ninth century. Al-Bīrunī (Sachau) gives this account of how the Hindu Śāhī won the throne occupied by the Turki Śāhī:

> The last king of this race [i.e. the race of the Turki Śāhī] was Lagatûrmân, and his vazir was Kallar, a Brahman. The latter had been fortunate, insofar as he had found by accident hidden treasures, which gave much influence and power. In consequence, the last king of this Tibetan house, after it had held the royal palace for so long a period, let it by degree slip from his hands. Besides, Lagatûrmân had bad manners and the worst behavior, on account of which people complained of him greatly to the vazir. Now the vazir put him in chains and imprisoned him for correction, but then he himself found ruling sweet. His riches enabled him to carry out his plans and so he occupied the royal throne.

Perhaps it was the extravagant expenditures by the Turkic kings on Buddhist institutions described by Huichao in the eighth century which exhausted the good will of the people and paved the way for a Hindu "takeover" in the ninth century. Göbl's historical reconstruction (1967:II,79 *passim*) based on numismatic evidence may provide an historical framework for the Hindu patrons. His hypothesis, that the so-called "Alxon" or "Indian Huns" spread from the area of Zabulistan (Ghaznī) to Kāpiśa-Kabul during the seventh and early eighth centuries also coincides with the evidence for Indian artistic influence in the region.[4]

It has been argued that the demise of Buddhism in eastern Afghanistan started in the fifth century as a result of the destruction of monasteries and settlements by the Hephthalites and the Western Turks.

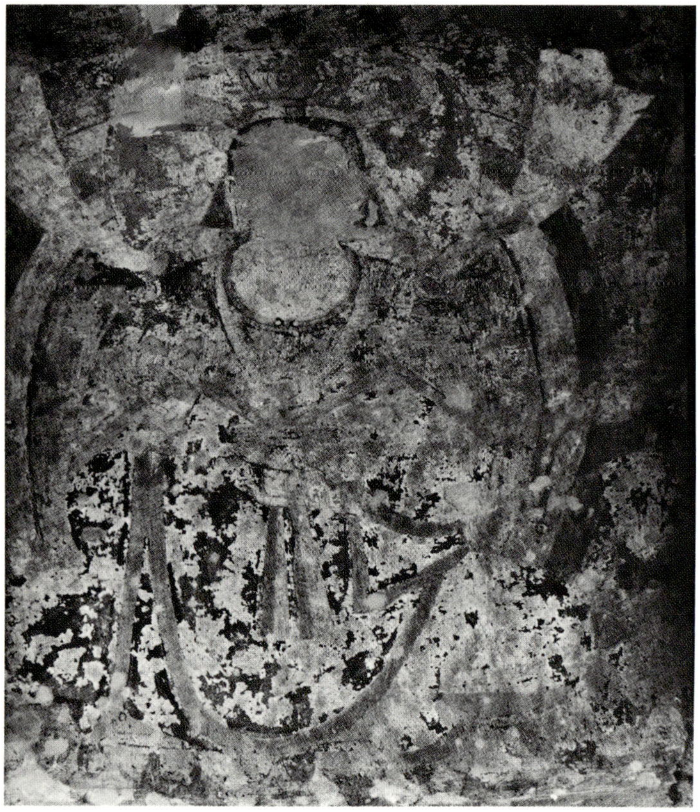

28. 38 meter Buddha donor figures, Bāmiyān.

The abandonment of monasteries in eastern Afghanistan in the fifth and sixth centuries has been used as evidence for this view; however, a recent study of these sites has demonstrated that there is no evidence of violent destruction (Fussman and Le Berre 1976). The evidence rather suggests that the monasteries were gradually abandoned as a result of the increased importance of Hinduism under the Śāhī rulers. The demise of Buddhism in historical northwest India was apparently a later event, caused by economic and political changes brought about by first Hindu and then Islamic rulers.

ŚĀHĪ ART OF AFGHANISTAN AND NORTH PAKISTAN, SIXTH TO NINTH CENTURIES

The art which originated in Afghanistan in about the sixth century under Śāhī patronage and had spread throughout north Pakistan by the ninth century can also be understood as developing, in part, from the local traditions established in Afghanistan and Central Asia during the Kuṣāṇa period (Klimburg-Salter in press). Kuṣāṇa Buddhist and dynastic arts affected the later Buddhist arts of the region, as Soviet scholars have already suggested (Belenitsky 1968). Hindu arts appear to have been more indebted to Gupta traditions.

The Kuṣāṇa traditions together with the Gupta art of northern India had an enormous impact on the later arts of Asia, including the art of historical northwest India. The Gupta style of Mathura—the simplified modeling of the torso; the longer, more slender proportions of the body; simplified drapery; and simple jewelry (such as a single bead necklace)—was particularly notable in the arts of Kashmir and, to a lesser degree, northern Pakistan. In Afghanistan a more typical Gandhāran style remained in vogue throughout the sixth century. A striking example of the survival of the distinctive formal characteristics of the Gandhāran Buddha image can be seen here in the bronze Buddha image from Kāpiśa, ca. sixth century A.D. (Pl. 2). The continued popularity of the Gandhāran-style Buddha is perhaps the most striking example of a phenomenon which is also identifiable in other iconographic types, such as female figures. The hairstyle and head jewelry of the figure depicted on the small bronze plaque (Pl. 25), are similar to that shown on the Umā seated with Maheśvara from Tepe Sikandar, ca. seventh century. Both this Kāpiśa image and a Kashmiri sculpture of the Hindu goddess (Pl. 41) depict the goddess with a broad face and thick features. The same hairstyle is also shown on a clay head from Tepe Sardar (Taddei 1978b: fig. 232). This Buddhist image has the narrow face of the women in Pl. 25.

In the Hindu and Buddhist arts of the ninth century, particularly in Śāhī territory in Pakistan, there are stylistic elements similar to those which appear in earlier works from Afghanistan. These elements, which include a coarsening of the features and a greater stiffness in the body and drapery, also appear in the very rare examples of ninth-century Buddhist images made of the white calciferous stone often used for Hindu images (Pl. 8). In Kashmiri art produced during this period, there appears to be no important stylistic or technical difference between the arts of the two religious groups, but a distinctive style does seem to emerge in the eighth and ninth century Hindu art of Afghanistan and Pakistan. This style, represented by the Śiva-liṅga (Pl. 24) from the Metropolitan Museum, is characterized by rather large facial features, a distinctive hairstyle, carving in very high relief and, above all, the use of white marble. As we have noted, marble is not used in Afghanistan prior to the sixth century. When it does appear, it is used exclusively for Hindu cult figures.

KASHMIR AND ITS ART

"As the country is protected by a dragon, it has always assumed superiority among neighboring peoples" (Beal 1884:II,148).

Thus Beal chose to explain the abundance of natural and material riches he found in seventh-century Kashmir, then ruled by the powerful Kārkoṭa Dynasty.

Kashmir always had an original, independent culture reflecting its relative isolation inside the northwestern mountains of the subcontinent. At the same time, because it borders the Himalayas, northern India, and Central Asia, Kashmir has received, summarized, and ultimately transformed the artistic experiences of its neighbors. The mediaeval arts retain elements of Gandhāran and post-Gupta art and also show evidence of influence from Central Asia, then under the domination of Tang China. Even today, Kashmir continues to be known for the extraordinary richness and diversity of its arts.

We know from literary sources that Kashmir was an early center for the practice of Buddhism, a role it continued to play throughout the life of the Buddhist community in India. Unfortunately, evidence for the material culture prior to the seventh century is rare. This is in part due to the fact that there have been no full-scale excavations; we must, therefore, rely almost totally on random finds and the remains of a few ruined monuments.

In the mid-seventh century four powers were established in the region: the Western Turks in east Afghanistan and western Central Asia; Harṣa of Kanauj in north India; the dynasty of the "first religious kings" in Tibet; and the Kārkoṭa of Kashmir. Each of these dynasties had a significant impact on the development of Buddhist art within their realm. As a result of their power struggles, these kingdoms had extensive contact with each other and with China and Nepal as well. Because of Kashmir's central location, it became a conduit of diverse cultural influences. In Kashmir, many of these ideas were grafted onto a northern Indian artistic heritage, which included the Kuṣāṇa, Gupta, and Śāhī legacies. As active patrons of both Buddhist and Hindu art, the Kārkoṭas had a particularly important role in the propagation and diffusion of Kashmiri culture.

Under the Kārkoṭa kings, a strong central government with a complex bureaucracy existed and the land-owning aristocracy was responsible for administration at the local level. According to the *Rājataranginī* (a chronicle of kings), written by Kalhaṇa in the twelfth century, state ceremonials were a means of socially integrating the large number of military and civil servants and feudal lords. These rites took place in monumental architectural complexes, both Hindu and Buddhist, constructed by the Kārkoṭa. Both in their use of state ceremony and in the form of their administrative system, the Kārkota continued ancient

Indian traditions which had been effectively revitalized by the Guptas. The religious syncretism that characterized both the rituals and the arts occurs elsewhere in Indian cultural history and has already been discussed in Chapter III.

The most famous of the Kārkoṭa kings was Lalitāditya. In addition to his impressive military exploits he was also an important patron of Buddhist and Hindu monumental architecture and art. Near the capital, he built a Buddhist monument, Parihāspura, which also served as a theater for state ceremonials (Kalhaṇa, trans. Stein 1900). It was, thus, comparable to the Buddhist complex at Bāmiyān in the Hindu Kush, which was also the scene of a royal ceremonial in the guise of a Buddhist ritual. In a ceremony similar to the Pāñcavarṣika described by Huichao in Pakistan, and Xuanzang in Bāmiyān, Kāpiśa, and Kanauj, the Kārkoṭa ruler distributed surplus wealth to the Buddhist monastic community (*saṅgha*) and the Buddhist faithful (Klimburg-Salter 1981).

Bāmiyān and Parihāspura were both located along the trade routes that connected India, Central Asia, and China. At both sites the main icons were colossal images of the Buddha, and at both sites the fusion of royal and secular functions was manifested both through the main ceremony performed at the site and by a jeweled Buddha wearing a crown and a three-pointed jeweled cape (Pl. 1).

In the eighth century Lalitāditya also built the great sun temple at Martand on an earlier sixth-century foundation. At Martand, regal and religious imagery merged with solar symbolism, as they had during the Kuṣāṇa period. The magnificent eighth-century sculpture of the sun god from the Cleveland Museum collection (Pl. 39) might suggest the style and appearance of the central cult image once worshipped at Martand. The existence of solar cults during the Śāhī period in Afghanistan and Pakistan is well known (Il. 21).

Many smaller stone temples were built in Kashmir between the eighth and thirteenth centuries and dedicated to forms of Śiva and, to a lesser degree, Viṣṇu. In many cases these were not royal foundations. Śiva was worshipped in the form of a *liṅga* (Pl. 40) or phallus, which is the most direct symbol of Śiva's essential characteristic energy. Śiva represents the primal force of the universe, but he may take many forms in the act of creation or destruction. When this energy is turned inward, it is a powerful meditative force and the god appears in the role of an ascetic. The duality of sexuality and asceticism is thus characteristic of Śiva. Śiva is also represented with his consort (Pl. 41). Like him, she has both passive and active aspects and is both wrathful and benign. This goddess was worshipped throughout northern India as Durgā (Pl. 42), Umā (Pl. 41), Parvatī (Pl. 43), etc. Horrific forms of these divinities can be associated with both Hindu and Buddhist tantric practices. Figures represented in sexual embrace (*yab-yum* images) (Pl. 97) first appear in Kashmiri style in the western Himalayas in the tenth to eleventh centuries. Ritual practices associated with these images may have been disseminated by groups and individuals outside the realm of mainstream Buddhist institutions.

According to legend, Padmasaṃbhava, the magician-saint, is believed to have brought Esoteric Buddhism from northwest India (Uḍḍiyāna) to Tibet. The figure of Padmasaṃbhava summarizes the tradition of tantric masters that was current throughout northern India during this period. Although used predominantly by small groups and secret societies, tantric practices may also have been incorporated into official Buddhism by Lalitāditya's minister, Caṅkuṇa (Kalhaṇa trans. Stein 1900). These traditions were also important in northeast India. The eighth century was a particularly creative period for Tantric Buddhist literature in both the northeast and the northwest. Several of the major *tantras* were apparently written in historical northwest India during this time. Kashmiri Buddhism transmitted to Tibet the legacy of both state Buddhism and the anarchist, tantric magic.

The military campaigns of the Kārkoṭa kings and their extravagant investments in monumental constructions and ceremonies encouraged the rapid decline of the great dynasty. The succeeding Utpala Dynasty (856–939) was founded under Avantivārman. His administrative reforms restored a level of economic security to Kashmir, but the lands he inherited were much reduced from the days of Kārkoṭa glory. Under

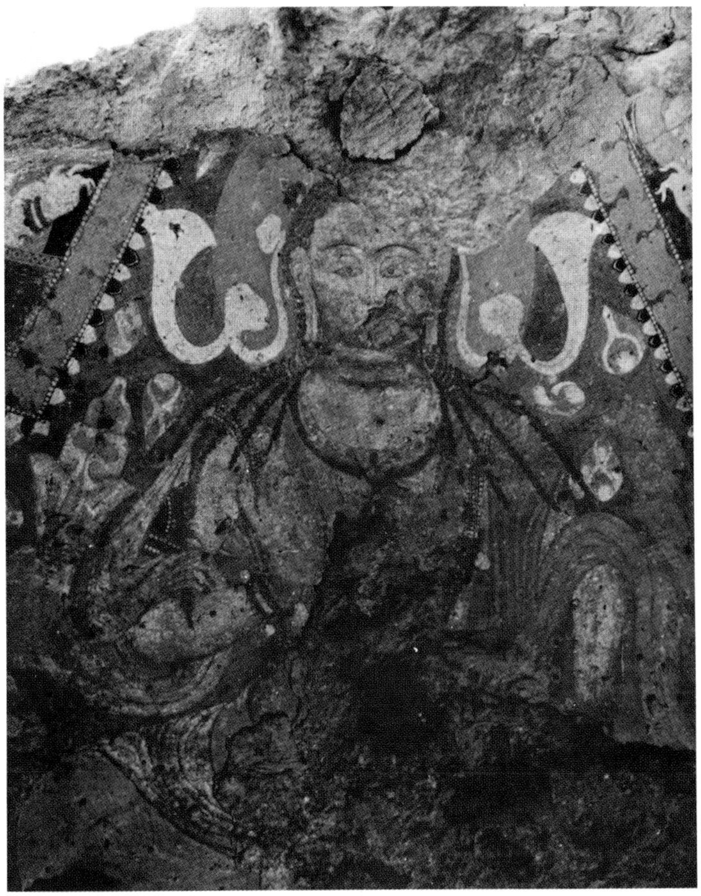

29. Niche "E" Bodhisattva, Bāmiyān.

his patronage several major monuments were constructed and all were dedicated to the Hindu gods he served. The significant amount of sculpture still remaining *in situ* at monuments at Avantipur allows us to understand both the form and content of Kashmir Hindu art produced during the later ninth and early tenth centuries. Comparison with Buddhist bronze sculpture shows that in this period, as in the preceding century, the stylistic attributes of Buddhist and Hindu sculptures were quite similar. The same artists probably created both Hindu and Buddhist bronzes, and we know that in many cases the same people patronized both Hinduism and Buddhism.

The Utpala kings were followed by the Lohara kings (1003–1101). During this period both economic prosperity and religious patronage declined. The advances of the Ghaznavid kings greatly reduced Kashmiri territory in the south and west, further isolating Kashmir from commerce and cultural interaction with neighboring territories. Particularly disastrous for the religious institutions was the reign of King Harṣa (1089–1101). In order to finance his costly military campaigns, this king ordered the looting of monasteries and the melting down of religious statues. It seems fair to assume that it is because of the desecration of sacred shrines at that time that so little remains of the great Kashmiri art of the early Middle Ages. Only two monumental Buddhist sculptures are reported to have survived Harṣa's onslaught. One was the famous colossal image (already referred to) at Parihāspura and the other was a huge image in the capital city of Śrīnagar.

The Islamic military conquests in northern India between the eleventh and fourteenth centuries had some economic repercussions in Kashmir, though the Muslims did not actually conquer the state until the fourteenth century.

Although only a small percentage of the Buddhist art produced in Kashmir between the eighth and fourteenth centuries has survived, the quality and range of the works (all three-dimensional objects) are aston-

30. Gilgit manuscript covers, Institute for Central Asian Studies, Śrīnagar, Kashmir.

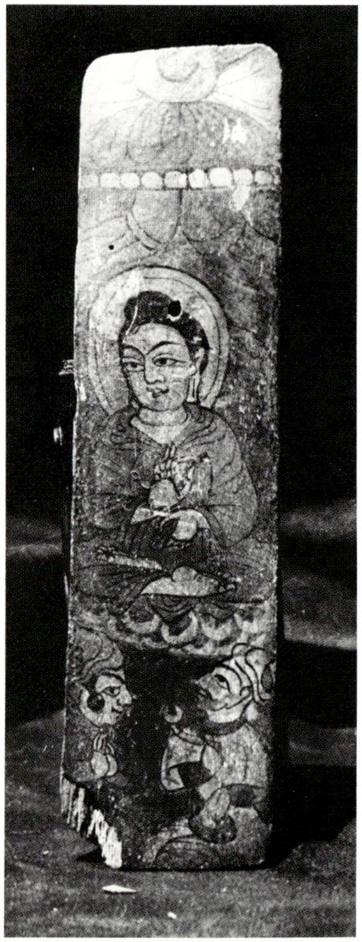

32. Gilgit manuscript covers, the Bodhisattva blesses a Śāhī donor. Institute for Central Asian Studies, Śrīnagar, Kashmir.

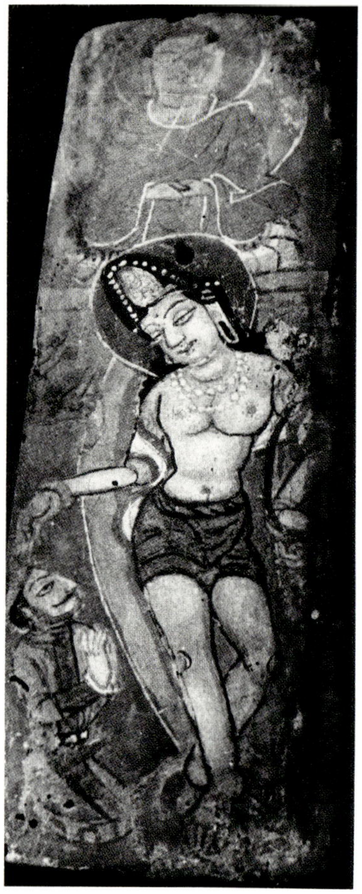

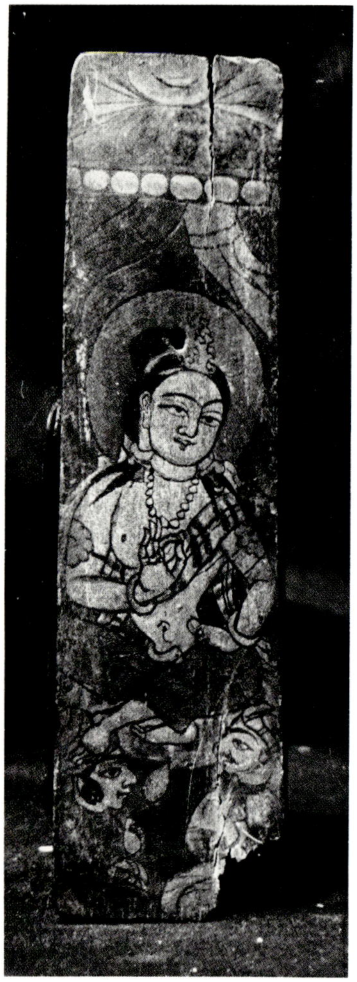

33. Gilgit manuscript covers, two Śāhī donors kneel before a preaching Bodhisattva. Institute for Central Asian Studies, Śrīnagar, Kashmir.

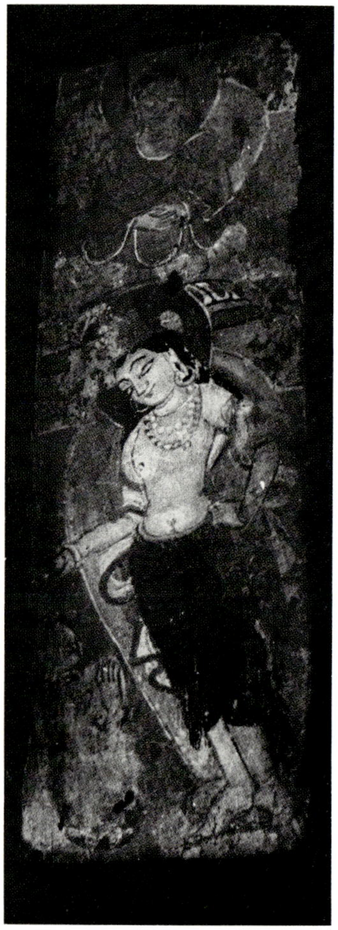

31. Gilgit manuscript covers, Institute for Central Asian Studies, Śrīnagar, Kashmir.

ishing. The skill of Kashmiri artists obviously justifies their enormous impact on the subsequent arts of the surrounding areas.

The Gilgit manuscript covers (Figs. 30–33) constitute the only surviving examples of Kashmiri-style painting. Nonetheless, their testimony combined with the evidence offered by murals from the Hindu Kush permits us to identify the eleventh-century murals from Ta-pho as a continuation of the now-lost school of tenth and eleventh century Kashmiri painting (Fig. 41).

No new Buddhist or Hindu monuments can be safely dated to the eleventh to fourteenth centuries, and few portable objects from this period are extant. It appears however, that in some techniques, particularly in bronze casting, the famous workshops of Kashmir continued to produce works of extraordinary quality. Perhaps the most famous example of work from this period is the large image of the Buddha from the Cleveland Museum (Pl. 27). It was probably made at the beginning of the eleventh century, and is therefore one of the largest and latest Buddhist bronzes of this quality attributed to Kashmir. It is significant that the inscription tells us that the image was commissioned by Lha-la-ma, a royal monk belonging to the dynasty of the kings of Western Tibet (Karmay 1975:61). Under the patronage of these kings, large-scale bronze icons were made in Kashmiri and western Himalayan workshops in the tenth and eleventh centuries. A single example serves to illustrate this point: an image like the Rockefeller Bodhisattva (Pl. 30), made by a Kashmiri artist, may well have served as a model for the Musée Guimet image (Pl. 92) produced in a western Himalayan monastic workshop in the tenth or eleventh century. In addition to the style, the large scale of the bronze images was clearly popular in the final phase of Kashmiri Buddhist art and this preference too continued in Ladakh. Portable bronze sculpture (Pl. 38) also affected monumental Ladakhi clay sculpture of the period (Fig. 21a).

One of the most interesting questions about Kashmir is the nature of its relationship with the surrounding area. It seems clear that Kashmir was always an important cultural center. The state "exported" both scholars and artists, and wealthy patrons from neighboring areas brought art and literary works from Kashmir into their homes and temples. It also seems clear that a close relationship existed between Kashmir and regions across the Himalayas, such as China and the city-states of Central Asia.

NORTHWEST INDIA AND CENTRAL ASIA

The relationship between Kashmir and Khotan, like that between Khotan and Gandhāra during an earlier period, is attested by numerous legends which have survived both in Khotanese texts and in the diaries of Chinese pilgrims. For instance, Xuanzang reports that a famous image of a crowned Buddha from Baghai was miraculously transported from Kashmir to Khotan where it became the icon of an important temple. It has been proposed elsewhere (Klimburg-Salter in press) that this type of crowned Buddha was peculiar to the cultural region now under discussion and might be identified as the *Abhiṣeka* (Consecration) of Śākyamuni (Pl. 9).

The legend of the Kashmiri image in Baghai belongs to the well-known story of the transmission of Buddhism from India to the Far East along the Trans-Himalayan trade routes. What is usually overlooked, however, is that this process, like all forms of human intercourse, must have been a dialogue in which elements of Central Asian and Chinese culture were also transmitted to India.

In the eighth century the Kashmiri and the Chinese exchanged diplomatic missions and the Chinese sent military and (perhaps) civil advisers to Kashmir. These exchanges cemented the alliance between Kashmir and China against the Arabs and Tibetans (Chavannes 1903b; 166–167,209; 1904:44,46,55,93)[5]

Trade and pilgrimage as well as official missions brought Central Asian and Chinese people to Afghanistan, Pakistan, and Kashmir. They undoubtedly brought with them from their homeland Buddhist images (icons, amulets, etc.) for their personal use. The rock carvings and inscriptions along the ancient pilgrimage and trade routes connecting northern Pakistan with Central Asia tend to confirm this theory. In fact, Jettmar's team has recently found a rock sculpture of a seated Buddha datable to the seventh–eighth century A.D. (Fig. 5). The thick proportions, drapery style, and facial features may be compared to rock-cut Buddha images of the Tang period from Central Asia. It has been suggested that after ca. 650 A.D. artists from Kucha may have influenced the mural painting of Bamiyan. Compare the Maitreya from Cave "K" (Fig. 27) with the painting of Maitreya from Kizil (Metropolitan Museum 1982: fig.27) (Klimburg-Salter in press). Some technical and stylistic relationships have been observed between the clay sculpture from Kucha (Pls. 51–52) and Fondukistan (Varma 1970:179). The sculptures from Kucha date to the first half of the seventh century, while the Fondukistan sculptures may be dated ca. seven hundred A.D. The eighth to ninth century sculpture uncovered at Tepe Sardar (Ghazni, Afghanistan) has also prompted the question of possible influence from either Sinkiang or Soviet Central Asia (Taddei 1978b:135). The excavators do not exclude the possibility that "Tapa Sardār's relation to Central Asia is that of a debtor rather than a creditor. The hypothesis of a return of the artistic trends that linked Afghanistan to Central Asia and China cannot be rejected before a thorough examination of all the available data has been made" *(ibid).*

This examination would involve a reevaluation of the long recognized relationship between certain sites in Central Asia and historical northwest India (Rhie 1974; 1976) in light of the later dates now proposed for several sites in northwest India.

The Chinese impact can also be seen in a very small number of sculptures from the seventh and eighth centuries. On the basis of their blackish color, technique, style, and individual motifs, these images can be attributed to northern Pakistan; but they also contain Sinicized features. An example of this phenomenon is the small figure of Avalokiteśvara (Pl. 13). This image shows some Sinicized facial features, such as eyes with an epicanthal fold; high, flat cheekbones; and a rather wide face. The slouched position, slight curvature of the stomach, the tilted head and movement of the shoulder are more easily associated with Chinese examples than with contemporaneous Indian sculpture. Other features, such as the hairstyle, point to northeast India. Another Bodhisattva figure from Pakistan still exhibits Sinicized features, but the style of this figure is more easily related to the prevailing eighth and ninth century Swat style (Pl. 15). Again, however, certain anomalies such as the slenderness of the lower half of the figure and the total lack of jewelry and the modeling of the torso suggest northeast Indian connections as well.

The Eilenberg Buddha represents a transition between the Sinicized Pakistani style and the eighth and ninth century Swat style (Pl. 5). In the eighth, ninth, and tenth centuries, Chinese influence can be identified in both Kashmiri art and the art of the western Himalayas produced under Kashmiri influence. Chinese influence can be detected in the pointed shape of the halo (Pl. 29); the tying of a scarf (Pl. 88); fleshy, broad faces (Pl. 89) and perhaps most important a new figure style. The voluptuous yet simple articulated torso construction notable at Tienlungxan can also be seen in Kashmir, and Kashmiri-style clay figures in Ta-pho monastery (Figs. 48, 49). There is also evidence of the influence of small-scale Chinese bronze sculptures on the portable arts of the western Himalayas. The eleven-headed Avalokiteśvara (Pl. 94) appears from the metal-working technique, particularly the summary treatment of the back, to have been made in the Himalayas; however, the style of the drapery and the pedestal clearly indicate that it was copied from a Chinese original of the Sui period (first quarter of the seventh century). A wooden image of a Amitābha (Pl. 85) must also have been made in the western Himalayas by the tenth century since it was originally part of the architectural decoration of Kyelong Monastery in Lahul. The shape of the eyes, the fleshy face, and the small mouth all hint at familiarity with Chinese art. But the drapery style is also seen in an eighth century Kashmiri ivory (Pal 1972: Pl. XXXVII).

The question of the influence of Chinese art on the art of historical northwest India is perhaps one of the most interesting of the many avenues one might pursue in a study of the evolution of Esoteric Buddhist art in northwest India. Now that recent Chinese excavations and publications are making more material known to us, critical and analytical studies on the Sino-Indian art occasionally found in India's inner Asian frontier regions should prove more fruitful. The examples which remain testify to a period when Chinese, Turkic, and Tibetan peoples frequently traveled through the mountain corridors connecting Central Asia with historical northwest India and the western Himalayas. The culture which they brought with them remained to affect subsequent generations of artists in the Trans-Himalaya.

Notes

1. Throughout the history of Buddhist art, changes in Buddhist doctrine appeared in literature sometime before the first date that these new ideas appeared in Buddhist iconography. The reasons for this "gap" are complex and not clearly understood. With regard to the specific case of the art of the Hindu Kush, this problem is discussed in my forthcoming publication (Klimburg-Salter in press).
2. The change in emphasis, from narrative scenes related to the life of Śākyamuni to iconic images used for devotional purposes, occurs in later Mahayāna art, as for example in the art of the Hindu Kush. However, narrative art continued to be important. In the *'du-khang,* Ta-pho monastery, Spiti, devotional images occupy the central position while wall paintings containing narrative scenes decorate the lower part of the wall (Figs. 49, 54). A similar format was maintained in later monasteries as well (Pls 105–108).
3. This alliance between Buddhist monastic and royal institutions did not preclude royal patronage of other religious cults as well. Earlier eminent Buddhist patrons such as Aśoka and Kaniṣka, as well as the contemporaneous Harṣa of Kanauj had also supported other cults. Indeed, the concept of a "king being Buddhist or Hindu is meaningless." See Staal for an extended discussion (Kosambi 1970:181).
4. Al-Birūni's statement that the Turki Ṣāhī were of Tibetan origin has several possible explanations. It would seem that the eleventh century Muslim scholar was aware that during the period of the western Turks (seventh to eighth century) the destinies of the Turkic and Tibetan rulers collided on the northeastern borders of the Western Turks' domains. I will discuss this passage in connection with another Arabic reference to the Ṣāhī in a forthcoming article.
5. A Chinese princess married to a Tibetan king was sufficiently certain of the good relations between Kashmir and China to propose seeking refuge at the Kashmiri court ca. 722 A.D. At the time she was reported as residing only seven days walk from Kashmir—i.e. in Ladakh (Chavannes 1900:204). This proposed escape appears not to have succeeded.

Catalogue Entries

Plates: 1 – 45

Pl. 1
Reliquary *Stūpa*
Gold and crystal, silver
Gandhāra
Undetermined date
H. 8.3 cm
Kreitman Gallery

This magnificent miniature *stūpa* originally may have been placed inside a silver *stūpa*, as indicated by traces of silver on the base. Early monumental *stūpas* were reliquary mounds which enshrined the relics of the Buddha and served as pilgrimage centers. Thousands of monumental *stūpas* were built throughout the Buddhist world. Later *stūpas* also contained fragments of sacred texts (*sūtras*) and other offerings, enshrined in the center of the *stūpa* inside reliquary containers which were usually made of precious materials. Small reliquary *stūpas* were meant to be placed on a shrine.

The simple shape of this *stūpa* with the round drum on a square base crowned with three umbrellas relates it to the earliest *stūpas* known from such diverse centers as Taxila in Pakistan and Sanchi in India. The archaic form is not necessarily indicative of the date of manufacture. From the precious minerals it is at least clear that the original reliquary belonged to an important personage, perhaps from the Gandhāran region where this *stūpa* was found. It is also indicative of the wealth enjoyed by the upper classes, which was in part obtained from the international trade. The exchange of luxury goods, such as gold from the Karakoram and precious gems from India, was a proportionately small but economically important component of this long distance trade.

Previously published: (Kreitman Gallery 1980:12, pl. 2).

(See Color Plate 1)

Pl. 2
Buddha Śākyamuni
Alloy containing copper, lead, zinc
Kāpiśa, Afghanistan—said to have been found in Gulbahār, Kāpiśa province
Ca. sixth century
H. 28.1 cm
Neil Kreitman
Inscription: "This is the pious gift of the Śākya Mon . . . an image of the Buddha, by Yaśonandinī . . . together with mother and father, most difficult . . . Buddha, by the teacher (Kreitman Gallery 1980:18)

This bronze image of Śākyamuni wears the traditional monastic robes draped in the style of Gandhāran Buddhas, and stands with his right hand raised in the gesture of "do not fear" (*abhya mudrā*). He has the marks and signs of a Buddha, such as the cranial protuberance (*uṣṇiṣa*) but no spot on the forehead (*urnā*). Somewhat unusual is the sign on the chest, here shaped as a sun. Such signs are found on Buddha images from Fondukistan and Bāmiyān, dated to the seventh century A.D., and may reflect influences from either Hinduism or Jainism, both of which were practiced in eastern Afghanistan from at least the sixth century A.D. While the inscription in punched Brahmī originally ran on all four sides of the high throne, only the front portion is now partially legible. The inscription contains no historical information, but stylistic factors—the somewhat long and slender figure, the rather simplified drapery, the deep V-neck collar, the oval face with long nose and arched brows, the hair which is arranged in parallel U forms (and which may be a later variant of the so-called Uḍḍiyāna hair style)—allow us to suggest a date in the sixth century A.D.

Stylistic features also allow us to suggest a possible origin in Kāpiśa where the image was said to have been found. Kāpiśa was the most important political center of eastern Afghanistan in the sixth and seventh centuries A.D. Comparisons can be drawn to stone Buddha images in the Kabul Museum, which were also found in Gulbahār, a modern city near ancient Begrām, and the capital of Kāpiśa in the pre-Islamic period. This important image may provide evidence for the metal workshops of Kāpiśa which fabricated the life-size silver Buddha image mentioned by Zuanxang (Huien-Tsang) in the seventh century. The famous Panshir silver mines and the copper mines of Logār and Ghorband, both traditionally under the control of Kāpiśa, would have been important resources for both the local mint (which was renowned in the Greco-Bactrian period) and the metal sculpture workshops. The importance of these workshops was recently recalled in an article attributing the Cleveland silver rhyton to eastern Afghanistan in 700 A.D. (Carter 1979).

Testing has revealed that the image and base were cast separately, and are made of different alloys. Both image and base contain a high percentage of lead. Although these images have been designated as bronzes for decades, in most cases this is not correct: indeed, most of the sculptures are in fact brass. However, there is some variability, as can be seen in this example. Therefore, we shall only adjust the terminology where we have scientific tests to demonstrate the actual metal composition.

Previously published: (Kreitman Gallery 1980:16, pl. 6; von Schroeder 1981:64)

Metal Content:
Buddha Figure: Copper 86.148; Zinc 13.290; Iron 0.304; Lead 0.196; Tin 0.060; Antimony 0.004; Silver 0.003; Arsenic 0.001; Bismuth 0.0003; Barium 0.0003; Manganese 0.0003; Gold 0.000009.
Base: Copper 59.384; Zinc 30.240; Lead 5.933; Iron 2.758; Tin 1.633; Silver 0.031; Manganese 0.008; Antimony 0.003; Barium 0.003; Arsenic 0.003; Gold 0.00008.

(See Color Plate 2)

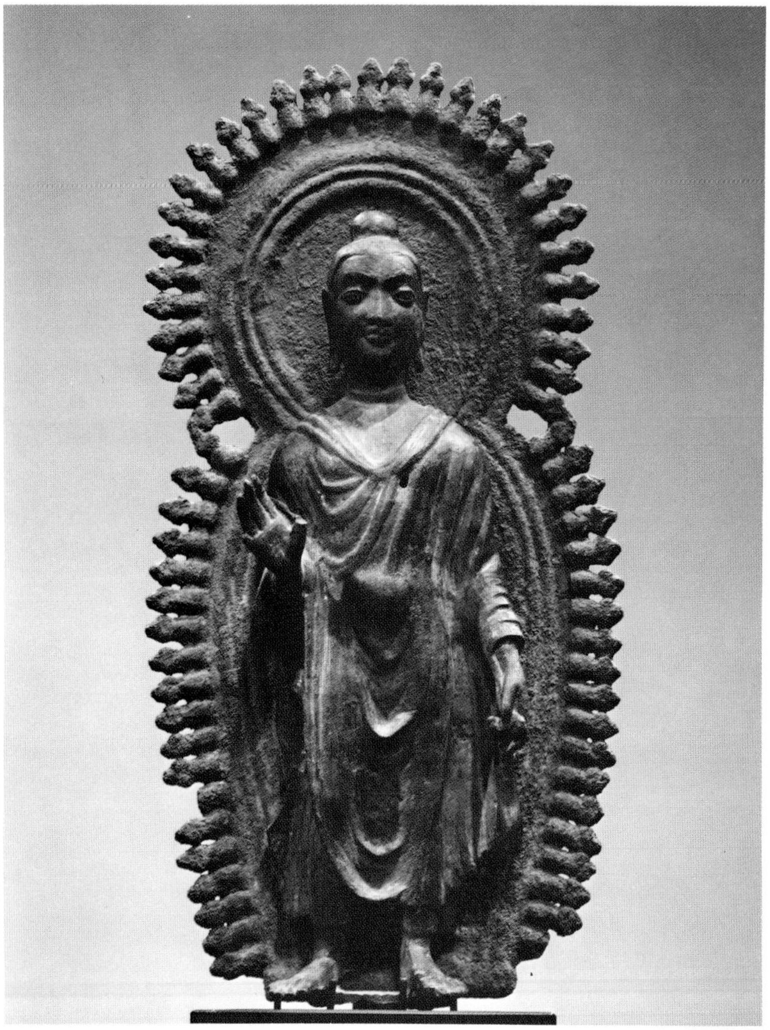

Pl. 4
Buddha Plaque
Embossed copper sheet
Afghanistan
Sixth-seventh century
Diameter 4.1 cm
The Brooklyn Museum. Lent by Dr. and Mrs. Robert Eisenberg. (L79.42.)

Despite the small size of the image, the Buddha figure conforms stylistically to other images from Afghanistan dating from the sixth to seventh centuries. The rather wide proportions of the neck, shoulders, and torso, the incised folds of the robe, and the rayed *mandorla* may be compared to architectural sculpture from Kāpiśa and wall paintings from the Hindu Kush. The bevelled edge indicates that the medallion was designed to be set into another component, perhaps a frame. Perhaps the image had been worn as an amulet.

Previously published: (von Schroeder 1981:78, fig. 3A).

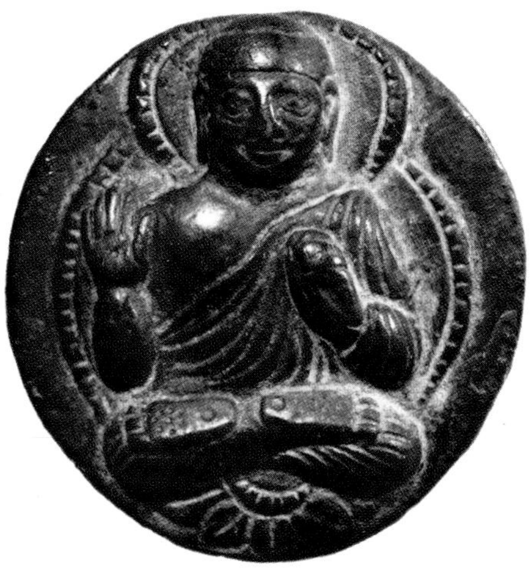

Pl. 3
Buddha Śākyamuni
Bronze
Sahri-Bahlol, Pakistan
Sixth-seventh century
H. 29.2 cm
The Metropolitan Museum of Art, New York. Edith Perry Chapman Fund, 1948. (48.66.)

This standing figure of Śākyamuni with combined halo and vesica belongs to a small group of standing bronze Buddha images from northwest Pakistan which, on stylistic grounds, is datable to the sixth-eighth centuries (see plates in von Schroeder 1981:72–73). While earlier scholarship dated this figure to the third-fourth century, more recently Barrett, followed by others, related its decorative motifs to post-Gandhāran art. The radiated halo and vesica with bead borders on the inner and outer edges may be compared to stucco forms from Cave G, Bāmiyān, datable to the late seventh century.

The heart-shaped ends of the drapery under the raised arm of the Buddha may be compared to similar forms from both the "Big Buddha" (53 m.) at Bāmiyān, and images from Tepe Sardār, Ghaznī. Other formal features which suggest a post-Gandhāran date are the rather simple yet still seminaturalistic treatment of the monastic robes and the deep V-necked collar. Both this image and two other similar bronzes appeared in the west at about the same time and were said to have been found at the partially excavated complex of Sahri-Bahlol which consisted of a monastery and fortified town. Fragments of marble Hindu sculpture and Śāhī coins suggest continuous operation until the tenth century A.D. At some time during the end of this period, the Buddhist monastery was abandoned and part of it was used as a Hindu temple. (ASI 1911–1912:115–119) The rather considerable evidence from this site needs to be carefully reevaluated in light of the large quantity of Śāhī marble sculpture which has only recently become known from Afghanistan and Pakistan.

It would appear that the Metropolitan Museum Buddha from northwest Pakistan and the Kreitman Buddha (Pl. 1) from Kāpiśa, in eastern Afghanistan, are both characterized by an international Buddhist style datable from the sixth to eighth centuries which was used from the Hindu Kush to Kashmir and which was contemporaneous with the first phase of Hindu sculpture from the same region. (Pls. 21–23)
Eve Dambra

Previously published: (Barrett 1960:fig. 30; Rowland 1963:no. 5; Hallade 1968:168, pl.128; Rowland 1970:143, pl. 86A; Lerner 1975:no. 1, pl. 1; von Schroeder 1981:72–73; 80–81, fig. 4A).

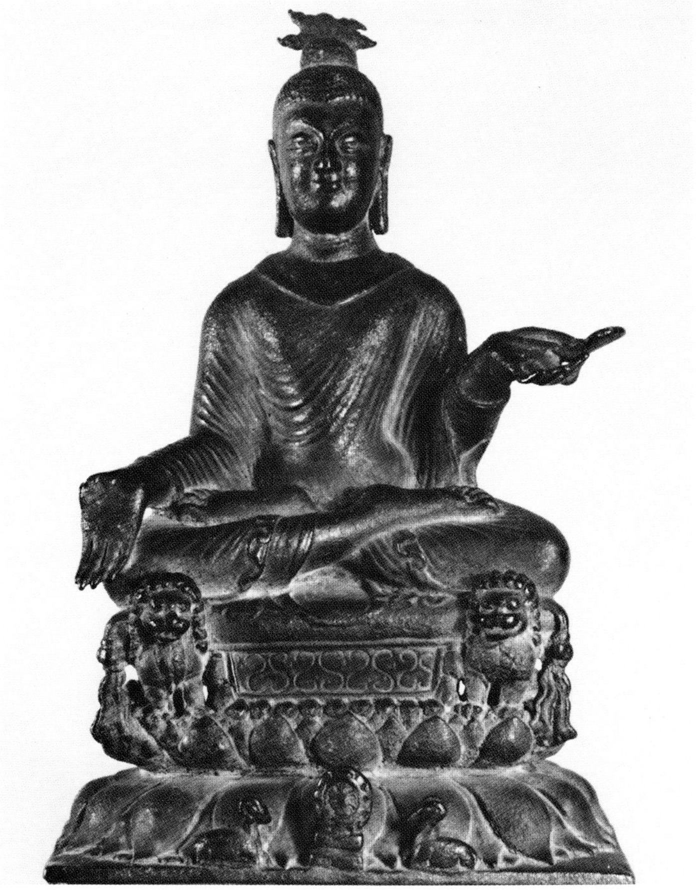

Pl. 5
Buddha
Bronze
Pakistan
Seventh century
H. 22.2 cm
Professor Samuel Eilenberg

The flowing incised folds of the Buddha's monastic robe merge with the incised petals of the lotus throne. The hair, arranged in incised rows of U-shaped curls, echoes the U-shaped pattern of the cloth folds across the chest. The hair on the back of the head is arranged in a U-shaped pattern as well—a mannerism also found in the sixth century Buddha from Kāpiśa (Pl. 2). This hairstyle also appears in a rock cut Tang-period Buddha from northern Pakistan (Fig. 5). There is a harmonious symmetry to the figure, both in the proportions of the figure and the throne, and in the incised lines which seem to flow across the surface of the image. This use of incised decor, and the slanted eyes, high cheekbones, and full lips relate this Buddha to the Ellsworth Avalokiteśvara (Pl. 15).

Previously published: (Lerner 1975:no. 6; Pal 1975b:no. 83; von Schroeder 1981:82, fig. 5F).

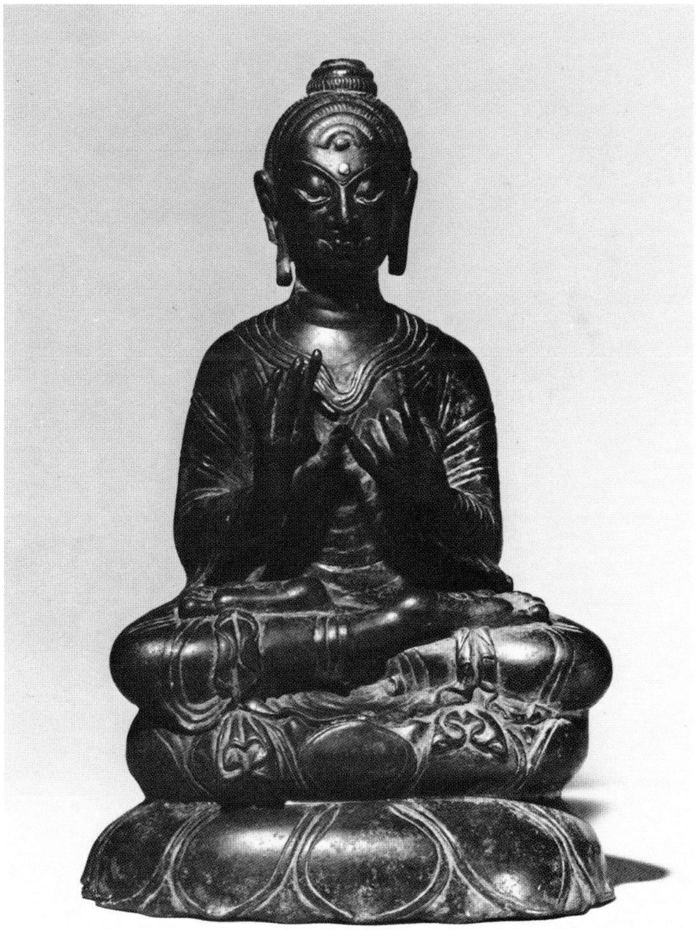

Pl. 6
Seated Buddha (not exhibited in Los Angeles)
Bronze
Afghanistan or Pakistan
Ninth century
H. 23.1 × W. 15 × D. 10 cm
Trustees of the British Museum, London. Gift of Louis Clark, Esq. (1957.2.12.1.)

At the beginning of the century, when this image was acquired from a Peshawar dealer, it was said that it had actually been found near the Helmand River, which flows from the Hindu Kush in a southwest direction towards Iran. The style of the Buddha figure permits an attribution to Afghanistan, but the style of the lotus throne also relates to the sculptures which are usually attributed to Pakistan. The unusual depiction of the lions is used with a Maitreya figure (also found near the Helmand River) in the British Museum. This image shares significant stylistic and iconographic features with the Buddha in the Ellsworth collection (Pl. 7).

Previously published: (Barrett 1962:37, pl. 33.3–4; Pal 1975b:no. 73; Snellgrove 1978:fig. 259; von Schroeder 1981:94, fig. 11E).

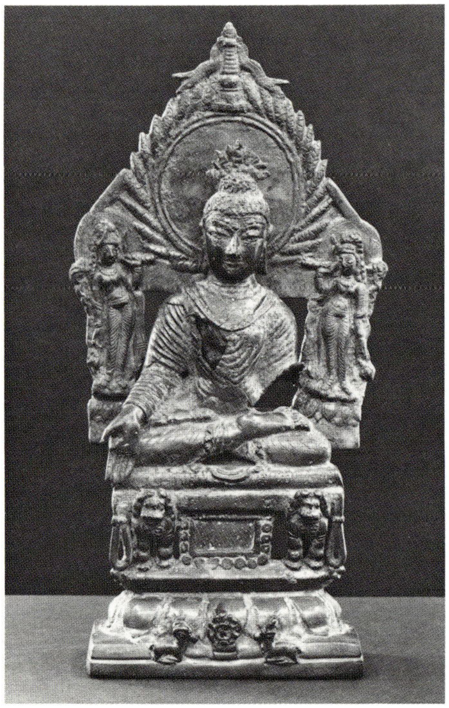

Pl. 7
Buddha with Female Attendants
Bronze
Swat Valley
Seventh-eighth century
H. 20.3 cm
Robert H. Ellsworth Limited

The Buddha is seated cross-legged on a lion throne which is supported by a single lotus pedestal, in front of which is a wheel flanked by two animals—a deer and an ibex. The Buddha's right hand is held in the gesture of charity, while the missing left hand would probably have held the folds of his garment in the same manner as is seen in a similar piece from the British Museum (Pl. 6). A strange, flame-like protuberance surmounts his *uṣṇīṣa* (the cranial bump). On the aureole fixed to a lug on the Buddha's back are included two female divinities holding ceremonial fly-whisks, a circular halo fringed with leaf-like elements, and a tiny *stūpa* with fluttering scarfs which tops the composition. Although it is possible that the easily removable aureole belonged originally to some other image, there is also much evidence to suggest that the two parts do belong together, such as great similarities in modelling, style and general craftsmanship, as well as the (visually) apparent closeness of the metal composition of the bronze used for each component.

That this is a rather provincial image is suggested by its relatively simple or crude craftsmanship: details added *after* casting by incision, anatomical features not worked out very correctly or thoroughly, and great use of shorthand in many of the designs (such as the snail-shell curls represented simply as concave circles). Both the *varadā-mudra* and the lion throne are associated with Kaśyapa Buddha, but as this *mudrā* appears so frequently with seated Buddha images of this period, it seems unlikely that such a specific reference is intended.

The female deities which flank the Buddha, albeit secondarily from their position on the aureole, are another perplexing item. In the art of historical northwest India, the Buddha is rarely represented as being flanked by female figures. An example of such a configuration in later art is found at Ta-pho Monastery, Spiti, where a statue of Amitābha Buddha is flanked by both clay Bodhisattvas and female figures which are painted on the wall beside the Bodhisattvas. The female deities here each stand on a lotus base, are provided with halos, elaborate crowns and incised *dhotis*, and a gently swaying pose. Each diety carries in her hand a *camara* or ceremonial fly-whisk.

Another peculiar detail occurs on the base, in the tiny composition which represents the occasion when Gautama Buddha delivered his first sermon at Sarnath—the "Turning of the Wheel of the Law"—usually symbolized by the wheel flanked by deer or antelope. Here, however, an ibex or mountain goat replaces the deer on our left, as can be ascertained from the clearly differentiated horn shapes of the two animals.

The ibex, or mountain goat, is often identified or associated with the gods and godlings of various local myths and ancient cults in the mountains of historical northwest India. Chitrali folklore is full of references to the ibex, such as that they are the cattle of the fairies or that fairies sometimes appear in the guise of an ibex and will punish the hunter who would fire at them. The Kafirs of the Hindu Kush also consider the mountain goat sacred to their female hunting deities. The myths and cults of the Dardic people associate this peak-dweller with the godlings of their pantheon. And there exists a cult of a goddess worshipped by hunters, the traces of which are still found from Gilgit to Swat (Jettmar 1975; Tucci 1963:153), in which this deity is believed to sometimes appear in the form of a she-ibex, and to require sacrifice of an ibex to herself. It is a cult restricted to women, and surely represents a survival of ancient ideas. Support for the animal's early importance comes also in the form of numerous rock carvings of ibexes found in northern Pakistan. In the cases known to me, the deities associated with the mountain goat are female. It is impossible to say if the function of the ibex and female divinities in local myths is related to their role in this Buddhist image. The impact of Hindu iconography on Buddhist iconography is well-known. However, too little is known about the impact of local belief systems on Mahāyāna iconography in Pakistan.
Barbara Paulson

Previously published: (Pal 1975b:no. 75; von Schroeder 1981:96–97, fig. 12E).

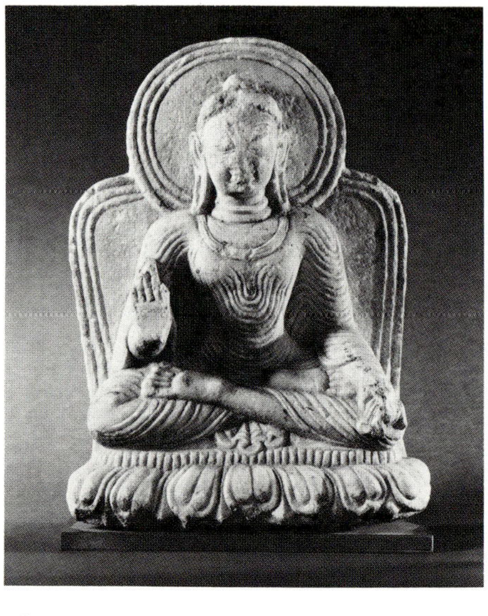

Pl. 8
Seated Buddha
White limestone
Pakistan
Ninth century
H. 44.5 cm
Los Angeles County Museum of Art. Anonymous gift. (M.78.135.)

The worship of Hindu gods increased in Afghanistan and Pakistan from the seventh century to the tenth century. These cult images were made in white limestone, usually marble. This figure is one of the few Buddhist images made in white stone. The large, rather coarse facial features are characteristic of Hindu Śāhī images from ninth century Pakistan (see Pl. 24). The shape of the *mandorla* also suggests a ninth or tenth century date. The posture, *mudrā* and dress of the figure are all characteristic of the Buddha image, although examples where the left leg is placed over the right are rare in northwest India at this time and found only infrequently in Central Asia. This may be one of a small group of Buddha images dating from this period in Pakistan. See also Fig. 3.

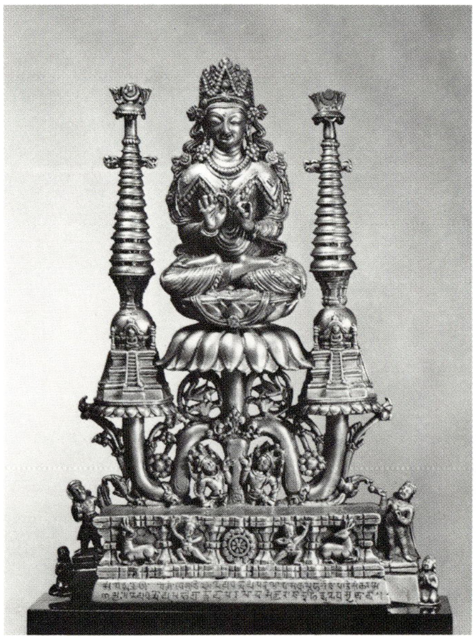

Pl. 9
Jeweled Śākyamuni (the Consecration of Śākyamuni)
Brass
Northern Pakistan (Gilgit?)
Eighth-early ninth century
H. 34.29 cm
The Asia Society: The Mr. and Mrs. John D. Rockefeller 3rd Collection (1979.44)
Inscription: "This is the pious gift of the devout Sankarasena, the great lord of the elephant brigade, and of the pure-minded and pious princess Devaśriya made in the year 3 or 8" (Pal 1975:106).

This extremely fine sculpture, a product of Kashmiri artistic traditions, may be attributed to eighth century northern Pakistan, perhaps Gilgit. This figure, a piece from the Norton Simon collection and the Ellsworth Buddha (Pl. 10) can be considered to form a group. Although this group has been attributed to Kashmir it has been suggested that the combination of Swat and Kashmiri stylistic features with Central Asian ornamentation may represent the work of a specific, and still unidentified school which flourished in the valleys of the western Himalayas (including those under Śāhī rule) (von Schroeder 1981:109). On the basis of the evidence obtained from the inscription on the Ellsworth bronze (Pl. 10), and the fact that the iconographic configuration found here appears limited to regions under the influence of Śāhī rulers, I have tentatively attributed these bronzes to a regional workshop under Kashmiri influence, perhaps in Gilgit. Such an attribution would accord well with the nature of artistic activity and the convergence of cultural influences in northern Pakistan during the eighth century (Jettmar 1980). The axis of the composition is a crowned Śākyamuni seated on a lotus supported by *nāga* kings emerging from the water. The jeweled and fringed three-pointed cape and shoulder effulgences which distinguish this image from other jeweled Buddha images (Pl. 10) assist us in providing a cultural and geographic context for the image. In addition to the five-pointed crown with side rosettes and long, flowing streamers, he wears long earrings, necklace and bracelets, and displays the teaching *mudrā*. Two smaller lotuses, each supporting a tall *stūpa*, spring from the main stem. The drum of each *stūpa*, known as the "descent from heaven" type (Fig. 9) is adorned by Buddhas seated under an arch crowned with crescents and floating streamers. On the base are male and female donors who wear Central Asian dress: the man carries a wreath; the woman, an incense burner. This configuration is the most complete example of a composition which appears earlier in the Hindu Kush in the famous sculptural group from Fondukistan (Niche D), dated circa 700 A.D. (Klimburg-Salter in press). I have proposed elsewhere that this image in the art of the Hindu Kush represents the consecration (*abhiṣeka*) of Śākyamuni in the Tuṣita Heaven (Klimburg-Salter in press). Most of the distinctive iconographic features—the crowned Buddha wearing a jeweled and fringed cape and having shoulder effulgences, the royal dress such as the woman's cape and the man's lapelled tunic and arms—appear in Bāmiyān (painting Niche 38m, Buddha; Ill. 1). However, it is only at Fondukistan that this variant of the jeweled Buddha appears seated on a lotus supported by *nāgas*, forming part of a pictorial composition with the Buddhas of the past and present (here symbolized by the *stūpas* to either side of Śākyamuni). A stylized form of this composition—rocky pedestal on lotus growing from a long stem and topped by a double-lotus base supporting a seated Śākyamuni—also appears in the portable wooden shrine from Central Asia (Pl. 54). A similar conjunction of symbolic forms may originally have been associated with the standing jeweled Buddha image in Tepe Sardār, Ghaznī.

This iconographic variant of the jeweled Buddha, which occurs only in historical northwest India, appears in all of the sites of the Hindu Kuṣh and appears to have originated there. The latest known examples are found in tenth-century Kashmiri bronze sculptures. This theme is particularly popular in the eighth century where it occurs in a stone sculpture from Parihāspura, Kashmir and a rock carving from the Gilgit Agency (Fig. 6), near Chilas, where it borders the Indus river south of the Gilgit-Karakoram range. Other distinctive features, such as the pedestal base with creatures wedged into the rock niches, appear in contemporaneous bronzes like that in the Norton Simon Museum. This motif may also have been used in the clay architectural decoration of chapels 23 and 37 Tepe Sardār (Taddei 1978:47–49).

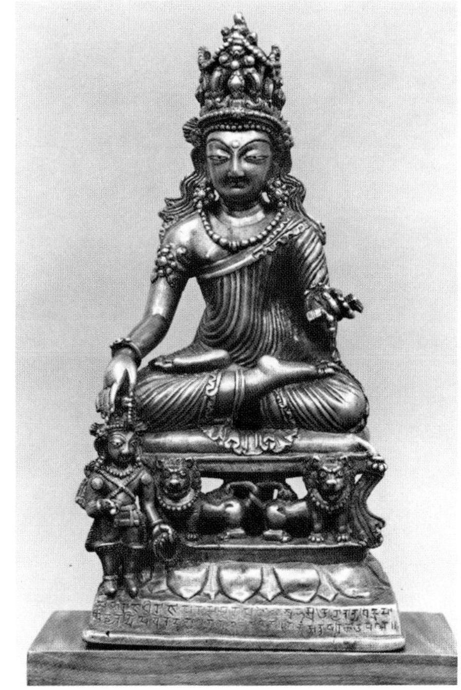

Pl. 10
Buddha Akṣobhya
Brass
Pedestal inscription states that in the year of an unknown era, the image was commissioned by King Nandi-Vikramāditya.
North Pakistan, Gilgit
Eighth century, perhaps 715 A.D.
H. 29.9 cm
Robert H. Ellsworth Limited

As one of the few bronze sculptures with an historical inscription, this example is particularly important because it contains both a date and the name of a king who might be identifiable from other historical sources. A new reading of the inscription (Jettmar 1980:190–91) gives 715 A.D. as the date of the donation of the bronze (615 A.D. is apparently also possible but less likely). The king's name, Nandi Vikramāditya, may indicate that he was Śrīdeva Śāhī Surendra Vikramāditya Nanda or, at least, that he was also a member of the Śāhī dynasty who ruled in the Gilgit region. The eighth century was a period of considerable economic and artistic activity in northern Pakistan (Jettmar 1980:191–194) and such a sophisticated image combining Kashmiri workmanship with secular and religious themes prevalent in Swat and Central Asia would seem to well express the cultural diversity of the time. Metal analysis and other technical studies should help us determine if there was an independent workshop in Gilgit or if this piece was produced in Kashmir for Gilgit patrons.

When a critical study of the newly discovered inscriptions is completed, it may be possible to define more precisely the patronage and production of art in the regions adjacent to, and under the influence of, Kashmiri artistic culture. This extraordinary body of material only recently uncovered along the trade routes of northern Pakistan consists of about 500 inscriptions in Kharosthi, Brahmī, Soghdian, Tibetan and even Chinese, in addition to innumerable Buddhist and non-Buddhist rock engravings (Jettmar 1977,1979,1980) (Figs. 2–6a).

At the present time, on the basis of the inscription, as well as the evidence of the other two sculptures which are related to this sculpture (Pl.9 and the Buddha image in the Norton Simon museum), we can tentatively suggest that this image represents a regional style of northern Pakistan. The fact that all three images depict donors dressed in the Turkic fashion of the period (Ill. 1) indicates that these donors probably belonged to the Śāhī elite ruling in one of the small principalities (Gilgit or Baltistan) which were intimately related to the history and culture of eastern Afghanistan, Kashmir and Ladakh.

Previously published: (Pal 1973a:Fig. 8; Pal 1975b:No. 31; Pal 1978a:No. 26; von Schroeder 1981:109,118–119,Fig.16c).

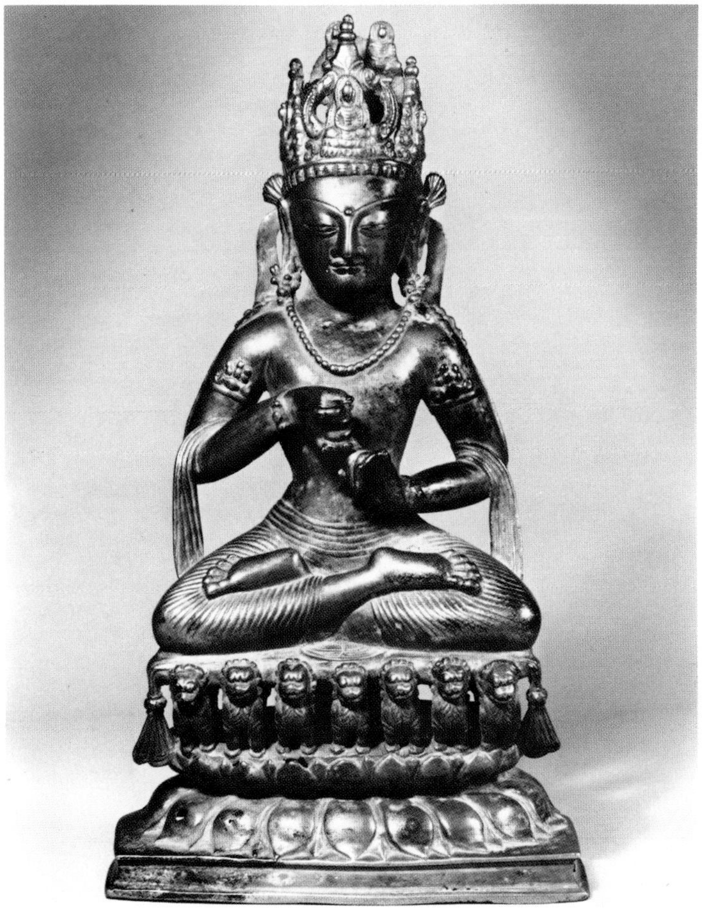

Pl. 11
Vairocana
Bronze
Northern Pakistan, perhaps Gilgit
Ca. ninth century
H. 33.2 cm
Professor Samuel Eilenberg

This image may be an early example of one of the Five Buddhas (Jina or Tathāgata) from historical northwest India. The arrangement of the crown with five Buddhas, the simplified Bodhisattva garments, and the figure style relate this Vairocana to depictions of the Five Buddhas from Dunhuang (Pls. 66, 67, 68). Stylistic features connect this image to the earlier bronze sculptures from Swat (the throne), and to the few sculptures attributable to Gilgit (the figure style and crown) (Pl. 10).

Previously published: (von Schroeder 1981:94–95, figs. 11G, 11I).

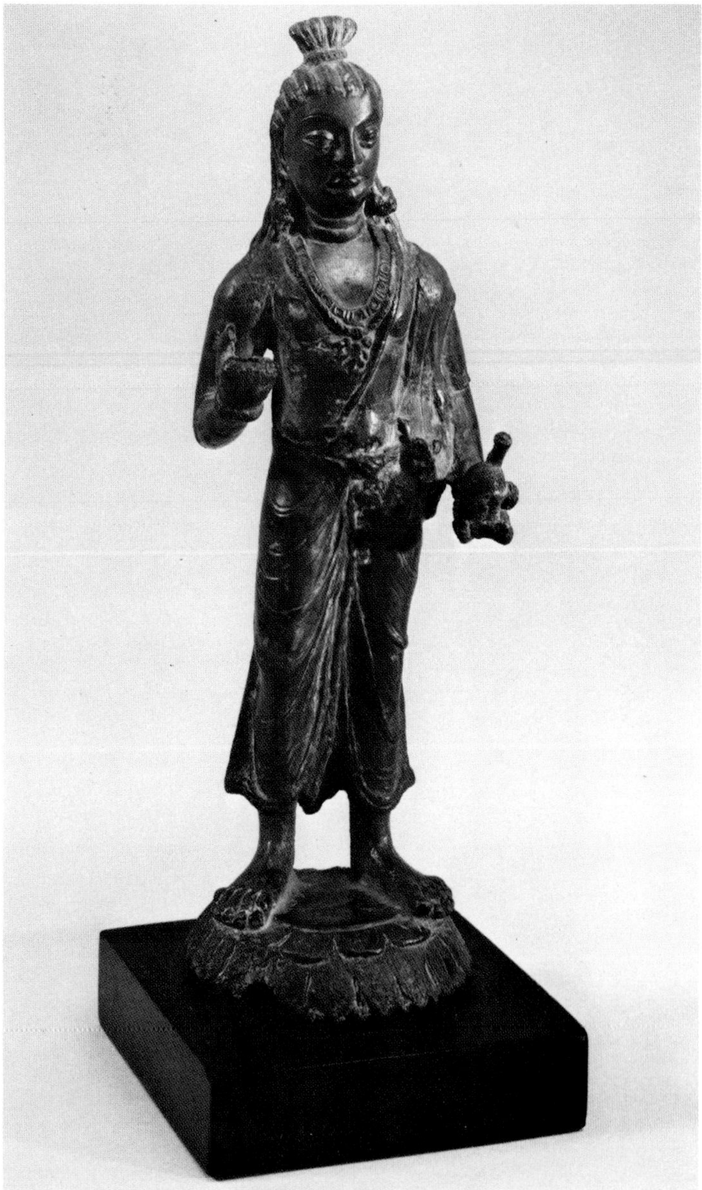

Pl. 12
Maitreya
Bronze
Pakistan
Fifth-sixth century
H. 26.7 cm
Los Angeles County Museum of Art. Nasli and Alice Heeramaneck Collection, Museum Associates Purchase. (M.69.15.2.)

Although considered unusual within the sculptural tradition of historical northwest India, this Maitreya figure can be compared to sixth and seventh century wall paintings from Kizil (Metropolitan Museum 1982,pl. 22). The style of the *dhotī* (skirt), the top knot, and the treatment of the figure are all found in Bodhisattva images from the Cave of the Musicians, to cite only one example. The mannerism of holding the water-pot in the palm of the left hand is also found in the Maitreya image painted in the center of the dome from Kakrak, Afghanistan, ca. late seventh century. (Klimburg-Salter in press). The right hand *mudrā* is also found in another early Maitreya figure from Swat (see Pl. 14). Both the characteristic black metal and the facial features suggest that this image was made in Swat.

Previously published: (Dohanian 1961:fig. 10; Glynn 1972:fig. 4; Pal 1973a:fig.10; Pal 1975b:no.38; Bhattacharya 1980:106, pl. VI.7; von Schroeder 1981:77–79, fig.3G).

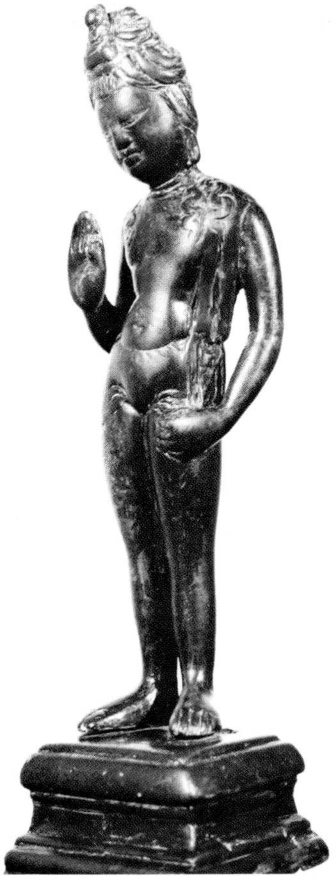

Pl. 13
Avalokiteśvara or Padmapāṇi
Brass
Northern Pakistan
Seventh-eighth century
H. 15.88 cm
Anonymous loan

This small delicate statue with its soft contours and unadorned youthful body combines stylistic influences of the Sarnath sixth century Gupta style—such as the treatment of the torso and the hair piled in loops cascading from the chignon—with somewhat sinicized features, such as the fleshy face, eyes with epicanthal folds, the slouch of the belly and the slight forward tilt of the head and shoulder. As with the Avalokiteśvara in Pl. 15, this Padmapāṇi wears no jewelry and even the image of Amitābha is not part of a crown but rather rests against the chignon. There appears to originally have been a stalk held in the left hand. This piece was said to have been found in Afghanistan and has been attributed to the Hindu Kush (von Schroeder 1981:72). Although other bronzes have also been found in Afghanistan (Pls. 2,6,25), their styles are so diverse and their numbers so limited that it is impossible at this point to define a distinctive style of Buddhist bronzes from Afghanistan. Furthermore, no other bronze is known to me which compares stylistically to this piece. Thus, an attribution to the Hindu Kush is only one of several possibilities. The blackish color of the image and the style of the base (although made of a very different alloy) as well as the contemporary cultural context also suggest that this piece may originally have come from Swat. " . . . As Swat was in the very middle of the Chinese-Tibetan quarrels for the control of the main routes connecting Central Asia with Kashmir and Northern India, in a general way, it is clear that we have to look to Swat with other eyes. A region, by its very geographical situation open to all sorts of trade and cultural influences; a fact which explains its wealth documented by the immense number of religious settlements and its high culture testified by the archeological discoveries . . ." (Tucci 1977:85).

Previously published: (von Schroeder 1981:72, 82–83, fig. 5A).
Metal content of figure: Copper 56.626%; Tin .89%; Lead 29.097%; Zinc 12.515%; Bismuth .002%; Gold .0002%; Tellurium .027%; Antimony .005%; Indium .003%; Silver .051%; Selenium .0004%; Arsenic .018%; Nickel .02%; Cobalt .013%; Iron .707%; Manganese .004%; Calcium .01%; Potassium .01%.
Metal content of base: Copper 43.303%; Tin .561%; Lead 6.119%; Zinc 39.983%; Iron 9.48%.

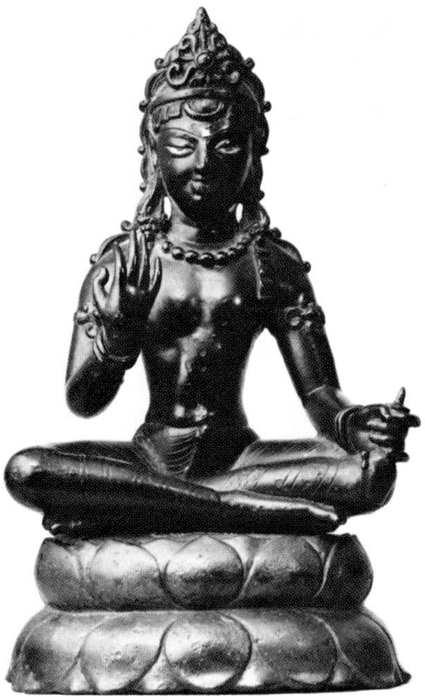

Pl. 14
Seated Maitreya
Bronze
Inscription on pedestal.
Pakistan
Seventh century
H. 18.1 cm
The Metropolitan Museum of Art, New York. Gift of Mr. and Mrs. Richard Benedek, 1978. (1978.536.)

The Bodhisattva Maitreya awaits his birth as the Buddha of the future in the inner court of the Tuṣita Heaven. Murals depicting this court as the northern paradise survive at Dunhuang. Paintings depicting the Bodhisattva Maitreya enthroned in the Tuṣita Heaven were popular in the sixth and seventh centuries in Kizil. Synoptic representations of this theme, which are derived from Kizil, were painted at all the sites of the Hindu Kush in the seventh and eighth centuries (Fig. 27). Sculpted representations were prominent in Kāpiśa in the fifth and sixth centuries A.D. In Japan, Maitreya remained important during the Nara period.

The worship of Amitābha and related deities such as Avalokiteśvara and his manifestations appears to have become more important in India and Central Asia from the seventh and eighth centuries.

This elegant sculpture has a glossy blue-black color. It integrates stylistic and iconographic elements from different sources while displaying typical seventh-century Swat features such as the simple double lotus throne with rounded petals, and the strictly frontal and symmetrical posture of the deity. The rounded modeling of the torso appears to derive from the Gupta-Sarnath school. Other features are more unusual; the manner of holding the water-pot and the single leaf crown also occurs in Japanese art. A whimsical version of this crown is also found at Fondukistan.

Previously published: (von Schroeder 1981:74, 82–83, fig. 5G).

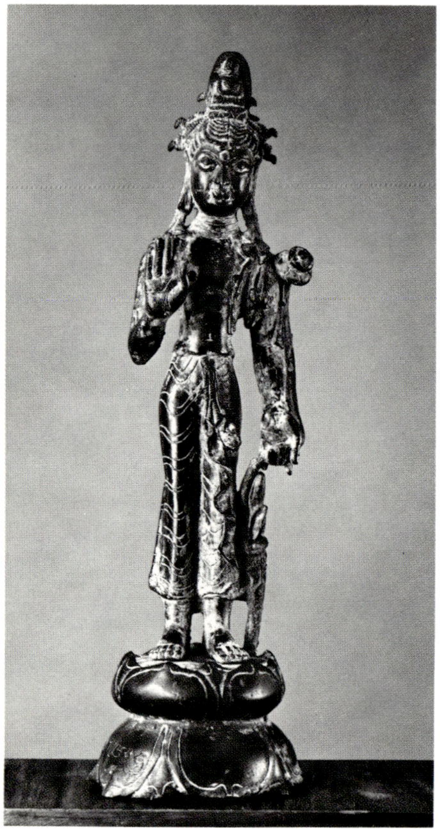

Pl. 15
Avalokiteśvara
Bronze
Pakistan
Seventh-eighth century
H. 29.2 cm
Robert H. Ellsworth Limited

Partly due to its "blackish" color, this sculpture of Avalokiteśvara has been attributed to Pakistan (Pal 1975:Fig.82). The unusual stylistic features distinguish this image from the earlier Gandhāran sculptures (Pl. 3) which were characterized by relatively broad shoulders on an articulated torso, swelling hips, and somewhat squarish faces with straight noses and regular features. This figure, in contrast, is quite slender with sloping shoulders, narrow hips and a relatively flat torso with little modeling. The face is also distinctive with its puffy cheeks and round bulging eyelids which curve upwards, and full lower lip. This new figure style occurred at a time when new iconographic themes, particularly associated with esoteric Buddhism, also appear. A small group of images, all of which represent either Avalokiteśvara or Maitreya, belong to this figural type. The Eilenberg Buddha (Pl. 5) has a similar treatment of the facial features, but a fuller figure style. The folds of the garment, the lotus petals, and the inscription are incised—features also found in Pl. 5. Another somewhat unusual feature is the total absence of jewelry: even the figure of Amitābha is not part of an elaborate crown, but rather rests against the unusual coiffure consisting of braid-like rows of hair. The Bodhisattva in Pl. 88, which is tentatively attributed to the eighth century and the western Himalayas, also wears no jewelry. Usually, although not always, Bodhisattva figures in historical northwest India are richly attired, while unadorned figures are found in the art of Central and Southeast Asia. The curious stippling of the lotus stalk is also a feature more frequently found in bronzes from northeast India.

Despite these unusual characteristics, however, the style of the figure, and particularly the somewhat Chinese features, can be related to a small group of bronzes generally attributed to the western Himalayas during the seventh and eighth centuries. These new stylistic trends have been identified in other media and sites as well, such as the clay sculptures from Fondukistan and the limestone reliefs from *Stūpa* A near Pandrethan. A relationship between these figures and the sandstone sculpture from Tianlongshan (Shanxi, 703–11 A.D.) has been established (Rhie 1974–75). The sculptures from Fondukistan and Pandrethan both appear to date from the first quarter of the eighth century (Goetz 1969; Klimburg-Salter in press). It has been suggested that the Ellsworth image is contemporaneous and that they derive from a common source (Spiro 1980, unpublished manuscript). This source may be either Indian or Chinese Central Asian, and is as yet unidentified. This image is one of several in this exhibition which have syncretic stylistic or iconographic features. Many of these objects serve to draw our attention to exchange between northern India, the Himalayas, and Chinese Central Asia during the seventh and eighth centuries. The manner in which this exchange occurred and the resulting dialogue which emerged in art and literature cannot yet be defined.

Previously published: (Pal 1975:no.210; Pal 1978a:no. 21; von Schroeder 1981:82–83, fig. 5C).

Pl. 17
Seated Bodhisattva
Limestone
Swat Valley, Pakistan
Seventh-eighth century
H. 78.7 × 48.3 × 10.8 cm
Mr. and Mrs. Robert L. Poster

This rock-cut image was carved into the rocks bordering the trade routes connecting Pakistan with Central Asia. A similar rock-cut image was photographed by Tucci on the road from Mingora to Kalam (Tucci 1958:295, fig. 10). The pioneering researches by Tucci and Stein (1942) have now been followed by a full-scale field survey to record and analyze these rock-cut engravings and sculptures (see bibliography under Jettmar) (Figs. 2–6a). Several of these images can be related to metal sculpture. Both the hairstyle and basket-like seat of this Avalokiteśvara are also found in bronze Kashmiri images of the eighth century (Pl. 28). Rock-cut sculptures bordering the trade routes appear to have been a phenomenon of the entire region from the Hindu Kush to Ladakh from the sixth to tenth centuries A.D. There are the colossal images, such as at Mulbek in Ladakh (Figs. 5 and 16), as well as the smaller scale images such as this Avalokiteśvara and the one shown in Pl. 18. The smaller scale images, which are more numerous, are generally sculpted in low relief, as the image shown on, or merely incised in the rock surface (Figs. 6, 6a). This custom of marking the route with rock-cut talismans is preserved today throughout the Himalayas. Rocks engraved with *mantras* and mystic signs are frequently found as part of stone prayer walls (*maṇi* walls). The earliest examples are the collossal Buddhas from Bāmiyān but these are actually stucco on a rock, core and are almost carved in the round, they therefore constitute a fourth technical group.

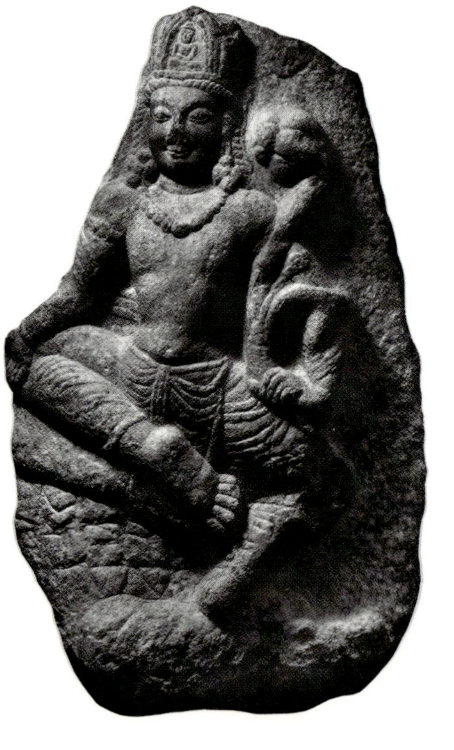

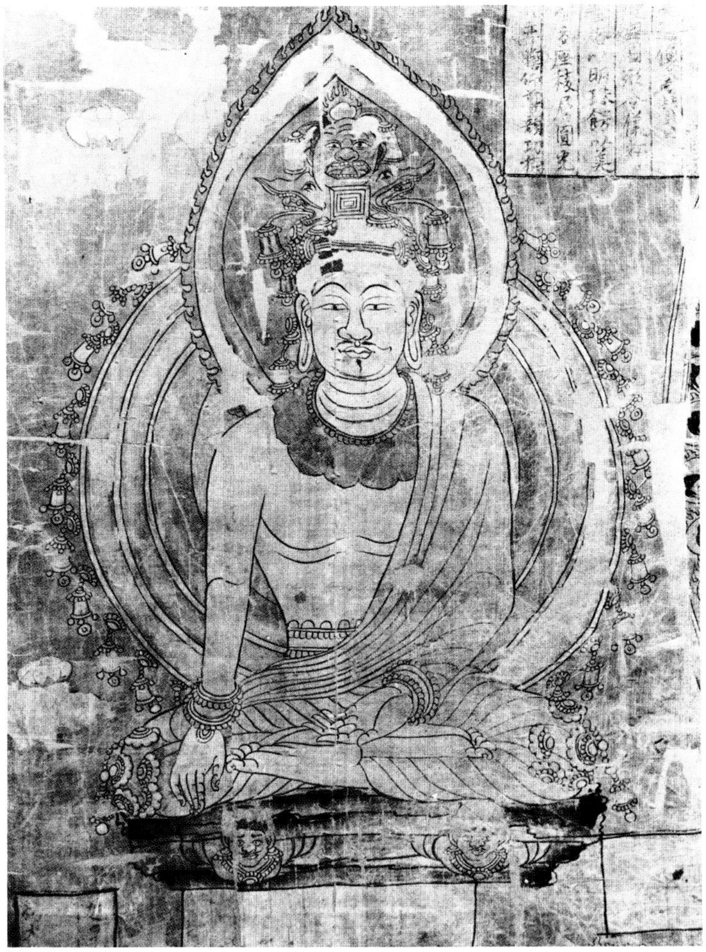

Pl. 16
Detail of Pl. 56
Iconographical Painting
Fragment of painting on silk
Dunhuang, Qianfodong
Seventh-eighth century
New Delhi National Museum

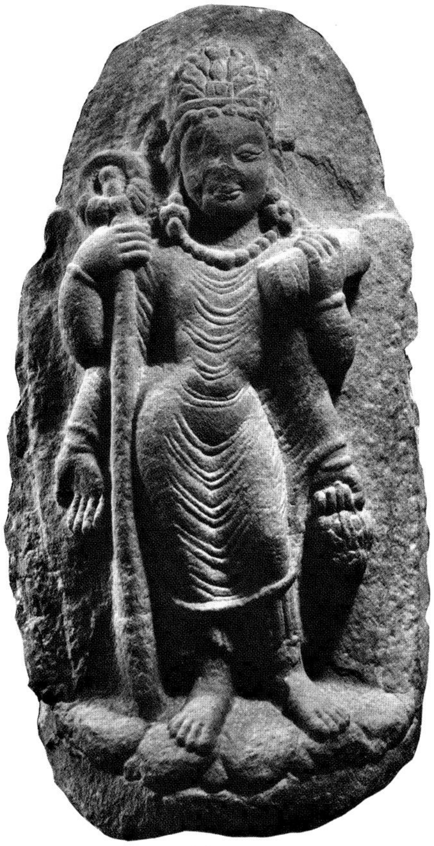

Pl. 18
Four-armed Brahmā
Limestone relief
Swat Valley, Pakistan
Seventh century
H. 72.4 × 43 × 20.3 cm (without frame)
H. 81.3 × 43.2 × 20.3 cm (with frame)
Shey Art Collection

The style of this unusual figure—the shape and features of the face, the Mediterranean-styled garment with symmetrical folds indicated by double incised lines and the slight relaxation of the figure—suggests a seventh century date for this limestone relief. This attribution is further confirmed by specific motifs such as the crown tied by a bow with streamers falling to each side of the head, the earrings, and hairstyle. The identification of the figure is problematic but it may represent Brahmā. (Unpublished paper by Nik Douglas.) A similar, although much worn, figure was photographed by Tucci in 1955 (Tucci 1958:307) and identified as Śiva by the *trisula* and a *damaru*. This appears to be a unique instance of a Hindu divinity among the many Buddhist divinities carved into cliffs bordering the trade routes of northern Pakistan. The attributes here are similar but the *trisula* is here a monk's staff and the upper left hand appears to carry a manuscript. The deity stands on a lotus.

The excavations at Tepe Sardār have demonstrated the syncretism of Hindu divinities with the Buddhist pantheon in northwest India, a phenomenon also well known in Central Asia. If this image is Brahmā, it might likewise have been seen as a Buddhist divinity, an interpretation recently proposed for the contemporaneous bronze image from the Indische Kunst Museum in West Berlin (Pal 1975:54). Four-armed divine images were rare in Pakistan at this time. The Hindu divinities among them typically wear Indian dress (Pl. 41). The monastic cloak draped in the heavy folds of the Gandhāran style and worn as shown here or covering only one shoulder, is usually associated with Buddhist figures. The latter fashion can be seen in Pl. 48. In another painting similar to the Smithsonian example, the walking monk carries the same type of staff represented here.

Pl. 19
Vajradharma Lokeśvara
Bronze
Swat Valley, Pakistan
Ninth century
H. 39.4 cm
The Metropolitan Museum of Art, New York. Gift of Mrs. John D. Rockefeller, Jr., 1942. 42.25.20.

This image of Vajradharma Lokeśvara is one of the largest and earliest known tantric images. As with most tantric figures of this period, the iconography deviates slightly from extant textual descriptions. The god is seated in meditation on a lotus throne supported by peacocks; he gently opens a lotus bud with his two lower hands. The seated image of Amitābha in his crown identifies him as a manifestation of Avalokiteśvara. Unusual are the two additional hands holding a bow and arrow—attributes of the Buddhist god Mañjuśrī and the Hindu god of love, Kāma (Pal 1975:206).

Previously published: (Barrett 1962:39–40, pl. 28.16; Lerner 1975:no.8, pl. 7; Pal 1975b:no. 79; von Schroeder 1981:74–75, 94, fig.11B).

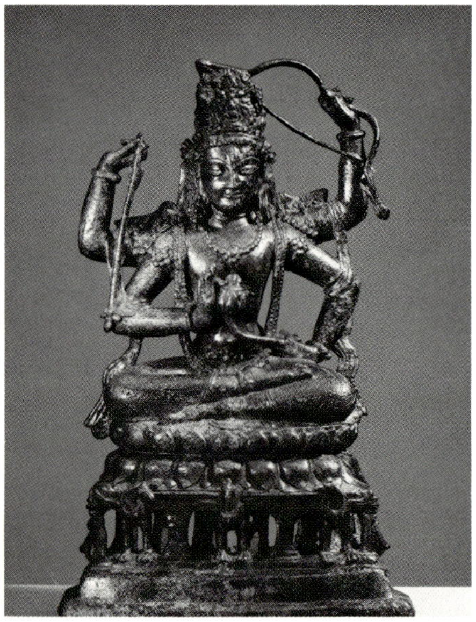

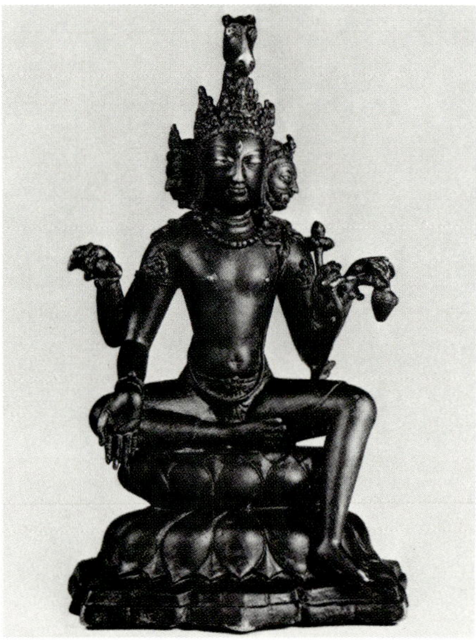

Pl. 20
Hayagrīva Lokeśvara
Bronze
Swat Valley, Pakistan
Eighth-ninth century
H. 21.2 cm
The St. Louis Art Museum. Gift of J. Lionberger Davis. (256:1955.)

According to the *Hayagrīvavidya* found among the famous Gilgit manuscript hoard (datable sixth-eighth century) recovered by Aurel Stein, the Hayagrīva has the following appearance: the center is Lokeśvara; on the right, Vajradhara; on the left, Avalokiteśvara; on the top is a horse-faced deity believed to be capable of destroying the evil effects of others' *mantras* (Dutt 1939–1953:vol.I, pp.61–62). Here the association with Avalokiteśvara is indicated by the presence of Amitābha seated in the crown. In his upper left hand he holds a *kamandalu*, in the lower left a lotus, the lower right is in *varadā-mudrā*, the upper right holds a *vajra*. Both the figure style and the combination lotus-throne with rock pedestal suggests an eighth-century date. Hayagrīva is frequently represented in paintings from both Dunhuang (Pl. 61) and Ta-pho.

Previously published: (Trubner 1950:87, no.143); Barrett 1962:fig.15; Art Institute of Chicago 1965:no.16; Museum of Art and Archaeology, University of Missouri 1969:46–47, fig.6; Pal 1975b:no.78; von Schroeder 1981:74, 92–93, fig.10F).

Pl. 21
Sūrya
Bronze
Pakistan
Seventh century
H. 13.33 cm
Professor Samuel Eilenberg

Textual sources give abundant evidence for the importance of Sun worship in historical northwest India during the Śāhī period. This is one of the few bronze sun gods known from the region. Both this image and the Sun God in the National Museum, New Delhi, wear the three-pointed, jewelled cape which may have been the coronation cape of the Śāhī dynasty (Klimburg-Salter in press) (Pl. 9). The flanking images of Daṇḍa and Piṅgala are badly eroded but they, like the main deity, appear to wear a Turkic style tunic and short dagger. The donor figures in Pls. 9–10 are dressed in similar fashion. These same Central Asian fashions are worn by the donors in the Bāmiyān painting (Ill. 1).

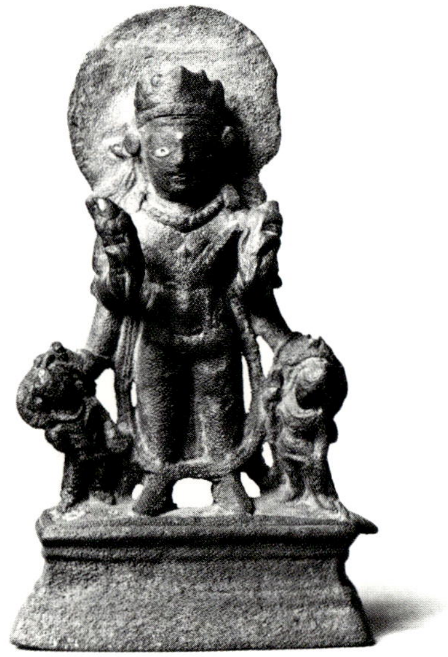

Pl. 23
Mahiśāsuramardinī
Yellow-white marble
Afghanistan
Eighth century
H. 26 × W. 35 × L. 17 cm
Property of Dottor Ferdinando Scorretti on loan to Museo Nazionale d'Arte Orientale, Roma

This figure is known as the "Scorretti Marble" (from the name of the man who acquired it in the Kabul Bazaar). This figure was at first thought to be related (Schlumberger 1955) to the Iranian god Mithra Tauroktonos. In recent decades, however, archaeologists have uncovered several Hindu shrines in Afghanistan dating to the Śāhī period. The goddess drags the bull's head back with her right hand while pinning him down with her foot and trident. The original composition of this image can be reconstructed on the basis of similar images, such as the Mahiśāsuramardinī white marble sculpture from Gardez now in the Kabul Museum and the seventh-century carving from Ellora (Goetz 1957:Fig. 2). The presence of the colossal clay image of Mahiśāsuramardinī in the Buddhist complex at Tepe Sardār demonstrates that this Śaivite goddess was integrated into Buddhist ritual practice in the Ghaznī region during the eighth century (Taddei 1978).

Previously published: (Schlumberger 1955; Goetz 1957:13–19; Taddei 1971; Taddei 1978a:137, fig.57).

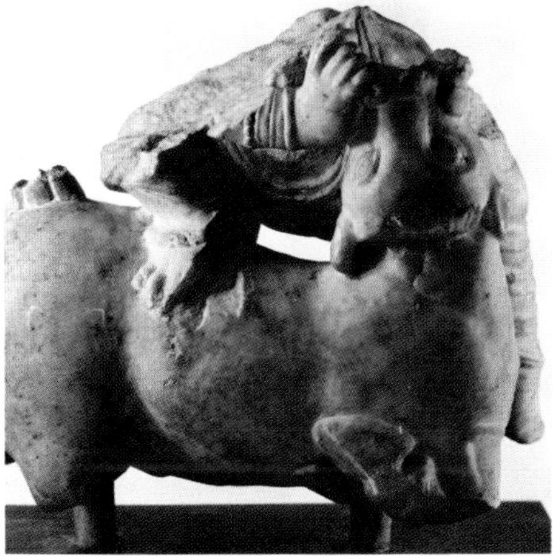

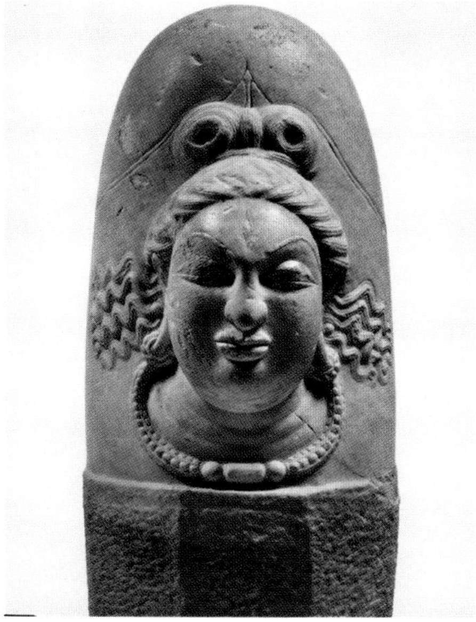

Pl. 24
Ekamukha-liṅga (One-faced *liṅga)*
White marble
Pakistan
Ninth century
H. 57 cm
Metropolitan Museum of Art, Rogers Fund, 1980 (1980.415)
(not exhibited in Los Angeles)

Śiva may be worshipped in various forms, but the *liṅga* or phallic emblem, prevails as his primary symbol. This monumental *liṅga* was once placed in the innermost sanctuary of a Śiva temple. A *liṅga* may be made of various types of material; however, many large-sized medieval examples from Afghanistan and Pakistan are sculpted in porous white stone. Śiva's face emerges from the polished upper portion of the *liṅga*. The lower, octagonal portion remains unworked, and was placed inside a square stone pedestal. Śiva's face as represented here is round and thick; the lips and eyes are bulging. The chin is doubled and a simple bead necklace adorns the thick neck. Four waves of hair, like serpents, flow outward onto the *liṅga*. On top of the head, the hair is combed and neatly spiraled into matted knots which are tied by another band of hair. The ears have elongated lobes pierced by earrings. The image has the characteristic iconographic features associated with Śiva—the crescent moon on the right knot of the hair and the vertical third eye on the forehead. A very similar *ekamukha-liṅga* was found in Pakistan and attributed to the region of the ancient Śāhī capital, Udabhāṇḍa, near modern Attock (Taddei 1962:288). Other *liṅgas* as well as marble sculptures with Hindu subjects have been found in that region. Both *ekamukha-liṅgas* are stylistically later than the white marble Hindu sculptures found in eastern Afghanistan which are dated for the most part to the seventh and eighth centuries (Kuwayama 1976) (see also Pl. 22). At present, material evidence for Turki and Hindu Śāhī culture comes primarily from random finds of Hindu sculptures. Careful art historical analysis of these objects combined with the limited archaeological documentation (Kuwayama 1972, 1974, 1975; Taddei 1968, 1971, 1972, 1978a, 1978b) is gradually allowing us to establish a relative chronology for the Hindu sculptures created under the Turki and Hindu Śāhī rulers.
Molly B. Alexander

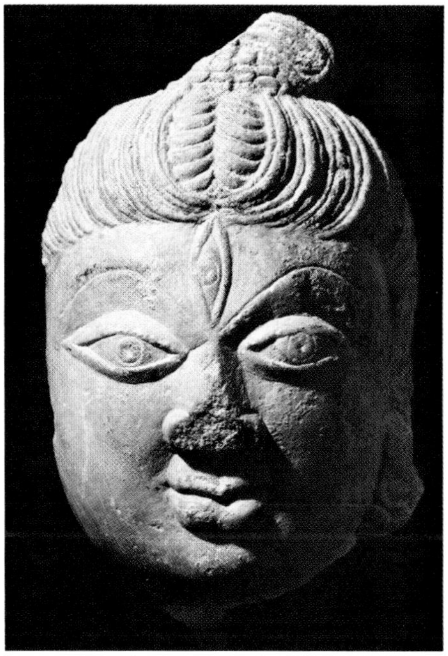

Pl. 22
Face from *Liṅga*
Marble
Afghanistan
Eighth century
H. 19.05 cm
Anonymous loan

The hairstyle and third eye identify this fragment as representing Śiva's face, originally part of an *ekamukha-liṅga* (one-faced *liṅga*) (Pl. 24). The shape of the head, eyes and mouth may be compared to the head of the great goddess Durgā excavated at Tepe Sardār, Ghaznī, Afghanistan and dated to the eighth century (Taddei 1978:Fig. 76–77). This hairstyle, however, is clearly associated with male figures. The hair parted in the center and then swept up on the sides into a topknot is found on other Śiva heads from this period.

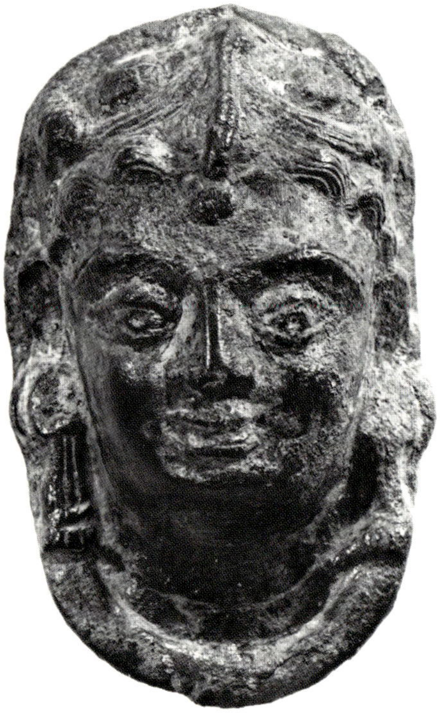

Pl. 25
Female Head
Bronze
Afghanistan
Ca. seventh century
H. 9 × 5.7 cm
The Brooklyn Museum. Lent by Dr. Bertram Schaffner (L80.47.1)

This small bronze repoussé plaque has a bevelled edge indicating that it was originally set into another element. It might have been placed in a frame in order to be worn as a broach or set into a larger metal container. The oval shape of the head and the regular Indo-European features are frequently encountered in Gandhāran art and also later such as at Tepe Sardar (Taddei 1978b:figs 232, 233). However, the headdress and hairstyle are closer to the feminine fashion of seventh and eighth century Hindu Śāhī sculpture. The hair, parted in the center, falls in even waves towards the back of the head. Placed on the crown of the head is a wreath, from the center of which hangs a chain; at the end of the chain, a circular ornament dangles, decorating the woman's forehead. Similar headdresses and coiffures are worn by Umā, in the sculpture depicting Umā-Maheśvara excavated at Tepe Sikandar, Kāpiśa, and by Durgā, in the sculpture excavated at the Buddhist complex of Tepe Sardār, Ghaznī. (Taddei 1978: pl. 77).

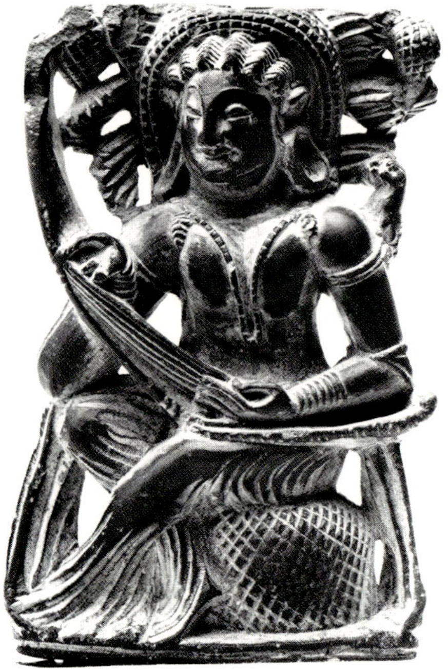

Pl. 26
Mirror Handle
Schist
Kashmir
Eighth century
H. 9.5 cm
Professor Samuel Eilenberg.

This stone mirror handle is an exquisite example of the little-known medieval Kashmiri decorative arts. The bottom of the lyre merges with the rounded arm of the chair and the overhanging branch in a smooth play of curving forms. The tightly bodiced gown and waved hairstyle is similar to that of the goddess Umā in Pl. 41.

Pl. 28
Seated Avalokiteśvara
Bronze
Tibetan inscription on petals
Kashmir
Eighth century
H. 20 cm
Mrs. John D. Rockefeller 3rd

The Bodhisattva sits in the posture of royal ease (*lalitāsana*), his right hand gracefully touching his cheek while the left holds a lotus. Both royal and divine images assume this pose in the wall paintings of Kizil. Only the sacred cord (*yajñopavita*) decorates the completely nude torso. The seated figure of Amitābha nestled against the crown identifies the Bodhisattva as belonging to the family of Avalokiteśvara. The soft, sweet expression in part results from the effacement of the facial features. Although this image has certain elements which relate it to Swat Valley sculpture (von Schroeder 1981: 84–85), the modeling and slightly longer proportions of the torso are more consistent with eighth-century Kashmiri sculpture. The presence of a Tibetan inscription suggests that at some indeterminate time this image was carried from Kashmir and reused in a Tibetan monastery.

Previously published: (Lee 1970:no.9; Pal 1975b:no.45; von Schroeder 1981:84–85, fig. 6I).

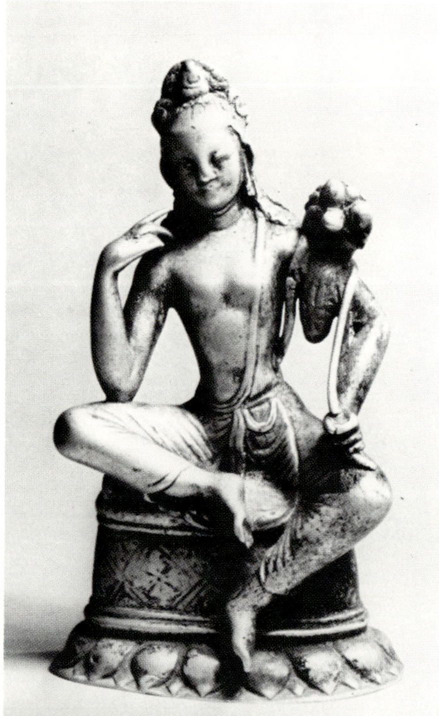

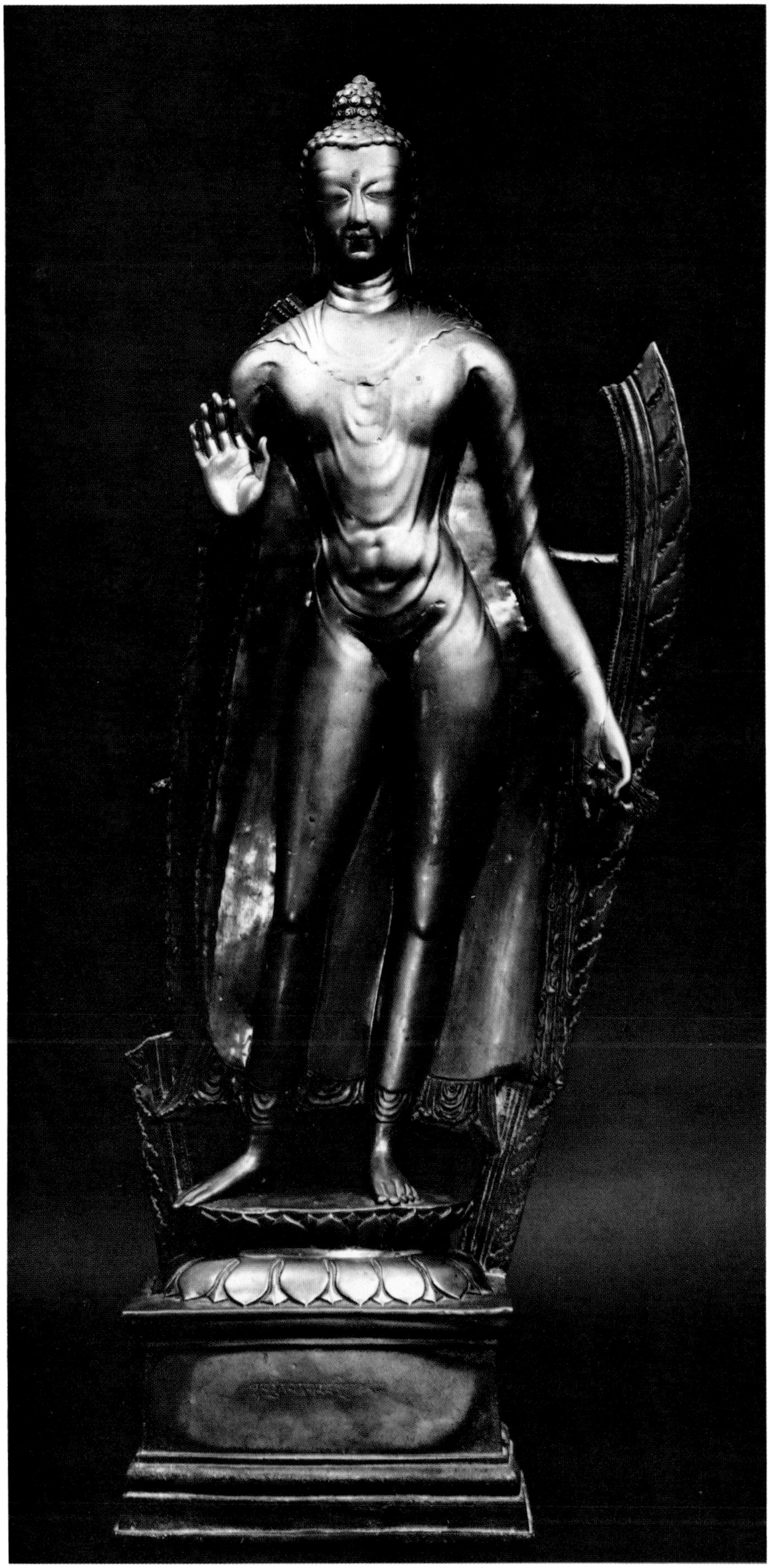

Pl. 27
Buddha (not exhibited in Los Angeles)
Brass
Tibetan inscription on pedestal: Lha-btsun-pa Na-ga-ra-dzahi thugs-dam "Priest (*Lha-btsun*) Nāgarāja's private image"
Kashmir
Tenth-eleventh century
H. 98.1 cm
The Cleveland Museum of Art. Purchase, John L. Severance Fund. (66.30.)

This imposing Buddha image is important not only for its extraordinary aesthetic appeal and technical accomplishment but because it is one of the few bronzes from historical northwest India with an inscription providing historical information. The long, elegant proportions of the figure and the clinging robe reflect the post-Gupta aesthetic of northern India while the undergarment follows the style of Central Asian images of the so-called Uḍḍiyāna type. Other details, such as the straited *mandorla*, the constricted double lotus pedestal, the high *uṣṇīśa* and the long second toe are also found in other tenth century sculptures from Kashmir. Medieval Kashmir's renowned metal technology is evidenced in the large size of this image. Even more impressive would have been such colossal images as the copper Buddha which Kalhāṇa reported had been enshrined in the royal foundation at Parihāspura. The Tibetan inscription on the pedestal "personal image of Lha-btsun Nāgarāja" has been interpreted by Heather Karmay (1975:29–30) as referring to Nāgarāja, the son of Lha-bla-ma Ye-śes'Öd who, like his father, had become a monk and who therefore would also have had the title Lha-btsun meaning god-monk. Lha-bla-ma Ye-śes'Öd was one of the kings of western Tibet (mNga'-ris) who, because of his devotion and patronage of Buddhism, was a significant figure in the period known as "the Second Propagation of Buddhism." Karmay has suggested that the inscription dates from the early eleventh century, a date which does not conflict with the style of the image. Although it seems clear that this image is the work of a Kashmiri artist, it is impossible to tell if it was fabricated in Kashmir or in one of the workshops in western Tibet where, in the eleventh century, Kashmiri artists participated in the fabrication of images and the decoration of many newly founded Buddhist temples.

Previously published: (Archaeology Vol. 19 (1966):279; Archives of Asian Art XXI, 1967-68:79, fig. 15; Burlington Magazine 1966:574, fig. 48; Bul. Cleveland Museum of Art 1966:250–251) Burton 1966:122–135, fig. 18; La Chronique des Arts 1966:8; Cleveland Museum of Art 1966:232; Lee 1967; Goetz 1969; Pal 1969:n. 41; Pal 1973a:745–746; Karmay 1975:29–30; Musée Guimet 1977:no. 36; von Schroeder 1981:122, fig. 18E).

Metal content: Copper 68.3%; Lead 11%; Zinc 20.2%.

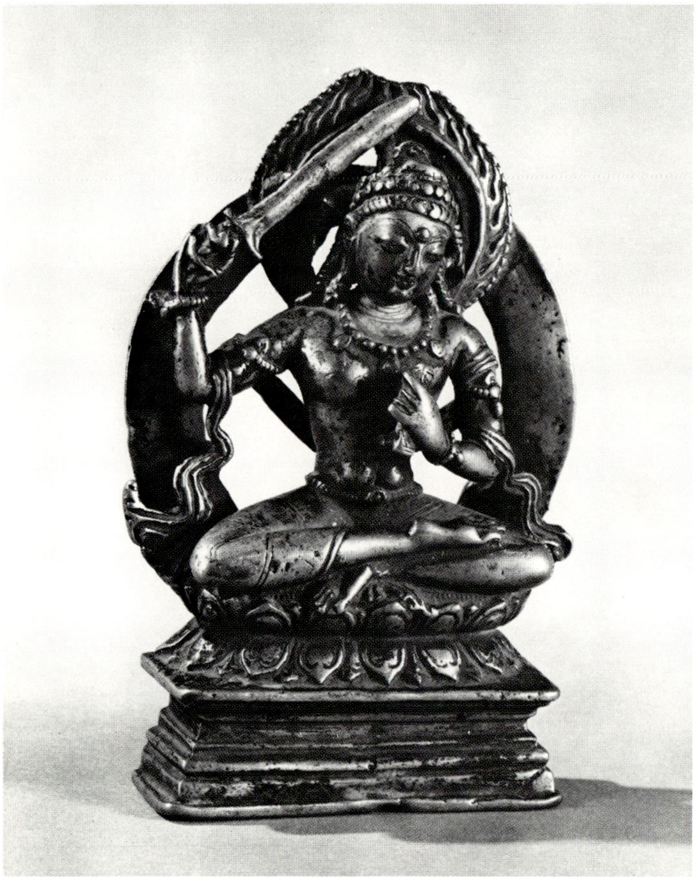

Pl. 29
Arapacana Mañjuśrī
Bronze
Kashmir
Eleventh century
H. 13 cm
Los Angeles County Museum of Art. Nasli and Alice Heeramaneck Collection, Museum Associates Purchase. (M.75.4.6.)

The Bodhisattva sits in *ārdhaparyaṅkāsana* and holds a sword in his right hand and a sacred text (*sūtra*) in the left. The figure style, incised lotus throne and pedestal suggest a Kashmiri attribution. The deeply incised flames on the halo and the fleshy Central Asian face may be compared to images from the western Himalayas. Indeed, several examples of this form of Mañjuśrī occur in the paintings from Ta-pho as well as in clay *ts'a-ts'a* from Ladakh.

Previously Published: (Museum of Fine Arts, Boston 1966:fig. 60; Pal 1975b:no.54).

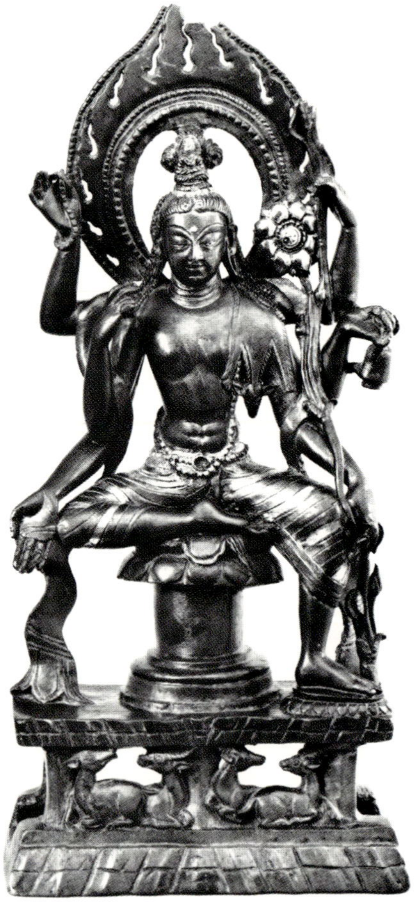

Pl. 30
Bodhisattva
Bronze
Kashmir
Ninth century
H. 69 cm
The Asia Society. Mr. and Mrs. John D. Rockefeller 3rd Collection. (1979.45.)

This large image is hollow-cast in one piece, inlaid with silver and copper, and embellished with incised decoration, and ornaments which were possibly precast. The metal is a dark, golden brown. The voluptuous modeling of the body and the elegantly controlled decoration combine to make this one of the finest surviving Kashmiri bronzes. The large crown, whose triple crescents each contain a large rosette with a jewel in the center, is attached to a band with rosettes standing out at a sharp angle from the head; the ties hang down from the rosettes over the shoulders. This crown type is first noted in Bāmiyān, but the triple-crescent crown with side rosettes as it appears here is characteristic of Kashmiri art in the eighth and ninth centuries. A more specific date for this crown is provided by the relief sculpture of a coronation theme from one of the temples at Avantipur, a major archaeological site outside. The *dhotī* (skirt) depicted as worn with one short leg and the sash hanging down between the flexed legs is a fashion which is also prominent in Kashmiri art of this period. From Kashmir, this fashion was transferred to early western Himalayan sculptures such as the Bodhisattva from Ta-pho (Fig. 42). There are several examples of large-size Kashmiri Padmapāṇi. This type of image continued to be produced in the following century in the western Himalayas. An example is Pl. 92 from the Musée Guimet, which appears to have been copied from such a Kashmiri image.

Previously published: (Handbook of the Mr. and Mrs. John D. Rockefeller 3rd Collection n.d.:23, fig.1; Lee 1970:no.10; Pal 1975b:no.30; von Schroeder 1981:107–109, 118, fig. 16B).

(See Color Plate 30)

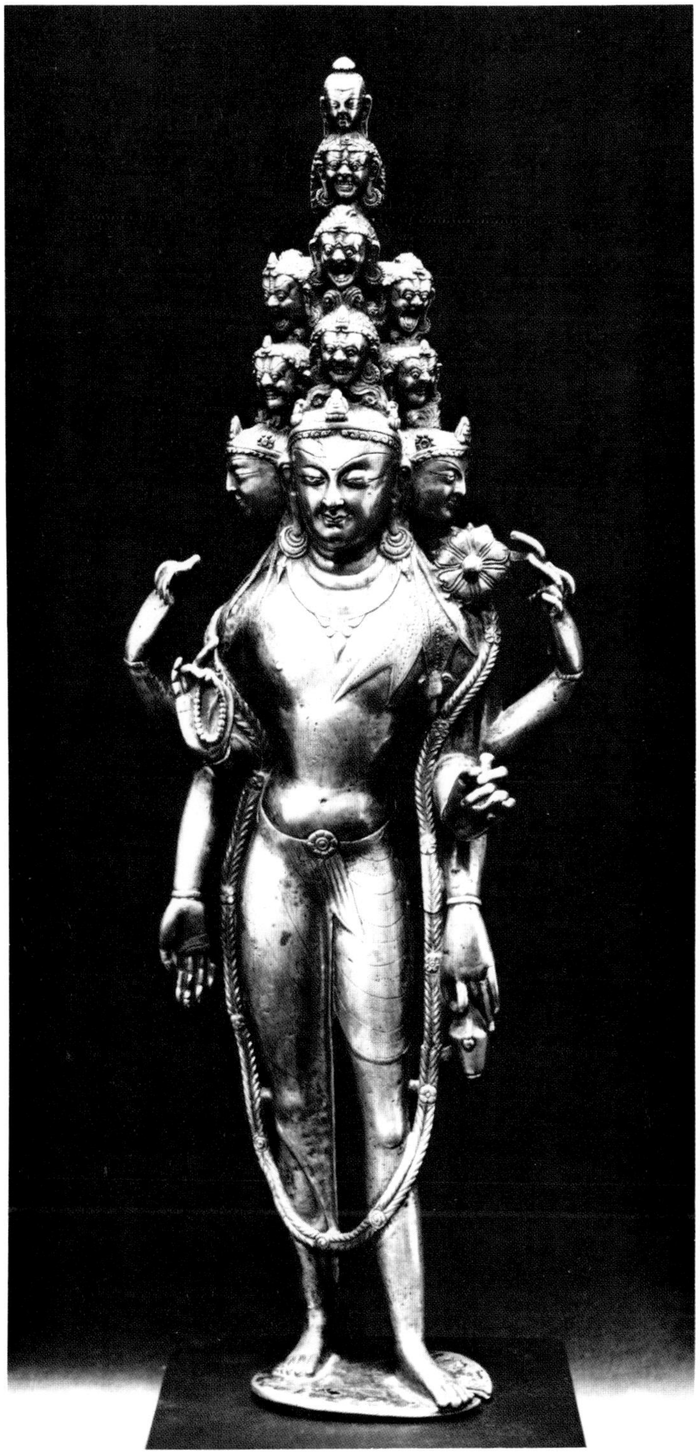

Pl. 31
Six-armed Lokeśvara
Bronze
Kashmir
Tenth-eleventh century
H. 24 × W. 10.5 × D. 5.5 cm
Trustees of the British Museum, London.
Brooke Sewell Fund. (1969.11.3.1.)

This six-armed deity is associated with the family of the Buddha Amitābha, seated on the Bodhisattva's topknot; the antelope skin on the left shoulder is also associated with the principal Bodhisattva of this family, Avalokiteśvara. In addition to its aesthetic appeal, this figure is important because of its close relationship to the "Queen Diddā" bronze in the Śrī Pratāp Singh Museum in Śrīnagar, Kashmir, dated by inscription to the reign of Queen Diddā, 980–1003 A.D. Because of its status as a dated image, the latter sculpture serves as a benchmark for the chronology of Kashmiri metal work. The exaggerated pedestal throne of the British museum piece may be compared to the thrones of the clay figures at Ta-pho (Figs. 48, 49). The prototype for this type of throne may have been in the cave temples of Central Asia, which in turn may have derived from simpler Gandhāran forms.

Previously published: (Snellgrove 1978:fig.261; von Schroeder 1981:128, fig. 21A).

Pl. 32
Eleven-headed Avalokiteśvara (Ekadaśamukha)
Bronze
Kashmir
Tenth century
H. 39.4 cm
The Cleveland Museum of Art. Purchase, Andrew R. and Martha Holden Jennings Fund. (75.101.)

Although rare in India (see Pl. 94), the Eleven-headed Avalokiteśvara is known from several examples in Central Asia prior to the tenth century and, from the eleventh century onward, becomes extremely popular in the mural art of western Himalayan monasteries. There are numerous representations of this image in the later arts of Nepal and Tibet. This extraordinarily fine image provides evidence of the cult of this deity in Kashmir as well. Many of the Ladakhi examples are also represented standing, although in Central Asia the seated form is preferred (see Pls. 70 and 95). The fact that seven of the eleven heads are in the terrifying aspect is somewhat unusual (see Pl. 95). The artist invests each of these faces with a powerful individuality. The elegant treatment of the long figure and graceful hands, as well as the facial type, suggests a tenth century date. The unfinished back, somewhat surprising in an image of this quality, was probably originally covered by a *mandorla*.

Previously published: (Handbook of the Cleveland Museum of Art 1978:293; Pal 1975a:36; Archives of Asian Art 1976–1977:110; National Museum of Western Art, Tokyo 1976; von Schroeder 1981:122–123, fig. 18C; Pal 1982).

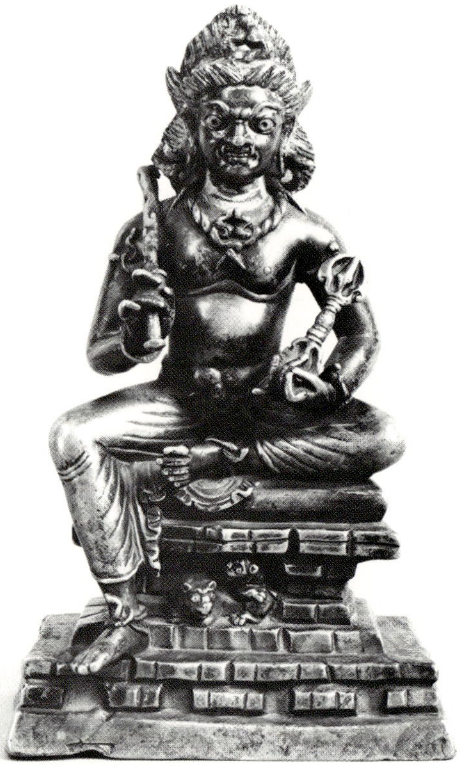

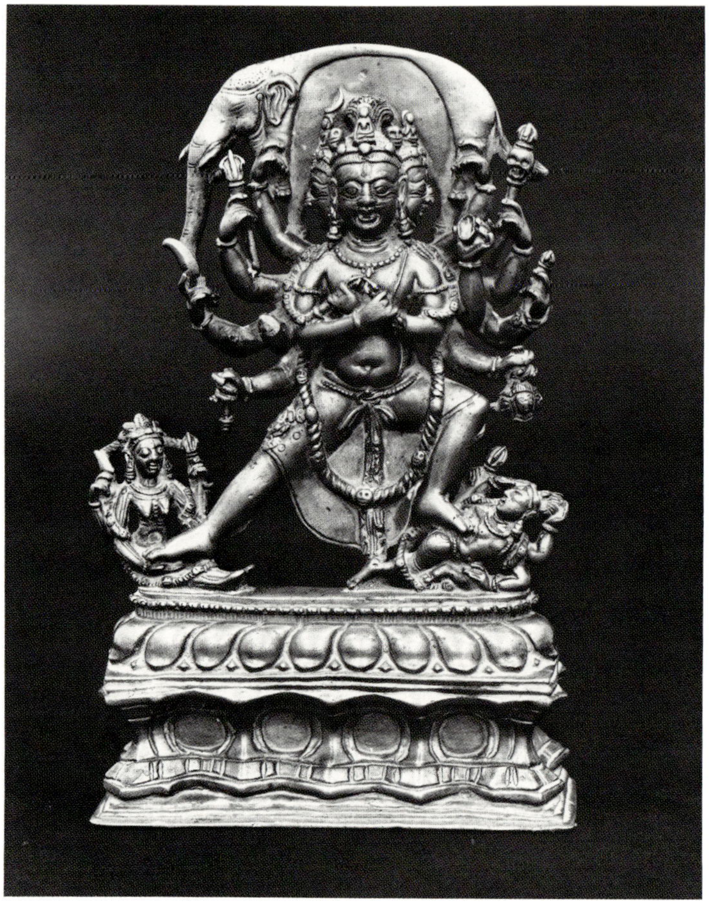

Pl. 33
Bhairava
Brass
Kashmir
Eighth-ninth century
H. 22.2 cm
The Cleveland Museum of Art. Purchase from the J. H. Wade Fund. (71.14.)

This extremely fine image had previously been identified as a representation of Vajrapāṇi. Recently, a plausible identification as Bhairava has been proposed (Pal 1981:44) which better explains certain iconographic peculiarities of the image, such as the erect phallus tied with a serpent. In the Vajrayāna pantheon, Bhairava, or Vajrabhairava, is a ferocious manifestation of Mañjuśrī. The lions within the mountain throne and the *vajra* would be appropriate in this context. In later Himalayan art, this deity is multi-limbed and bull-headed, but human-headed images are also known (Getty 1962:164). An important problem for the history of Buddhist philosophy is what function Śaivite images performed within a Buddhist ritual context in Kashmir and Central Asia (Granoff 1979,1981).

Previously published: (Archives of Asian Art 1972:81, fig. 14; Pal 1973a:747–748, fig.16; Pal 1975b:no. 60; Musée Guimet 1977:88; von Schroeder 1981:122–123, fig. 18B).

Pl. 34
Śaṃvara
Brass
Kashmir
Tenth century
H. 21.6 × W. 14 × D. 5.5 cm
Los Angeles County Museum of Art. Nasli and Alice Heeramaneck Collection. (L.69.24.288.)

This sculpture of Śaṃvara, which is an emanation of the Buddha Akṣobhya who is seated in the crown, is perhaps one of the earliest known Kashmiri icons representing a Vajrayāna deity. The elegant figure style and stylized rock base (see Pl. 9) combined with lotus pedestal suggest a tenth to eleventh century date. Śaṃvara is particularly popular in Tibet and Nepal (Pl. 111). Numerous iconographic details are borrowed from Śaivite iconography: the elephant skin, trident, crescent, third eye, skull cup, and tiger's skin. Vajrayāna iconography frequently borrowed elements from the Hindu pantheon, while also maintaining the superiority of Buddhist philosophy. Here this theme is expressed by the prostrate figures of Bhairava (a form of Śiva) and Cāmuṇḍā (or Kālī) being trampled by Śaṃvara, who holds the severed head of Brahmā in one of his left hands.

Previously published: (Museum of Fine Arts, Boston 1966:no.50; Pal 1975b:no.64; Musée Guimet 1977:no.38; von Schroeder 1981: 126–127, fig. 20F).

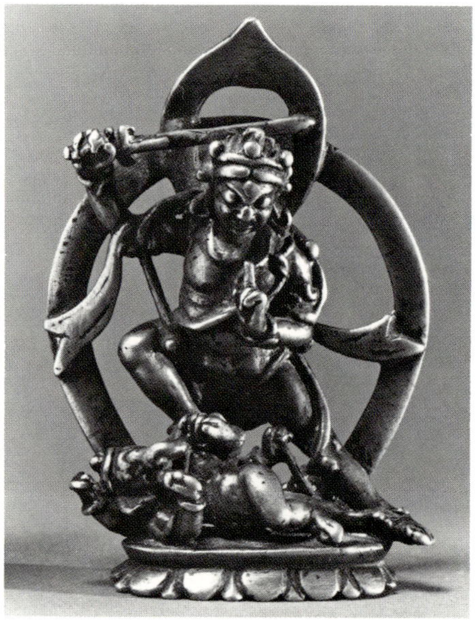

Pl. 36
Yama or Yamāri
Brass
Kashmir
Tenth century
H. 10.2 cm
Robert H. Ellsworth Limited

This three-headed, six-armed (the upper left arm is broken) figure appears to be Yama or Yamāri, as suggested by the buffalo, or perhaps he is another ferocious manifestation of Mañjuśrī. The association with Mañjuśrī is indicated by the sword, as is also the case with Guhya-Mañjuvajra in Pl. 37. As with other Kashmiri bronzes of this period, the figures are rendered in an animated and seminaturalistic style.

Previously published: (Pal 1973a:fig. 15; Pal 1975b:no.62; von Schroeder 1981:124–125, fig. 19G).

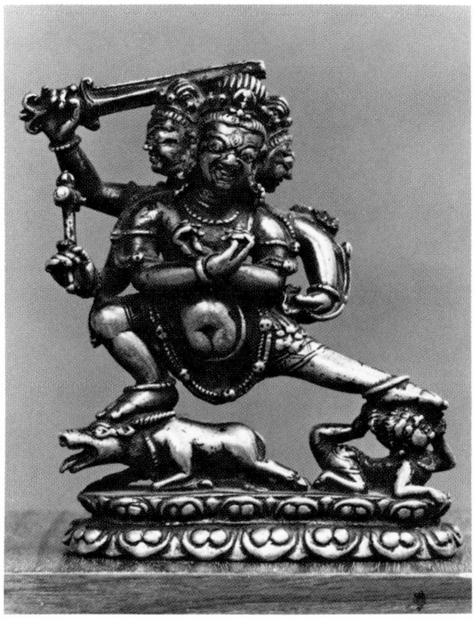

Pl. 35
Vighnāntaka
Bronze
Kashmir
Tenth century
H. 0.099 mm
Robert H. Ellsworth Limited

The ferocious deity, Vighnāntaka is shown subduing the elephant-headed god Gaṇeśa. Like the latter, he is considered the "remover of obstacles." He is an emanation of Akṣobhya. The left hand makes the gesture of admonition (*tarjanimudrā*) or threatening, while the right brandishes a sword. The treatment of the almost-naked torso and the animated style of the Gaṇeśa figure suggest Kashmiri workmanship, while the simple lotus base and shape of the combined halo-*mandorla* are usually associated with the western Himalayan sculpture of the eleventh century.

Previously published: (Pal 1975:Fig. 61; von Schroeder 1981:142,150, fig. 27F).

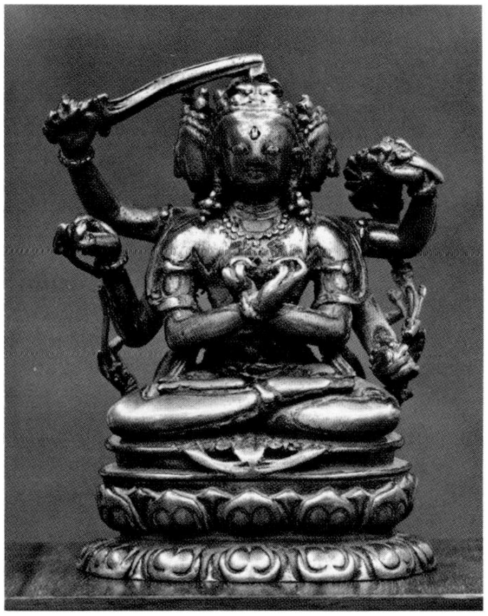

Pl. 37
Guhya-Mañjuvajra
Brass
Kashmir
Tenth-eleventh century
H. 14.3 × 10.8 × 6 cm
Robert H. Ellsworth Limited

Related to the family of Mañjuśrī, Guhya-Mañjuvajra has three heads and six arms and is seated in meditative posture. He holds a sword, arrow, bow and lotus. According to the *Sādhanamālā*, this deity should also be embracing his consort with his two principal hands, which here make the gesture of *vajrahūṅkāra mudrā*. The iconography of the contemporaneous Kashmiri sculpture of Śaṃvara (Pl. 34) also conforms to textual descriptions except for the omission of the female consort. Indeed, as we have noted, *yab-yum* figures are rare in early Vajrayāna art from historical northwest India.

Previously published: (Fong 1971:no.3; Pal 1975b:no.57; von Schroeder 1981:124–125, fig. 19F).

Pl. 38
Vajrasattva and Consort
Brass
Kashmir
Eleventh century
H. 14.3 cm
Robert H. Ellsworth Limited

This exceptional bronze depicts the Buddhist divinity, Vajrasattva, seated with his consort on his knee. Both the theme and the style may be compared to the Musée Guimet painting in Pl. 110. Both divinities hold bell and thunderbolt (*rdo-rje*). The extremely fine detailing of the facial features, hairdress, and crown containing images of the Five Buddhas, can be related to the clay sculpture of Maitreya in the Sum-tsek Chapel at Alchi Monastery in Ladakh (Fig. 21a).

Previously published: (Pal 1978a:no.29; von Schroeder 1981:126, fig. 20C).

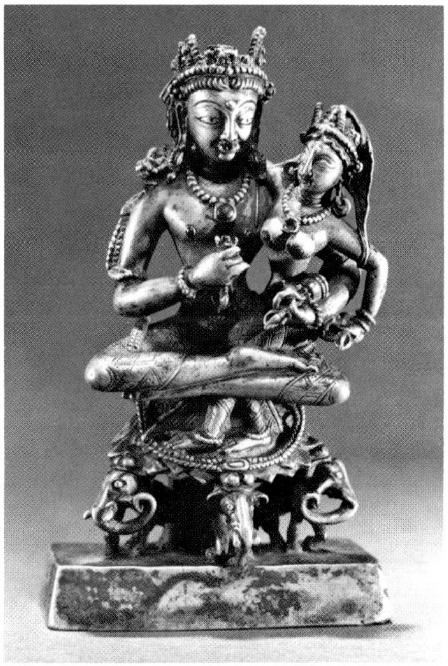

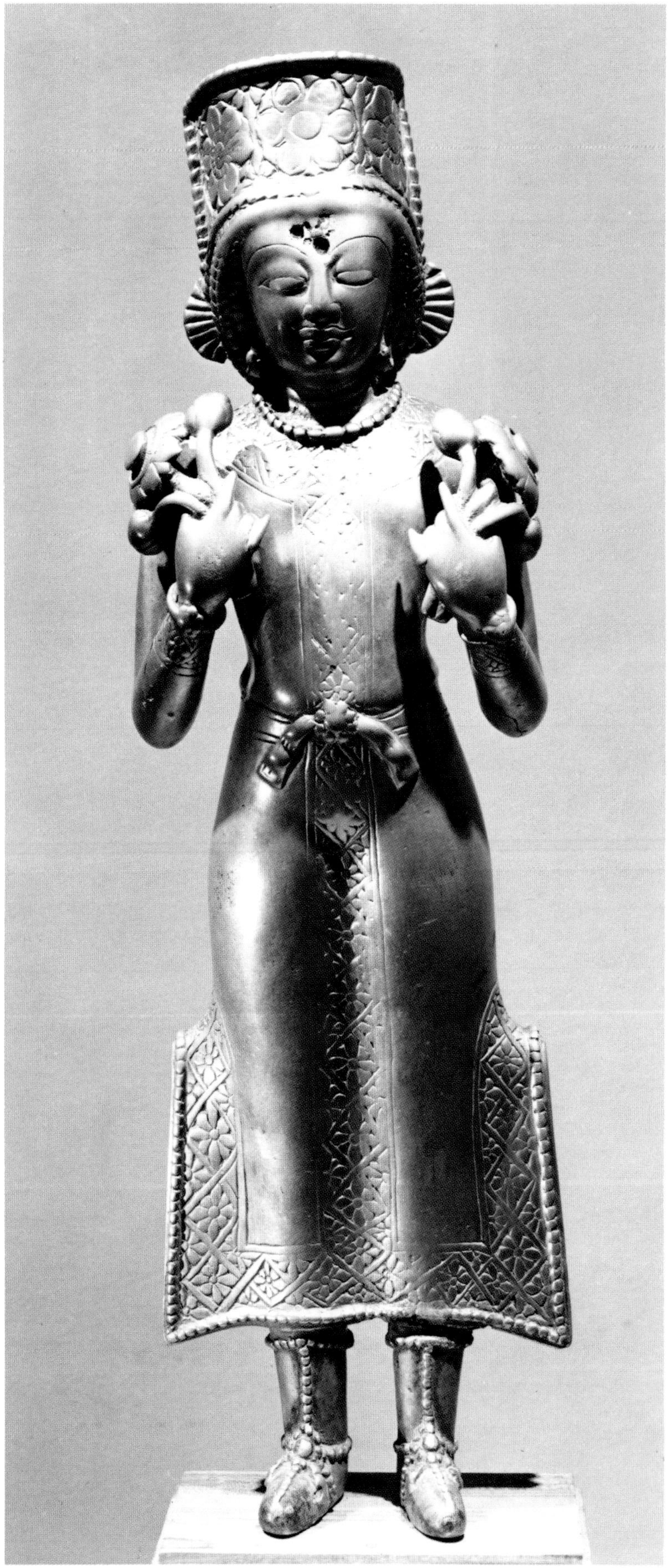

Pl. 39
Sūrya (not exhibited in Los Angeles)
Brass
Kashmir
Eighth century
H. 50.3 cm
The Cleveland Museum of Art. Gift of Katherine Holden Thayer. (65.557.)

The size and quality of this image suggest that it may have been the main icon in an important Kashmiri temple. The most important Kashmiri temple during the eighth century was the royal foundation at Martand; moreover, there were several important temples dedicated to Surya worship elsewhere in northwest India. The Chinese traveler Xuanzang, who visited the famous sun temple at Multan, Pakistan in the seventh century, described it as follows: "There is a temple dedicated to the sun, very magnificent and profusely decorated. The image of the Sun-dêva is cast in yellow gold and ornamented with rare gems. Its divine insight is mysteriously manifested and its spiritual power made plain to all. Women play their music, light their torches, offer their flowers and perfumes to honor it. This custom has been continued from the very first. The kings and high families of the five Indies never fail to make their offerings of gems and precious stones (to this Dêva). They have founded a house of mercy (happiness), in which they provide food, and drink, and medicines for the poor and sick, affording succour and sustenance. Men from all countries come here to offer up their prayers. There are always some thousands doing so. On the four sides of the temple are tanks with flowering groves where one can wander about without restraint." (Trans. by Beal II:274–5). The long tunic and soft high boots with beaded trim are also worn by the marble Sūrya figure from Khair Khana near Kabul.

Previously published: (Archives of Asian Art 1966–1967:88, fig. 13; Cleveland Museum of Art Bulletin 1966:255, no.158; Handbook of Cleveland Museum of Art 1978:293; Lee 1967:42–64, figs. 5,6; Pal 1975b:no.17, von Schroeder 1981:104,112–113, fig. 13F).

Metal content: Copper 78.1%; Zinc 18.7%; Lead 2.7%.

Pl. 41
Umā-Maheśvara
Schist
Kashmir
Seventh-eighth century
H. 8.3 × W. 5.4 cm
Professor Samuel Eilenberg

A three-faced Śiva stands before the bull, Nandi, and next to his consort, Umā. The style of this elegant small icon in fine-grained green stone reflects the heritage of late Gandhāran art as well as the contemporaneous Hindu Śāhī art of Pakistan. Śaivism became increasingly important in northwest India from the sixth century onward, and we have several representations of this theme, although the iconographic details of Śaivite images vary widely. (Barrett 1957; figs. 10 and 12). Hindu images were produced in the same medium and in similar styles as contemporaneous Buddhist icons; indeed, there was frequent syncretism of Buddhist and Hindu iconographic forms during this period. (Granoff 1978,1981; Pal 1981).

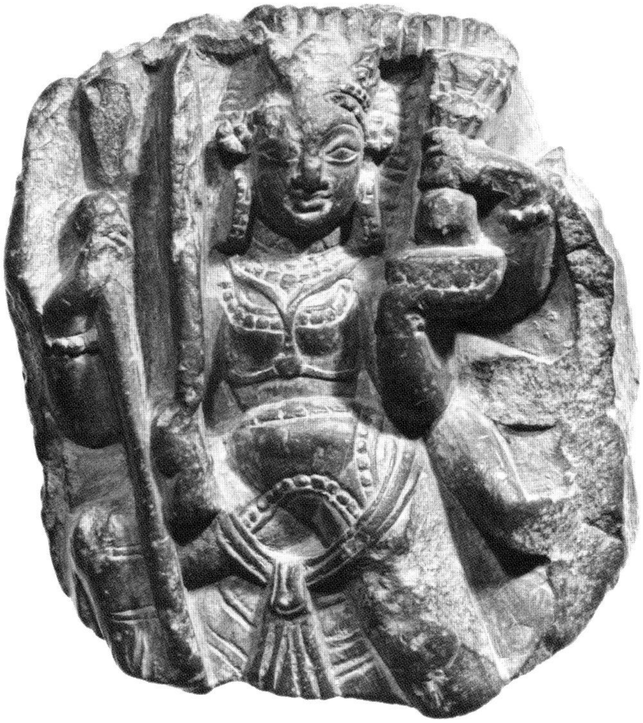

Pl. 42
Durgā Mahiśāsuramardinī
Carved green schist plaque
Kashmir
Eighth century
Diameter 9.5 cm.
The Brooklyn Museum. Lent by Professor Samuel Eilenberg. (L80.22.3.)

This small stone carving depicts a multi-armed Durgā triumphantly pinioning the bull (now lost) with her right foot and a spear held in her main right hand. The scalloped tunic and enormous circular earrings are typical of divine and royal female apparel in Kashmiri art of the eighth through tenth centuries.

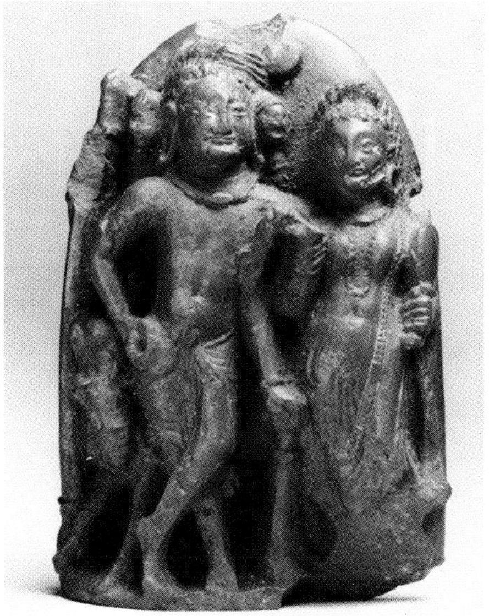

Pl. 40
***Ekamukhalinga* (One-faced *Liṅga*) (not exhibited in Los Angeles)**
Schist
Kashmir
Seventh-eighth century
H. 8.9 × W. 6 × D. 6.5 cm
Trustees of the British Museum, London. Given by Major-General W. Scott Cole.
(1959.10.13.1)

Unlike the other one-faced *liṅga* (Pl. 24), this small icon would have been placed on a shrine. The delicately carved image is stylistically related to Pl. 41: both sculptures have large facial features, long, protruding eyes, full lips, and similar hairstyles. These rather exaggerated facial features relate these Kashmiri images to Hindu Śāhī sculpture from Pakistan. The more typical Kashmiri-style sculptures, both stone (Pl. 43) and metal (Pl. 30), have smaller, more delicate features which are frequently associated with Swat sculpture. These same stylistic contrasts occur in the Hindu (Pl. 24) and Buddhist (Pl. 8) sculptures attributable to the period of the Śāhī dynasties in Northern Pakistan. There is a third facial type specific to Kashmiri sculpture of the eighth to ninth centuries (Pal. 1975:pl. 47), characterized by a more fleshy face with full cheeks, flat nose, and less elongated eyes.

Previously published: (Barrett 1962).

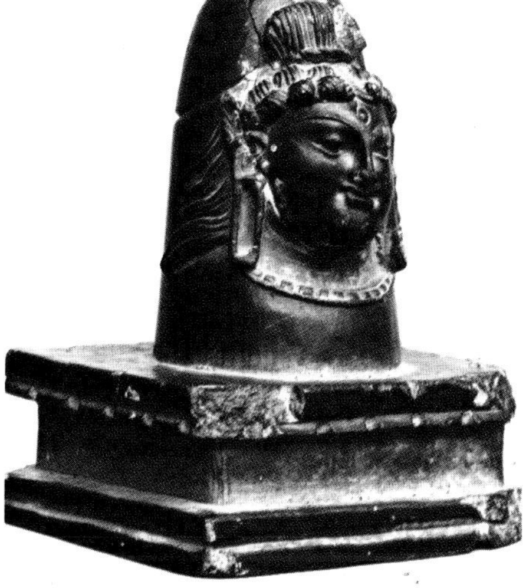

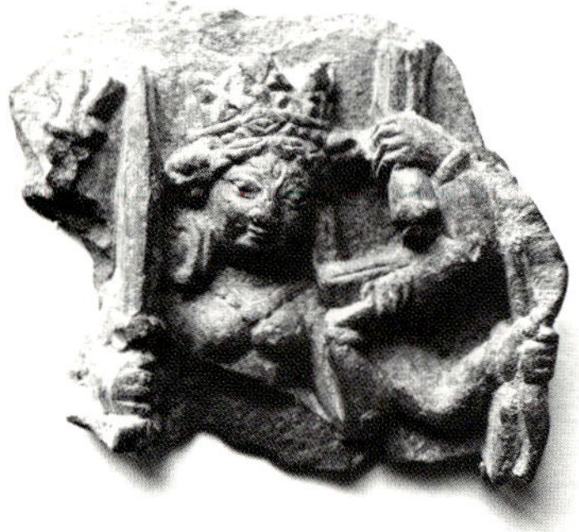

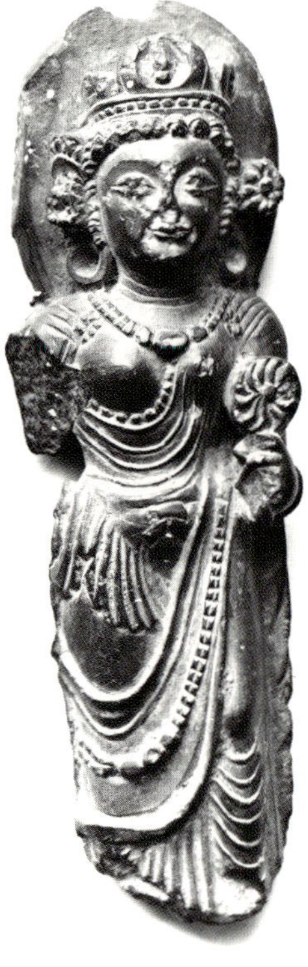

Pl. 43
Parvatī (not exhibited in Los Angeles)
Potstone
Kashmir
Eighth century
H. 15.5 × W. 5 × D. 2.8 cm
Trustees of the British Museum, London.
(1898.6.27.6).

Acquired in the late nineteenth century from the Yusufzai district in north Pakistan, this image is characteristic of a group of small-scale Hindu images in fine-grained stone from Kashmir and Pakistan, datable to the seventh to tenth centuries. Although attributed to Kashmir (Barrett 1957:58), certain features of this image can be compared to another representation of the goddess also found in Pakistan. (Barrett 1957:fig. 10: British Museum No. 1939:1–19, 17). In both cases, the goddess wears a crown with crescents, carries a disc in the left hand and wears a gown draped in a stylized Hellenistic manner. This gown is found earlier on Gandhāran figures and a ca. sixth century sculpture from Vijabror in Kashmir (Śrī Pratāp Singh Museum 1923:Ab.1). The unusual attribute of a disc is also held by a three-headed Śiva in two eighth century paintings from the Khotan region (Pal 1973: 41, Figs. 14, 15).

Previously published: (Barrett 1957:58, fig. 9).

Pl. 44 Female Head
Pl. 45 Male Head
Clay
Northwest India
Early seventh century;
Seventh-eighth century
H. 14.3 cm. (each)
The Metropolitan Museum of Art.
Plate 44: Gift of Mr. and Mrs. William Spielman, 1980 (1980.525).
Plate 45: Gift of Mr. and Mrs. Guy Weill, 1975 (1975.414)

These two clay heads from the Metropolitan Museum, one female (Pl. 44) and one male (Pl. 45), represent an important group of clay sculptures, which at present can best be designated as coming from nrothwest India (Taddei 1978: Pl. 71). This group was previously designated as terra-cotta but Varma (1970: 1334) says the pieces are dried clay, some of which were later accidentally fired.

Remains of terra-cotta Buddhist sculptures have been found in Gandhāra as early as the second century A.D. but it was not until ca. the sixth century A.D. that clay became the preferred medium of artistic expression in eastern Afghanistan and Pakistan. Similar techniques of manufacturing of clay sculptures were used in Afghanistan, Central Asia (Varma), and the western Himalayas (where large scale clay images were constructed on wooden armatures). See Sengupta for this technique in the eleventh century sculpture from Ta-pho. The clay sculpture of historical northwest India, however, would appear to relate to the Gupta terracotta sculpture of northern India and this Gupta influence can be appreciated in the style of the figures as well. The female head from the Metropolitan Museum with its soft round contours and gentle smile is an excellent example of this relationship to the earlier Gupta terracotta sculptures.

The largest collections of northwest Indian so-called terra-cottas are in the Śrī Pratāp Singh Museum in Śrīnagar, in the Museum at Lahore, Pakistan, and in the British Museum. Of these, only the fragments in the Śrīnagar Museum have a known provenance (Archaeological Survey of India 1915–16). This record assists us in identifying the fragments from Ushkur near Baramula and from Harwan (Kak 1925). The Ushkur sculptures came from the *Vihāra* probably built by Lalitāditya Muktapīda and may therefore be dated to the second quarter of the eighth century. Some of these sculptures can be compared stylistically and iconographically to the clay sculptures from Fondukistan attributed to the first quarter of the eighth century (Klimburg-Salter in press). This Ushkur-Fondukistan group can be distinguished stylistically from the Lahore (so-called Akhnur-style) group. Most of the fragments recorded by Fabri in public and private collections in Lahore were purchased from a dealer in Rawalpindi but Fabri believed that they came from Jammu (1955:61). He located a field in the village of Pambarvan with a large number of fragments and the remains of a wall with clay architectural decoration similar to the one uncovered at Ushkur (Fabri 1955). The nearest town to this field was Akhnur, nineteen miles northwest of Jammu city. Hence, the designation Akhnur does not derive from an archaeological site but is merely a convenient term by which to refer to the Lahore figures which were for the most part purchased

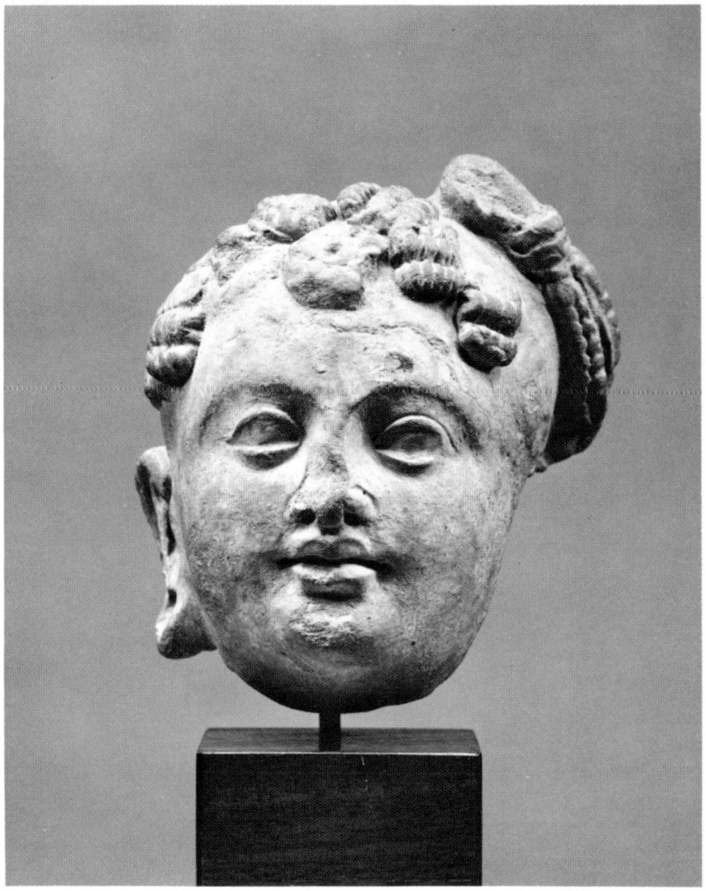

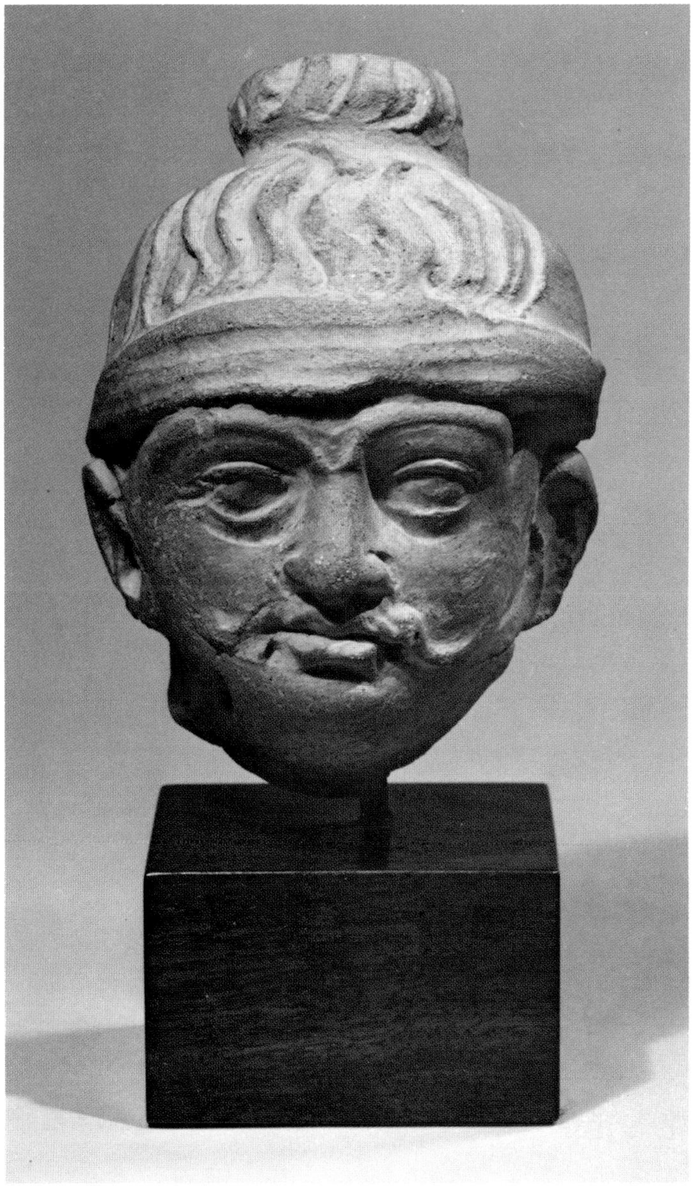

in Rawalpindi. Closely related to the Lahore, Akhnur-style, group is a collection of heads purchased in Peshawar, which the British Museum obtained in 1861. This group may havew come from the northwest frontier region, perhaps from Shah ji-ki Dheri (Barrett 1957:58), a site with a long history of occupation (Archaeological Survey of India, Annual Report 1908–09). Thus we have little archaeological data to assist us in an analysis of these sculptures.

On stylistic grounds, the Metropolitan Museum heads may be grouped with the heads from Lahore (Fabri 1955:61, fig. 12) but the male head (Pl. 45) is also comparable to the head in the British Museum (Barrett 1957:56 fig. 6). If we consider the "Akhnur style" Metropolitan heads both in relation to the Ushkur pieces, and to the later Gupta terra-cotta heads to which they appear stylistically related, we may suggest an early seventh century date.

(b) Reflections from along the Silk Route — Seventh to Tenth Centuries

Central Asia is a geographical area with no universally recognized boundaries. One usually defines the area as bounded on the north by Siberia and on the south by Iran, Afghanistan, Pakistan, and Tibet; by the Caspian Sea in the west; and Mongolia in the northeast. From the geographical perspective, northern Afghanistan should also be considered a part of Central Asia. Within the context of cultural history, Tibet and other Himalayan countries are sometimes included.

It is here, in the midst of the greatest land mass on earth, far removed from the seas, that the great civilizations of Asia converge. A region of great aridity (except for the substantial precipitation on the Pamirs, Alai and Tianshan Mountains), Central Asia has always supported two types of economic specialization—irrigation agriculture along the river valleys and pastoralism on the steppes, steppe-like deserts, and mountains.

Both the ecology and the social systems of eastern and western Central Asia are quite different from one another. The economy of western Central Asia, traditionally based on agriculture rather than pastoralism, promoted the development of small feudal kingdoms which each had an urbanized core. The urban populations coexisted with the nomadic pastoralists, and as the centuries passed many of these nomads adopted a more sedentary way of life (Fig. 34).

Western Central Asia, also known as West Turkestan or Soviet Central Asia (and northern Afghanistan), lay within the eastern Iranian cultural sphere. During the first millennium A.D., rich literary traditions in several Indo-European languages developed; Indian philosophical systems, of which Buddhism was by far the most prominent, made a substantial impact on the area; and influences from Iran and the Mediterranean world also affected cultural and religious institutions. These various influences were gradually transformed into a distinctive artistic culture in which Iranian epic and religious themes predominated. The urban centers of Sogdiana—which were ruled by feudal lords and owed their prosperity, in part, to enterprising merchants—are particularly interesting to a cultural historian. Both the local aristocracy and wealthy merchant families were important patrons of the arts (Azarpay 1981), and the Sogdian monumental art which they commissioned contained a variety of themes. These included: local cult figures, ancestor cult figures, and syncretized cult images which embraced elements from Indian religions (Belenitsky 1968:214–219).

The ecology of the eastern zone of Central Asia was affected by the scarcity of water resources. These steppe-desert regions, bordering the great deserts of inner Asia, were, therefore, more suitable for a pastoral economy than for the sedentary lifestyle which had earlier evolved in the west. As a consequence, these eastern zones were dominated far longer than the western regions by the great steppe empires which grew up and were maintained on the borders of the Taklamakan deserts. While the population in the eastern zone also had an Iranian component, in time it came to be dominated by the Chinese, Turks, and Mongols.

Prior to the Tang period the culture of eastern Central Asia, particularly the region known as East Turkestan, Chinese Central Asia, was also influenced by India and Iran. In addition, the influence of the steppe nomads and of China was important. The influence of Chinese civilization was felt in various stages in Central Asia from the period of the Han Dynasty, and it became increasingly important after the beginning of the Tang period in the seventh century.

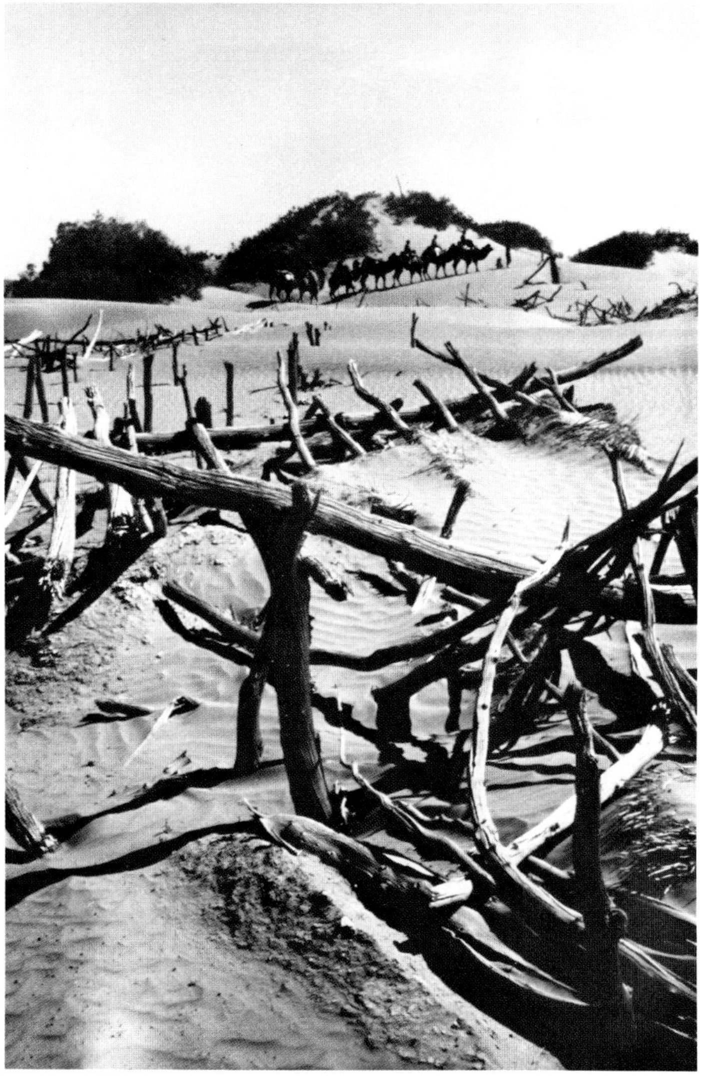

34. Central Asian ruins.

Since the eastern region could only support a limited population, the income derived from long distance trade was an essential component of the economy .The trade between the Turkic or Mongol steppe empires and China was particularly important, and the maintenance of this trade was the primary activity of the nomadic rulers who dominated Central Asia during the mediaeval period. Trade between China and the peoples of Central Asia was accomplished through an institutionalized system of coercion, tribute, and exchange (Fig. 35).

Traditionally, pastoralism has been associated with trade and these economies have always been interdependent. By the beginning of the first millennium A.D., an exchange network had developed across

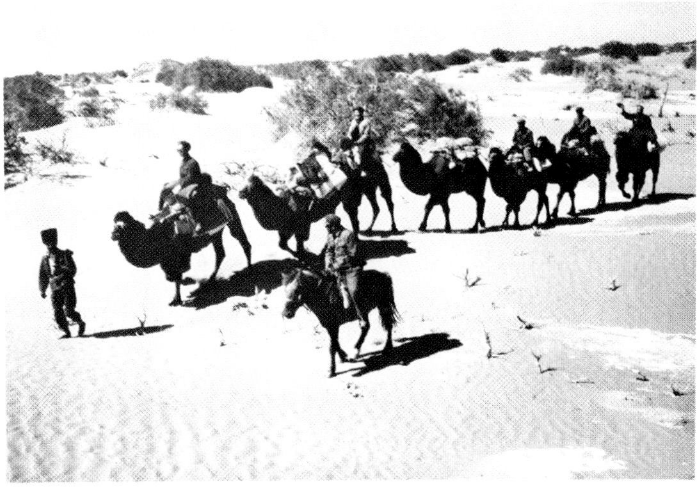

35. Central Asian caravan.

inner Asia; and the oasis towns and city states served as the economic nodes of this network. Interdependent institutions developed which linked the merchants, pastoralists, and agriculturalists of Central Asia with communities in adjacent countries—India, China, and Iran. By the seventh century A.D., the cities of Central Asia located in oases and along the river valleys had become cosmopolitan centers which served not only as relay points in the international trade system, but also as manufacturing centers. Trade essentially financed the political and religious centers which clustered along these international trade routes, and each center evolved a cultural synthesis resulting from the particular ecological, historical, and philosophical features of the area (Figs. 36–39).

The trade routes attracted adventurous merchants throughout the centuries. The Venetian Marco Polo is only one of the latest and in the West most famous; his fame rests not on the fact that his voyage was unique, but on the fact that he returned to tell about it, in vivid and perceptive detail. Marco Polo dared to travel to China, but the majority of the mediaeval travelers were content to stay within one of the regional sectors into which the routes between China, India, and the Mediterranean were divided. Different social connections, linguistic skills, and other adaptive mechanisms were needed to deal with the special dangers inherent in each part of the long journey. Very rarely did a man who began the journey in China ever see the Mediterranean.

There was more direct interaction between the trade centers of India and China. Not only was the cultural and geographical distance shorter, but the pilgrimage places of India served as a powerful magnet for Central and East Asian Buddhists.

EARLY ESOTERIC BUDDHIST ART IN CENTRAL ASIA

Scholars have discussed the obvious relationship between the Buddhist art of Central Asia and northern India for decades. While the process of cultural contact and change is complex and obscure, it has always been assumed that the art of India influenced the art of Central Asia at several stages (Rowland 1974:27–32). In this study we suggest that at certain times the art of Central Asia also influenced the art of northwest India and the western Himalayas (Taddei 1978b:134–135). It is impossible to prove this hypothesis here; rather, our purpose is to assemble some of the artistic evidence that would permit a comparative study of the themes and forms which contributed to early Vajrayāna art. I believe that a comparative analysis will demonstrate that the process of cultural transformation which resulted in the monastic art of the western Trans-Himalayas involved periods in which a dialectic occurred between the arts of Central Asia and northern India (including the western Himalayas). A similar process can also be identified in the evolution of the belief systems and Buddhist literature of the region (Chs. III and IV).

The Buddhist art of Central Asia can be conveniently divided into two geographic groups: the art of western and eastern Central Asia. In both Soviet Central Asia and north Afghanistan, one can identify a renaissance of Buddhist art between the sixth and eighth centuries. During this time, artistic activity appears to have increased at Buddhist centers located in regions under the political overlordship of the Western Turks (Klimburg-Salter 1981). According to evidence uncovered by Soviet archaeologists, a distinctive western Central Asian style with post-Gandhāran stylistic tendencies can be identified. The continuity of themes established during the Kuṣāṇa period is particularly noticeable. It has, in fact, been established that the Kuṣāṇa culture was an important source for much of the later pre-Islamic art of western Central Asia. A common artistic style can be identified from Transoxiana to Ghazni in eastern Afghanistan. Examples are the eighth-century arts of Bāmiyān in the Hindu Kush and Tepe Sardār, in Ghazni. The art of these sites can be compared to the art from Adjina Tepe in the Soviet Union.

Farther to the east in Semirechiye (Belenitsky 1968:109–142), the artistic style during this period also shows evidence of contact with Chinese Central Asia. The bronze staff topped with a representation of seven seated Buddhas (Pl. 53) illustrates this style. It would seem that throughout western Central Asia both the formal and iconographic features of Buddhist art evolved from the art of the Kuṣāṇa period. In

36. Bust of Śiva clay sculpture, Karakhoto, Fogg Museum.

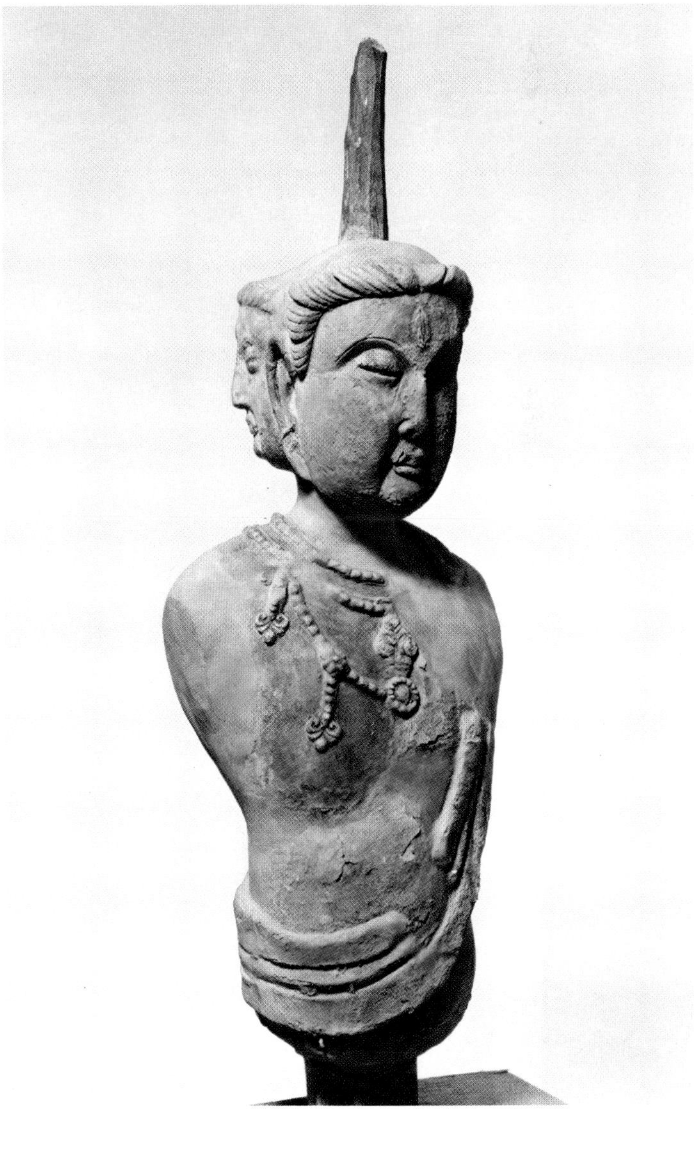

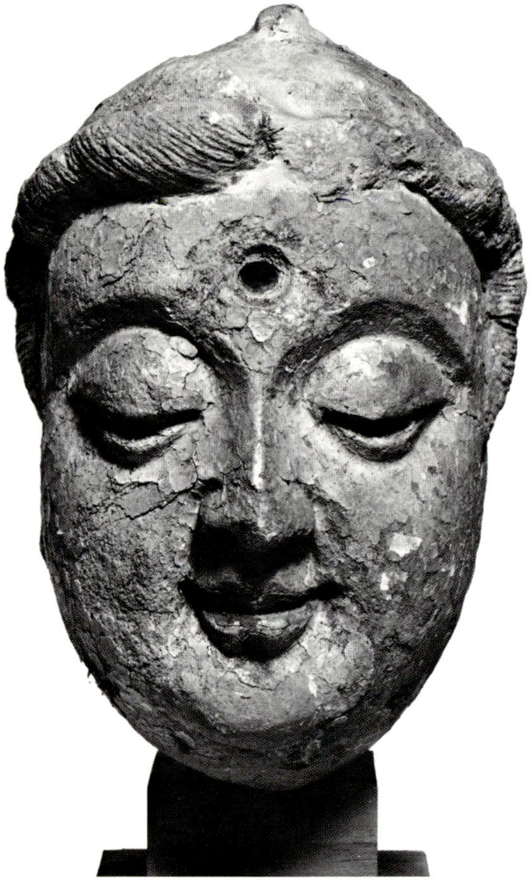

37. Buddha clay sculpture, Karakhoto, Fogg Museum.

Afghanistan, Indian—particularly Gupta—influence is more noticeable, while Chinese influence is naturally more apparent in the northeast in Chinese Turkestan.

CENTRAL ASIA AND NORTHWEST INDIA

We have selected objects which provide three types of art historical evidence for the study of the evolution of Trans-Himalayan art: (1) the art which might have influenced Indian and Tibetan artists, either in Central Asia or in their homeland, (2) evidence for early Tibetan art, the earliest of which has been preserved at Dunhuang in Central Asia and (3) evidence for the, now lost, Esoteric art of India which would have been one source of the Vajrayāna monastic art of the western Trans-Himalayas.

We have little textual information about sectarian affiliations, and the artistic evidence does not allow us to identify which sects patronized particular art forms; however, we do know that there was a gradual transition to Mahāyāna practices and eventually to Vajrayāna by the seventh century A.D. The early stages in Esoteric Buddhist practice were associated with secret rites and composite iconographic images. These features can be identified in the art of historical northwest India and Central Asia only from about the seventh century A.D.; however, on the basis of literary documents it is clear that these Esoteric Buddhist practices existed in India before this time.

The monasteries of the large oases of Kucha and Khotan were important in the development and diffusion of Vajrayāna art in the Trans-Himalaya. The economic and cultural connections between historical northwest India and Central Asia, particularly Kucha and Khotan, have already been discussed in Chapters II and VIa. Part of this process of cultural interaction was the development of shared belief systems and visual themes which allowed artists to seek employment at various monastic centers along the trade routes. It is within this pattern that the importance of the art of Kizil to the art of the Hindu Kush in the second half of the seventh century can be understood.

As we have already noted, the earliest esoteric themes identifiable in historical northwest India, such as the *maṇḍala* and a set of Five Buddhas, can also be identified in the seventh- and eighth-century art of the Hindu Kush. It is possible that certain components of this iconography (as in the case of certain stylistic features at Bāmiyān) were derived from Central Asia—to some degree from Khotan, but more specifically from Kizil. It may be suggested that artists from Kizil influenced and contributed to the art of Bāmiyān in the second half of the seventh century. In the mid-seventh century, the Chinese conquered Kucha, where an administrative center was established which was also (nominally) responsible for the Hindu Kush. Prior to this time, both Kucha and most of northern and eastern Afghanistan had been under the indirect rule of the confederation of the Western Turks (Pls. 46–50).

The arts produced at Kucha, particularly the wall paintings of the extensive Buddhist center at Kizil, have a complex chronology. For our purposes, the art can be simply divided into an "Indo-Iranian" phase before and a more Sinicized phase after the Chinese conquest in the mid-seventh century (Klimburg: 1970, 1974). The art of Kizil appears to have been dedicated to traditional Buddhist themes common to both Hīnayāna and Mahāyāna sects. Stories of the life and previous lives of the Buddha are particularly prevalent (Pls. 105–107), as are scenes of the preaching Buddha Śākyamuni (Pl. 48). In the late sixth and seventh centuries, other themes, which can be associated

38. Bodhisattva clay sculpture, Karakhoto, Fogg Museum.

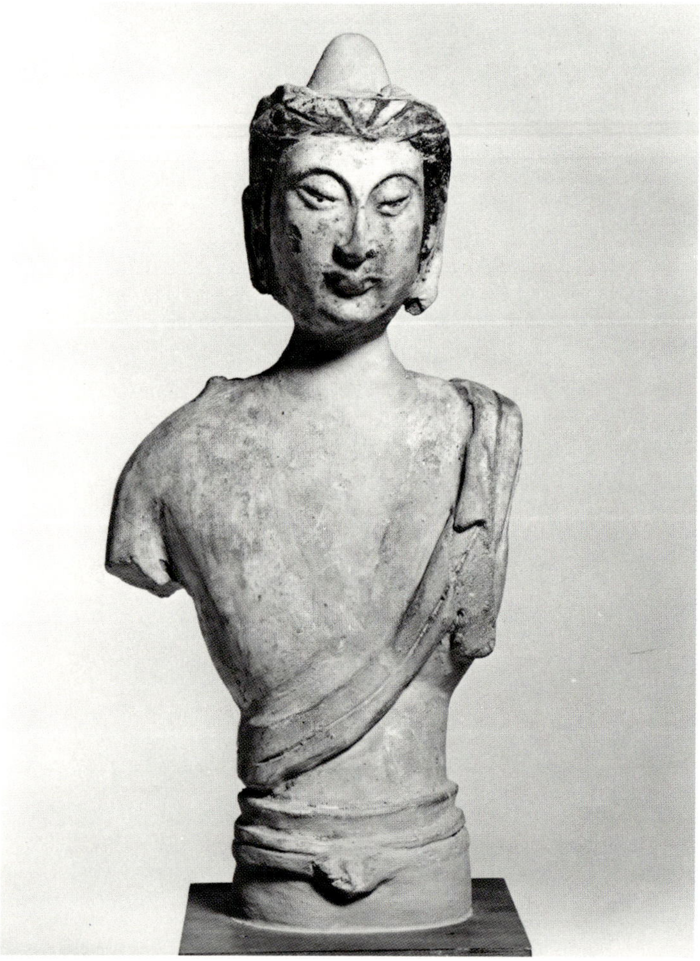

with esoteric ideas, began to emerge (Nagai 1977:160). It is this art which can be directly related stylistically and iconographically to the late seventh-century art at Bāmiyān.

A particularly interesting motif which I have already discussed in Chapter VIa is the Bodhisattva Maitreya, the Buddha of the Future, enthroned amidst his entourage in the Tuṣita heaven. This figure became the center of an early proto-*maṇḍala* in the Hindu Kush (Klimburg-Salter in press). The earliest truly developed *maṇḍalas* only survive in the eighth- to ninth-century paintings from Dunhuang. In India, the earliest surviving examples of the fully developed artistic representation of the *maṇḍala* appear in the art of Ta-pho, ca. 1000 A.D.

There are a number of similar stylistic features in the wall paintings at Kizil and the Hindu Kush. Artists in both places used white lines to highlight the contours of dark-skinned figures, and this technique was frequently employed in the eighth- to ninth-century paintings at Foladi in the Bāmiyān area. This highly stylized conception of the human body is also seen in the paintings at Ta-pho (Figs. 58, 59).

Chinese Central Asian stylistic influences also appear in the art of historical northwest India (Chapter VIa). A small group of portable bronze sculptures, assigned to the eighth-century art of Swat (northern Pakistan), shows a Sinicized treatment of facial features (broad cheeks, small noses, and epicanthal folds of the eyes) which is probably a result of cultural contacts with China. The influence of Chinese modes of dress can be discerned in ninth to twelfth-century images from the western Himalayas, particularly from Kashmir. The Kreitman eleven-headed Avalokiteśvara (Pl. 94), which seems to copy the costume and drapery style of a Sui period image (first quarter of the seventh century), is the most extraordinary example of this amalgam of Chinese and Indian features. Other elements borrowed from China, such as the pointed halo (Pl. 35) or the knot under the right breast (Pl. 89), are integrated into the prevailing Indian modes of presentation. As these features seem to appear first in portable rather than monumental art, it can be suggested that originally the more typically Chinese features were used in sculptures produced for a specialized clientele.

39. Guardian figure clay sculpture, Karakhoto, Fogg Museum.

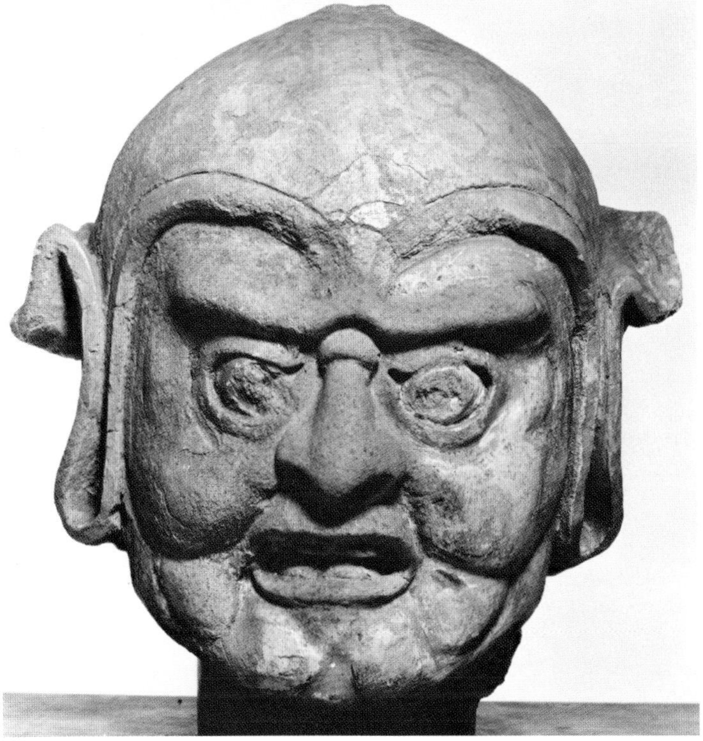

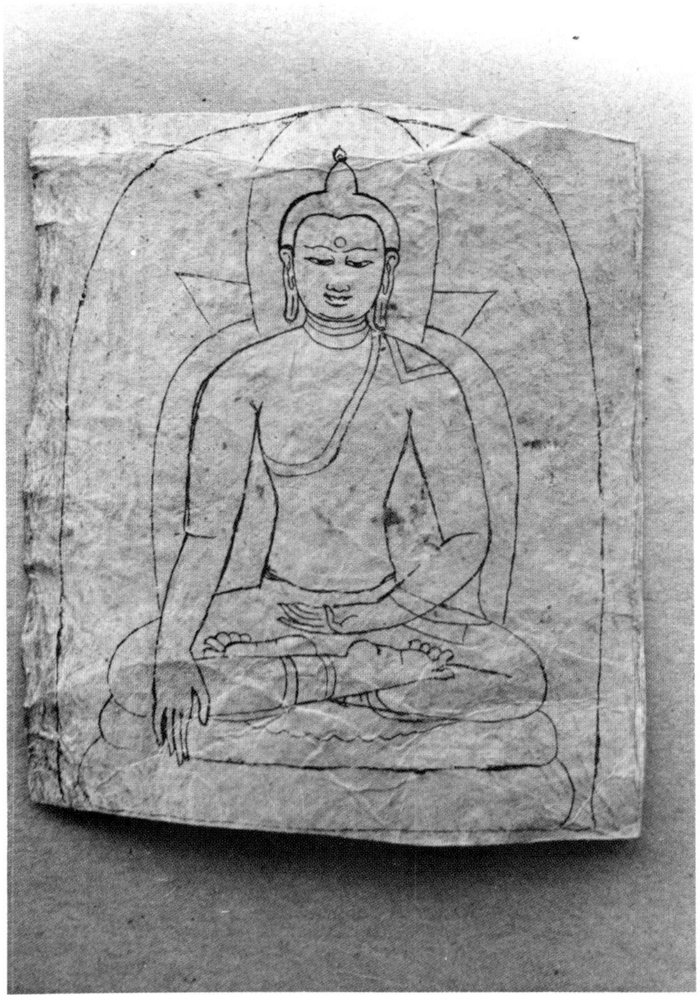

40. Drawing from Hatt Chörten, Newark Museum.

The presence of Chinese stylistic features in the western Trans-Himalayas increased from the eighth century. At the same time, the iconographic variations expanded enormously with the production of an increased number of tantric images. Both these artistic features were probably related to the intensified cultural contact resulting from the Tibetan advance into Central Asia in the seventh century and the adoption of Buddhism as the Tibetan state religion in the eighth century. Also caravan traffic increased as the routes via Ladakh became more important. Chaio Yi-Liang 1944–45:60).

REFLECTIONS OF INDIAN ESOTERIC BUDDHIST ART IN CENTRAL ASIA

In *ca.* 666 A.D., when the Tibetans conquered Khotan, Karashar, Kucha, and Kashgar, Esoteric Buddhist practices were already known in Khotan (Williams 1973). Esoteric forms of Buddhist deities and several Hindu deities (which had been integrated into the Buddhist pantheon) appear in both literature and art found at Khotan. Although the first Tibetan occupation lasted only until *ca.* 692 A.D., the Tibetans retained their connection to the Buddhist centers there.

We know, for instance, that in the eighth century the king of Tibet offered sanctuary to monks fleeing from Khotan, most likely in the wake of the Arab victory over the Chinese at Talas in Central Asia. In the following century, an artist from Khotan came to Tibet in order to decorate Buddhist temples. We know little about the artistic style imported from Khotan to Tibet in the ninth century, but the ideological content of the art must, by that time, have resembled the fully developed Vajrayāna art created in Dunhuang during that period. The con-

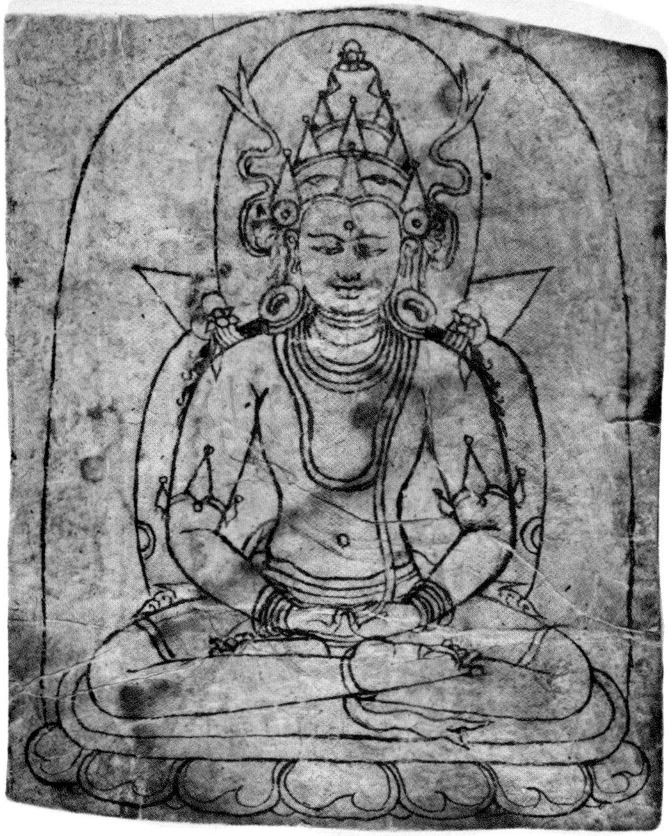

40a. Drawing from Hatt Chörten, Newark Museum.

tent and style of Esoteric Buddhist art from the eighth to tenth centuries can best be understood through an examination of the works preserved at Dunhuang. It should, however, be noted that although an exceedingly large number of relevant artistic and literary documents were preserved at this site (see Chapter IV), individual remains from other sites in Central Asia also provide evidence for an early stage of Esoteric Buddhism. An important example is the wooden shrine which depicts the *maṇḍala* of the eight Bodhisattvas (Pl. 54).

We have frequently remarked in this study that the earliest extant examples of fully developed *maṇḍalas* come from Dunhuang. One of the earliest of these may be represented in the fragments from a painting on paper now in the Central Asian collection of the National Museum in New Delhi. The Jinas represented in the two examples shown here (Pls. 66, 67) were originally part of a *maṇḍala* whose center configuration was a five-pointed star with one Jina depicted in each triangle. Two other *maṇḍalas* are partially represented by the fragments seen in Pls. 63–65. These brilliantly colored images appear to have been part of large *maṇḍalas* which included secondary divinities and guardian figures. Some idea of the original appearance of these *maṇḍalas* can be obtained from the British Museum sketch (Pl. 69) and the two *maṇḍalas* from the Musée Guimet (Pls. 61, 68). A similar concept also appears in an example of local "folk art" (Pl. 72).

These early *maṇḍalas* appear to focus on the five Jinas. In the tenth-century *maṇḍalas* from the Musée Guimet, Lokeśvara (Pl. 68), a tantric manifestation of Avalokiteśvara, is placed at the center of the *maṇḍala*. Both Lokeśvara (Pl. 19) and other individual tantric forms of Avalokiteśvara—such as Hayagrīva (Pl. 72)—found in this painting appeared almost two hundred years earlier in historical northwest India. However, no complete iconographic representation of these or other tantric divinities and their retinues is preserved in India prior to the eleventh century. The Jinas (Five Buddhas, Tathāgatha) (Pl. 69) and also other divinities, are each placed within the point of a star. This star, which occupies the center of the *maṇḍala*, is then enclosed in a circle, which is in turn surrounded by a square with four "doors." Each of these gateways is protected by the guardian deity of that particular direction. This square composition with four doors enclosing a geometrically ordered assembly of deities is sometimes called a *maṇḍala*-palace composition. It is this type which adorns the walls of the Sum-tsek Temple, Alchi (Figs. 22, 23). It does not appear at Ta-pho or in the earlier art of the western Himalayas. But other earlier *maṇḍala* compositions are known in India, such as the *maṇḍala* of the eight Bodhisattvas (Pl. 54), where the Bodhisattvas form a simple square around the central divinity. The round *maṇḍala*-like compositions in the Hindu-Kush may represent another variety (Fig. 27). The common theme is the geometric ordering of the divinities according to consistent spatial and philosophical relationships so that there is an integrated center and a periphery.

A *maṇḍala* can be dedicated to one of many deities. The art of Central Asia preserves many iconographic representations based on the *yoga-tantras*. This form of Vajrayāna was particularly important in the western Trans-Himalaya during the eleventh to thirteenth century (see Snellgrove Ch V).

Other tantric deities represented by earlier individual sculptures from historical northwest India (Pl. 20) are clearly integrated into the Vajrayāna pantheon in the art of Dunhuang. In the works from Dunhuang, some Hindu divinities, such as Indra (Pl. 60), appear as guardian figures; but, in some instances, Hindu gods and Buddhist divinities have been syncretized to form tantric images, such as the deity Amoghapāśa, who can be associated with an aspect of Maheśvara, the great god Śiva (Pl. 70; Nicolas-Vandier 1976:xiii). Other deities found at Dunhuang, such as Bhaiṣajyaguru, are not important in the earlier art of historical northwest India but are very popular in the Vajrayāna art of the western Trans-Himalaya. There are two chapels dedicated to Bhaiṣajyaguru at Ta-pho.

At least one iconographic theme which occurs both in Central Asia and historical northwest India in the eighth century appears to be related to the impact of the Western Turks who were the dominant political power in much of Central Asia in the sixth and seventh centuries. This theme involves the depiction of the guardian figure of the north, Vaiśravaṇa, as conceived in Dunhuang (Pl. 59). This depiction is distinguished from other representations of the same deity elsewhere. The distinctive features of this type of Vaiśrāvaṇa are the shoulder flames and Kuṣāṇa warrior's dress. This type of Vaiśrāvaṇa, derived from the image of a divinized Kuṣāṇa emperor, appears first in northern Pakistan and Afghanistan in the seventh to eighth centuries. However, given our limited documentation, it would not be correct to attribute any of this art directly to the exclusive patronage of the Western Turks. It is more likely that both Hephthalite and Turkic local rulers, who belonged to the confederation of the Western Turks, developed a shared political and artistic vocabulary—especially in relation to dynastic

41. Wall painting, Buddha, *'du-khang,* Ta-pho.

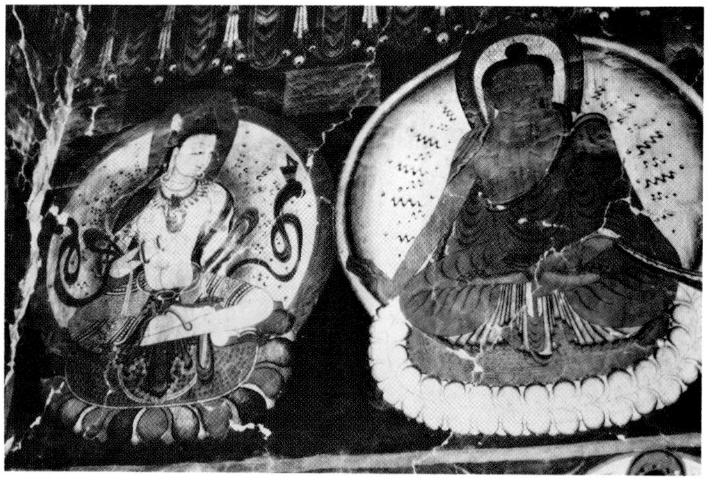

subjects. This vocabulary can be traced back to the dynastic arts of the Kuṣāṇas (Klimburg-Salter 1981a:260).

THE ART OF DUNHUANG

We have exceedingly limited information about the production of works of art and the role of the artist in the western Himalayas during the mediaeval period. The sacred art of the Himalayas is essentially anonymous. A work of art is rarely signed and, in fact, may have resulted from the combined efforts of several people. It is an art which is not meant to express the individual will of the artist, nor of the patron who commissioned it; rather, it is an art meant to serve a particular sacred function. The correct rendering of every detail, therefore, is necessary if the work is to fulfill its devotional and magical function.

The traditional, doctrinally prescribed manner of depicting an image was maintained through the rigorous process of apprenticeship and through the use of various mechanical aids. Each master and family carefully guarded these preliminary tools—pounces, stencils, or sketchbooks—in order to ensure continued observance of the established standards. Few of these have survived from the early periods of Buddhist art in the western Himalayas and for this reason the aids, preliminary drawings, and other types of unfinished works of art found in Cave 17 at Dunhuang are particularly valuable. Two examples, a stencil and a sketchbook, are reproduced here. The stencil (Pl. 74) was used to transfer a painted image of a Bodhisattva to paper or silk. This technique produced a bold image consisting of broad bands of color, outlined in black, and accented by the whitish background. The stylistic characteristics of this kind of stenciled image can be seen in the seated Buddha between sun and moon (Pl. 76) from Dunhuang. Other motifs such as the halo decorated with triangular forms can be seen in Pl. 70.

42. Clay sculptures, *'du-khang* apse, Ta-pho.

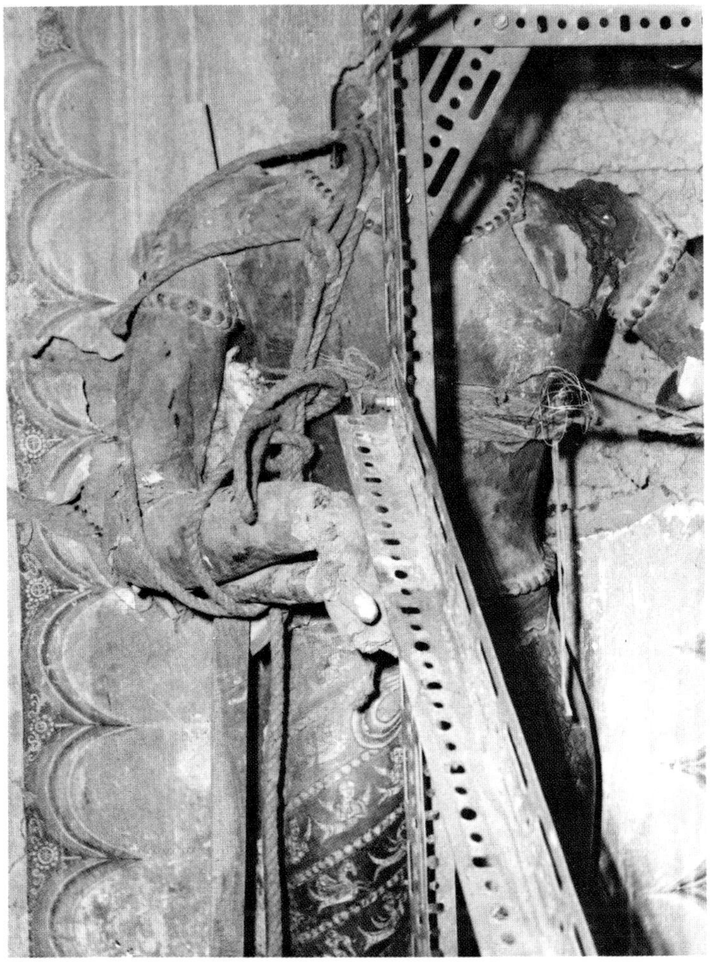

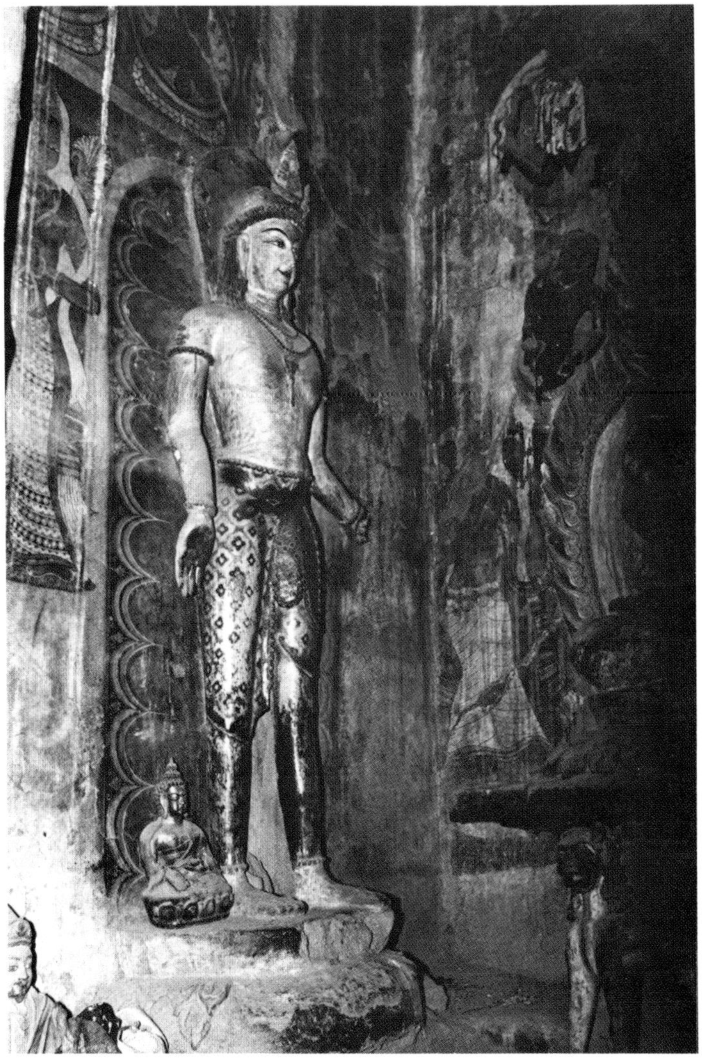

43. Clay sculpture, *'du-khang* apse, Ta-pho.

Even an extremely complex image could be reproduced precisely over hundreds of years by following directions such as those in this sketchbook or instruction manual.

The art of Dunhuang is also important for the study of the development of Tibetan Buddhist art. As noted in Chapter I, the earliest evidence of Buddhist art made for, or by, Tibetans (Pl. 58) was preserved at Dunhuang. The Tibetan inscription on one of the paintings and the distinctive style (Pl. 58) show that these works were produced by Tibetan craftsmen or intended for a Tibetan audience. A slightly later variant of this style is found in the *maṇḍalas* we discussed above. This style is both simpler and more two-dimensional than the well-known Chinese style associated with Dunhuang (Pl. 70). The figures are slightly heavier in the shoulders, but very slender in the waist; the facial features are sketchily drawn and the eyes are large and extended. The figures always wear Indian dress—the upper body naked, the shoulders covered with a thin scarf. The hairstyle is Indian, rather than Chinese. This style appears in the Tang period paintings at Dunhuang. Sometimes all the figures in a painting are represented in this way, but individual figures of this type may appear in paintings that also contain figures depicted in a Chinese style (Pl. 70).Another style which has been classified as "Himalayan" (Nicolas-Vandier 1976:xviii) has slightly different characteristics, and is particularly marked by a more rigid treatment of the figures. Here, too, Himalayan and Chinese features are found together in the same composition (Pl. 68).

These three variants of the Himalayan style at Dunhuang can be

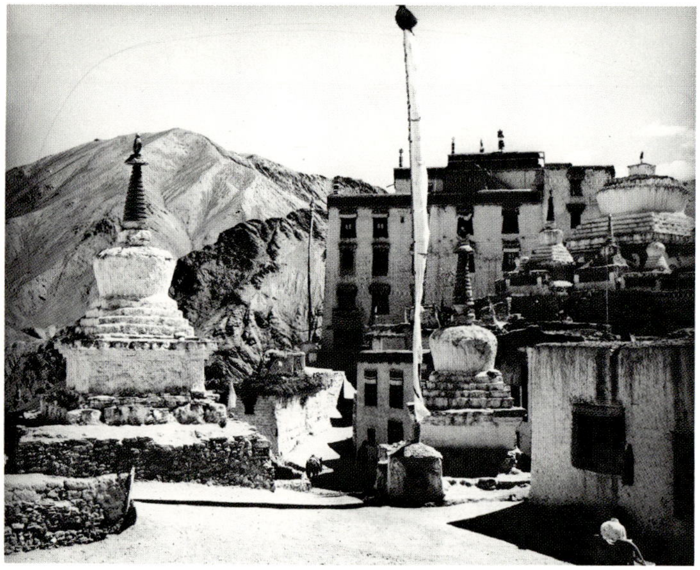

44. Lamayuru Monastery, Ladakh.

summarized as follows:

a) (Pl. 58) simple linear style may be the earliest or a provincial version, same stylistic elements but less refined use of line and color than
b) (Pls. 63, 66); this variant is the most frequently encountered, like a) has been found in paintings with Tibetan inscriptions (Karmay 1975:9–13);
c) (Pl. 68) more rigid and frontal, mixture of Chinese dress with some Himalayan components such as the "helmet crown," may be contemporaneous with variants a) and b).

The Himalayan styles a) and b), as well as the iconographic components of all three variants, are found throughout the area of the western Trans-Himalaya from the eleventh to thirteenth centuries, as well as in the art of Nepal. These features (which are discussed in greater detail in connection with the plates) are:

1) A linear two-dimensional style; usually a single even line describes a graceful, languid pose (compare Pl. 62 and Fig. 41 from Ta-pho monastery).
2) The straight-sided halo; the exact shape varies but in all cases the sides are flat and in variant b) it also has a slightly pointed top. The straight-sided halo is always used in Dunhuang with the Himalayan style. It is found in Ta-pho (Figs. 42, 43) and in most of the painted scrolls of the period (Pl. 108).
3) Specific forms of dress, most notably the crowns; the Five Buddha crown used in b) has a similar outline to the "helmet crown" in c). Only one example is known to me of the five-Buddha crown in the earlier art of northwest India (Pl. 11). The "helmet crown" occurs in several examples from the twelfth century onward (Pl. 109; Fig. 40a). Only the three-pointed crown worn by figures depicted in the stylistic variant a) is commonly found in the earlier art of the western Himalayas.
4) A variant of the "vajra fist" mudrā (Pl. 101). This unusual mudrā has so far only been identified in paintings in Dunhuang in the Himalayan style (Pl. 60) and the art of the western Trans-Himalaya, eleventh to thirteenth century (Fig. 41).

There are relatively few paintings containing images in the Himalayan style from Dunhuang; some of these have Tibetan inscriptions and many of them can be dated to the period of Tibetan occupation of Dunhuang. The characteristic stylistic and iconographic features of the Himalayan style are always used together, even when they occur in paintings in the Chinese style (Karmay 1975:1–12). Because both the stylistic and iconographic features of this Himalayan style are so widespread in Himalayan art, it seems reasonable to conclude that this mode of representation in Dunhuang and the Trans-Himalaya originated in an earlier, and now lost, type of painting which existed in northern India (Fig. 33). Such a conclusion is confirmed by the presence of similar features in the surviving three-dimensional art of the western Himalayans (Pls. 28, 33, 88) and numerous examples in Nepal as well (Kramrisch 1964; Pal 1975a; 1978). Even the variant "a" may be preserved in a group of Ladakhi images (Pl. 90). These images may have been produced in a deliberately archaic style, preserving an earlier, and now lost, style of the western Himalayas.

Mural paintings at Dunhuang from the Yuan period (Pelliot 1914–15:VI, pls.CCCXLVII–CCCLI) also contain images painted in a Himalayan style which also appear in the twelfth century in the western Trans-Himalaya. A famous example of this relationship is the painting from the Musée Guimet (Pl. 110; Karmay 1975:20).

THE CITY OF KARAKHOTO

The eastern-most evidence for a relationship between the arts of Central Asia and the western Himalayas has survived in the city of Karakhoto. This frontier outpost of the Hsi Hsia state, once used as a place of exile for political prisoners, was destroyed by the Mongols in 1227 A.D. (Karmay 1975:35). The considerable body of artistic evidence—painting, sculpture, wood-block prints, and manuscripts—obtained from this site may provide the necessary clues to an understanding of its Buddhist culture. In addition to the Buddhist paintings and sculpture, Stein found several fragments from Tibetan manuscripts (Pl. 77) which also appear to have dealt with Buddhist subjects. The degree

45. Wall painting, Lhakhang, Soma, Alchi, 12th–13th centuries.

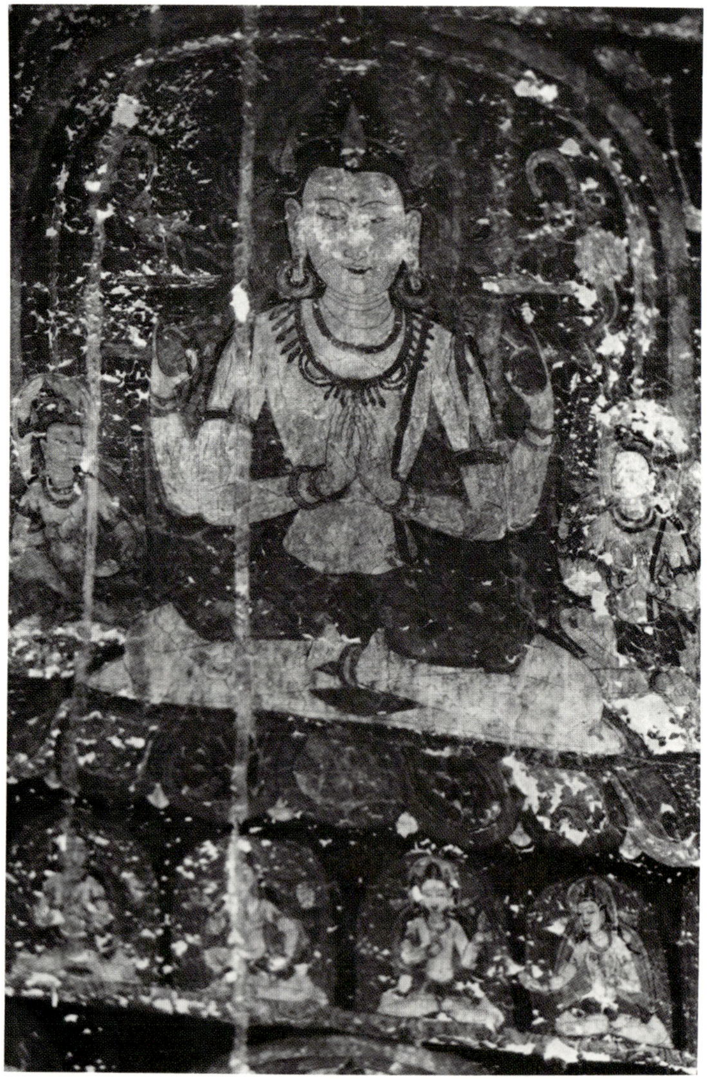

of influence of Tibetan culture on Hsi Hsia culture is still a subject of scholarly debate (Kwanten, Snellgrove and Richardson 1968:111).

The problems one encounters in a study of Karakhoto culture are similar to the problems involved in the study of other archaeological centers in Central Asia. Inadequate literary sources lead to conflicting hypotheses derived from existing numismatic, epigraphic, and archaeological evidence. Hence, while there are clear stylistic and iconographic similarities between the hanging scroll paintings from Karakhoto (Musée Guimet 1977:76–85) and the wall paintings from Alchi in Ladakh (in particular in the Lhakhang Soma) (Figs. 17, 17a) as well as isolated paintings on cloth in Western collections (Pls. 109, 112), the process of artistic interaction is unclear. None of these paintings can be firmly dated. Furthermore, the body of material is too small for establishing a relative chronology based on formal analysis. We can only say, for example, that the long bodies, large heads, and narrow waists of the figures in the mural paintings from Luk Monastery in western Tibet (Pl. 105) indicate a later date for those paintings than for the Alchi murals containing similar figures (Fig. 17). The Ladakh paintings appear to have been made between the twelfth and thirteenth centuries. The Karakhoto paintings may have been made somewhat earlier, perhaps in the late twelfth or early thirteenth century. However, the most interesting question remains unanswered: how is it possible that wall paintings in a monastery in Ladakh can relate so strongly to images painted on cloth and preserved in a *stūpa* in Karakhoto more than one thousand miles away in the Gobi Desert?

One might be tempted to think that the paintings of Karakhoto are the works of western Himalayan artists preserved by chance and the dry climate of the Central Asian deserts; however, the fragile clay sculptures retrieved from Karakhoto by Langdon Warner and preserved in the Fogg Museum (Figs. 36–39) suggest that these artists must have been working in Karakhoto itself. Such clay sculpture is known throughout Central Asian centers, where it is always part of the architectural decoration of a Buddhist shrine. The arrangement of the life-size sculptures at Karakhoto which appears in the report published by Oldenburg also suggests an original function similar to that of the life-size clay sculptures in Ta-pho (Oldenburg 1914:90.).

These Fogg Museum clay sculptures, while much decayed, are stylistically similar to the Karakhoto paintings. Furthermore, their technique, function, and style can be compared to that of the clay sculptures which still survive at Alchi and Lamayuru in Ladakh (Fig. 44). This correlation is all the more interesting when one notes that the slightly earlier clay sculptures from Ta-pho do not belong to this stylistic group. The fuller, more balanced proportions and the smooth, voluptuous transitions of the Ta-pho figures are closely related to monumental clay sculptures from the Tang period in central Asia and the clay images surviving in the Jokhang at Lhasa, and to Kashmiri bronzes. The evidence for the existence of a common style in Ladakh and Karakhoto is strengthened by a group of bronzes thought to be from the western Trans-Himalaya. Once again the same stylistic features are present: the extremely elongated torso, narrow hips, flat abdomen; the relatively large shoulders and large head with large ears and eyes (Pl. 82); and the high cranial protuberance (*uṣṇīṣa*). The height of the wooden armature protruding from the Karakhoto sculptures indicates that they also had the characteristic high *uṣṇīṣa* (Pl. 38).

Similar iconographic themes are also found at Karakhoto and in the western Trans-Himalaya. There is an emphasis on tantric themes, and these themes are expressed in a number of paintings with Vajrayāna subjects (Musée Guimet 1977:78–85) and in the Fogg sculpture of a three-headed male figure which can be identified as Śiva (Fig. 47). At both Karakhoto and the Lhakhang Soma chapel (Fig. 45) at Alchi—and in the western Trans-Himalaya, generally (Pls. 111,112)—there is a preference for images of Śaṃvara or his consort Vajrayoginī. This doctrinal interest continues in the contemporary practices of the Karma Kagyud (Pl. 128; Fig. 53; see Chapter VII).

The complex artistic relations which evolved between the two remote Buddhist centers in Ladakh and Karakhoto, separated by the most formidable deserts and mountains in the world, remain unknown. However, once again, it is significant that these centers are linked by Trans-Himalayan trade routes, and that their cultures are related by a common ideology and economic system. The social structure of both centers was conditioned by Buddhist institutions and a stratified society shaped by dependence on long-distance trade and pastoralism. Furthermore, the entire region shared a common history shaped by the Chinese, Turkic, and Tibetan peoples moving across this vast and formidable landscape as merchants, missionaries, or military men. These shared cultural and historical factors allow us to explain how the art of Karakhoto and Ladakh might have evolved similar features, but the correspondence between specific motifs (such as the triangular jewelry), individual mannerisms (such as the pigeon-toed Bodhisattvas), and the similar iconography suggest the possibility of related patronage groups. For example, it has recently been noted (Karmay 1975:42) that six monks of the Dri-gung-pa (a particularly prominent branch of the Kagyud-pa *(bka'-brgyud-pa)* sect then present in the western Trans-Himalaya) were also in Karakhoto in 1222. It is possible that the Trans-Himalayan Indo-Tibetan art found at this city may have resulted from Dri-gung-pa patronage.

The process of cultural transformation is perhaps nowhere more complex and enigmatic than in Central Asia (Chapter IV), and this is especially true of the cultural and economic interactions which occurred in the monastic centers along the trade routes of the Trans-Himalaya. Although stylistic and iconographic relationships between the art of Dunhuang and distant centers in India can be identified, the processes by which this cross-fertilization occurred are still obscure. This study is meant to provide an opportunity to analyze and compare works from Central Asia and the western Trans-Himalaya, and to assist us in understanding the role of Central Asia in the evolution of Esoteric Buddhist art.

Catalogue Entries

Plates: 46 – 77

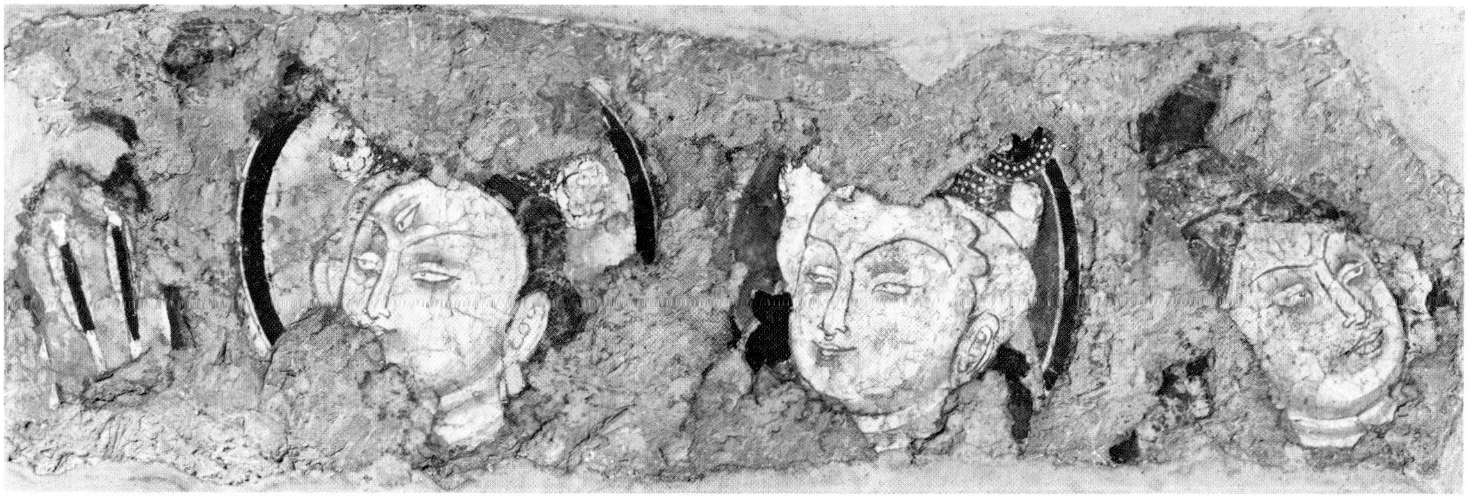

Pl. 46
Three Heads
Fragment of wall painting
Kizil (Turfan), Maya Cave III
Ca. 625–650 A.D.
H. 18.73 × 48.26 cm with frame
National Museum of American Art, Smithsonian Institution
Gift of John Gellatly (1929.8.325.6)

Pl. 48
Standing Monk in Patched Robe; Group of Heavenly Attendants
Fragment of wall painting
Kizil (Turfan), Maya Cave III
Ca. 625–650 A.D.
H. 82.87 × 72.71 × 7.94 cm (with frame)
National Museum of American Art, Smithsonian Institution
Gift of John Gellatly (1929.8.325.5)

(See Color Plate 48)

Pl. 47
Assembly Listening to the Buddha Preaching
Fragment of wall painting
Kizil (Turfan), Maya Cave III
Ca. 625–650 A.D.
H. 67.31 × 36.61 cm (with frame)
National Museum of American Art, Smithsonian Institution
Gift of John Gellatly (1929.8.325.0)

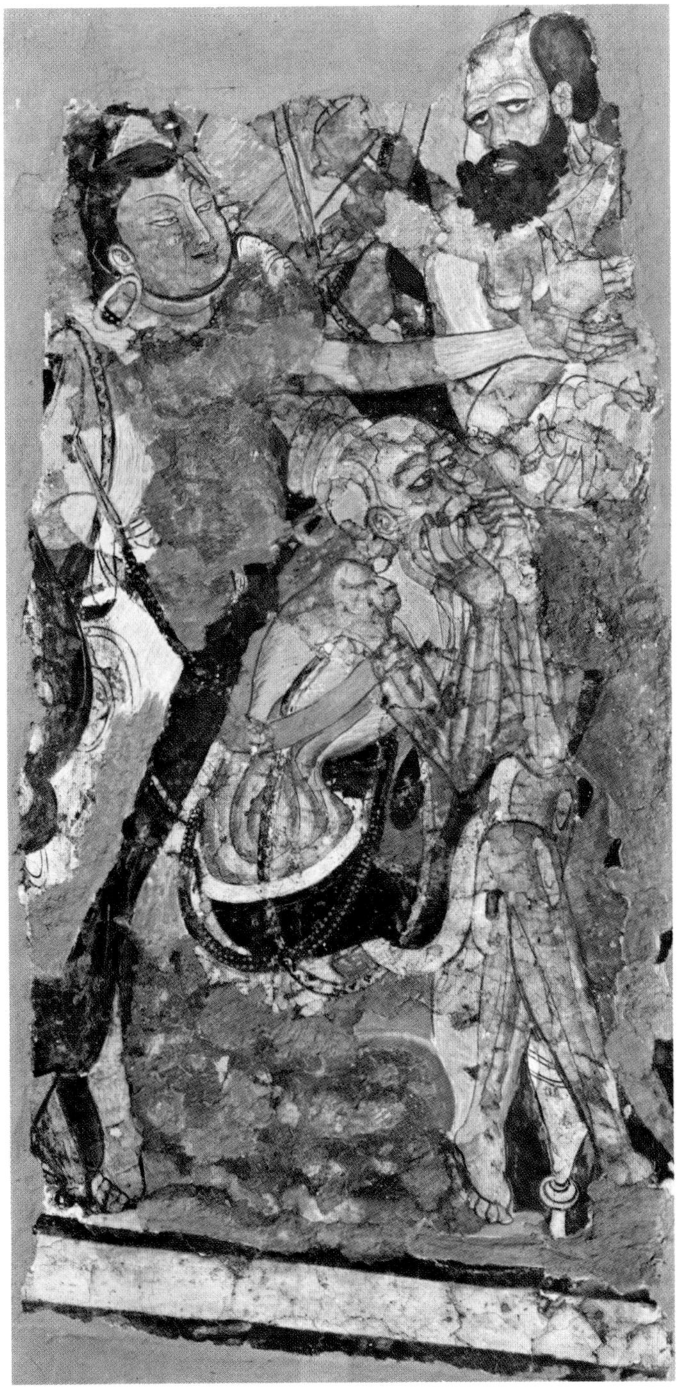

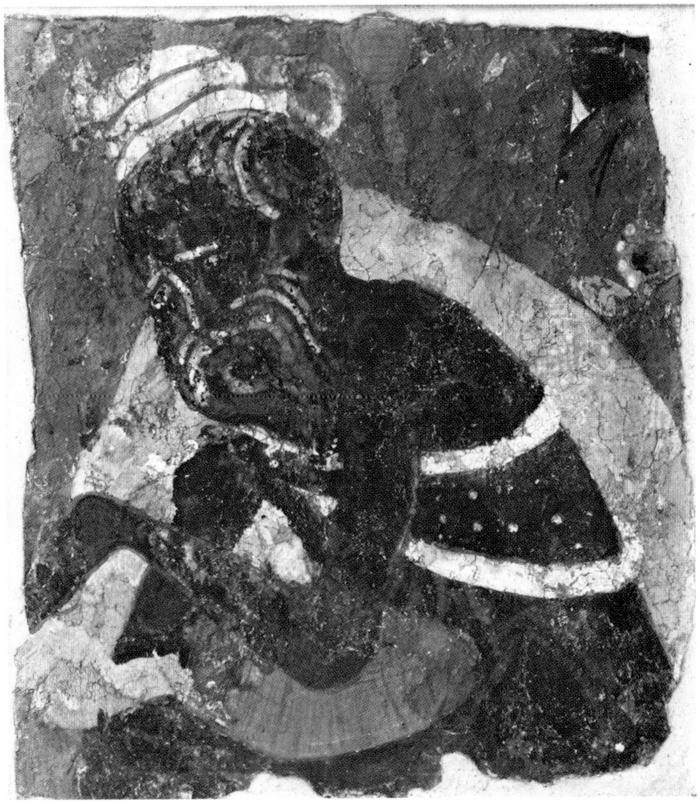

Pl. 49
Hermit in Cave
Fragment of wall painting
Kizil (Turfan), Maya Cave III
Ca. 625–650 A.D.
H. 20.02 × 18.415 × 5.08 cm (with frame)
National Museum of American Art, Smithsonian Institution
Gift of John Gellatly (1929.8.325.3)

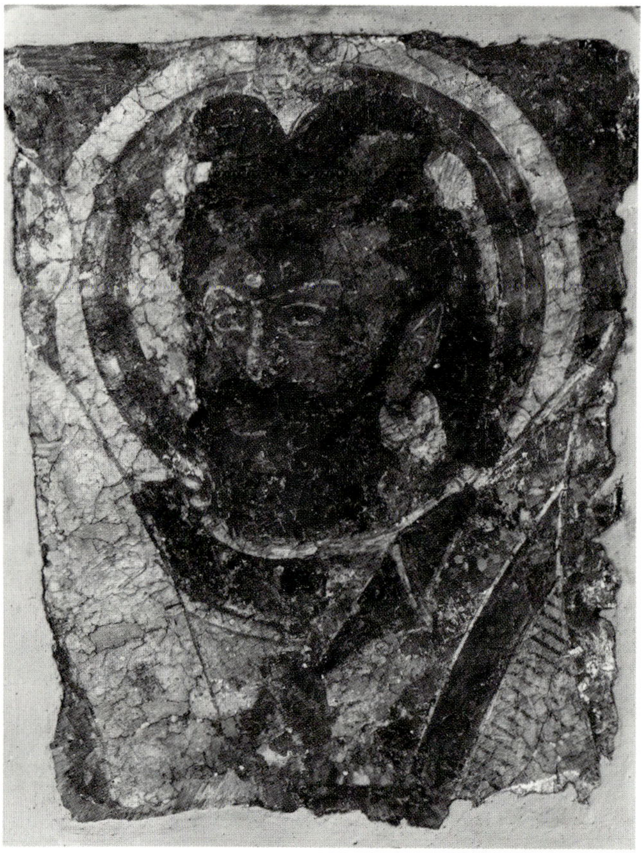

Pl. 50
Head of Devatā
Fragment of wall painting
Kizil (Turfan), Maya Cave III
Ca. 625–650 A.D.
H. 42.88 × 34.61 × 7.62 cm (with frame)
National Museum of American Art, Smithsonian Institution
Gift of John Gellatly (1929.8.325.3)

These little-known fragments from the Smithsonian Institution have been chosen because of the long-acknowledged relationship between the art of Kucha and historical northwest India. It had, for instance, been suggested several times that the Buddhist wall painting of the Hindu Kush influenced the wall painting of Kizil. However, in recent decades, art historical studies have redated the art of many trade centers in both greater India and Central Asia. As a result, the clear progression of Buddhist art from the earlier artistic centers in Gandhāra and Afghanistan to Central Asia and beyond can no longer be maintained. In fact, Buddhist art continued to be produced in Afghanistan and Pakistan until the eighth and probably also the ninth centuries. Thus, some sites such as Bāmiyān or Tepe Sardār in Ghaznī were contemporaneous with the silk route sites such as Kizil and Khotan. In contrast to earlier opinions, it now appears that the seventh-century art of Kizil (the approximate date of all four fragments) influenced the art of Bāmiyān dating to the late seventh century (Klimburg-Salter in press). Recent studies on Kizil (Nagai 1977), Khotan (Williams 1973), and the Hindu Kush (Klimburg-Salter 1976, 1980), as well as the iconography of Central Asia in general (Gaulier et al. 1976), have established an interest in late Mahāyāna and tantric iconographic themes at these Buddhist centers.

It has been established (Uyeno 1980) that the Smithsonian fragments came from Maya Cave III, and the Cave of the Musicians. This places their date of manufacture between 625–650 A.D. and relates them to the latest phase of the Indo-Iranian style (Klimburg 1970; 1974). Unfortunately, the exact placement of these paintings within the murals is impossible to identify because many of the field notes recorded during the fourth German Central Asian expedition were lost. Some paintings, however, still have notes written on the back.

The iconography of Kizil is, however, extremely repetitive and the compositions remain constant within the different chronological groups. Thus, the themes of these fragments can be inferred, by comparison, to more complete paintings.

Pl. 46: These three heads may belong to a divine assembly listening to the Buddha preach. The head with the third eye (Indra?) is next to three arrows. Thus, this scene may belong to a narrative where Buddha is offered arrows (Jera-Bezard 1980:42). The third head to the right looks in another direction and belongs to another scene.

Pl. 47: In the center of the composition is seated the expressively painted figure of an *arhat*. Behind him are another *arhat* and a monk.

Pl. 48: This painting may actually contain fragments of two scenes. To the left is a divine assembly listening to the Buddha preach. To the right, two monks in patched robes, one carrying a long staff, are surrounded by divine beings. These monks are always treated in a semi-naturalistic style (Bussagli 1979). The ribs and musculature, as well as the facial features, are carefully delineated. In contrast, other figures show an extreme schematization. The use of dark figures with white outlines is a unique theme from Kizil. The same theme is found in Niche H at Bāmiyān and must derive from Kizil (Klimburg-Salter in press). The black figures with white outlines at Foladi (Fig. 40) are a development of the Kizil style. The last phase of this schematic and diagrammatic rendering of the human body may be seen at Ta-pho (Fig. 58).

Pl. 49: This dark-skinned figure is shown seated with his expressive face drawn in white. The setting may be a cave, the dark skin resulting from ashes. Thus, this figure may be a hermit in a cave. That the scene is a part of a Jātaka or Avadana story is also suggested by landscape details in the background. Xuanzang reports both Jain and Śaivite worshippers in Afghanistan who smeared their bodies with ashes. The latter were certainly also known in Central Asia in the seventh century.

Pl. 50: This dark-skinned person with his red hair caught in an ascetic's topknot has the Indo-European facial features frequently remarked upon in the paintings from Kizil. He stands between two large body *mandorlas* which belong to two Buddha figures.

Previously published: (Jera-Bezard 1980:fig.10; Uyeno 1980:Part I and II, pl.VII C; Uyeno 1980).

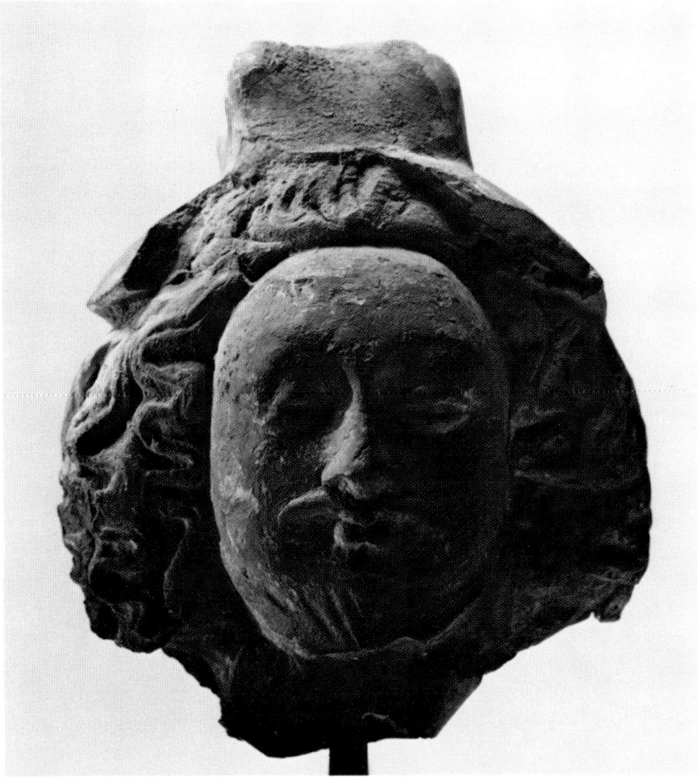

Pl. 51
Central Asian Male Head
Clay
Kucha
Sixth-seventh century
H. 15 × 12.2 cm
George P. Bickford Collection on loan to The Cleveland Museum of Art

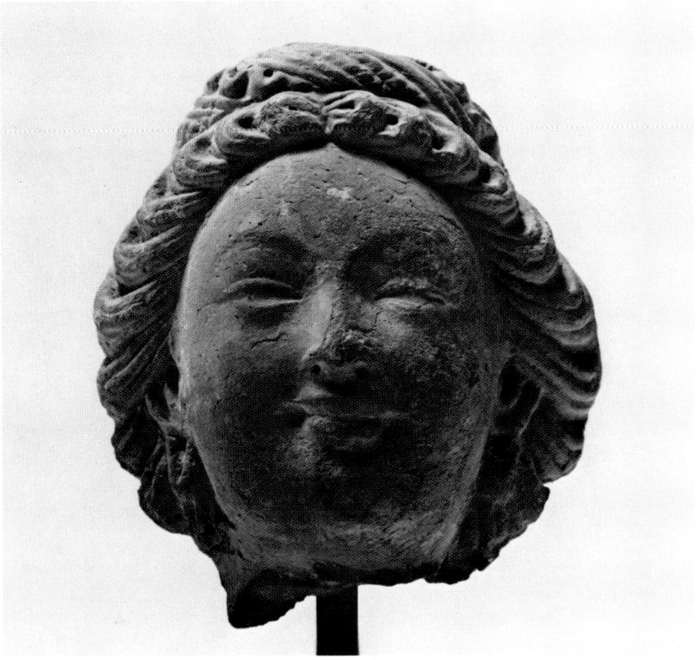

Pl. 52
Central Asian Female Head
Clay
Kucha
Sixth-seventh century
H. 10.5 × 9.7 cm
George P. Bickford Collection on loan to The Cleveland Museum of Art

These small sculptures are made of clay mixed with organic materials and covered with a coating of clay and stucco which was then painted. The fleshy faces, mask-like expressions and stylized hair composed of repetitive loops or S-forms relate these heads to others found in the Kucha region and now in the collections of the Indische Kunst Museum, West Berlin (Metropolitan Museum 1982) and the Musée Guimet, Paris (Musée Guimet 1966, fig. 199). These pieces, once in the Hackin collection, were previously attributed to Fondukistan (Cleveland Museum, 1975). The similarity of the techniques employed in the clay sculpture of Fondukistan and Kucha is discussed in the text. (See Varma 1970:179)

Previously published: (Cleveland Museum 1975:fig.11).

Pl. 53
Finial with Nine Buddhas
Bronze
Central Asia
Ca. sixth-seventh centuries
H. 21.3 × 8.9 cm
Michael Phillips

Nine identical Buddhas are seated in meditation, with the symmetrical U-shaped folds of the monastic garment completely covering both shoulders, hands, and feet. The wide rounded collar of the gown, the wide shoulders of the image and the simple lotus throne relate this figure to stone Buddha images from north India in the sixth century. The shape of the face with rather bloated cheeks and a low *uṣṇīṣa* as well as the pointed *mandorla* indicate the influence of Chinese Central Asian art. The combination of Chinese and Indian stylistic elements suggests a Central Asian origin for this unusual bronze sculpture whose original function is uncertain. Small gilded bronze plaques in different styles, but also combining Chinese and Indian stylistic features, were found at Ak-Beshim in Semirechye in the Kirghiz Republic, U.S.S.R. (Belenitsky 1959) and in Kucha, (for an example of the latter, see Metropolitan Museum 1982:pl. 103).

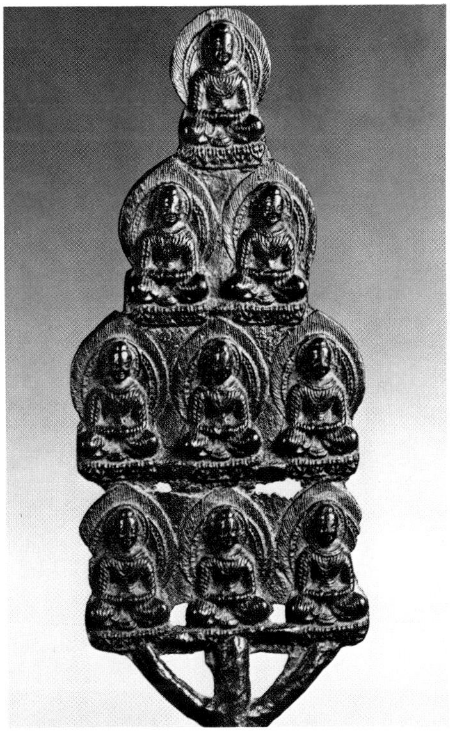

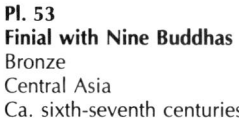

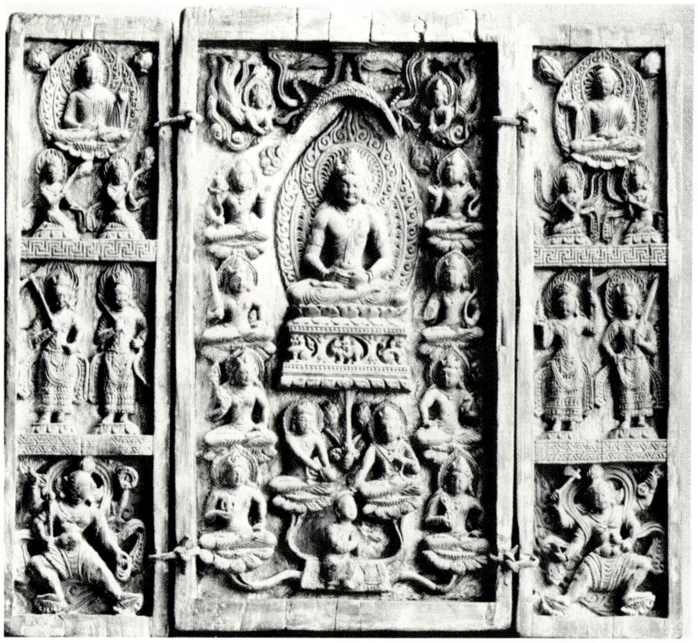

Pl. 54
Traveling Shrine
Sandalwood, traces of red and green colors. Ink inscription on reverse in Tibetan: *"byaṅ chub sems (dpa')*," i.e., Bodhisattva.
Central Asia
Ninth century
H. 30.8 × 35.5 cm (when opened)
Nelson Gallery, Atkins Museum

This exceptional image has frequently been used to illustrate the "close relationship between the arts of Central Asia and those of Kashmir" (Pal 1975:248). The treatment of the crowns and the Buddha's combined pedestal and lotus throne indicate that the Central Asian artist was familiar with Kashmiri bronzes. Indeed, such shrines were meant to be used by travelers and could easily have been carried to northwest India; and thus, portable images like these would have in turn contributed to the exchange of artistic influence between these contiguous areas. The identification of the composition as the *maṇḍala* of the eighth Bodhisattvas, and the occurrence of this theme in India and Dunhuang, have been thoroughly discussed (Granoff 1968–1969). The vertical axis of the entire configuration is a jeweled and crowned image of Śākyamuni seated in meditation. Canopy and banners are suspended over his head suggesting the consecration (*abhiṣeka*) of Śākyamuni as described in the *Mañjuśrīmūlakalpa* (McDonald 1962). Two levels of meaning attached to the *abhiseka* ceremony in Vajrayāna Buddhism (see Ch. VII by Trungpa, Rinpoche) are graphically expressed here: the consecration of Śākyamuni to Buddhahood (*Mahāvastu* as translated by Jones 1900) and the consecration of the initiate. The latter theme is treated at the bottom of the central panel where two Bodhisattvas are consecrating a monk.

Previously published: (Granoff 1968; Handbook of the Collections in the William Rockhill Nelson Gallery of Art and Mary Atkins Museum of Fine Arts, Kansas City, Missouri 2: Art of the Orient 1973:129; Pal 1975b:no.102; Klimburg-Salter in press).

Pl. 55
Buddha
Painting on paper
Qianfodong
Ca. seventh-eighth century A.D.
H. 30 cm
National Museum, New Delhi (Ch. 00296 c.)

Rectangular piece of brown paper with a seated Buddha figure painted on its right side. The left end of the paper had a stick attached to it. According to Stein, such a painting was "probably pasted at the beginning of manuscript rolls, as one end always shows signs of pasting, and the other is sometimes stiffened by gumming round a strip of bamboo. The paper is the same as used in Ch'ien-fo-tung MSS of the T'ang period" (Stein 1921:997). Buddha is seated in *vajraparyaṅkāsana* on a lotus-seat. His right hand is in *vyākhyānamudrā* and the left hand on the lap holds a red lotus-bud. Behind him a circular aureole and a round *mandorla* are seen. Above his head is a stylized canopy. The black *uṣṇīṣa* of the Buddha is shaped like a trefoil. Below the top-knot a white circular jewel outlined in black is seen. He has a slightly square-shaped face. The facile features are drawn by very fine black lines, ears are long, color of the flesh is dark-buff, shading is done with light-buff color. A green *antaravāsaka*, with a border painted black and white, passes horizontally across his chest. Over the *antaravāsaka* he wears an *uttarāsaṅga*, which is painted red on the outside and grey on its reverse. The *uttarāsaṅga* is worn like a sacred thread but part of it is seen over his right shoulder. Folds of the robe are shown by thin black lines. The aureole and *mandorla* are designed with concentric bands.

The canopy is shown by two curved white bands; the ends of each band are voluted. Between the two volutes a flaming jewel is seen. In the middle of the band there is a dome-shaped object surmounted by a flaming jewel with a lotus base. On either side of the central jewel there are small elliptical red jewels. From the curved canopy hang four pairs of long streamers tied into large bow-knots. Below the central large jewel of the canopy hangs a rosette with a pendent green gem. The throne of the Buddha is raised high by an ornamental stand with a lotus-base. The painting is well-preserved and the colors look very fresh. Outlines of the painting seem to be drawn by a master-hand but shading of the skin is crudely accomplished.
Chhaya Bhattacharya

Published in: Andrews 1935:232; Stein 1921:996–997; Waley 1931:246.

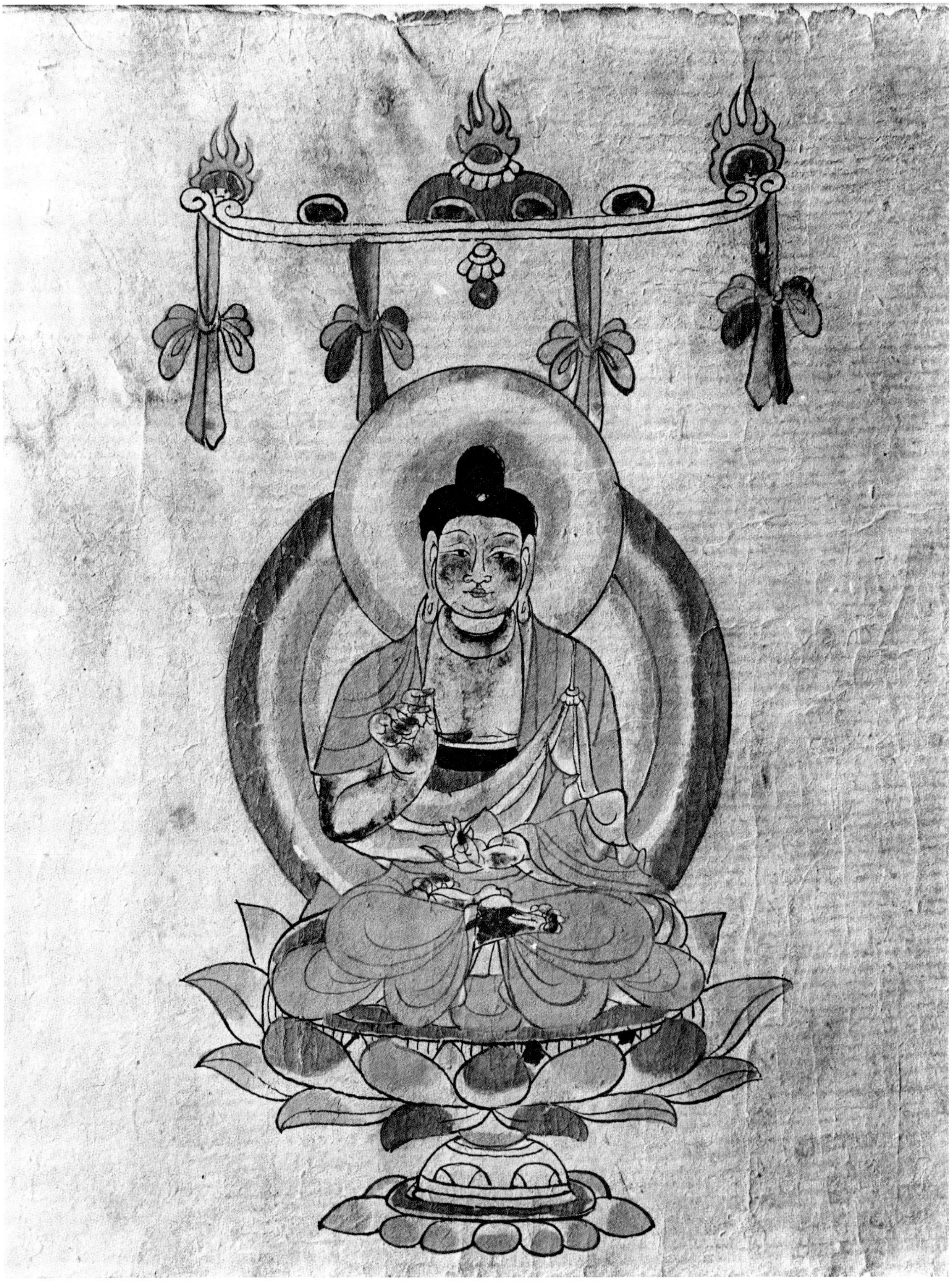

Pl. 56
Iconographic Painting/Representations of Famous Buddha Images
Fragments of ink and colors on silk
Dunhuang, Qianfodong, Cave 17
Tang dynasty, eighth century
Original painting approx. H. 310 × 200 cm
The Trustees of the British Museum, London.

In the division of the Stein collection by Raphael Petrucci, he recognized the outstanding importance of this painting for its associations with India, and the major part of the painting is therefore lent to this exhibition by the National Museum of India. Various fragments remaining were assembled on a panel and were assigned to the British Museum. Professor Alexander Soper has studied and reproduced them in an article in *Artibus Asiae* (vol. 27, 1967 pp 349–364). For the present exhibition these fragments have been remounted so that they can better be seen in relation to the New Delhi portion of the painting.

The whole painting originally consisted of four rows of images, here referred to as A, B, C, and D. The largest British Museum fragment is from row A at the top of the painting, with a very small piece of purple silk border defining the left edge of the painting. This fragment shows two Buddhas standing side by side beneath canopies, followed by a large seated Buddha in a red robe, also under a canopy, and attended by monks, only one of whom survives. Of the next scene only two figures with a ladder remain, with the bare feet of another, on the opposite side of the missing central image.

The second fragment in the British Museum may also come from row A, from the extreme right since it shows traces of the right hand border. If it does, then the painting was originally made up of three and a half widths of silk approximately, each width about 59–60 cm wide, the extra half width being at the left. This second fragment comprises a large garlanded Bodhisattva, and a standing figure holding a sun disc in his raised right hand.

The Delhi portion is less fragmentary, continuing down the left side of the painting with rows B, C, and D. One seated figure has been moved from the end of row C into a space at the end of row B. Its present place there rightly belongs to the third of the British Museum fragments, showing a Buddha seated in western fashion with legs pendent, with multiple small figures in the aureole, which has a top section of musicians. Next to this Buddha is the lower half of a standing Buddha in a red robe.

The British Museum also has the inscription panel, probably from row E below the lowest figures in rocky settings, and part of the figure of an eighth century donor. Until recently this fragment was mounted upside down. Finally, a narrow strip preserves a *stūpa* and a lance, enough to identify their holders as two guardian kings. The position of these in the original composition must await the possible identification of further fragments from the painting, some of which are believed to be in the Hermitage, Leningrad (personal communication from Mme. Krishna Riboud).

Evidence for the dating of the *Famous Images* painting is both iconographical and stylistic, with both elements suggesting a date earlier than most of the rest of the paintings from Dunhuang. In his article in *Artibus Asiae,* Propfessor Soper has already drawn attention to the Buddha or Bodhisattva in row C, immediately to the right of the four smaller configurations in the New Delhi portion. This figure "has a flaming aureole surrounded by musician angels in flight, and topped by a small reliquary *stupa:* a combination whose only known source is the purely Chinese repertory of the sixth century Wei style." He goes on to note the "authentic Chinese dragon" of the same figure's throne, but he might also have noticed that the jewellery worn by the figure itself has its origins in the art of Gandhara. We may begin with the elaborate pendant suspended on the chest: although it contains Chinese elements such as the dragon heads, the whole pendant with its two central figures is extraordinarily close to a Bodhisattva in the Musée Guimet (Madeleine Hallade, *The Gandhara Style,* London 1968 Pl. 68). That same Gandhāra Bodhisattva also provides the explanation for the curious little animal seen emerging from the ear of the same figure in the New Delhi painting: in the stone sculpture both ears wear heavy pendants in the form of the bust and forelegs of a small, possibly winged, animal. Of the headdress itself only a large rosette and one edge of a rectangular panel remain in the painting to suggest that this too may have resembled the sculpture. Other ornaments such as the armband worn above the elbow, or the double bracelet on the left arm, confirm the close kinship of the painted figure with its sculptural prototype.

This iconographical evidence for an early date, before such features were modified and absorbed into the Chinese tradition, is confirmed when we examine the stylistic qualities of line and structure in the same figure. The means of depiction used throughout is a fine, continuous and sensitively modulated brush line; such colours as remain are principally used for the ornamental parts, such as the dragon throne, the collar, and the figures in the aureole. This brush line is equally able to render both drapery folds and the features of the figure itself: as an example we may take the fairly complex delineation of the lips, closely resembling the formula still current in the early eighth century, and made up of at least five separate strokes. By the early tenth century, the mouth could be rendered in just three strokes, with a single straight line dividing the lips and ending in pronounced hooks that no longer imply the depressions at either side of the mouth. This loss of three-dimensional effect is matched in the quality of line seen in tenth-century paintings, generally short and with abrupt changes in thickness.

Further evidence of early date for the *Famous Images* painting may be found in many of its features, for example the canopies, especially those in the British Museum fragment from row A at the top of the painting: their clear three-dimensionality, emphasised by the curled-up ends of the ribs or the segmental panels of contrasting colour between them, finds its closest parallel in such wall-paintings as those of the early Tang in Cave 322, or those of the High Tang in Cave 45 at Dunhuang (*Makkōkutsu,* vol. 3, pls. 18, 135). Indeed, the closer one examines the surviving parts of this outstanding painting, the more one is led to conclude that it is possibly a seventh-century work, and certainly no later than the eighth century.

Roderick Whitfield

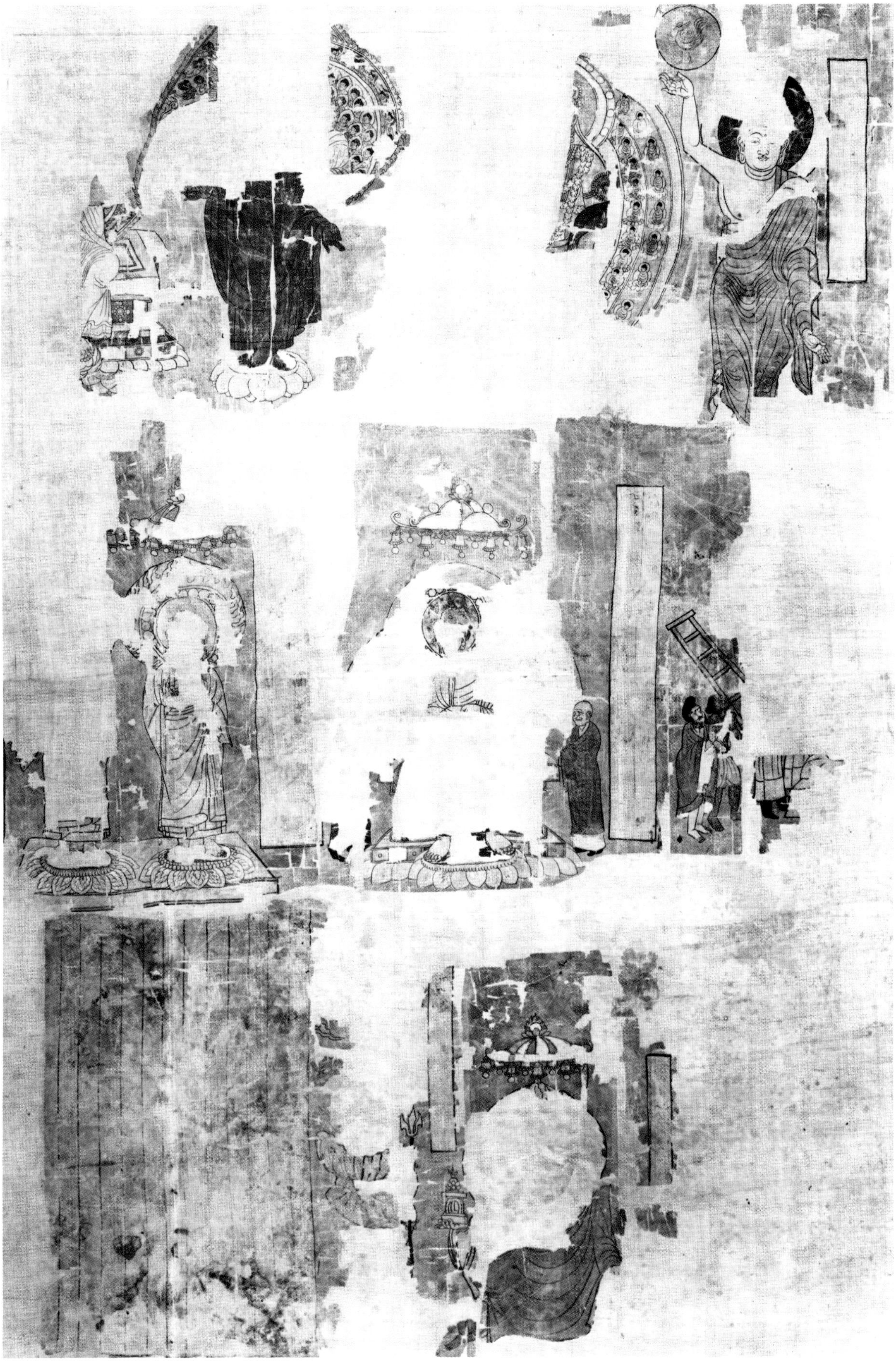

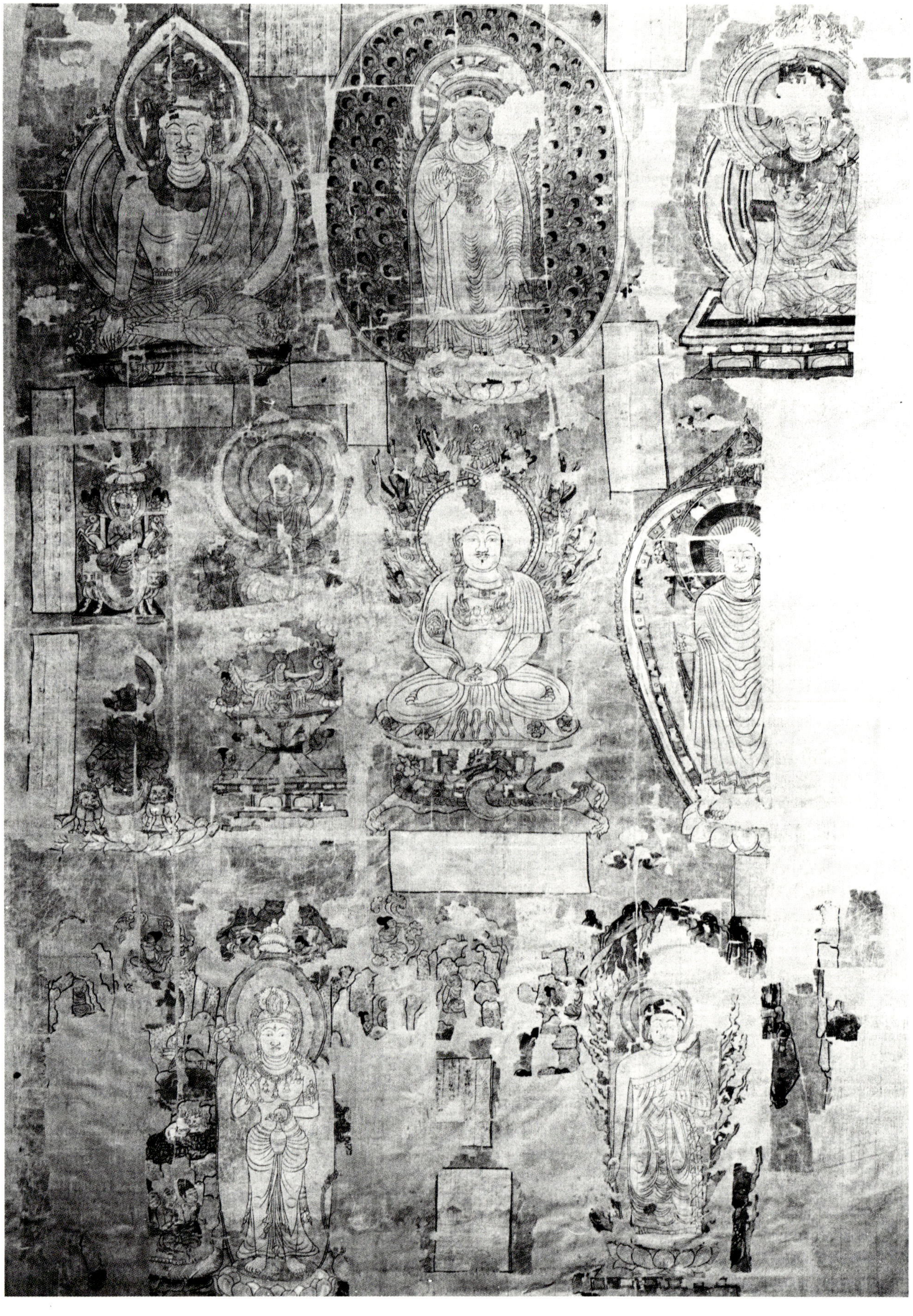

Pl. 57
Copies of Buddha and Bodhisattva Images from India
Paint on silk
Dunhuang, Qianfodong
Ca. seventh-eighth century
H. 60 × W. 90 cm
National Museum, New Delhi (Ch. XXII.0023)

This fragment of the large banner shows reproductions of famous Buddha and Bodhisattva figures in different postures and *mudrās* worshipped at various sacred places in India. They are arranged in three rows. The inscriptions in cartouches in Chinese characters and the clear iconographic indications help to identify the figures represented in the painting. (See Waley 1931:268–271; Stein 1921:877–879, 1024–1026; Rowland 1947:5–20; Soper 1964).

On the top row, left corner, a bejeweled Buddha (No. 1) is seated in *vajraparyaṅkāsana* on a flat rock supported by two grotesque human figures with heads emerging in front. His right hand is in *bhūmisparṣamudrā*. The crown is decorated with a three-headed demon. The demon and the hand touching the earth symbolize his victory over Māra, an event which took place before his Enlightenment. He is ornamented with a heavy necklace and wristlets. His knees are covered with jewels. He has a thin beard and moustache. The circular *mandorla* is decorated with bell-shaped tassels and rosettes as borders. The pipal-leaf shaped aureole has a flaming border. The cartouche on his left bears an inscription in Chinese characters which is translated by Waley as "Country of Magadha, light-emitting magical image. The eulogy of the picture says: This pictured form is noble and dignified. The head is spangled with bright pearls and adorned with lovely jewels. Square throne, cornered tiers, halo . . . the merit of looking up at the Blessed One's face" (Waley 1931:268). This represents "a statue in the Kingdom of Magadha," which may be identified with the "Vajrasana of Mahā-bodhi" (Stein 1921b:1025).

Next to figure No. 1, the figure of a Buddha (No. 2) is seen standing on a lotus. His right hand is in *abhayamudrā* and his left hand is pendent. Radiating bursts of small Buddha figures decorate the elliptical *mandorla* behind him. Each of these small figures has a circular aureole with flames on top. Flames are also seen shooting up like wings at the edges of the head-scarf which is the same as found on the heads of Kṣitigarbha figures from Central Asia. This drawing represents the episode "Great Miracle of Śrāvastī." A similar sculptural representation was unearthed by Stein at the Rawak *vihara* in Khotan (Stein 1921b:figs. 63,64).

On the left of figure No. 2, another seated figure (No.3) is seen, in the same attitude as figure No. 1. Stein says this figure is misplaced (Stein 1921b:1025). The figure is framed by a circular aureole and a *mandorla* with flaming borders. On either side of his head a crescent of moon is seen. The figure may represent Bodhisattva Chandraprabhā: Light of the Moon, he is white in colour and holds a moon disc on a lotus (Bhattacharyya 1968 89). Usually the banners from Central Asia represent the Sun and Moon Bodhisattvas (Jāliniprabhā and Chandraprabhā) against red and white discs respectively (cf. Ch.XXVIII.006, Stein 1921b:pl.LXIV).

In the beginning of the middle row, four smaller Buddha figures are seen. Fig. No. 4 is seen seated in *vajraparyaṅkāsana* on a high throne supported by lions. The hands near his chest show palms outwards. Above his head a well-decorated canopy is visible. Over his throne, busts of two figures hold fly whisks and either side of his throne is decorated with grotesque animal figures having wings and prominent beaks. A much-effaced inscription in Chinese characters is translated by Waley as follows: "Kapilāvastu . . . silver image. The eulogy of the picture says . . . true appearance . . . image . . . then . . . merit" (Waley 1931:269).

On the left of figure No. 4 another small Buddha figure, perhaps Amitābha, (No. 5), is seen seated in *dhyānāsana* on a lotus with everted lotus petals. Behind his body there is a large circular *mandorla* with a flaming border. A dancing Bodhisatta is shown holding a long lotus stalk with a small Dhyāni Buddha on the lotus at bottom on his right, perhaps Avalokiteśvara.

Below figure No. 5, a small Buddha (No. 6) is seen seated on a triple elephant head rested on a *ḍamaru*-shaped throne which in turn is placed on a raised platform similar to the seat of figure No.3. Two elephant heads on the sides emit two lotuses, each with one of the Five Buddhas seated on it. In the middle of the *ḍamaru*-shaped throne upper portions of two small human figures are seen as if trying to climb up with great difficulty. Below on the platform two devotees are seen with hands in *añjalimudrā*. This representation seems to depict the Subjugation of Elephant Nālāgiri by Lord Buddha.

The Buddha figure (No.7) is seen seated on a high throne supported by two lions below figure No. 4. Underneath the throne, a lotus base is visible. The Buddha is seated in *dhyānāsana* with his right hand over his right knee and left hand in *abhayamudrā* is raised near his chest.

On the left of the group of four Buddhas described above is a figure of a Bodhisattva (No. 8) in *vajraparyaṅkāsana* on a raised throne borne by a dragon. According to Rowland "this may be a replica of the image of Buddha subduing the dragon of Nagarahara, which was among the trophies brought to China by Hsüan-tsang" (Rowland 1947:12). His hands, with fingers interlaced and thumbs joined at tips, are on his lap. He is richly adorned with ornaments, *viz.*, a heavy necklace with two lion heads as spacers and two dragon-heads (*makara*), each with an opened jaw as if ready to swallow the two small figures (Buddha figures?) as pendants. The border of the aureola is embellished with a beaded band and flaming tongues of fire. Right above his crown is a *stūpa*. On the flaming border divine musicians and devotees are seen. The figure may be identified as Bodhisattva Maitreya, the Future Buddha (Bhattacharyya 1968:80). The joyous scene on the flaming border may suggest the descent of the Future Buddha from the Tusita heaven to the Earth.

On the left of figure No. 8, a standing Buddha (No. 9) is seen framed against a circular aureole and an oval *mandorla*. The top of the *mandorla* is again extended to form an ogee-top. The Buddha stands on a lotus. His right arm is held out sideways and the hand is opened. The ogee-top probably represents the scene of the First Sermon of the Buddha in the Deer Park at Sārnāth. The small figure of the Buddha seated in *dhyānāsana* shows his right hand in *vyākhyānamudrā*. He sits on a high lotus throne. On each side, a standing Bodhisattva figure is seen together with a kneeling deer near the lower legs of the extant Bodhisattva.

Below figure No. 6, a bejeweled three-eyed Avalokiteśvara (No. 10) stands on a lotus, his crown embellished with a standing Buddha figure, a long lotus stalk in his right hand, an *amṛta kalaśa* in his left hand, and his hair matted in the manner of Lord Śiva. Above his aureole, two flying figures amidst three bears carry the crown of Avalokiteśvara. On his right, at the bottom of a group of three devotees is seen. Above this group, a relaxing lion is depicted. Above the lion, a Garuda plays a lute. The effaced inscription in Chinese characters is translated by Waley as "Middle (India) Varanasi (Benares) country, Deer Park . . . image. The eulogy of the picture says . . ." (Waley 1931:270; Soper 1964:362).

On the left of figure No. 10, there is a rocky landscape which represents the Gṛdhakuta hill. In the grotto, Śākyamuṇi (No. 11) stands on a lotus in *samapādabhanga* pose. His right hand, pendent, is in *varadāmudrā*.

This painting is highly interesting not only because of its iconography and the valuable inscriptional information but also for its style. The Chinese pilgrims to India made drawings of important Buddha figures with the intention to reproduce them in their country. The Chinese artists were more concerned with the general proportion and attributes of the icons than the peculiarities in style. However, some of their paintings or sculptures show remarkably faithful reproductions of the Indian originals. Figure Nos. 8 and 10 are the best examples. They show a strong Gandhāra influence in their treatment, e.g. the ornaments (*makara* type pendant of a necklace), moustache and folds of garments.

Chhaya Bhattacharya

Previously published: (Stein 1921a:26–28, pl.LXX; Stein 1921b:877–879, pl.XIV; Waley 1931:268–271; Andrews 1935: 224; Rowland 1947:5–20, figs.1,2,4,7,13,16; Soper 1967).

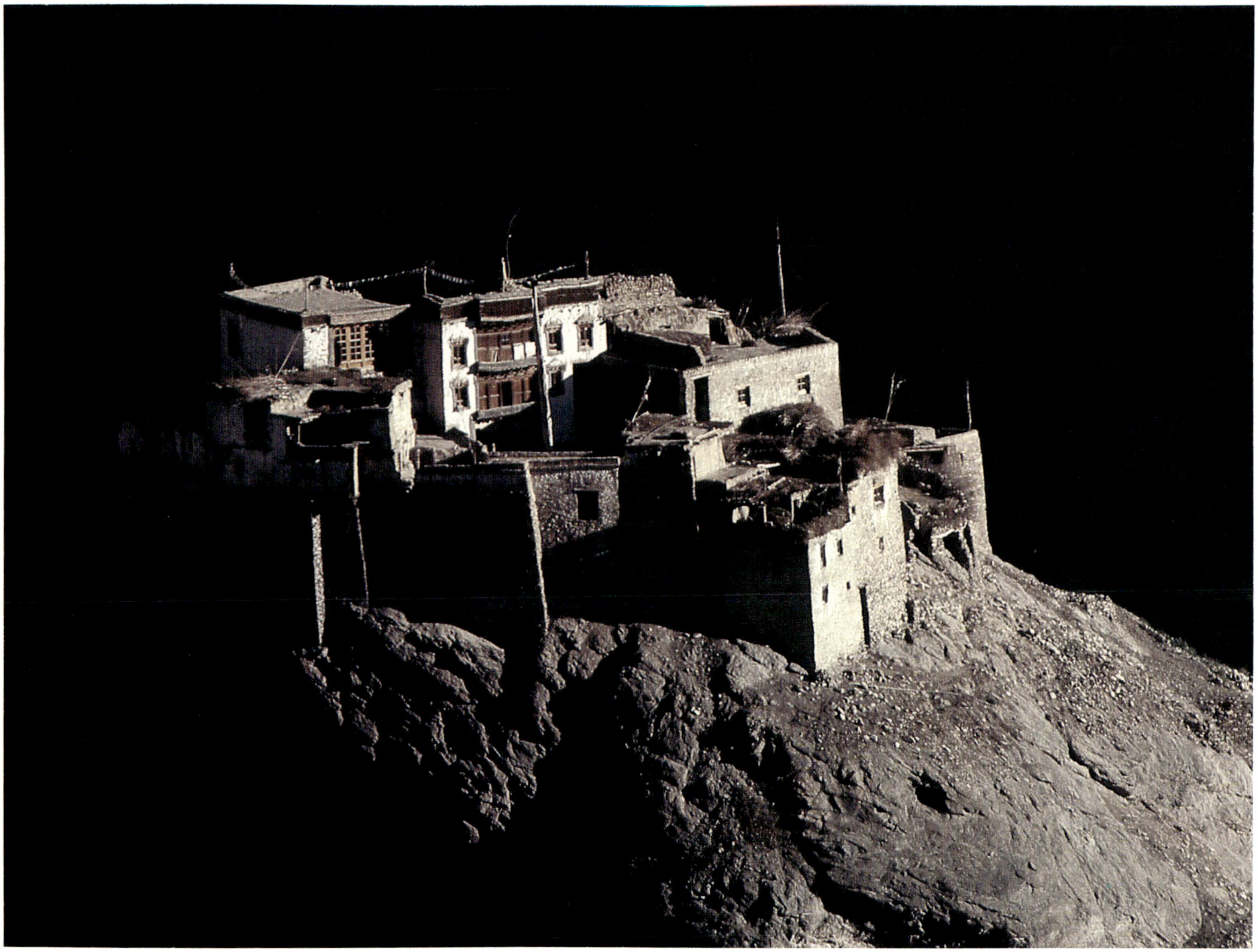

Fig. 7

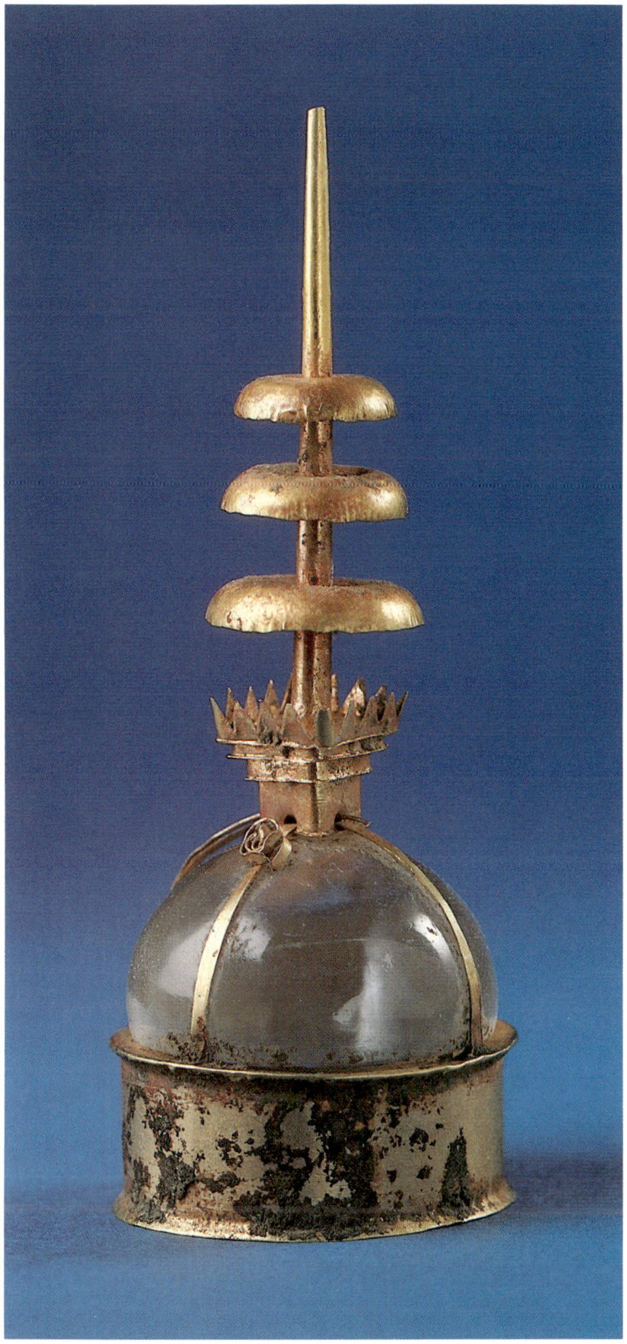

Pl. 1

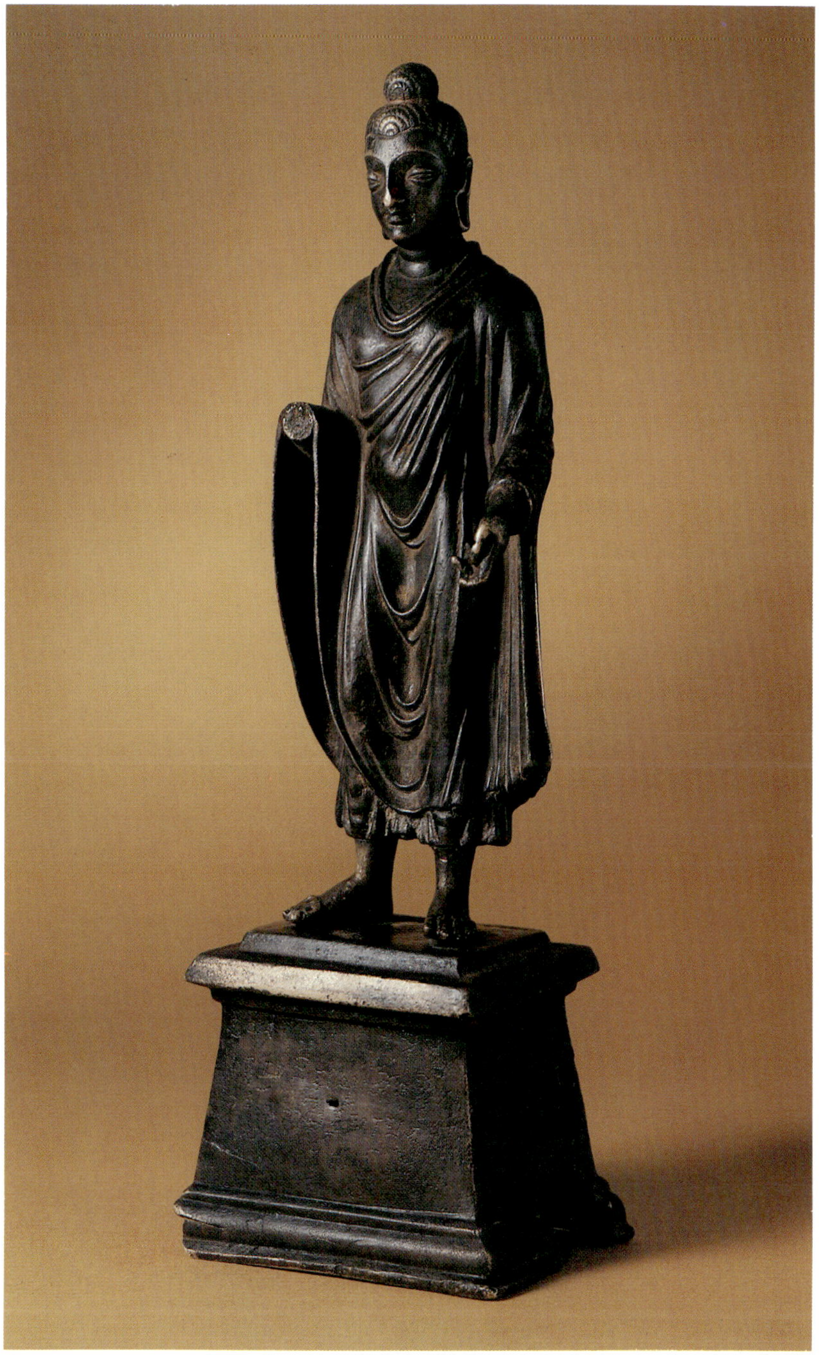

Pl. 2

Pl. 58
Mañjuśrī
Painting on silk
Dunhuang, Qianfodong
Ca. ninth-tenth century
H. 53.4 × 14.6 cm
National Museum, New Delhi (Ch.lvi.005)

Stein identified this figure as Mañjuśrī with a question mark (Stein 1921b:1074). Waley simply described the figure as a Bodhisattva (Waley 1931:302). But on the basis of the golden complexion and the *pothī* (*Prajñāpāramitā* manuscript) on the lotus, he may be identified as Mañjuśrī (Bhattacharyya 1968:104,115–117).

A narrow rectangular banner shows the Bodhisattva Mañjuśrī standing in *samapādabhaṅga* on a lotus pedestal, his right hand holding a spotted object which Stein describes as a "lemon" (Stein 1921b:1074). A long lotus-stalk is seen behind his left hand. The lotus, carrying a *pothī*, is visible over his left shoulder; above his head are the remains of a canopy. All other accessories are lost, *viz.*, the triangular headpiece, side and bottom streamers. He wears a three-pronged crown which is elaborately studded with precious stones. Part of his black hair is tied into a high knot and the rest of the hair falls over his shoulders in the form of narrow wavy locks. He wears large ear ornaments, a necklace and a pair of wristlets which are profusely studded with varied precious stones. The upper part of his body is unclothed except for a long narrow stole painted green, with pale pink lining which falls symmetrically over his shoulders. He wears a short *dhotī*. The treatment of the yellow flesh color gives a metallic effect to the figure, reminiscent of Tibetan and Nepalese bronzes. The lotus petals with the *Prajñāpāramitā* text on it are painted pale pink. The shape of the aureole, patterned after a stylized lotus petal, also displays Nepalese characteristics. On the whole, the figure is very crude. The proportion of the body is not well-balanced; his legs look like logs and the feet are shapeless. A thin border is stitched along the longer edges of the banner. There are ten similar banners (Ch.lvi.001–0010 in the British Museum Stein 101–103) which form a distinct group. All of them are more or less the same size and were found in one bundle, which suggests that they were painted by the same artist and were intended as a set. According to Stein, "In style of design, treatment of garment, ornaments, etc., they show the closest resemblance to the miniatures illustrating Bodhisattvas in two Nepalese manuscripts of the eleventh century. . . . they must have been painted under the direct influence of that late Buddhist pictorial art of India which prevailed in the Gangetic plains. That this influence reached Dun-huang straight from the south, i.e., through Tibet, is *a priori* highly probable, and the occurrence of a short Tibetan inscription on one of these (Ch.lvi.004) banners and of a similar one in Brahmī on another confirms this" (Stein 1921b:862). More recently scholars have considered this group to represent the earliest known example of paintings made for or by Tibetans (Pal 1969 figs 11–12).
Chhaya Bhattacharya

Previously published: Stein 1921b:863–865, 1073–1074; Waley 1931:302–303, no.DXXX; Andrews 1935:228; Matsumoto 1937:II, pl.CCII.b)

(See Color Plate 58)

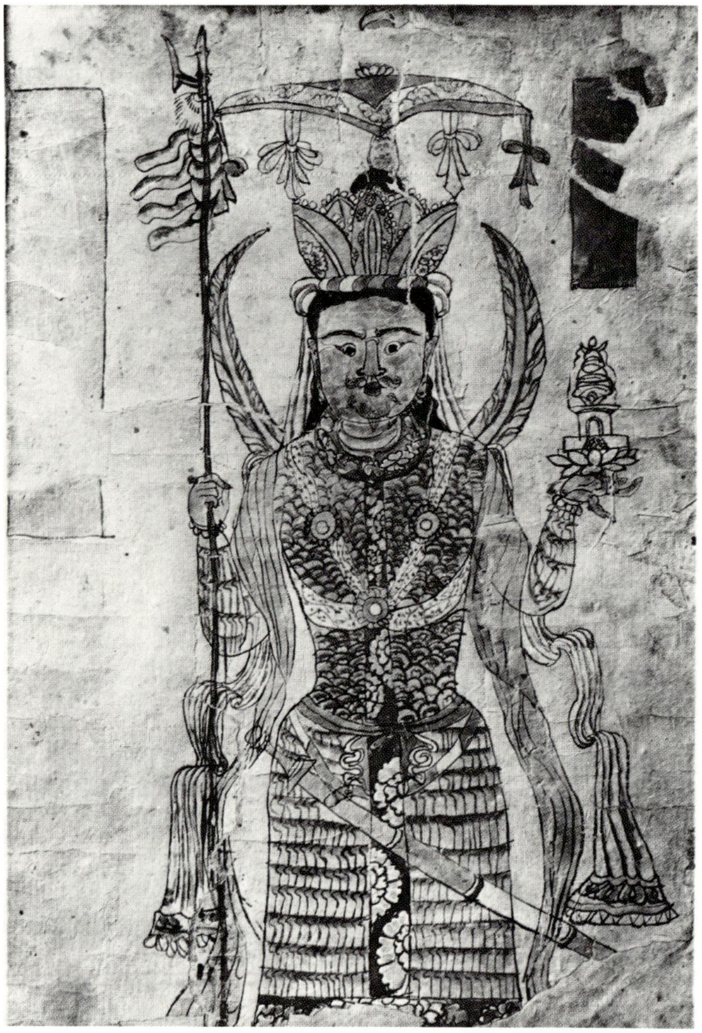

Pl. 59
Vaiśravana
Painting on paper
Dunhuang
Ninth-tenth century
H. 40 × 27 cm
Musée Guimet, Paris

This Vaiśravana stands in a strictly frontal and immobile position underneath a small canopy. His black hair is piled in a very high chignon surrounded by a five-pointed crown tied by streamers on either side of his head; long black curls fall down his back. He has heavy brows, slanted eyes and a moustache and beard. The skin is painted in flesh tones and the military costume drawn in black and colored in yellow, brown and red. He wears a long scarf around his shoulders and a suit of armour with two rondels at the breast and a third in the middle of his chest. He carries a banner in his right hand, a small *stūpa* in his left and a long sword is suspended from his belt. His most distinctive feature is the long arches representing flames rising from his shoulders. The iconographic origins and significance of this form of Vaiśravaṇa have recently been much debated. The iconography appears to have originated from the variant of the Kuṣāṇa royal portrait which represents the king with flaming shoulders. The Vaiśravaṇa type represented here appears to have become prominent after the sixth century A.D. in those regions of Afghanistan and northern Pakistan which were under the influence of the Western Turks (Klimburg-Salter 1981). This would explain the observation (Jera-Bezard 1976) that this form of Vaiśravaṇa with flaming shoulders does not appear at Dunhuang before the beginning of the Tang period. In Khotan, Vaiśravaṇa was associated with a cult of dynastic worship (Granoff 1973). The form of Vaiśravana represented here may form the basis of one of the two aspects of Vaiśravaṇa represented in Tibetan art. (Tucci 1949:II,578–578). This aspect Tucci identified as both the god of war and the divine king. At that time he noted that "in some Buddhist traditions he is already identified with the Turks, Ge sar's Hor" (1949:II,574). The Tibetans briefly occupied both Dunhuang and Khotan and thus could easily have adopted this variant of Vaiśravaṇa during that time.

Previously published: (Matsumoto 1937:418–420; Lalou 1946:103, pl.3; Pelliot (Mission) 1947: no.188; Hallade and Hambis 1956: no.178; Granoff 1970).

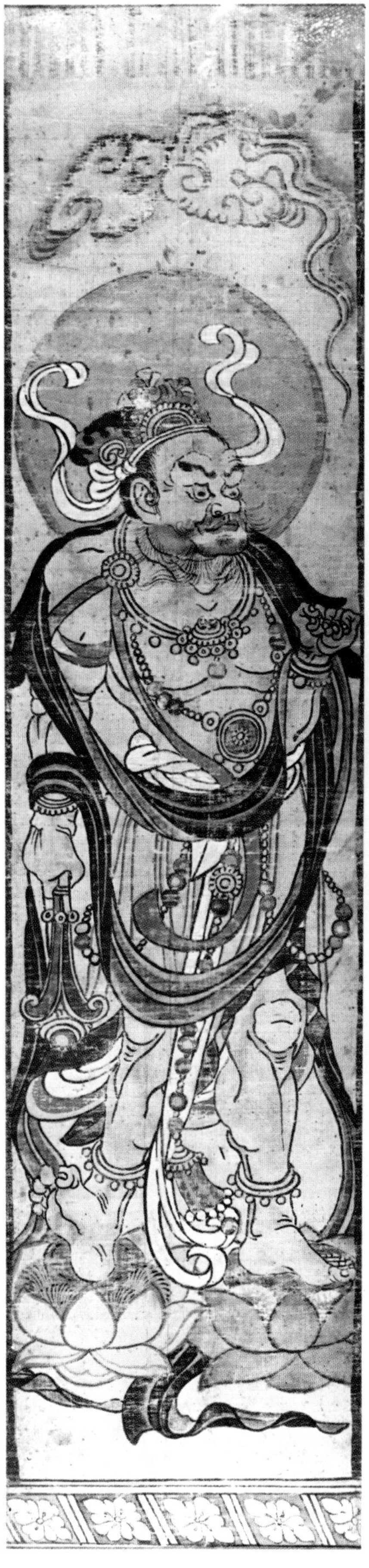

Pl. 60
Indra
Painting on silk
Dunhuang
Ninth century
H. 71 × 17 cm
Musée Guimet, Paris (EO 11726)

This image of the guardian king Kin-Kang Li-Che (Jen Wang), a form of the Hindu god, Indra, provides an interesting contrast to Pl. 59. Although contemporaneous, the paintings are completely different stylistically. Here the god Indra is depicted in three-quarter view wearing the princely garments of India and a diadem tied with flying Sasanian-like ribbons. The luxurious movement of the brown scarf and white drapery, and the flexed right foot poised on the red lotus contrast with the frontal symmetry of the Vaiśravaṇa figure (Pl. 59). The fluid lines of Indra's garments, cloud forms and lotus relate this painting to the Chinese style of ninth-century Dunhuang. But the heavy musculature of the legs and chest are reminiscent of a much earlier depiction of Indra Vajrapāṇi as Hercules found at Hada, Afghanistan. This tradition of pictorial realism is frequently found in Gandharan art associated with certain classes of figures including Vajrapaṇi. The dynamic treatment of the figure and the posture are characteristic of the Tang style (Musée Guimet 1976:68)

Previously published: (Nicholas-Vandier 1954:I,380, II,no.199; *L'Arte del Gandhāra* 1958:no.58; *1,000 (Tausend) Jahrè Chinesische Maleri* 1959:6,no.5).

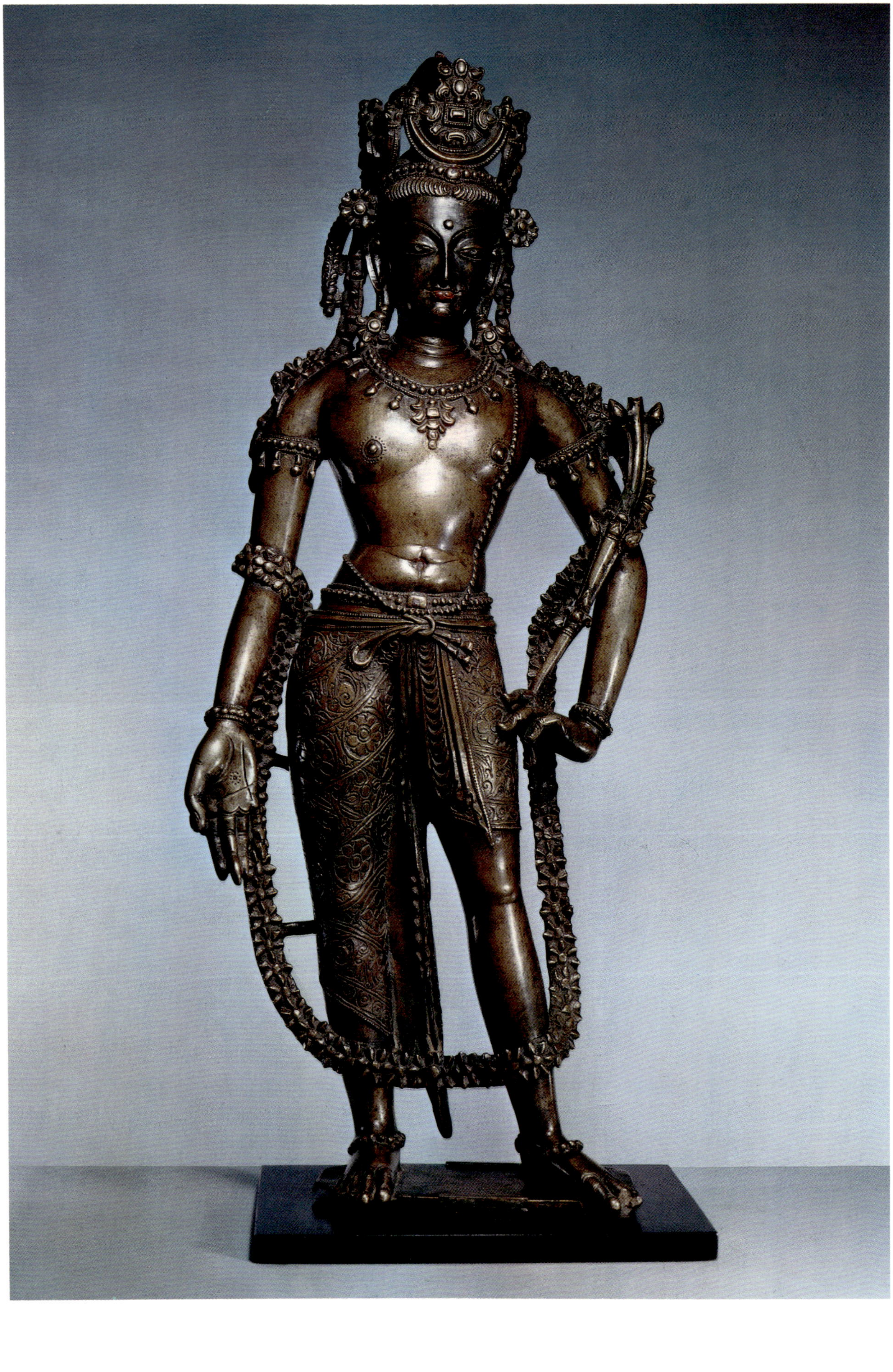

Pl. 30

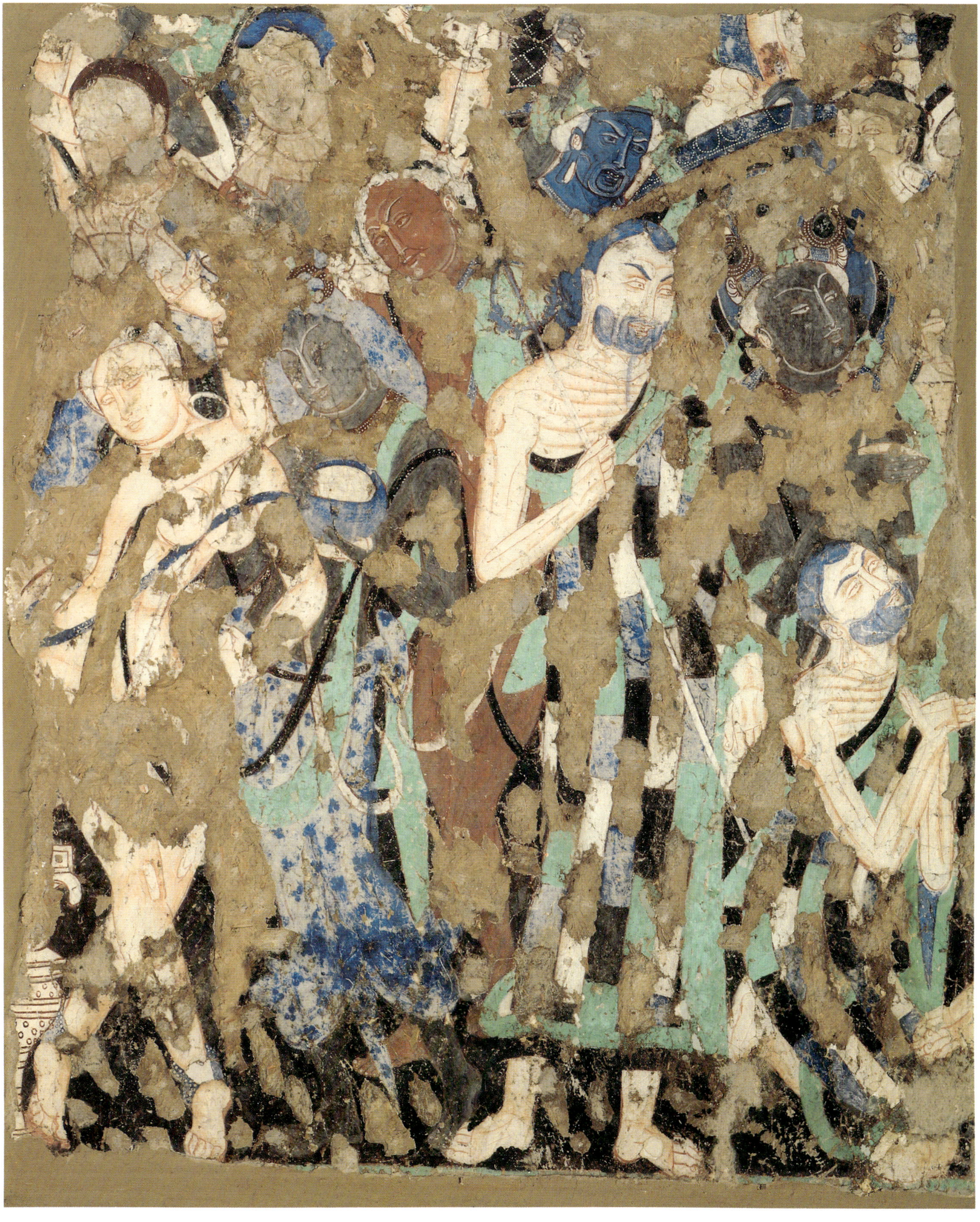

Pl. 48

Pl. 61
Maṇḍala of Avalokiteśvara (Guanyin)
Painting on silk
Dunhuang, Qianfodong
Tenth century
H. 90 × 63 cm
Musée Guimet, Paris (EO 3579)

Despite its size, this painting is depicted with an extraordinary refinement both in line and purity of color. There are three registers. The center contains the *maṇḍala* of the four-armed Avalokiteśvara (at the center-Av.); the upper register, the five Jina (Five Buddhas); and the lower register, donor figures. It is interesting to compare the stylistic and iconographic variations between related motifs in this painting and others from Dunhuang. The small fragment of the center of the *maṇḍala* in Pl. 64 appears quite similar to the central configuration of this *maṇḍala*, but figures in the border area are totally different. In Pl. 66 and Pl. 67, Vairocana and Amoghasiddhi hold their attributes in their right hands, while in this painting and in Pl. 69, the attributes are held in the left hand. Here the animals associated with each guardian figure (14, 13, 16, 15) are almost trampled underfoot while, in Pl. 69, they are given a prominent placement. The circular border of black *vajras* here and in Pl. 64 is missing in Pl. 69. This same border surrounds the clay deities, at Ta-pho (Fig. 28).

The date of this painting can be inferred from the donor figures, the decorative forms between the divinities and other elements such as the pedestals. The deities themselves, however, are represented in an earlier "Himalayan" style datable to ca. ninth century A.D. (Pl. 62). There are several representations of this type of mandala composition (Pls. 64, 69, 72) in which the divinities are ordered into a geometric pattern, then inscribed in a circle which is surrounded by a square with four doors (see also Bhattacharya's entry for Pl. 72). Similar maṇḍalas must also have been known in northern India for by the second half of the eleventh century they are widely used in the western Trans-Himalaya (Figs. 21, 22) In these somewhat more elaborate examples such as in the Sum-tsek in Alchi, the circle encloses the square. It is this latter type which is widely found in later Tibetan art (Pl. 127) A similar history can be proposed for individual motifs such as the "helmet crown." This crown consists of five points which cluster to form a dome or helmet; each point is topped with a medallion containing a Buddha. This crown may have derived from the type of crown illustrated in Pl. 11 and is known in several variants in the Trans-Himalaya (Figs 17 and 40a; Pls. 109, 110, 111).

A diagram of the painting follows:

Upper register:
I. Vairocana
II. Ratnasaṃbhava
III. Akṣobhya
IV. Amitabha
V. Amoghasiddhi
VI. Cintamaṇicakra
VII. 1,000-armed Avalokiteśvara

Center panel:
Av. 4-armed Avalokiteśvara
1. Hayagriva
2. Hayagriva
5. Avalokiteśvara
2,4,6,8 = 4 Bodhisattavas of offering
9,10,11,12 = 4 Bodhisattvas of offering
Four guardians:
13 vajraphota
14 vajravesa
15 vajrankusa
16 vajrapasa

Previously published: (Matsumoto 1937:pl. 65; Musée Guimet 1947:31; Vandier-Nicolas 1954:I, 216–225, II, no. 104; Hallade and Hambis 1956:no. 168; Mallmann 1964:pl. 16.)

Upper register:
I. Vairocana, holds a wheel, throne with lion.
II. Ratnasaṃbhava, holds a *vajra,* throne with elephant.
III. Akṣobhya, holds a flaming jewel, throne with horse.
IV. Amitābha, holds a lotus, a throne with swans.
V. Amoghasiddhi, holds a double *vajra*, throne with garuḍa.
VI. Cintamaṇicakra with six arms.
VII. Thousand-armed Avalokiteśvara.

Central register:
1 and 3 forms of Hayagrīva; 5 and 7 forms of Avalokiteśvara. Bodhisattvas of offering: 8 = Vajralasyā, 2 = Vajramālā, 4 = Vajragītā; 6 = Vajraurṭyā; 9 = Vajradhūpā; 10 = Vajrapuṣpā; 11 = Vajrālokā; 12 = Vajragandhā.

Guardians: 13 = Vajrasphōta; 14 = Vajravesa; 15 = Vajrāṇkusa; 16 = Vajrapāsá.

Lower register: donor figures

This description is condensed from Vandier-Nicholas 1976:II, 216–225.

(See Color Plate 61)

					W					
			III				**IV**			
	VI				**I**				**VII**	
			II				**V**			
					13					
		10						**11**		
					3					
				2		**4**				
S	**16**	**1**			Av.			**5**	**14**	**N**
				8		**6**				
					7					
		9						**12**		
					15					
					E					

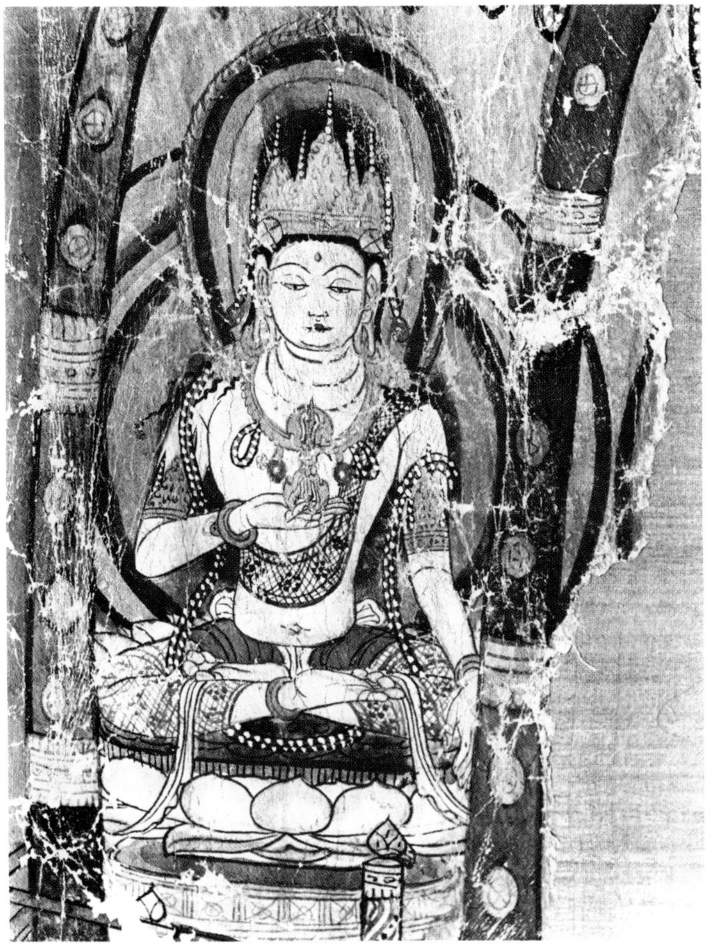

Pls. 62, 63
Fragment of a Maṇḍala with Bodhisattva Figures
Painting on paper
Qianfodong, cave 17, Dunhuang
Ca. Eighth-ninth century
H. 30 × 104.5 cm
National Museum, New Delhi (Ch. 00383 c.)

A horizontal strip of a large painting consists of fragments now mounted together. Two of these fragments show a group of similar Bodhisattva figures while the third fragment, mounted on the extreme left, shows three smaller Bodhisattva figures seated one above the other. Though fragmentary, the painting seems to be part of a large *maṇḍala*. A number of banners painted on silk and ramie depict the theme "*Maṇḍala* of Avalokiteśvara" in which the main figure is surrounded by many Bodhisattva figures in a fashion similar to that in this painting. Here, the central figure can be hypothesized on the basis of the remains of the borders of a *mandorla* within an arch-shaped structure, The *mandorla* of the missing figure is flanked by six Bodhisattva figures, three on each side. Except for the attributes, the group of three Bodhisattvas on each side is executed in the same manner. To the left of the central figure, two figures of Bodhisattva Padmapāṇi are seen on the top row and the bust of Bodhisattva Mañjuśrī appears below. One of the two figures of Bodhisattva Padmapāṇi holds a lotus in his right hand near the chest, and the left hand is placed on his lap. He is seated in *vajraparyaṅkāsana* between the two richly decorated arched pillars of the niche. He is heavily adorned with a three-pronged golden crown, necklaces, armlets, bracelets and anklets. His complexion is orange, tinged with red. He wears a stole like a sacred-thread and an orange *dhotī* with criss-cross designs. Above his head, beaded garlands hang in loops from the canopy and a round *mandorla*. The other Bodhisattva Padmapāṇi is seated in *ardhaparyaṅkāsana* on a white lotus shaded with blue. He holds a long lotus-stalk. His right hand is in *vyākhyānamudrā*. He wears an ear-stud in his right ear and a decorative pendant attached to a ring in his left ear. Similar ear ornaments are also worn by Bodhisattva Mañjuśrī below him, Bodhisattva Vajrapāṇi painted on the extreme right of the fragment, and the Bodhisattva figure below him. Above his head remains of the lotus-seat of another Bodhisattva figure are visible. On the right of the missing central figure are two figures of Bodhisattva Vajrapāṇi. One of them is seen between two elaborately decorated pillars of the niche, adjacent to Bodhisattva Padmapāṇi. Except for his complexion, attribute and position of the left hand, this Bodhisattva Vajrapāṇi figure is painted in the same manner as the Bodhisattva Padmapāṇi opposite him. His complexion is white. He holds a *vajra* in his right hand. The figure on Varjrapāṇi's right is also that of Bodhisattva Vajrapāṇi. He is seated in *mahārājalīlāsana* (or *lalitāsana*) on a white lotus. Each figure has a blank cartouche painted light green and yellow, and outlined in black.

The three, small, seated Bodhisattva figures on the extreme left of the mount appear one above the other. These figures no doubt belong to this style but certainly not to this painting. Of the three figures, two are complete and the third figure, on top, is seen only from the abdomen up. The small figure on the extreme left of the figures in the main part has been identified by Waley and Stein as a Bodhisattva (Waley 1931:242; Stein 1921:995). The figure appears to be that of Vajradhara. He may be shown seated in *vajraparyaṅkāsana* with hands in *vajrahūṅkāramudrā* holding a *vajra* in each hand (Bhattacharyya 1968:43). It is not clear if he holds *vajras* in his hands. He is heavily ornamented and his complexion is white. The figure below him sits on his knees turning three-quarters to his left. He holds a long red stalk with three lotuses. He may be identified as Bodhisattva Mahāsthāmaprāpta. According to Bhattacharyya, the complexion of Mahāsthāmaprāpta is either white or yellow and he holds six lotuses in his hand, and is bedecked in the same way as the figure above. The figures in this painting remind one of Tibetan and Kashmiri art. Both the figure style and the three-pronged crown appear in the art of Kashmir.
Chhaya Bhattacharya

Previously published: (Stein 1921b:II, 865, 995; Waley 1931:170–173, no. 366; 242, no. 367).

(See Color Plate 63)

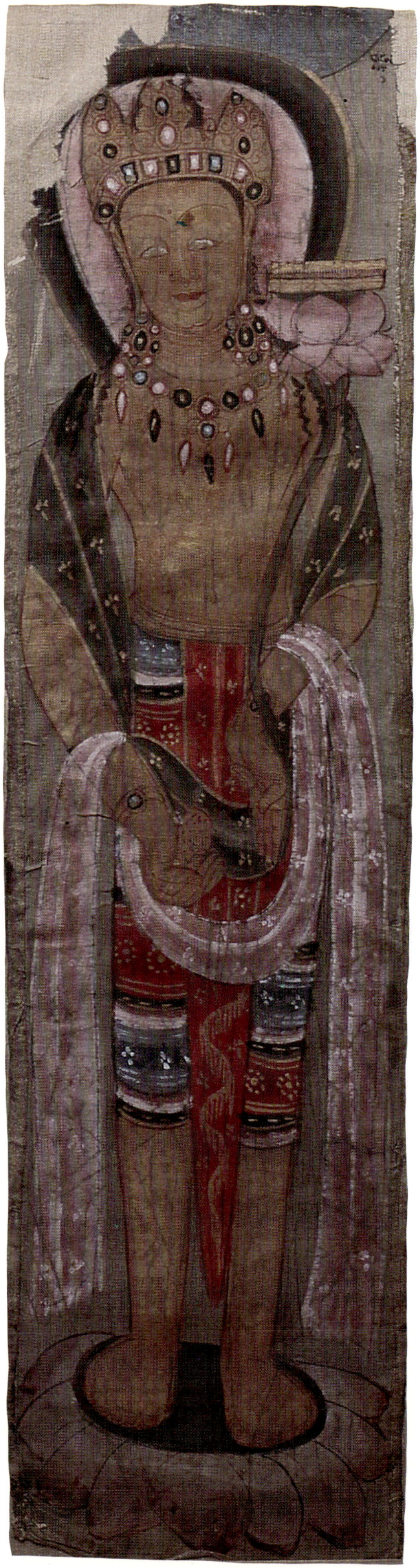

Pl. 58

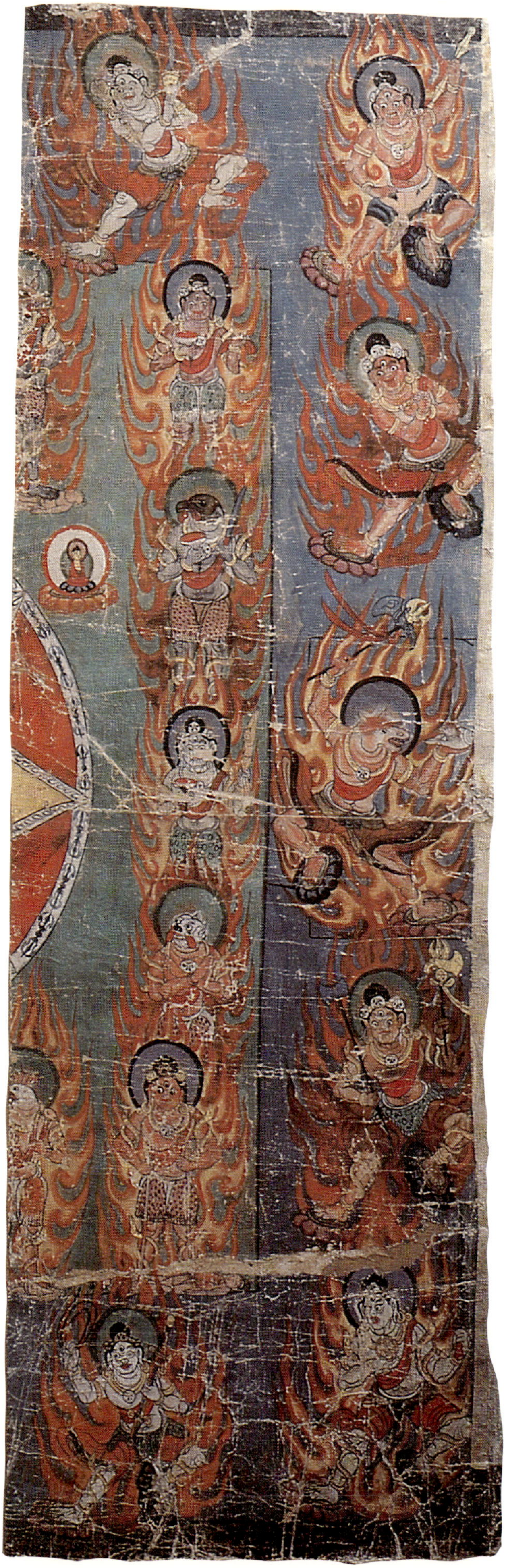

Pl. 64

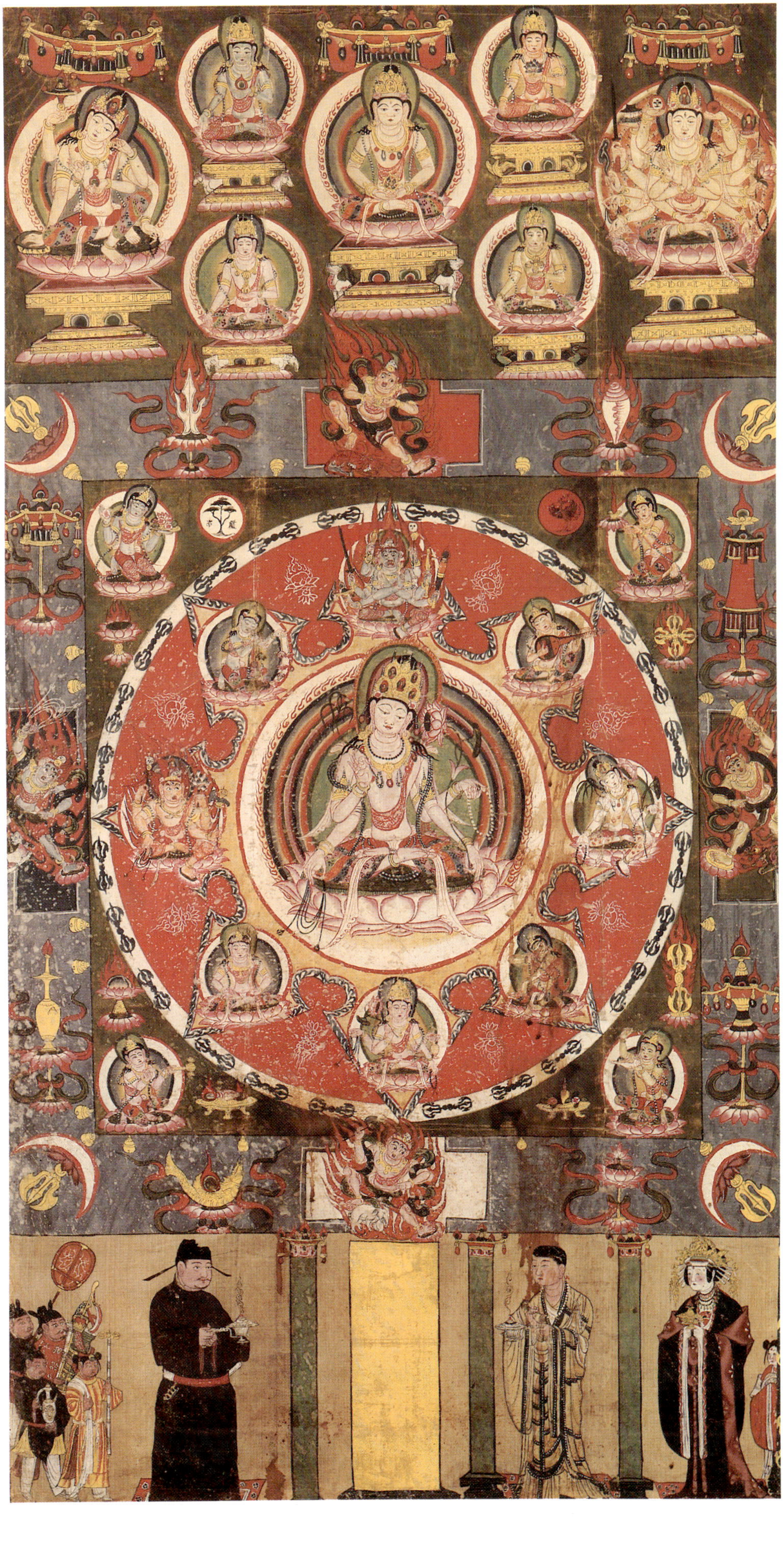

Pl. 61

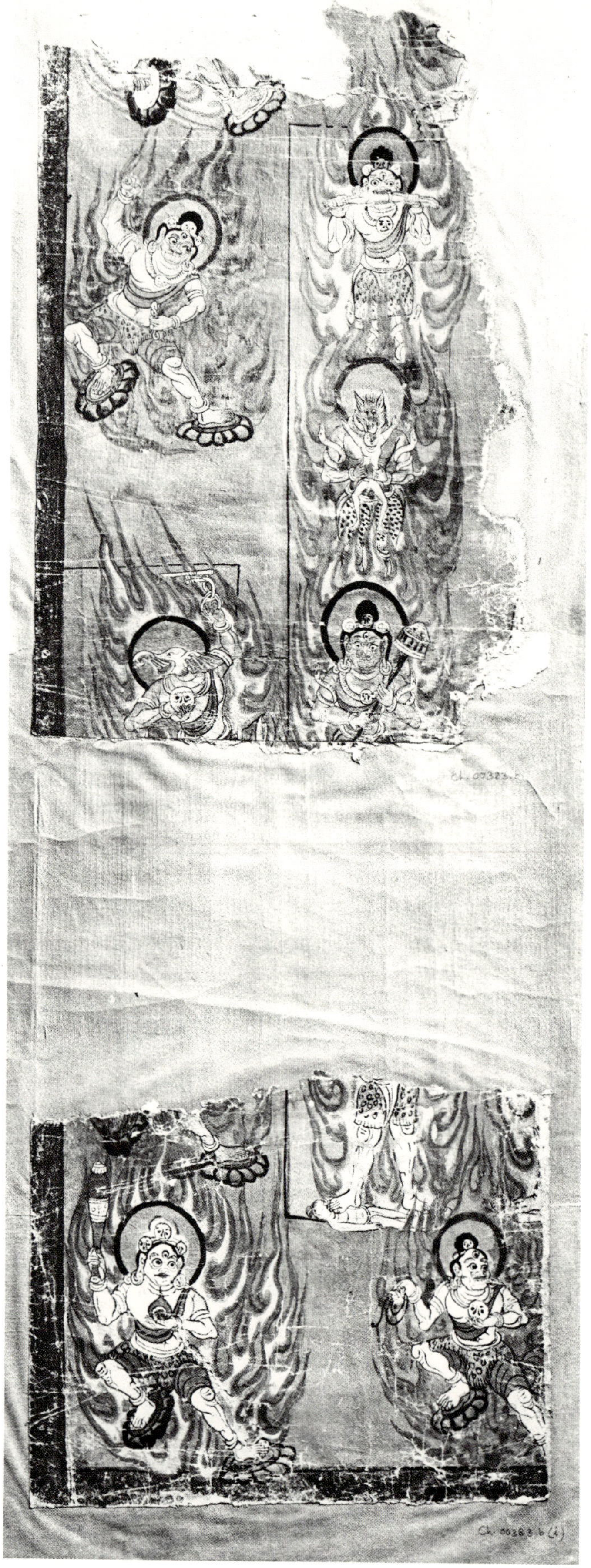

Pls. 64, 65
"Child Protecting" (?) Maṇḍala
Paint on paper
Qianfodong, Dunhuang
(a) H. 95 × 31.4 cm
(b) H. 92 × 30 cm
Eighth-ninth century
National Museum, New Delhi (Ch. 00383 a and b)

These plates represent two fragments of a *maṇḍala* with a T-shaped space outlined in black in the middle of each slate blue colored band. The original form of the *maṇḍala* seems to be oblong. The central part of the *maṇḍala* is missing but a segment of a disc is seen in the center. Next to this border there is a thick slate blue band. The field of the oblong *maṇḍala* and the disc in the center are painted bright green and red, respectively. Here, twenty-four figures with grotesque human and animal heads are represented. All the figures on the slate blue band stand in a vigorous pose (*ālīḍha*) while those on the bright green field stand in *samapādabhaṅga* pose. The upper parts of their bodies are without garments except for a narrow stole passing across their bodies like a sacred thread. Each of them wears a short *dhotī* and a leopard skin over it. They also wear ornaments made of skulls and snakes. Deification of the figures is indicated by the haloes behind their heads, orange flames around their bodies, and lotuses beneath their feet. They hold various attributes, e.g., mace, flaming jewel, noose, skull, *vajra,* sword, *cakra,* axe, *triśūla* with an axe and a skull tied to it, *triśūla* with an axe tied to it, and a conch shell containing a horse head. The figures on the bright green field are shown one above the other as if they were connected by a chain of flames. The supporting figures below stand on human beings. A few of these figures are shown either holding a child, or tearing out the belly of a child, or eating a child (it is impossible to determine exactly). All of these children are naked. Of these twenty-four figures, seven have animal heads, viz., elephant, wolf, cow, crow (?), horse, dog and cock. A segment of the red disc in the center shows a yellow pointed blade and tips of two similar blades touching the border which is decorated with three-pronged *vajras.* The shape of the blade with flaming borders and the tips of the blades at a regular distance clearly suggest that the central disc was adorned with similar *vajras* (four in all) as seen in Pl.73. Between the cow-headed figure and the remaining segment of the disc, there is a small figure of a Buddha seated in *dhyānāsana.* According to Waley, the small Buddha may be "one of the Buddhas of the Ten Quarters, who are to be invoked before reciting the dharani prescribed in the Sutra" (Waley 1931:241).

Stein simply describes the two fragments in the following words: "paper painting in Tibetan style: (a) and (b) belonging to same picture, prob. a *Maṇḍala*" (Stein 1921:995). Both Andrews (1935:232) and Waley (1931:170–173, 241) identify the *maṇḍala* as a "Child-Protecting *Maṇḍala*." On the basis of figures painted on the obverse and reverse of three pothi leaves with inscriptions both in Chinese and Khotanese, describing the painted figures, Waley identifies these animal-headed figures as female demons who prey upon children and he identifies them as *Mukhamaṇḍikā* (wolf-demon), *Pūtanā* (calf-demon), *Śaknī* (crow-

demon), *Revatī* (dog-demon) and *Kānthapāninī* (cock-demon). About the horse-headed and elephant-headed figures on the T-shaped spaces of the mandala, he says that these "outer demons are the divinities who, led by the Gandharva King Candana, put the child-devouring spirits to flight" (*ibid.*). Two points are to be noted in this regard. First, the divinities are not female and second, none of the extant figures has an inscription to support the identification. The animal-headed figures in the *maṇḍala* remind one of the *bar-do maṇḍala* (Pott 1976:193, pl. 72). Though crudely made, the figures, especially those on the slate blue band, are drawn with force. The figures in *ālīḍha* pose are typically Tibetan in style.
Chhaya Bhattacharya

Previously published: (Stein 1921:865, 995; Waley 1931:170–173, 241; Andrews 1935:232).

(See Color Plate 64)

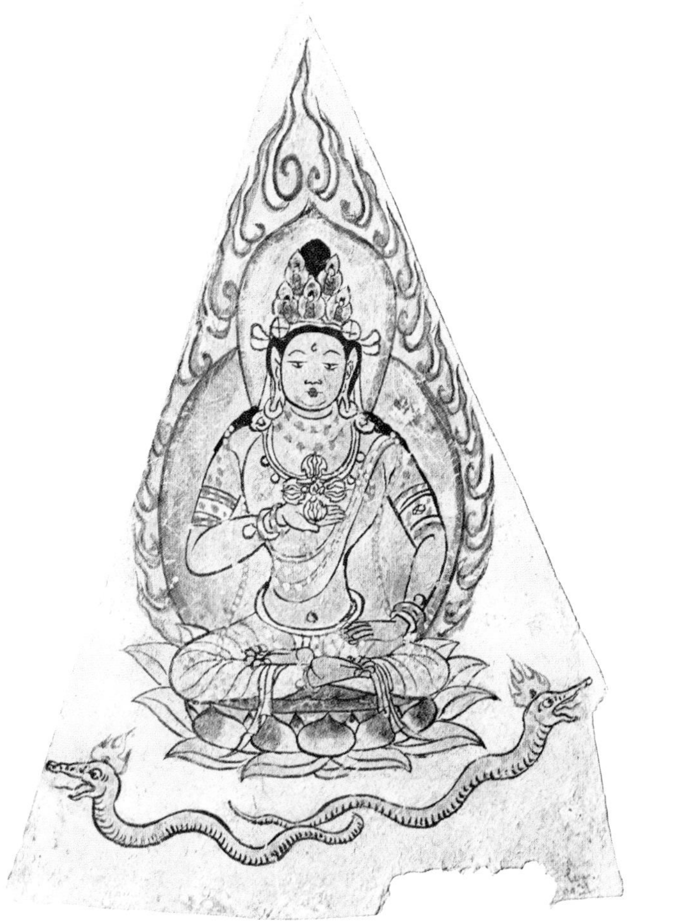

Pl. 66
Deity with Five Buddhas on Crown
Paint on paper
Qianfodong, Dunhuang
Ca. eighth-ninth century, A.D.
H. 26.5 cm
National Museum, New Delhi (Ch.lvi.0027)

This fragment of a painting on paper shows a Bodhisattva-like figure seated *vajraparyaṅkāsana* on a fully blossomed lotus. Behind his head a lotus petal-shaped aureole and a round *mandorla* are seen. Above his aureole a flaming jewel on a lotus is visible. He is framed between two flaming bands which gradually taper upwards to form a triangle. Traces of similar painting are seen pasted along the edge of this painting. There are four similar triangular fragments (Cf. Ch. lvi. 0028–0031) which probably were meant to form the center of a *maṇḍala* (see Pl. 69).

The upper part of the Bodhisattva's body is slightly tilted to his left. Traces of his originally blue complexion remain. Shading is done in orange. His black hair is tied into a high knot by a white fillet, which extends on either side of his head. He wears a crown decorated with Five Buddhas. Both Andrews (1935: 234) and Waley (1931:309), describe the five figures (Ch. lvi. 0027–0031) as "Five Divine Bodhisattvas," and identify this particular figure as Samantabhadra, the emanation of Vairocana. But Stein (1921: 1079, 1080) describes them as the Five Dhyāni Buddhas or Jinas. This particular figure is identified by Stein as Vairocana, with a flaming jewel above his head and *cakra* in his hand. The celestial Jinas or Buddhas may wear crown and jewels like the Bodhisattvas but they are not known to have "Dhyāni" Buddhas on their crowns (see Pls. 11 and 61). This figure may represent Vajradharma, who is one of the fifteen forms of Avalokiteśvara emanating from Buddha Amitābha, and is said to have Five Buddhas on his crown. According to Bhattacharyya, "such images are popular both in Tibet as well as in China" (1968:125). His other ornaments, i.e., armlets, bracelets, anklets and ear-ornaments, are shown by simple bands and circles which are painted orange and outlined in black. He is decorated with a *rudrākṣa*-like necklace close to his neck, besides two other necklaces. He wears a long *dhotī* painted buff with criss-cross and dot motifs in orange. A narrow stole, painted brown with yellow dots, passes across his bare body. His right hand holds an eight-spoked *cakra* close to his chest and the left hand forms an unusual *mudra*. [Ed. note: this *mudrā* has until now only been identified in Dunhuang and the western Himalaya in the eleventh and twelfth centuries.]
Chhaya Bhattacharya

Previously published: (Stein 1921b:II,360,n.3, 1079–1080, IV, pl.SCII; Waley 1931:309,no.DXLII; Andrews 1935:234; Matsumoto 1937:II,pl.CXCVI.).

(See Color Plate 66)

Pl. 67
Deity with Five Buddhas on Crown
Painting on paper
Quianfodong, Dunhuang
Ca. eighth-ninth century
H. 25.5 cm
National Museum, New Delhi

This triangular fragment shows a Bodhisattva-like figure similar to that in Pl. 66, with slight variations in ornaments and attribute. This painting and Pl. 66 belong to the same series and both of them show Indian elements in their dresses and ornaments. His green complexion has mostly faded away. He holds a *viśvavajra* in his right hand and his left hand, with palm inward, is placed on his left thigh. He has Five Buddhas on his crown. Considering his attribute, i.e., the *viśvavajra* and his green complexion, he may be identified as Bodhisattva Viśvapāṇi, who is an emanation of Buddha Amoghasiddhi (Bhattacharyya 1968:73). Waley also identifies him as Viśvapāṇi (1931:309). Below the lotus-seat are two flame-crested snakes whose jaws are opened to reveal their flame-like tongues. Pl. 66 and 67 also may be early representations of the Five Buddhas, hence this figure could be Amoghasiddhi and Pl. 66 would be Vairocana (see Pl. 69).

Previously published: (Stein 1921a:1079–1080, pl. XCII; Waley 1931:309; Andrews 1935:234).

Pl. 63

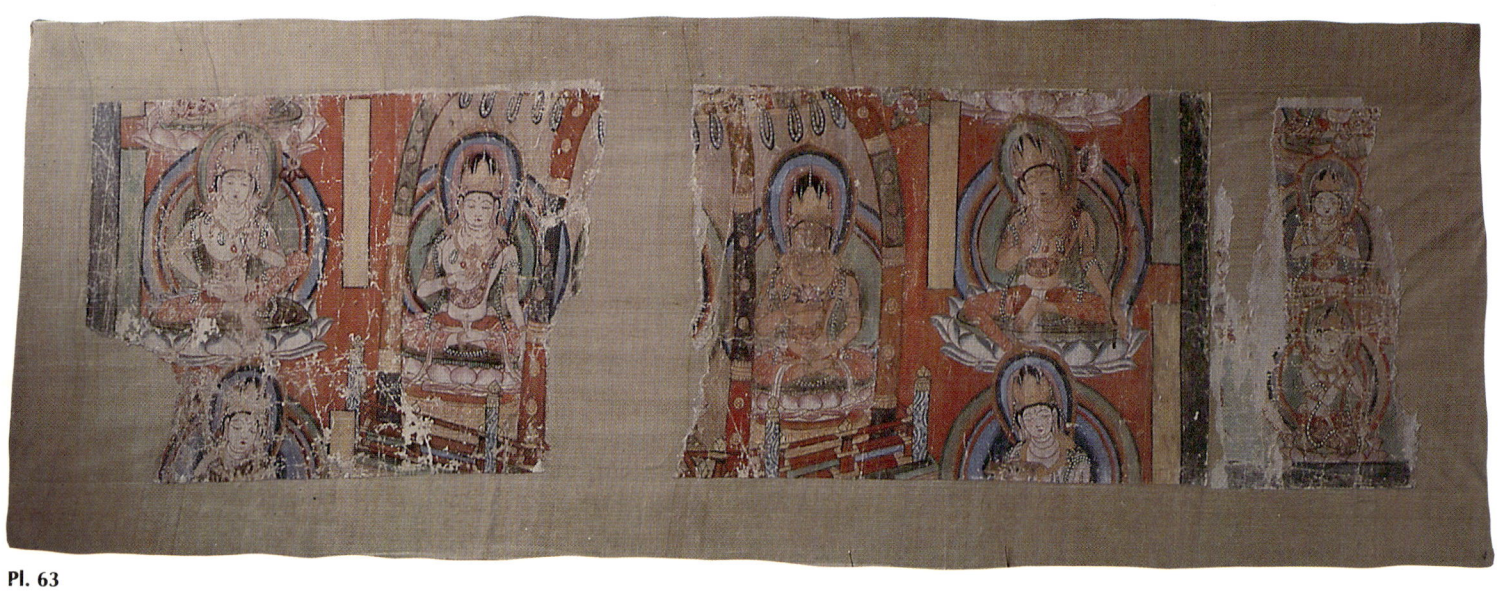

Pl. 70
Amoghapāśa
Painting on silk
Dunhuang
Ninth century
H. 85.5 × 66 cm
Musée Guimet, Paris (MG 23.076)

Amoghapāśa is one of the many tantric forms of Avalokiteśvara (Lokeśvara) and is distinguished by the lasso he carries. He is related to other forms of Avalokiteśvara by such details as the Amitābha image seated in the crown and the antelope skin, here represented as a black cape with a white design. The *Sādhanamālā* (Bhattacharyya 1968: 418 and 428) describes Amoghapāśa Lokeśvara as standing and having four heads and eight arms. (See Kramrisch 1964:Pl.84 for a Nepalese painting of this divinity). Indeed, in Indian and Himalayan art Lokeśvara images are more commonly represented standing (Pls. 32, 122) while in Dunhuang, as here, they are generally seated. The seated eleven-headed figure representing either Avalokiteśvara or a Bön deity (Pls. 32, 122) is an example of the continuation of this tradition in the western Himalayas.

Himalayan paintings depicting Amoghapāśa frequently show him attended by guardian divinities and other Bodhisattvas, as is seen here. A comparison of the style of this painting and the Buddha figure in Pl. 55 with Pls. 68, 66, and 58 allows us to contrast the three variants of the HJimalayan style dated from the eighth to tenth centuries with examples of divinities in the Chinese style depicted in paintings from the same period.

1a Dhṛtarāṣṭra
1b Virūpākṣa
2a Cintamaṇicakra
2b, 4a, 5a, 5b Bodhisattvas
3a perhaps Subhūti
3b Perhaps Śāriputra
(Nicolas-Vandier Vol.II, 1976:156–158)

	1a	1b	
2a	3a	3b	2b
	Amoghapāśa		
	4a	4b	
	5a	5b	

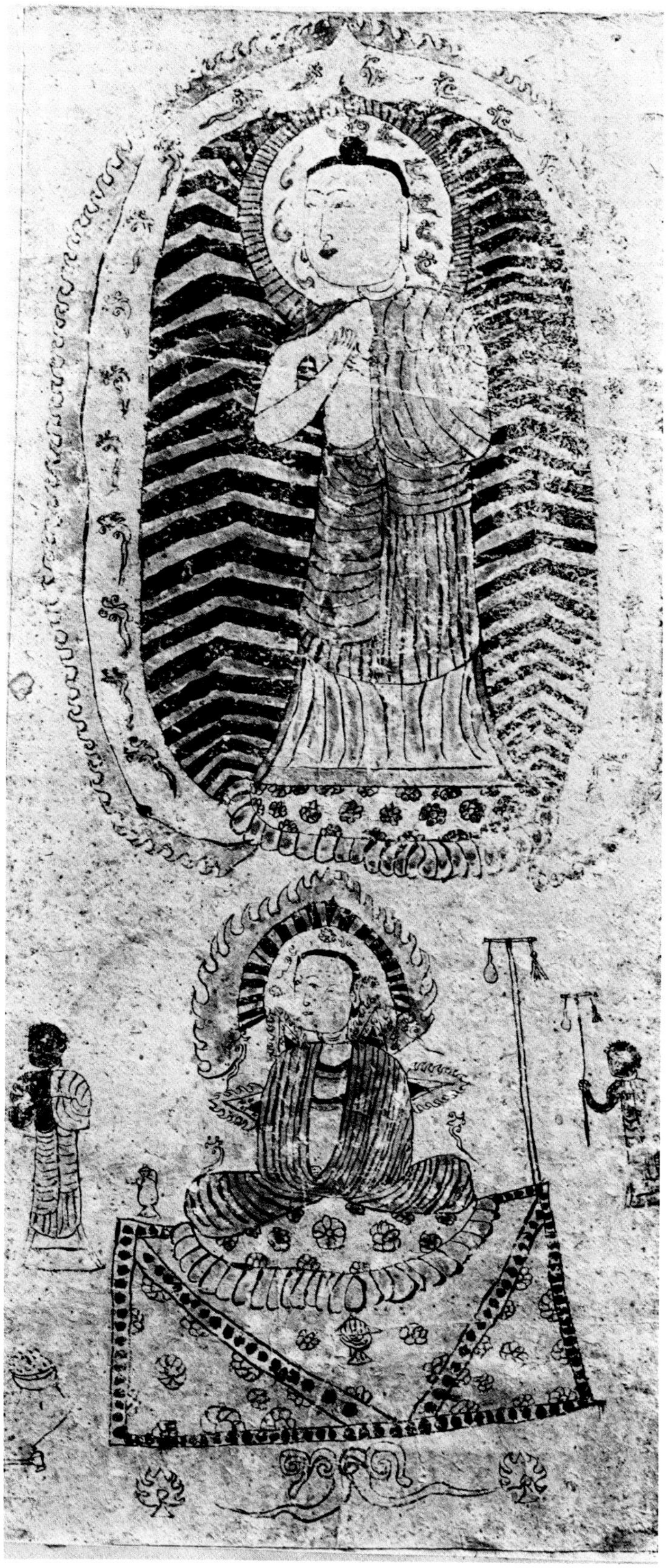

Previously published: (Hallada and Hambis 1956:no.166; *L'Arte del Gandhāra* 1958:no.237,pl.61; Nicolas-Vandier 1976:I,156–158; II, pl. 85.)

(See Color Plate 70)

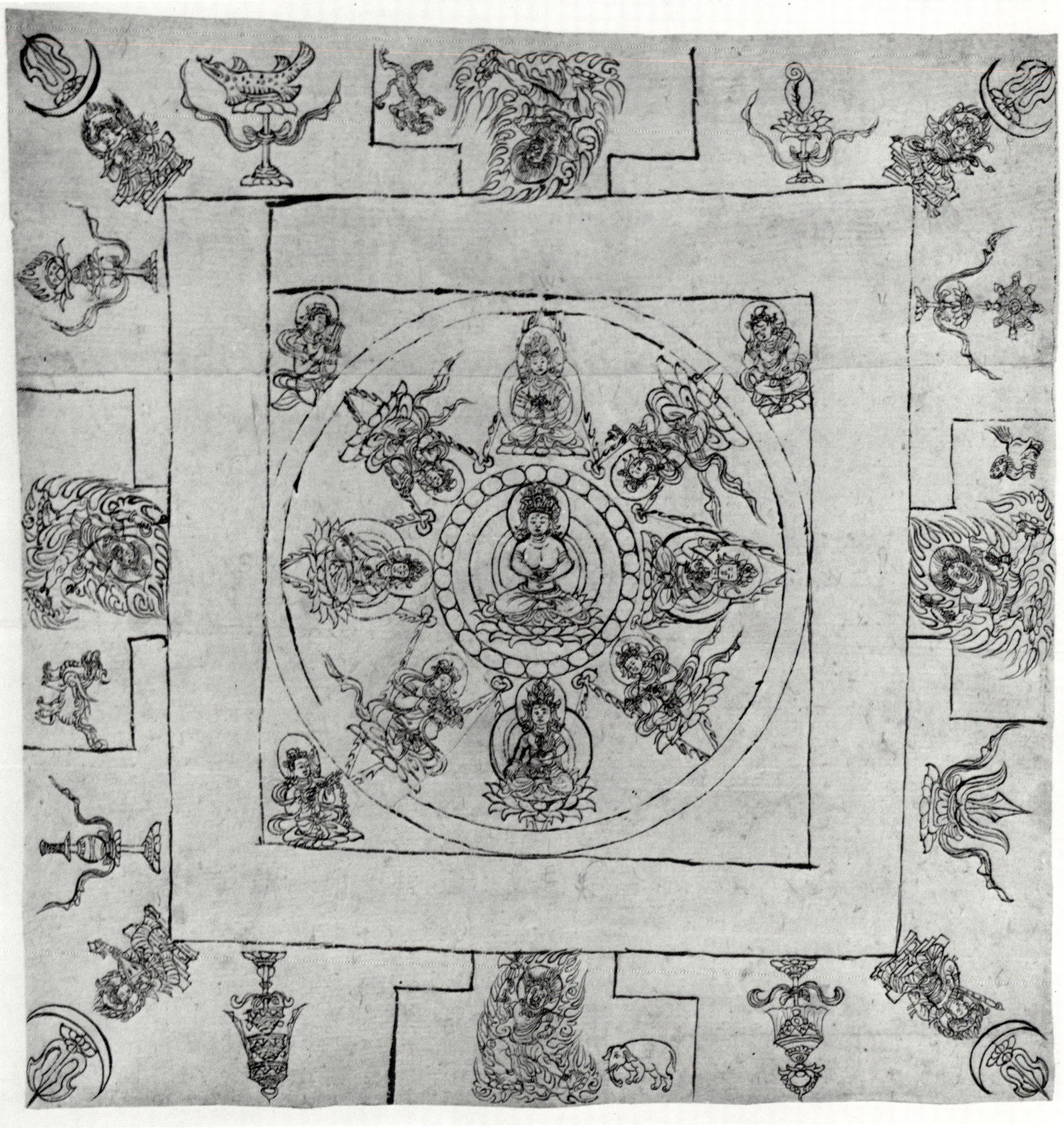

Pl. 68
***Maṇḍala* of the Five Jinas (The Five Buddhas)**
Painting on silk
Dunhuang
Ninth century
H. 103 × 62 cm
Musée Guimet, Paris (MG 17.780)

This extremely fine painting on silk is an important document for the history of Buddhist painting and the representations of the *Vajradhātu-maṇḍala*. Representations of this *maṇḍala* were important not only in the western Trans-Himalayan monasteries founded by Rin-chen bZang-po (Fig. 49), but also among certain sects of Japanese Buddhism. The mixture of stylistic features has prompted scholars to date this painting from the eighth-ninth centuries (Karmay 1975:9) to the tenth century (Vandier-Nicolas 1976:58), and to discuss artistic connections with early Tibetan painting (Karmay 1975:8) and paintings from Khotan and the Horyuji in Japan (Hackin 1928:243). The images of the Five Buddhas have been considered representative of an Himalayan style. While the proportions and strict frontality of the Buddha figures, and the color scheme and composition clearly distinguish this painting from the Dunhuang paintings in the Chinese manner (Pl. 70), these same features also distinguish this painting from a group of painted banners in the National Museum, New Delhi (Pl. 58), which have long been considered to represent examples of Tibetan painting, and which also seem more clearly related to Khotanese paintings (Gropp 1974). The Bodhisattva in Pl. 58 may represent the earliest phase of Tibetan painting at Dunhuang. How are we to relate this manner to the third variant of the Himalayan style, also represented at Dunhuang (Pl. 62, 66, 67), which has been associated with Tibetan painting there, as well as to the different styles found in this painting? (See Karmay 1975:5–14, for a discussion of this third stylistic type which appears in a painting, Stein Collection 32, in the British Museum, datable from its Chinese and Tibetan inscriptions to 836 A.D.) A careful study of Esoteric Buddhist art in Japan from the eighth through tenth centuries should prove helpful in clarifying these three stylistic groups.

This *maṇḍala* consists of 25 personages beneath which appear seven donor figures and three dedicatory inscriptions in Chinese. The central figure, the (I) Jina (Buddha) Vairocana, is distinguished from the other four Buddhas by his slightly different garments and larger size; he holds a wheel and is seated on a throne supported by eight lions. Standing dragons support the back of his throne (see Pl. 108 for a later variant of this theme). All five Buddhas (Jinas) wear the crown of the Five Buddhas (*pañcabuddha-mukuṭa*); (II) Ratnasaṃbhava holds a jewel and has winged horses in his throne base; (III) Amitābha is depicted with lotus and peacocks; (IV) Akṣobhya is depicted with a *vajra* and elephants; (V) Amoghasiddhi is depicted with a *vajra* and *garuḍa*. The Bodhisattvas of offering are figures *a* through *h*. The ground between the deities is strewn with symbols of the "seven jewels" and the "eight auspicious signs."

The seven personages at the bottom of the painting are members of the donor's family, both living and dead, as well as retainers. (See Vandier-Nicolas 1976:58–61 for the complete description). **(See Color Plate 68)**

II III
I
b e f c
IV V
h a d g

Previously published: (Gime Tōyō bijutsu-kan 1968:172; Hackin Asiatique Mythologie: 243 ff.) Hackin 1911 6asc. 2 no. 8: 12-13; Hackin 1928; 218; Mission Paul Pelliot 1947:30; Vandier-Nicolas 1976 Vol. I: 58-61; Vol. II: Pl. 28; Musée Guimet 1976:60)

Pl. 69
The Five Dhyāni Buddhas
Ink on Paper
Dunhuang
Late ninth century A.D.
H. 44.8 cm × 43.2 cm
Trustees of the British Museum, London (1919.1.1.0173)

The drawing is on two sheets of the usual fairly thick paper used and perhaps made at Dunhuang. Perhaps because of some defect in the paper, or as a result of a pentimento, one of the four kneeling Bodhisattvas surrounding the central figure of Vairocana has been drawn on a piece of paper stuck in place after the circles had been drawn. As a result the festoon of flame surrounding him extends somewhat further than the rest. To the right there is no figure in the fourth corner outside the circle.

The impression gained from the whole is that of a sketch or preparatory layout rather than a finished painting. It is exactly comparable in style to some of the booklets, illustrating the *Diamond Sūtra* in 32 sections or the chapter on Avalokiteśvara from the *Lotus Sūtra* (British Library, Stein 5646, 6983). These booklets were intended for personal use, being small enough to carry about in the pocket. Those of the *Diamond Sūtra* may have illustrations of the eight *vajra* kings, executed in ink, but probably with a reed pen as first proposed by Professor Akira Fujida, rather than with a brush. The resulting lines are relatively short, as can be seen from the frequent fresh starts in the boundary lines, but they can still be surprisingly fine, and the figures capable of lively expression, as can be seen from the fiery *vajra* figures at the cardinal points.

The probable date for the booklets of this kind is circa A.D. 900, and it therefore seems likely that this painting too is from this time, at the very end of the Tang dynasty. Confirmation for this hypothesis may be sought in the form of the lotus petals in the *padmāsana* of Vairocana, or Akṣobya beneath him, and of Ratnasaṃbhava to the left (the rest are more summarily depicted). The lotus petals of earlier thrones (for instance those in the 8th century Representations of Famous Images) do not have the same pointed, outward-splayed form; instead they tend to surround the figure they support with swelling petals as those of an actual flower surround the central stems and future seed-head.
Roderick Whitfield

Previously published: (Stein 1921b:Ch.00428, p. 999; Waley 1931:168, CLXXIII; Whitfield 1982:fig. 78).

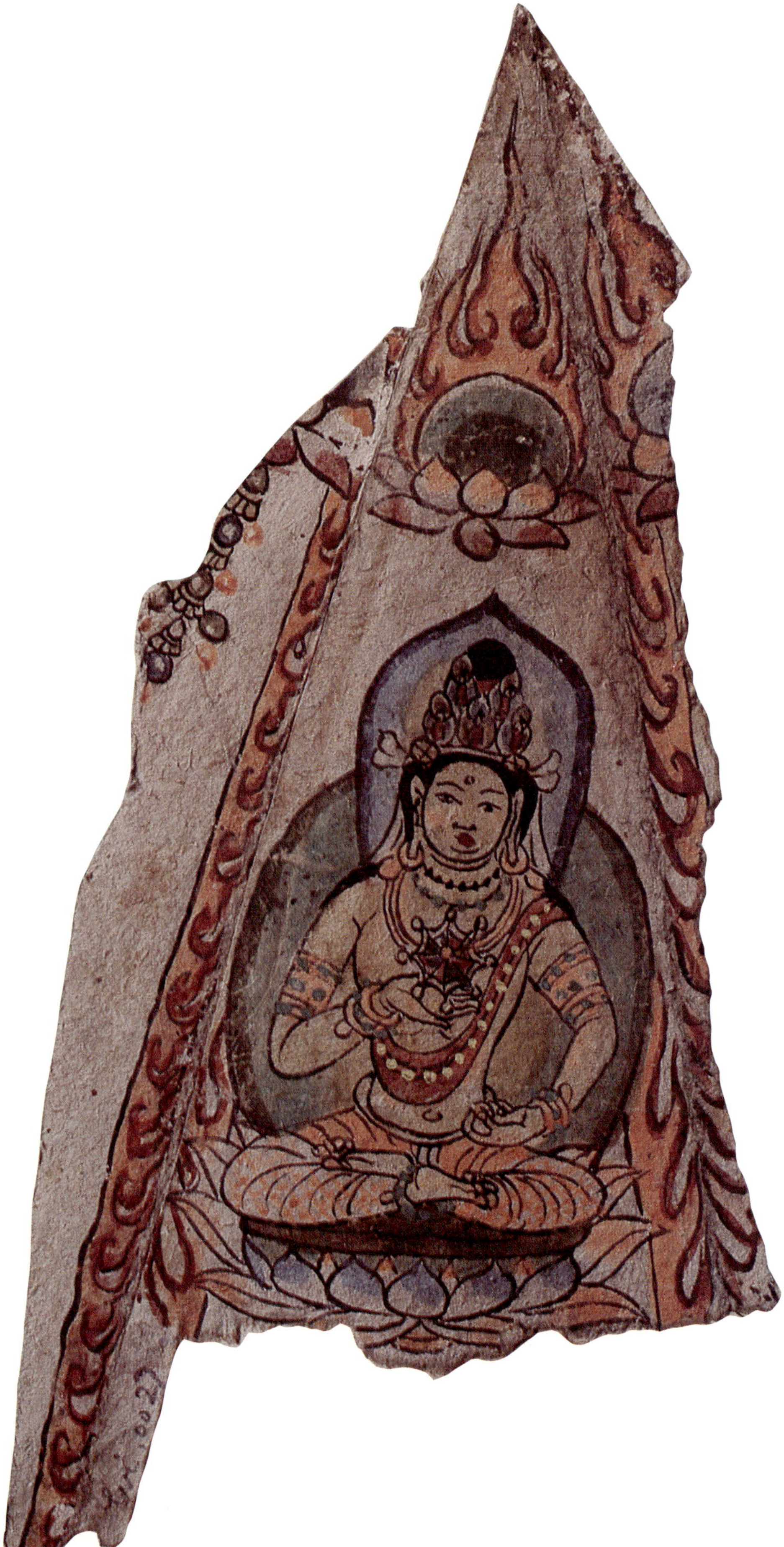

Pl. 66

Pl. 71
Two Buddha Figures
Black and light red ink on paper
Dunhuang, Qianfodong
Ca. seventh-eighth century
H. 44.3 × 19.8 cm
National Museum, New Delhi. (Ch. 00378)

The Buddha on top is standing on a lotus. An elliptical *mandorla* surrounds his body and a circular aureole. His face is turned three-quarters to his right, while his body remains frontal. His right hand with opened palm is shown over the fingers of the left hand. His *uṣṇīṣa* shows a thin strip of black hair with a round top-knot. He wears an *antaravāsaka* which covers his feet and an *uttarāsaṅga* which is seen around his waist and knees. It covers his left shoulder, half of his chest, left arm and part of his right shoulder. The field of his *mandorla* shows undulating rays which may suggest the lineage of the Buddha. He belonged to the family of the *Ikśvākus* and his *gotra* was *Āditya* or the Sun.

Below the standing Buddha on a lotus, another Buddha figure is seen seated on a carpet in *dhyānāsana* on a lotus-seat. Except for the *uṣṇīṣa*, the figure exhibits all the characteristics of a Buddha figure. Waley describes this figure as "the transformation of a Buddha into a priest or hermit" (1931:240). In front of the lotus-seat an incense-burner (perhaps) is visible. Above his shoulders and on either side of his upper arms, small triangular flames shoot upwards and sideways, respectively. Also shown are two monks, who may be the two chief disciples of the Buddha known as Śāriputra and Maudgalyāyana of Rājagṛha. One makes the gesture of devotion, another holds a T-shaped staff. From the cross-piece of the staff hang a pot and a tassel. There is also a similar staff at the corner of the carpet, as well as a flask, a bowl with tripod containing offerings, and an incense-burner. Flames or Chinese clouds and a flaming jewel further decorate the scene. The painting is crudely made and may be the work of a devotee who painted it for his personal use, perhaps while traveling.
Chhaya Bhattacharya

Previously published: (Stein 1921b:994; Waley 1931:240, no. CCCLXIV; Andrews 1935:232).

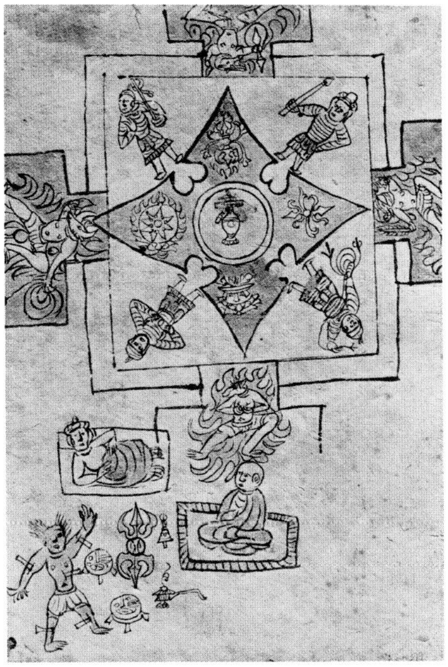

Pl. 72
***Maṇḍala* with Healing Scene**
Paint on paper
Dunhuang, Qianfodang
Ca. ninth-tenth century A.D.
H. 42.8 × 30.1 cm
National Museum, New Delhi (Ch.00379)

This painting on a rectangular piece of paper shows a *maṇḍala* probably used for healing the sick. The shape of the *maṇḍala* is roughly square, with a T-shaped space in the center of each side. The square frame represents the four walls of the sanctuary with four doors opened to the four quarters. The central part of the sanctuary is meant for the seat of the "Chosen Deity" (*iṣṭadevatā*) In the present case, the vase seems to represent the Bodhisattva Maitreya, the Future Buddha, as the *iṣṭadevatā*. The four doors are guarded by the demonic figures with animal heads (see Pls. 62–64) and the rest of the four quarters are guarded by the four Lokapālas. Within each T-shaped space, an animal-headed figure is seen in *ālīḍha* posture against a flaming background. The figures on the top and below have a horse head and an unidentified animal head, respectively. According to Stein it is a "dragon head" (1921:994), while to Waley and Andrews it is a "tiger head" (Waley 1931:241; Andrews 1935:232). On the left of the painting the figures have an elephant-head and a cow-head; according to Stein, Waley and Andrews, it is an ox-head (*ibid.*). The horse-headed figure holds a *vajra* in his right hand and an unidentified object in his left hand. The elephant-headed figure holds a flaming sword in his right hand and what may be a wheel in his left hand. The figure opposite the horse-headed figure is shown with hands clasped near his chest and the cow-headed figure holds a noose in his left hand and an unidentified object in his right hand. Each of the four figures wears a short white *dhotī*. Their breasts and navels are prominently shown by small circles. All the heads are shown in profile turning to their right.

Within the *maṇḍala*, a large *viśvavajra* is drawn with thick black outline. On each of the spearhead-shaped arms of the *viśvavajra*, a *vajra* with three-pronged ends and flames on the tips, a *vajra* with *triśūla*-type ends, an eight-spoked wheel with a flaming border resting upon the tip of a *triśūla* and a plate over a tripod with floral offerings are shown. The plate with tripod is placed upon a fully blossomed lotus. These are the symbols representing the divine treasures. (See Pl. 73.) In the center of the large *vajra*, a vase, which is the same as the *amṛtakalaśa* of Bodhisattva Maitreya or Avalokiteśvara, is seen within a circle. Four corners of the *maṇḍala* are filled by four armored figures standing diagonally who seem to represent the Lokapālas, or Dharmapālas, of four directions. Three of them hold attributes, *viz.*, staff, flaming torch and noose. The fourth places his hands near his belly as if tearing something apart. Except for one with the flaming torch, all others wear helmets. The figure with a flaming torch wears a type of crown which is usually worn by Lokapāla Vaiśravaṇa as he is represented in the art of Central Asia. A monk is seen seated on a prayer-mat right below the unidentified animal-headed figure. On his right, a figure wearing a red lower garment lies on a mat. He holds his stomach as if to comfort his pain. Below, a figure wearing a short *dhotī* stretches his arms and legs apart. His hair stands on end and his body, arms and legs are transfixed with knives. This grotesque figure surely personifies the disease of the sick man. The disease has been arrested by means of charms performed by the monk or the priest. Between him and the monk's prayer-mat, a large *vajra* with triple-forked ends, a *vajra-ghaṇṭā*, incense-burner and two circular plates containing what may be cowrie, and other unidentified objects with tripods are portrayed.

The *maṇḍala* which is crudely drawn may be considered an example of the medieval "folk art" of Central Asia.
Chhaya Bhattacharya

Previously published: (Stein 1921b:994, Waley 1931:241, no. CCLXV; Andrews 1935:232; Matsumoto 1937: pl.CLXIII.a).

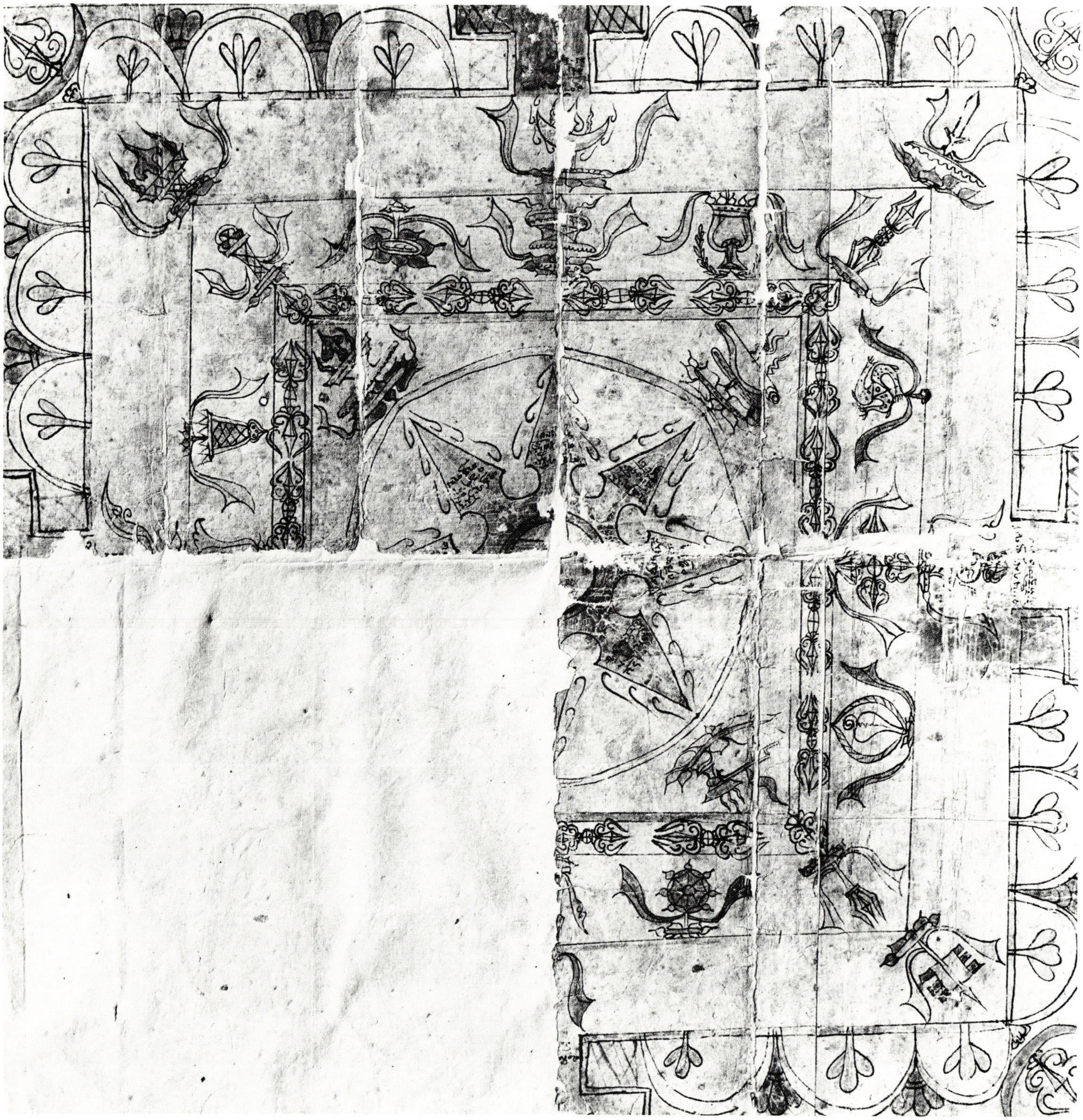

Pl. 73
Diagram for *Maṇḍala* of Uṣṇīṣavijāyā
Black ink on paper, traces of red and yellow coloring. Tibetan inscription. Painting on paper
Dunhuang, Qiafodong
Ninth-tenth century
H. 57.79 × 58 cm
National Museum, New Delhi (Ch.00398)

Almost a square paper with a Buddhist magic diagram drawn on it in black lines, it was folded into four and one quarter of it is missing. At places it is filled with red and dark buff colors. It contains a combination of some *mantras* written in cursive Tibetan; various symbols are arranged all around the *maṇḍala*, and no divine figure is visible except for a head near the northern opening (T-shaped) on the outer square of the *maṇḍala*.

A *maṇḍala* is "the systematic arrangement of symbols on which the process of visualization is based. It is generally built upon the shape of a four-, eight-, or sixteen-petalled lotus-blossom (*padma*) which forms the visible starting-point of meditation. . . . In a *maṇḍala* . . . the rays or spokes of the *Vajra*, converging upon the axis, can be raised four to eight . . ." (Govinda, 1977: 64, 92). In this *maṇḍala* instead of lotus petals the blades of the *vajra* are arranged in the centre like spokes. *Vajra* means diamond, which, though colorless, is able to produce all colors. It is the most appropriate symbol to signify the transcendental state of "voidness" (*śūnyatā*). The diagram is made of five squares and an octagon with a circle in its centre. The squares are schematically filled with various symbols and the octagon is decorated with four *vajras* with a small circle in the centre. Spearhead-like blades of the *vajras* are arranged like spokes of a wheel; the tip of each blade touches the joints of the octagon. Tapering edges of the blades have flames as borders. On each of the eight blades (three are damaged) a *mantra* is written in Tibetan script. This diagram should be held in a way so that the missing portion remains on the left lower corner of the spectator. In a Tibetan *maṇḍala*, the directions of space are arranged in the following manner: west is placed on the top and east below. North and south directions are to be seen on the right and left of the spectator. In this *maṇḍala*, the northern direction is indicated by the inscription written on the T-shaped space on the outer square of the *maṇḍala*.

The central part of the octagon shows a small circle with red border outlined in black. Field of the circle shows part of a thin black line only.

The three corners corresponding to the tips of blades *ii, iv,* and *vi* are filled with the following symbols: flaming jewel—Stein describes it as an "arrow-head" (Stein 1921b:997)—upon a dish stand, *śaṁkha*—according to Stein it is a "bow." Though crudely drawn, it is a conch seen in profile—with flames on a lotus leaf (?) and an incense burner respectively. The inner square is distinguished by a band which is decorated with a row of horizontal *vajras*. The second band above this is broader than the band with *vajra* decorations. The corners of this band corresponding to the tips of the blades of *vajras ii, iv,* and *vi* are shown with "tribolate jewel," *vajra* and *triśūla* respectively. Other symbols drawn on the band from left to right are: *chatra*—according to Stein it is "rice-cake" symbolizing the Universe (1921b:997) (umbrella), lotus, vase with offering, *purṇaghaṭa* or vase with willow-like foliage, fish—Stein thinks it to be a three-armed symbol resembling the Manx emblem (1921b:997). But they seem to be fish. There are three fishes with one head. Their tails and fins are clearly recognized, as well as *víśvavára, śaṁkha* and *cakra*. The third band above is also decorated with symbols. Three corners corresponding to the tips of the blades of the *vajras* in the center (ii, iv, and vi) show a flaming jewel on a pot with stand, a sword and a flag (prayer-banner) respectively. Between the flaming jewel and the sword, a crescent-shaped flaming vase containing flames is seen just below the northern doorway. Stein was unable to identify these objects.

Between the sword and the prayer-banner, a round human face with a flaming *vajra* above his head is visible. Each of the symbols resting on a lotus base is shown between two fluttering streamers.

The outer frame of the square is decorated with arch-shaped designs and each of them is again decorated with a trefoil-shape, perhaps lotus buds painted a dark buff color. Between the joints of two arches a similar trefoil-shaped lotus bud is painted red.

At the centre of each outer frame, a T-shaped space, or doorway, is made. The doorway on the west, which is painted red and decorated with criss-cross designs, bears an inscription in Tibetan. Although the inscription is not very clear, it is apparent that this T-shaped space represents the western gate. The other T-shaped space on its right should be the northern gate.

On each of the three corners of the outer frame, the head of a *vajra* rests on a red crescent.

The painting appears to be either a study made by the artist, or instructions for work to be completed by another craftsman.

Tibetan inscription seems to read:

ii. *uṣṇīṣa* of *jālaka*
iii. *uṣṇīṣa*
iv. *uṣṇīṣa* of *padma*
v. *uṣṇīṣa* (of *Cakravartin*)
vi. *uṣṇīṣa* of truth (pure light)

Chhaya Bhattacharya

Previously published: (Stein 1921b:II,997; Andrews 1935:232; Matsumoto 1937:II, pl.154).

Pl. 74
Bodhisattva Padmapāṇi
Paper stencil
Dunhuang, Qianfodong
Ca. eighth century ?
H. 47.5 × W. 27 cm
National Museum, New Delhi (Ch. 00425)

This fragment of a rectangular paper stencil shows a Bodhisattva Padmapāṇi figure. The edges of the paper are left as borders and the details of the figure are cut out. The lower portion of the figure is damaged, and parts of the figure are missing. The Bodhisattva stands with his face turned three-quarters to his right. His right arm is pendent; his left arm is bent at the elbow, and the hand holding a lotus is placed near his chest. His head is placed against an aureole elaborately decorated with spear-head and dot motifs. Above his right shoulder, a lotus-stalk shoots up along the curve of the aureole. A fluttering banner, with a loop at the apex of its triangular headpiece, is suspended from the stalk. The Bodhisattva is elaborately ornamented with jewels, but the upper part of his body is devoid of any garment. A long, narrow stole is shown meandering symmetrically from his shoulders to the lower part of his body. He wears a long *dhotī* and a skirt over it; a sash ties into a bow over the skirt.

The stencil is well-made. The figure and other details were drawn first by a master hand and then the relevant portions were cut out.

Quite a few stencils from Dunhuang have been found. It is apparent that such stencils were used as simple aids to paint banners for mass production. Probably, they were also used to paint the walls of the caves. The image achieved by such a stencil would resemble Pl. 76 in its use of broad monochromatic bands and Pl. 70 in the decorative details of the mandorla.

Chhaya Bhattacharya

Previously published: (Stein 1921b: II, 892–893, 999; Waley 1931:247, no. CCCLXXXVI; Andrews 1035:233).

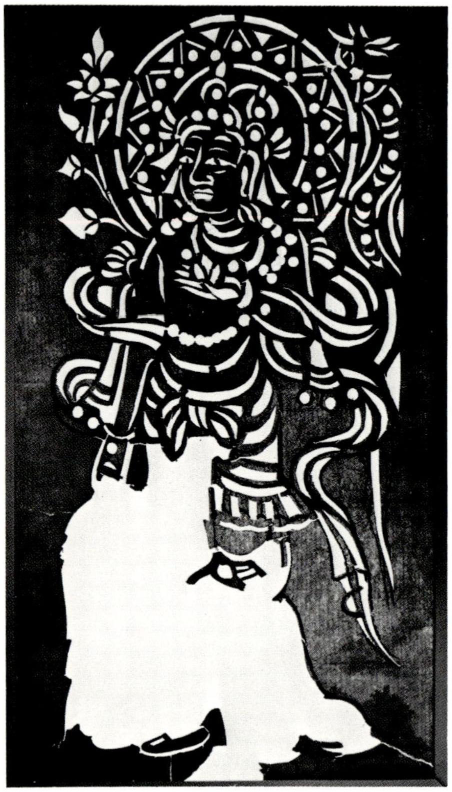

Pl. 75
Mudrās of the Thousand-armed Avalokiteśvara
Ink on paper
Dunhuang, Qianfodong
Ca. eighth or ninth century
H. 20.32 × 33.02 cm
National Museum, New Delhi (Ch.00146)

Although the manuscripts and drawings found in the cave at Dunhuang by Sir Aurel Stein cover a wide timespan, Stein places those on coarser paper with a grayish tint in the period of Tibetan occupation (759 A.D. to 850 A.D.) (Stein 1921:II,812; a study in preparation by Akira Fujieda should clarify this point). Thus, according to Stein, this drawing can be attributed to the Tibetan period, although Chinese influences can clearly be seen in some of the objects, and the inscriptions show that the drawing was meant to be used by people literate in Chinese.

The drawing can be identified as an illustration of hands and objects belonging to the Thousand-armed Avalokiteśvara. The majority of these hands and objects correspond to those associated with this same deity in many paintings found at Dunhuang. On the front of the drawing are: two hands in *vitarka mudrā*; two hands in *añjali mudrā*; two hands in *siṃhamukha mudrā*; two forms of vase, one probably a water vase and the other an *amṛta* vase; two types of sword or knife; a trident; a skull-topped staff; a conch shell; a staff; seated Buddha, probably Amitābha; a shield; prayer beads; two types of *vajra*; an arrow; sacred grass; a fly whisk; a *stūpa*; a mirror; a flower; a book; a scroll; rays of light; a seal with swastika impression; a coin of the type common in Dunhuang during the Tibetan period; a bow; a set square; grains of rice or wheat; a *vajra*-topped bell; a jewel; and a bowl. The Chinese inscriptions show *yin shou* (*mudrā* category), *chi shou* (*mudrā* category), *ch'ih shou* (vermilion category), and *gong shu* (bow category). On the reverse side are additional objects: two discs (sun and moon); a cloud; a flaming jewel; a lotus bud; a canopy; and a *vajra*-topped bell. There is also a faded bell, which is the only object represented by itself. There is a Chinese inscription on this side which is faded and difficult to read, but appears to be random jottings.

This drawing differs from other *mudrā* manuals found at Dunhuang and elsewhere in that the hands are not organized in straight rows. This may indicate that it was not meant to be a formal, permanent iconographic manual. However, it does not appear to be merely a random sketch or practice drawing, since each type of object is drawn only once, all objects are related to Avalokiteśvara, and the hands and objects appear to be well-executed. Thus, it may be a sketch which served as an aid for constructing one painting or for a group of paintings.

An additional point of interest about this drawing is that although the objects held are generally similar to those found in many Thousand-armed Avalokiteśvara images from Dunhuang, the *mudrās* used to hold the objects here and in the paintings vary throughout the site. Thus, it appears that in the Thousand-armed Avalokiteśvara image of Dunhuang, the objects were depicted more precisely than the *mudrās* for holding them.
Chandra Reedy

Previously published: (Stein 1921b:II, p.892, 967; IV, pl. XCVII; Stein 1921c:pl.XVIII; Waley 1931:233, No.CCXLIX; Matsumoto 1937:II, pl. CLXXV.b.)

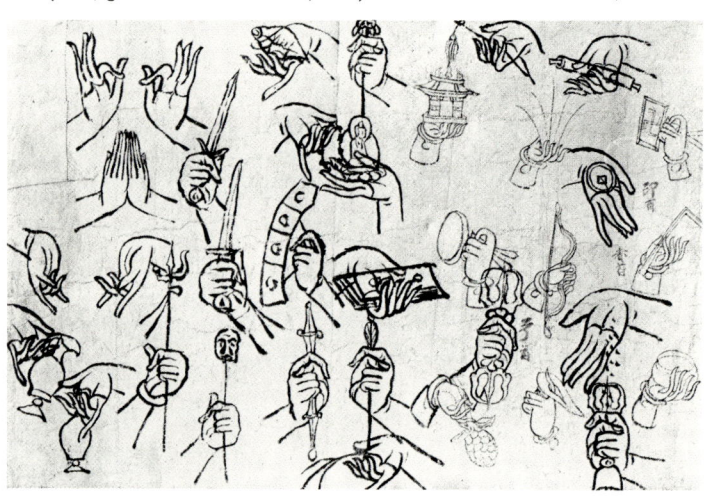

Pl. 76
Avalokiteśvara
Painting on paper
Dunhuang, Qianfodong
Ca. seventh-eighth century
H. 50.5 × W. 37.8 cm
National Museum, New Delhi (Ch. 00395)

This four-armed Avalokiteśvara is seated in *vajraparyaṅkāsana* on a large lotus with his upper pair of arms raised. His right upper hand holds a moon disc while the left upper hand holds a sun disc. The sun disc here, as always, painted red, shows a three-legged phoenix with a crest and outspread wings curled upward. The moon disc, which is always painted white, displays a tree of immortality flanked by a hare and a frog. The hare is usually depicted pounding the drug of immortality in a mortar (Stein 1921b:958). The other pair of Avalokiteśvara's hands, placed on either side of his chest, is in *vitarkamudrā* and he is framed by a circular aureole and *mandorla*. Andrews identifies the figure as "eleven-headed Avalokiteśvara" which is not correct (Andrews 1935:232).

He is richly ornamented with a three-pronged crown, elaborately designed with circular, trefoil and rosette motifs. Similar crowns are observed in the sixth and seventh century art of Kashmir and also in Tibetan and Nepalese art of a later period.

The upper part of his body is bare and shows a prominent navel. He wears only a narrow stole across his torso like a sacred thread; another stole, very long and narrow, falls symmetrically in loops from his shoulders to his knees. His long *dhotī* is tied by a sash whose terminal staves appear over his lower legs and the lotus seat. Each petal of the lotus seat is boldly distinguished by thick black lines and the tips are prominently painted in red. This painting is basically a sketch in bold black outline drawn by a master artist. This image, as with similar individual figures of Avalokiteśvara and other Bodhisattvas, is painted on silk and ramie and was used either for banners or votive offerings by devotees.
Chhaya Bhattacharya

Previously published: (Stein 1921b:868, 996; Waley 1931:243, no.CCCLXXI; Andrews 1935:232).

Pl. 77
Riders on Horse and Yak
Sketches in ink on paper
Karakhoto
Ca. seventh-eighth century
H. 21 × 35 cm
National Museum, New Delhi (K.K.11.0313A)

This fragment of a sketch on paper shows two riders on horse and yak drawn with pen-and-ink.

Although the heads of both figures are missing, the dress and part of an aureole suggest the rider on horseback to be either a divine or a princely figure, and the figure on yak-back, an attendant. The figure on horseback wears a tight-fitting tunic with simple ornamentations on his lower arms which Stein thinks may be embroidery (Stein 1921a:497). It may be armor. His loose trouser is gathered below the right knee, either tucked together or held in place by a garter. He wears a simple boot which is fastened to the saddle. His left hand holds the reins tightly. His right hand, holding a flower between the thumb and index finger, rests on his right thigh. A long stole flutters in large, waving loops. Of the ornaments only the rosette-like ear ornament and a pair of bracelets on each wrist are visible. Part of a simple aureole, recognizable only by its curved line, appears over his left shoulder. The horseback rider is turned to the front while the galloping horse is seen in profile. Probably the rider looks at the other figure. The speed of the galloping horse is shown by the erect streaming mane and ears pressed forward. A neck-band, probably with bells, decorates the horse's neck.

The figure on yak-back wears a long stole across his bare, muscular body like a sacred thread, and a short *dhotī* tied with a sash. Usually the Lokapālas drawn on banners show this type of muscular body structure. The yak-rider's arm is missing; his left hand, which rests on his left thigh, probably holds the reins. The head of the yak, turned three-quarters to its right, exhibits a fearful expression on its face. The figures seem to ride through scrolls which are suggestive of clouds. The drawing is forceful and shows the graceful movements of the figures. [Ed. note: the style clearly suggests Chinese influences, and the subject matter may relate to Chinese astrological themes where Saturn is sometimes depicted as an old man on an ox and Mars as a warrior with a horse; e.g. Rosenfield and ten Grotenhuis 1979:10.)
Chhaya Bhattacharya

Previously published: (Stein 1928:I,497–498, II, Pl.60; Andrews 1935:261–262).

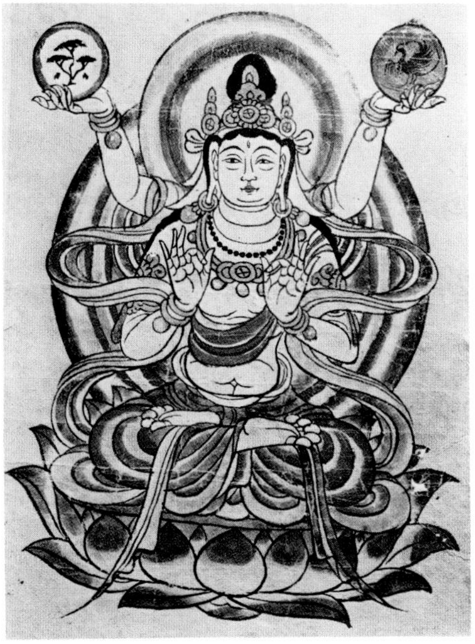

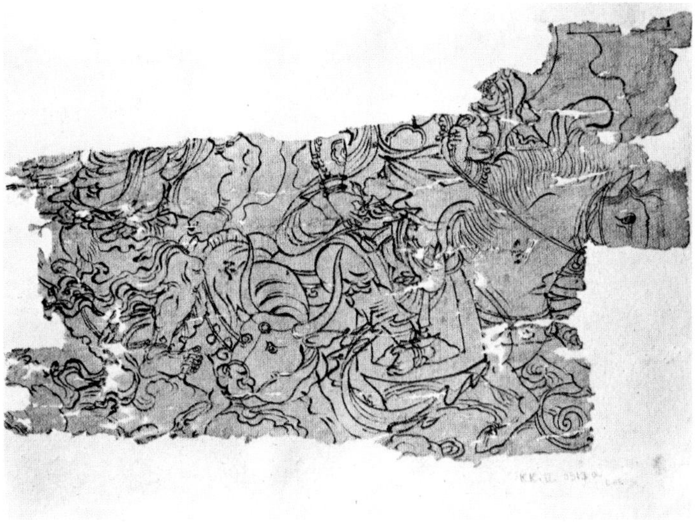

(c) Monastic Art of the Western Trans-Himalayas: Seventh to Seventeenth Centuries

The region we call the "western Himalayas" was never a unified political entity. It presently includes areas in west Tibet, northwest India, and north Pakistan. The part of this region located to the north of the Great Himalayan Mountain Range, from Mt. Kailāsa in the east to the Gilgit Agency in the west, is called the western Trans-Himalaya. For short periods in the tenth and eleventh centuries, and again in the sixteenth century, this area was politically unified.

In the tenth to eleventh centuries the "Kings of Western Tibet," also known as the "Kings of Gu-ge" (mNga-ris Gyalpo), controlled an area which comprised Gu-ge in west Tibet, Ladakh (with Nubra and Zaṇgskar) in northwest India, and Purang, which extends into Nepal. Also included were some Cis-Himalayan areas and valleys, such as Lahul and Spiti in Himachal Pradesh (India), which thus became part of the Trans-Himalayan cultural zone. It was at that time that the cultural Tibetinization of the western Trans-Himalaya became widespread, combined with a revival of Buddhist monasticism under the patronage of the kings of western Tibet. As a result, the most active period of art production in the western Trans-Himalaya lasted from the eleventh to thirteenth centuries, followed by a second period of intensive artistic activity from the late fifteenth to early sixteenth centuries. These art historical phases are well documented in the monasteries of Ladakh, Zangskar, Lahul, and Spiti.

HISTORICAL BACKGROUND

Toward the close of the seventh century, two powerful new forces began to conquer northwest India and Central Asia. Arab armies (from the west) invaded Afghanistan and Central Asia while, at the same time, a unified Tibet emerged as a major military power in the Trans-Himalaya. Both these powers coveted the lucrative trade carried across Inner Asia along the so-called silk routes; both had a substantial impact on the economic, social, and political life of the area; and both left a permanent mark on the cultural history of the region.

In western Central Asia, including northern Afghanistan, the Muslim impact on the local political scene was immediate, but the invaders had little effect on political events in the western Trans-Himalaya until a Muslim dynasty came to power in Kashmir in the fourteenth century. Nonetheless, the repercussions of the Arab conquests on the economic life of the region began centuries earlier. Fighting in western Central Asia and northern Afghanistan lasted for more than one hundred years (into the eighth century), and disrupted the traditional exchange systems across present-day Soviet Central Asia, northern Afghanistan, and the Hindu Kush. Merchants who wanted access to the lucrative markets of India were forced to find alternative routes (Xi Liang Chou: 1944–45). Most of these alternative routes crossed the Pamirs, though in later years the Karakoram routes became more popular (see Chapter II). This expansion of the Pamir-Karakoram trade stimulated the economies of northern Pakistan and Kashmir, and helped finance art production in those countries in the seventh and eighth centuries (see Chapter VIa).

Thanks to a flourishing economy and the military and administrative genius of Lalitāditya (ca. 701–738 A.D.), the greatest of the Kārkoṭa kings, Kashmir became the dominant power in historical northwest India. In the years that followed, the Kārkoṭa kings of Kashmir attempted (with Chinese help) to maintain a balance of power in the Trans-Himalayan region. The possibility of warfare with Tibet was an ever-present threat. To cope with that threat, the Kārkoṭa kings formed an alliance with China that lasted throughout the eighth century.

During this period, the Chinese were battling for their Central Asian garrisons at Karashahr, Khotan, Kashgar, and Kucha, which Tibet first conquered about 649–676 A.D. The Tibetan-Chinese struggle of the seventh to eighth centuries centered in three areas: Sichuan, to the east of Tibet; Tsinghai and Ganzu (to the northeast); and Chinese Turkestan in the northwest. In order to gain control of the Chinese Four Garrisons, Tibet had to control the western Himalayas and the routes connecting Tibet with Chinese Turkestan[1]. In the eighth century the power struggle centered along the Baltistan, Ladakh, and Chinese-Turkestan borders, where today, once again, military troops face each other across ceasefire lines.

In 783 and 822, China and Tibet signed peace treaties which are still preserved. A comparison of these treaties shows that there were significant changes in Tibetan society during that period, particularly with regard to the increased importance of Buddhism. Despite the fact that these treaties acknowledged the Tibetan position in Central Asia, the inevitable geopolitical tensions with China continued. There was, in fact, little ground for the optimistic view of perpetual peace proclaimed in the treaty of 821–822, inscribed on the west side of a monolith in Lhasa:

> The Divine King of Miracles, Khri Gtsug Lde Btsan and the Chinese King Bhun Bhu He-hu Tig Hvan Te, Nephew and Uncle, with far reaching wisdom, guarding against anything that may harm the

good of their countries at present or in the future . . . have made this great treaty.

Tibet and China shall keep the frontier of which they now hold possession. All to the east is the country of Great China. All to the west is assuredly the country of Great Tibet. Henceforth, on either side, there shall be no emnity, no making of war and no seizure of territory. . . . (Richardson 1952:71)

By the end of the ninth century, Tibet had lost its Central Asian possessions to the Chinese and the Uighurs, and the history of Buddhism in Tibet should be viewed against the background of the Sino-Tibetan power struggle outlined above.

The introduction of Buddhism to Tibet occurred at the same time as the Tibetan expansion into Central Asia. In Tibet, Buddhism was first propagated in the seventh and eighth centuries under the patronage of the "Religious (Buddhist) Kings" (Srong tsan Gam-po 620–649; Tri-srong De-tsan 755–797; Tri-tsug De-tsan Ralpachan 815–838. Legends describe the importation of Mahāyāna Buddhism through the agency of the Nepalese and Chinese princesses married to Srong-tsan Gam-po and the introduction of Indian tantric Buddhist practices in the eighth century, but the true story of the Tibetan conversion to Buddhism is more complex than the fabric of legend allows. The influence of Chinese Buddhism undoubtedly increased following the Tibetan conquest of Central Asia (649–676).

Buddhism appears to have taken hold gradually. We do know that for several hundred years following the seventh century, Buddhism was practiced primarily by some groups in the upper classes. The vast majority of the population and those aristocratic families who were allied to Bön institutions continued their traditional spiritual practices. By the end of the eighth century, Buddhism was recognized as the state religion by King Tri-srong De-tsan. The great monastery of Sam-ye was founded at this time (ca. 775 A.D.) By the mid-ninth century, Buddhist monastic institutions had become an important economic and political force in central and eastern Tibet. We have little direct information about these institutions, but the available evidence suggests that these monasteries, like their counterparts in India and Central Asia, owned land, possessed servants, and were involved in trade and banking. Monks were exempt from military service. Monasteries were exempt from taxation, and as these institutions acquired more land there was a concurrent reduction in tax revenues (Tucci 1980:11–12). In Tibet, the chief monastic official was appointed by the king and thus the monastic community was independent of the feudal aristocracy. Bitter conflicts erupted as monks and aristocrats vied for influence at court, and by the mid-ninth century, it seemed the existence of monastic institutions had begun to threaten the stability of the state. It was at this point that one can see a direct repercussion of the Sino-Tibetan power struggle on the history of Tibetan Buddhism. To mount a successful campaign against the Chinese in Central Asia, the government needed money and military forces. King Lang dar ma (838–842) resolved this problem by destroying the Buddhist monasteries and seizing their treasure (Tucci 1980:12).

We do not know what happened to the Buddhist monks and their texts during this period of persecution and civil chaos. Deprived of official patronage, monasteries fell victim to neglect, but more unconventional Buddhist practices continued. In the more remote areas mainstream Buddhism kept its position, as in particular in the eastern areas, and somewhat later in the newly established kingdoms in the west. In the tenth century Tibet was affected by the burst of missionary activity known as "the second diffusion of Buddhism." The principle impetus behind the revival of monasticism in western Tibet was the active patronage by the kings of western Tibert, descendants of the old royal dynasty of central Tibet who had founded several small kingdoms from Ladakh to Mustang (now in Nepal) in the tenth to eleventh centuries. The most important of the kings of western Tibet for the history of Buddhist art, were Ye śes 'Öd and Byang chub Öd, (Snellgrove and Richardson 1968:105–115). Tsaparang became the capital of the kings of western Tibet and the nearby monastery at T'oling (later inhabited by the Drugpa order) became an important center of philosophical and artistic activity.

Although born a king, Ye-śes 'Öd was so committed to the propagation of Buddhism that he became a monk and took the title "Lha-bla-ma," meaning "royal monk." His sons also entered religious orders. It would not, however, be correct to think of these kings as retreating to a cloistered life. Ye-śes 'Öd did not, it seems, actually abandon power; he appears rather to have redefined his role. The *Blue Annals* record that "Lha-bla-ma Ye-śes 'Öd, though he had given up his kingdom, continued to act as commander of the troops. While fighting the Garlog (Qarluq), he suffered defeat, and was thrown into prison (by them)." (*Blue Annals* trans. by Roerich 1976:244.)

We will probably never understand the complex personality of this religious king-monk or all the socioeconomic factors he manipulated in the process of creating his regional kingdom. We do know, however, that the kings of Western Tibet (Ye-śes 'Öd's dynasty) were successful largely because they were able to unify political, economic, and religious institutions (Tucci 1980:25). As we have seen in earlier sections, there was ample precedent for this tactic; and, in fact, Buddhism had been the state religion in historical northwest India under the Śāhī kings in the seventh and eighth centuries and had held the same status in Tibet in the ninth century. I have suggested that a form of state Buddhism and a related social structure in the Hindu Kush influenced the development of the "Royal Buddha" figure and elaborate Buddhist ceremonies. A similar union of religious and political institutions in Western Tibet is graphically expressed by the eleventh-century paintings of "Royal Buddha" images in the Sum-tsek Chapel at Alchi, Ladakh (Fig. 46).

THE INTRODUCTION OF BUDDHIST MONASTICISM

Under the kings of western Tibet, the propagation of Buddhism and the establishment of Buddhist institutions were effective tools for economic, social, and cultural change (Fig. 44). The alliance between

46. Wall painting, crowned Buddha, Alchi, Ladakh.

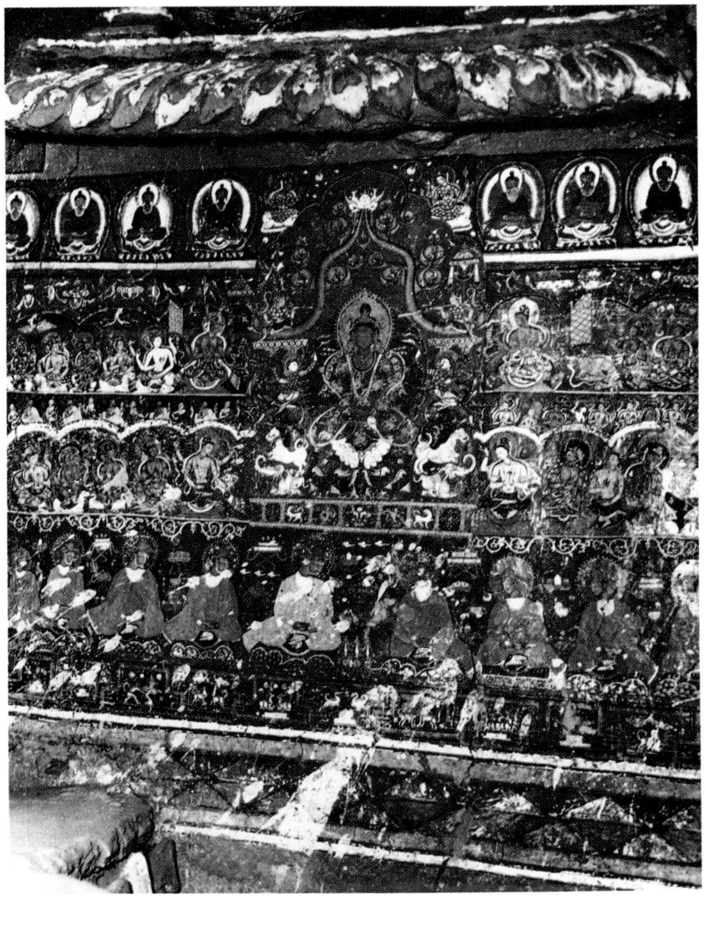

the kings and the Buddhist institutions and their inevitable conflict with the land-owning aristocracy must have been similar to the situation which existed under the first "Religious Kings" in central Tibet (Tucci 1980:20–21).

The founding of so many monasteries, each with lands and peasants attached to it (see below), profoundly influenced the traditional peasant-landlord relationships. This change in the traditional feudal structure must have occurred at a time when the society was already in the process of social change. In addition to the political impact of the new dynasty from central Tibet, there was also an influx of Tibetan immigrants from Central Asia in the second half of the ninth century. These Tibetan laymen, monks, merchants, and officials (Tucci 1980:19) had surely adopted the urban Buddhist culture of Central Asia; and their more sophisticated skills, particularly their knowledge of the long distance trade network of the Trans-Himalaya were an important component of the expanding economy (Hudūd al'Ālam, trans. Minorsky: 1970:92ff).

It is difficult to detail the role of the monasteries in the political and economic development of the western Trans-Himalaya. Recent research has demonstrated how, in the Tang period, decentralized monastic treasuries were used in the development of regional economies in Inner Asia (Gernet 1956), and it has been pointed out that the model for this economic pattern existed earlier in India (Miller 1960–61). The location of all the monasteries at important trade junctions and Ye-śes 'Öd's continued involvement in secular affairs suggest that the monasteries played an important role in the economic and cultural changes which occurred in the area from the eleventh to thirteenth centuries.

HISTORICAL ROOTS OF BUDDHIST MONASTICISM

Changes in settlement patterns and class relationships in the feudal society of northern India from the sixth century onward (Kosambi 1977:176–187) are reflected in the patronage of Buddhist and Hindu institutions. In the period between the second and sixth centuries, members of the merchant class were important supporters of Buddhist institutions, and numerous inscriptions dating from this period record donations from a variety of individuals and guilds; but this diversity of patronage disappeared as feudalism became entrenched. The middle class continued to support Buddhist institutions, but the aristocracy became a main source of patronage.

In the ensuing centuries, certain royal houses increased their patronage of Buddhism, and Buddhist institutions in these areas flourished. Entire Buddhist complexes, such as Bāmiyān, resulted from the patronage of a single dynasty; and this was also the case in China. Under the sponsorship of the regional aristocracy, the monastic centers of northeast India expanded and became centers for the study and dissemination of Buddhist philosophy. The description of Nālandā, in northeast India, written by Xuanzang in the mid-seventh century gives us some idea of the tradition of royal patronage at the monastery, which was an important training center for Tibetan Buddhists in the eleventh and twelfth centuries:

> Six kings built as many monasteries, one after the other, and an enclosure was made with bricks to make all the buildings into one great monastery with one entrance for them all. There were many courtyards and they were divided into eight departments. Precious terraces, spread like stars and jade pavilions, were spired like peaks. The temples arose into the mists and the shrine halls stood high above the clouds. . . . The king gave them (the monks) the revenues of more than 100 villages to support them, and each of the villages had 200 families who daily offered several hundred *tan* of rice, butter and milk. Thus, the students could have the requisite (clothing, food, shelter, and medicine) sufficient for their needs without going to beg for them. It was because of this support that they had achieved so much in learning (as quoted by Kosambi 1970:176–177. See also translation by Beal 1911 for the full passage pps. 111–113).

The system of endowments at Nālandā described by Xuanzang was not unusual in India. Likewise, in the western Trans-Himalaya and Tibet monastic institutions established by royal decree were provided with extensive lands and peasants. From the eighth century on, monasteries in Tibet played an increasingly important role in economic and political affairs. Although we know little about these institutions and their socioeconomic function in the period of Rinchen Zangpo, an examination of the sites and architecture of the monasteries he founded provides certain clues. These buildings are distinguished by size and location from monasteries founded later, after the advent of Mongol influence. All early monasteries were built on valley floors near rivers and other principal trade routes. The buildings that remain, such as Ta-pho and the early chapels at Alchi and Lamayuru in Ladakh, are relatively small structures. They do not have elaborate exteriors, and are built of mud and timber on stone foundations (Fig. 19). This suggests that the monastic community itself was not too large, and that Buddhist institutions were comfortably integrated into the agricultural communities which they owned and served (see Chapter V).

As time went on, monasteries played an increasingly important role in Tibetan political and economic life. In the thirteenth century, for example, the Tibetan monastic orders became involved in the international power plays of the Mongol steppe empires. In response to these events, monasteries developed a more complex institutional and economic structure, and learned to defend militarily their political interests. Monastic architecture reflects these developments, and monasteries built from the fourteenth century onward were large, complex structures bristling with battlements, protected by heavy walls, and located—like fortresses—on mountain tops (Fig. 7).

BUDDHISM IN THE WESTERN TRANS-HIMALAYA

The story of the Tibetan Buddhist orders belongs for the most part to a later period. Our concern is the early period of monastic art in the western Trans-Himalaya, particularly the tenth to thirteenth centuries. Snellgrave has already briefly surveyed (Ch. V) the complex development of Buddhism in the western Trans-Himalayas. While the monasteries were founded under Tibetan patronage in the tenth-eleventh centuries, at that time Buddhism was still drawing on the living Buddhist traditions of India and therefore these monasteries can best be understood within the context of contemporaneous Indian Buddhism (Snellgrave and Skorupski 1977:105). Many of the renowned teachers who helped bring about the Buddhist renaissance in the western Himalayas and Tibet were trained in the monasteries of northeast India, Magadha, and Bengal. The most famous of these, Rinchen Zangpo (died 1055), Atīśa (also known as Dīpāṅkara; died 1054) and Dharmapāla (died 1013), were invited to Tibet by royal patrons, but many other important Buddhist teachers came of their own accord. A number of these scholars and monks were renowned for their teachings of the *tantras*, and many of the teachings and traditions they brought have been maintained in Tibet.

That there were a variety of views at that time concerning tantric practices is evident from a reported exchange between Ye-śes 'Öd and his nephew, Byaṅ-chub 'Öd. Ye-śes 'Öd and his family seem to have distrusted much of what they believed to be associated with tantric practices, and they wished to reassert more conventional Buddhist teaching. The *Blue Annals* attributes the following thoughts to Byan chub 'Öd: "Though many monks are found in the country of Tibet, there exist many wrong practices in respect of sByor (sexual practices) and sGrol (ritual murder) in the study of Tantra. Some, who had practiced these rites, preached extensively that one could obtain Enlightenment through (the mere acceptance of) the principle of Relativity (Śūnyata, stoṅ-pa-ñid) without practicing meritorious works. Though the doctrine of Prātimokṣa had spread (in Tibet), those who practiced the precepts of the Path of the Bodhisattva (Mahāyāna) had deteriorated. Now we desire to invite scholars who would remove these moral faults" (Roerich 1976:245).

The forms of Buddhism taught by the official guests, such as Rinchen Zangpo, are fairly well documented by contemporary literature and art. Rinchen Zangpo's doctrinal predilections are clearly reflected in the paintings and sculptures of the monasteries he founded. As we shall see, in the *'du-khang* (assembly hall) at Ta-pho in Spiti (Figs. 47, 48). The *Blue Annals* tells us that the "Great Translator" had "mastered and expounded all the basic texts of the *Prajñāpāramitā* and *tantra*

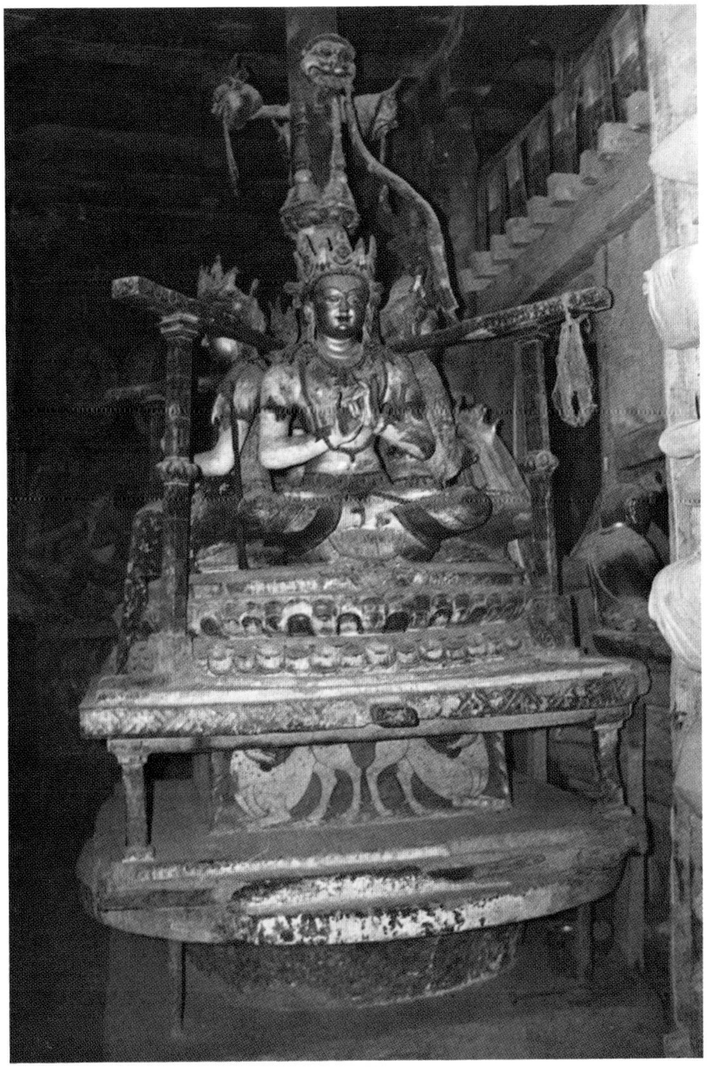

47. *'Du-khang*, Sarvavid Vairocana, sculpture, Ta-pho.

classes, has especially expounded the *yoga-tantras*." It goes on to say that Rinchen Zangpo, the "great Translator, on three occasions journeyed to Kasmira and there attended on many teachers. He also invited many paṇḍitas to Tibet and properly established the custom of preaching (the Yoga Tantras). (Roerich 1976:351–352). From the artistic remains, as confirmed by literary accounts, it appears that, of the *yoga-tantra* class, the *Sarva-tathāgatha-tattva-saṃgraha* (*STTS*) (translated by Rinchen Zangpo) and the *Durgati-pariśodhana* were particularly favored. In addition, there are the arts associated with the *sūtras* of the *Prajñāpāramitā* and *Avataṃsaka* groups (Pl. 101,102) (see Snellgrove's discussion, Ch. V).

There was no recognized Mahāyāna canon in northern India. At the same time in parts of northeast India, such as at the Vikramaśīla monastery, other literary traditions were also important. Other *tantras*, brought to Tibet by other Tibetan teachers, also formed the doctrinal foundation of early Tibetan orders. Two famous Tibetan scholars, 'Drog-mi (992–1072) and Mar-pa (1012–1092), spent many years studying the *tantras* in the monastic universities of northeast India. Upon their return, their teachings formed the foundation of Sakya and Kagyud orders respectively. Many ideas were current in India and the Himalayas and these diverse trends contributed to the philosophical ferment of the eleventh century. With the founding of the great monasteries came the establishment of institutional structures and hierarchies, and each center became the focal point of increasingly well-defined doctrines and practices. It was around these institutional cores that the Tibetan schools were formed.

ART HISTORICAL PROBLEMS

In the eleventh century, Muslim armies were pushing across northern India and the Kashmiri economy was in a state of decline. Patronage of Buddhist and Hindu institutions had diminished, and Kalhāṇa indicates that between 1003 and 1028 only one new Buddhist institution was established in that state (Stein 1900:II,121). As the Kashmiri economy deteriorated, however, the patronage of Buddhism in the western Himalayas increased. New monasteries were being built and the talents of skilled artisans were much in demand. Many Kashmiri translators, artists, and craftsmen traveled eastward to find work in the neighboring regions of Ladakh, Spiti, Lahul, and Gu-ge. Craftsmen also came from the Indian Hill States in Himachal Pradesh (Plate 96) and from more distant monastic centers in northeast India and Nepal; some may even have come from the renowned artistic centers of Khotan and Kashgar. In addition objects, even of colossal size, were brought into Ladakh.[3]

The available artistic remains allow us to distinguish five regional artistic styles in the western Himalayas. These regional centers can be identified as: 1) Baltistan, because Buddhist art in this region is earlier and falls within the sphere of Kashmiri influence, the art is treated in Ch. VIa; 2) the Hill States of Chamba, Kulu, Kangra, Manali; 3) Spiti-Lahul and Kunawar; 4) Ladakh, including Zangskar and Nubra; and 5) Gu-ge. Because the remains are unevenly clustered and no scientific archaeological excavation has taken place, it is not yet possible to precisely define either the regional schools or the process of artistic

48. *'Du-khang*, sculpture, Ta-pho.

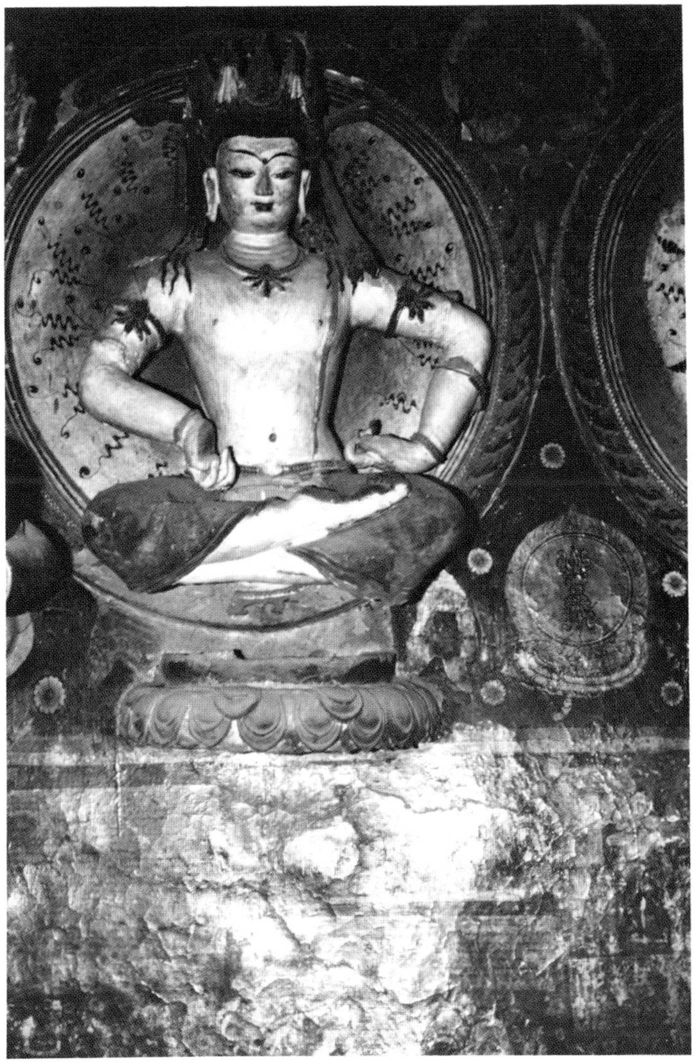

interaction between them. We know that some styles occur in several regions simultaneously because the regions were politically unified at the time, or because of the movement of artists throughout the area. There is such a strong resemblance between works executed in several regional centers at certain times that it is often difficult to identify the place of manufacture. Sculptures from Ladakh made about the tenth to eleventh centuries (Pls.81,89) are very strongly related to Kashmiri sculpture of about the tenth century. Manuscript painting from T'oling monastery in West Tibet ca. eleventh century (Pls. 101,102) is quite similar to the mural painting of Ta-pho at Spiti (eleventh century) and Alchi (eleventh-twelfth centuries) in Ladakh. The dependence on northeast Indian (Pl. 81) and Nepalese (Pl. 91) models is also apparent.

It has proved particularly difficult to attribute scroll paintings to specific artistic centers on the basis of stylistic indications alone. In the later periods of Tibetan art, the presence of historical personages is often the most reliable guide. In the earlier periods, such clues are usually no longer available or cannot be understood. As a result, an entire group of early western Himalayan *t'ang-kas*, several of which are exhibited here (Pl. 112), have previously been attributed to Nepalese artists. This overevaluation of the impact of Nepalese artists began in a period when the majority of early Esoteric Buddhist art from the Himalayas known in the West was, in fact, Nepalese. The terms "Nepali style" and "Tibeto-Nepalese" (Karmay 1975:12) were used to describe a variety of paintings, ranging from the eighth to ninth century images preserved at Dunhuang to Himalayan *t'ang-kas* made in the thirteenth to fourteenth centuries. There is no longer any justification for the use of these terms (Snellgrove 1977:16–17). Snellgrove and Tucci have more correctly employed the term "Indo-Tibetan" to describe the amalgam of northwest Indian and Tibetan cultural influences which we have been discussing here (Fig. 49). The abundant artistic evidence now available in monasteries from Ladakh to West Tibet allows us to say that a distinctive western Himalayan school of art existed from the eleventh to thirteenth centuries. Furthermore, in cases where portable arts can directly be compared to the painting or sculpture still located in monasteries, more specific regional designations, such as Ladakh, Spiti, etc., seem justified. The characteristics of these regional styles are discussed in the descriptions of the individual objects.

The Buddhist monasteries of Ladakh are presently the most accessible monuments for the study of Vajrayāna art in the western Trans-Himalaya. The study and publication of Ladakhi art has only just begun but there are enough extant mural paintings and architectural sculptures to allow us to define at least three distinctive Ladakhi styles (Pls. 82, 89, and 90).[4] in the twelfth through thirteenth centuries. It is thus possible to include individual bronze sculptures in the corpus of Ladakhi art. The stylistic features of this bronze Buddha (Pl. 82) can be compared to painted images from the Lhakung Soma, Alchi. Both show the characteristic long, slender torso; thick neck; shovel-shaped head with high forehead and hair arranged in rows of bead-like curls; and the high cranial protuberance (*uṣṇīṣa*) topped by an extra bump. The garment is treated in a similar way in both the painted and sculpted images: the monastic robe covers only the left shoulder and its presence is only indicated by the single fold across the chest and the folded ends on the left shoulder, the arm, and at both ankles. This same style can be identified as far west as Baltistan (Fig. 2).

The definition of regional styles is complicated by the fact that a number of extant mediaeval works may not have been made in principal centers of artistic production. In fact, many areas, such as Lahul and Chamba, which today are important for the history of Buddhist art, may have retained their mediaeval treasures precisely because their more isolated location protected them from invaders traveling over the main thoroughfares. As provincial centers, they also escaped the more well-intentioned destruction of mediaeval art brought about by successive generations of wealthy patrons who wished to donate better and newer offerings to the gods[5].

A thorough and detailed study of the remaining monuments should allow us to trace the movement of artists from one regional center to another. Tucci has frequently noted that the monasteries of the western Himalayas contain the sole surviving records of Kashmiri painting prior

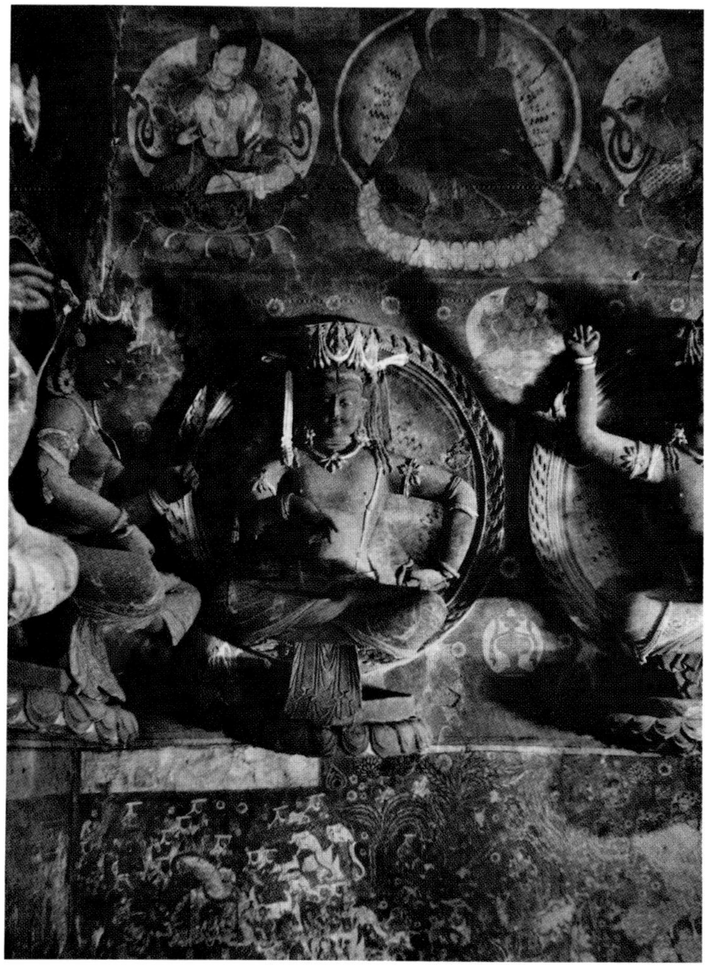

49. *'Du-khang*, sculpture, Ta-pho.

to the eleventh century. By the same token, a comparative analysis of the surviving wood sculpture and architectural decoration in Chamba and Kulu would testify to the importation of artists from these areas to Alchi and Lamayuru during the eleventh and twelfth centuries when Ladakh controlled Kulu and Chamba. An example of wooden sculpture from the British Museum also testifies to the presence of other artistic influences; for example, this rare large-scale wooden architectural sculpture from Kyelong monastery in Lahul (Pl. 85) clearly shows evidence of Central Asian influence combined with eighth century Kashmiri stylistic features.[6]

Medieval bronzes from Chamba and Kulu allow us to understand the role of certain iconographic themes in western Himalayan art. Female divinities appear to have been particularly important. The goddess was worshipped in both Hindu and Buddhist settings, frequently in tantric forms (Pl. 96). Multiarmed female divinities, such as Prajñāpāramitā (Pl. 101) and Uṣṇīṣavijayā (Pl. 97) appear frequently in the wall paintings at Ta-pho and Alchi and are also depicted in small devotional images. As we noted in Chapter VIa the worship of the goddess, even in Buddhist sanctuaries, became widespread in historical northwest India from the Śāhī period and may be attributed to the impact of Hinduism throughout the area (Pl. 41). Devotional paintings dedicated to the goddess (Pl. 112) are among the earliest surviving devotional paintings from the western Himalayas. Some early depictions of Buddhist divinities and their consorts were undoubtedly based on representations of Hindu deities and their consorts (Pl. 110).

The compositions of these early devotional paintings are relatively simple. Female divinities in later Tibetan devotional paintings occupy the center of diverse symbolic compositions. Here we find manifestations of Vajrayoginī in the center of a star (Pl. 128) or a palace-like *maṇḍala* (Pl. 125). While the liturgy of Vajrayoginī, on which these paintings are based, claims that the goddess originated in Uḍḍiyāna (Swat), her widespread worship throughout the Himalayas is accompanied by visual representations which resulted from diverse sources.

As the mural paintings help to provide a chronological and geographical context for the *t'angkas* and manuscript paintings, surviving architectural sculpture should provide a chronological framework for portable sculpture, and the combined evidence should allow us to understand the characteristics of regional artistic centers. Excavations and more detailed art historical analysis of the post-Gupta (Pls. 78, 79) Hindu monuments of greater Kashmir and Himachal Pradesh should allow us to better define the bronze sculptures of the eighth to eleventh centuries which have been preserved in western Himalayan and Tibetan monasteries. Laboratory and technical analysis of sculptures in Western collections should eventually permit the definition of regional metal-working schools.

TA-PHO: A CASE STUDY

The art of the western Himalayas reflects not only the artistic traditions of northwest India and Central Asia but also those of northeast India and Nepal. In the eleventh century, the political and economic center for the western Himalayas was located in the ancient region of Gu-ge.

Tucci studied the early monasteries such as mang-hang, T'oling, and Tsaparang and compared them to the important early monasteries of the Tsang region such as Iwang and Samada (Tucci 1932–41:Vols 2 and 4). The art produced in the great monasteries of Tsang (central-west Tibet) shared many characteristics with the art of central Tibet and Nepal. By the fourteenth century, the interregional trade within Tibet (in which monasteries often served as economic links) as well as, to a certain degree, the standardization of Buddhist texts and iconography, had resulted in a more unified artistic production in all of the major monastic centers.

In India, the most important documents of the evolution of Esoteric Buddhist art are the magnificently decorated temples created in the late tenth and early eleventh centuries. Among the earliest examples are Ta-pho in Spiti, the Sum-tsek in Alchi, and *du 'Kang*at Sumda in Zangskar. Of these, the earliest is undoubtedly Ta-pho, and a careful examination of its artistic remains will allow us to understand the evolution of Buddhist art and the philosophical currents of the time.

Ta-pho is located in the village by that name on the steep banks of the Spiti River. The people of the region are ethnically Tibetan or Bhotia. Spiti became part of India in the middle of the nineteenth century, but the close proximity of Hindus, Sikhs, and Muslims has only recently begun to affect the traditional lifestyle of the villagers. A newly built military road has brought bus service, postal deliveries, education, and health care to the area, and both the monastery and the village are now about to enter the twentieth century.

Ta-pho was visited by three scholars earlier in the century and each published an account: Francke in 1909, Tucci in 1933, and Snellgrove in 1953. Each was overwhelmed by both the historical importance of the monastery and the physical beauty of its art. It was with sadness that Snellgrove wrote, "The whole place is in process of sad decay, for the few monks that now care for it have neither the will nor the means to carry out the necessary preservation" (Snellgrove 1957:183). At that time, monks no longer lived within the enclosure, although the prescribed chants to the protective deity, Vajrabhairava, were faithfully performed by the Ge-lug-pa lamas living in the village. In the last ten years, Ta-pho has been revived, thanks to the efforts of the Indian government and the Archaeological Survey of India.

The magnificent assembly hall (*'du-khang*) of Ta-pho stands in stark contrast to the mud huts in the contemporary small village. Despite the Indian government's effort to introduce new food crops and poultry farming, people here remain pitifully poor. The altitude and harsh climate must always have limited the available agricultural resources, but in the past tariffs on trade and travel must have provided considerable revenue and would explain the higher standard of living implied by the well-endowed chapels. When Ta-pho was built, ca. 996 A.D., the village lay across the main thoroughfare between Tsaparang (the capital of Gu-ge), Ladakh, and Central Asia. Later, trade patterns and political alliances changed. The nearby border now isolates "Indian-Tibet" (as Francke called Spiti-Lahul) from Tibet. No longer a cross-roads, for centuries Ta-pho has been a dead end.

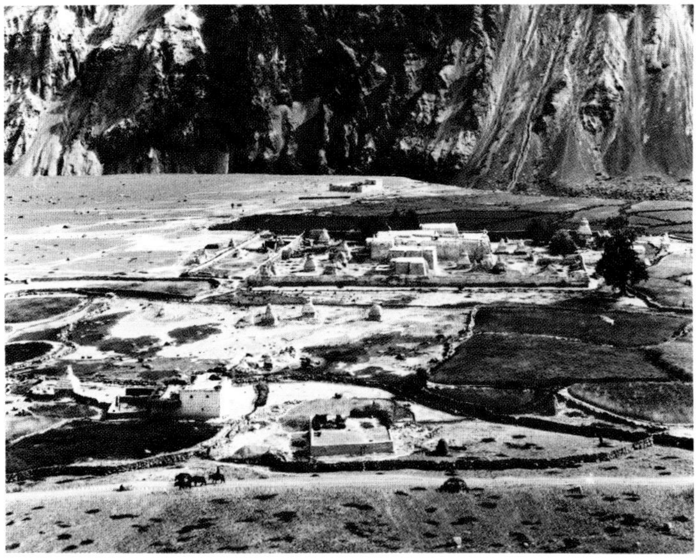

50. *Chos-'khor*, Ta-pho.

The *chos-'khor* (sacred enclosure) occupies a large area in the middle of a cultivated field south of the village. The enclosure is surrounded by a mud wall which is approximately 280 by 250 feet. Inside the enclosure, there are eight free-standing chapels including one that touches the west boundary wall (Fig. 50). This structure is a later addition.

The Buddhist structures belong to at least three periods. The *'du-khang*, still used as the main assembly hall, dates from the tenth to eleventh centuries. Seven other chapels are decorated with paintings that appear to have been executed in the fifteenth or sixteenth century. Seven of these chapels are located in the sacred enclosure and the eighth can be found in a cave high above the monastery. The small chapel which may date to the sixteenth or seventeenth century is located in the western wall of the sacred enclosure.

The *'Du-khang* (Assembly Hall)

The oldest building is without doubt the main assembly hall (*'du-khang*), and it alone can be attributed to the time of Rinchen Zangpo. An inscription records that King Byaṅ-chub 'Öd repaired the monastery forty-six years after it was founded by Ye-śes 'Öd. It is likely, therefore, that the institution was established in 996 (or 1008 A.D. as calculated by Snellgrove 1957:184), and was one of the monasteries founded by Rinchen Zangpo under Ye-śes 'Öd's patronage. Rinchen Zangpo's biography lends credence to this theory, for Ta-pho is listed among the institutions founded by the "Great Translator." In addition, the style of the paintings and sculptures and the theme, a *vajradhātu-maṇḍala* with the four-fold (Sarvavid) Vairocana at the center, confirms the connection of the Ta-pho *'du-khang* with other chapels founded by Rinchen Zangpo.

The *'du-khang* faces east and is on the medial east-west axis, almost in the center of the compound. The main hall stands in the center of a building which also houses two smaller halls or chapels. Two other smaller chapels are located behind the building (Plan 1). The entire enclosure is dotted with *chörtens*, (*stūpas*, or reliquary mounds), many of quite ancient date. Behind the rear northwest wall, one can still see the walls of the monastic cells. Originally, as at other monastic complexes in northwest India, such cells must originally have lined the inside perimeters of the enclosure.

Later additions have obscured the original three-part ground plan of the *'du-khang*, which was similar to that of other Tibetan monasteries of this period. It consists basically of the vestibule, the main assembly

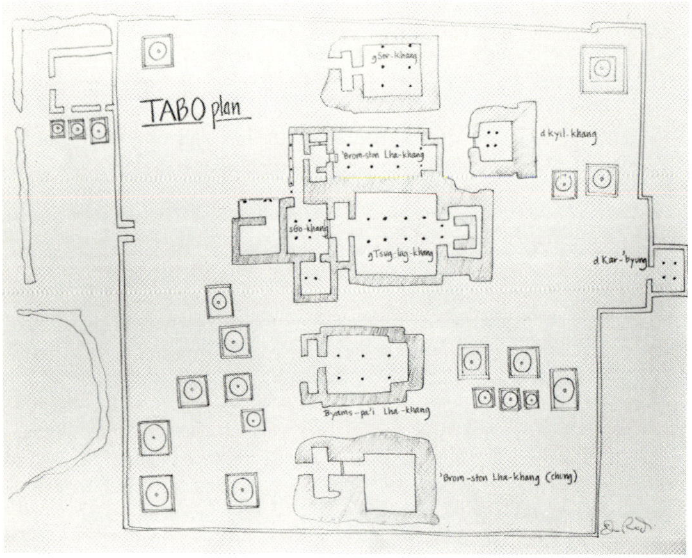

Plan 1 — Ta-pho Monastery.

hall, and the cella or apse. The vestibule, called by monks the *go-khang*, appears to be a later addition to the original structure and is decorated with twentieth-century paintings. Here one finds the usual iconography, representations of Tsong-kha-pa, and representations of the divinity Guhyasamāja in *yab-yum*.

If the vestibule, *go-khang*, was not part of the original plan, then the original entrance would have been on the main axis of the entire sacred complex. To one side of this vestibule is the *mgon-khang*, the shrine room of the guardian deities. It is possible that this room was not to be seen by Tucci when he made his visit (Tucci: 1935:VIII/i). This shrine is used for the performance of the Mahākāla liturgy (*sādhana*), a rite performed each morning and evening in order to propitiate the guardian deity of the temple, Vajrabhairava. The paintings in the shrine room are extraordinarily expressive and appear to date from about the fifteenth or sixteenth century (Fig. 51). A complete set of religious dance masks (cham) are kept in the *mgon-khang* because these masks are thought to symbolize the deities. The masks (Fig. 52) are of equally fine quality, and are used in religious dances performed at Ta-pho.

The main assembly hall (*'du-khang*) measures 40 feet by 36 feet and is divided into four unequal bays, the largest being in the center. The wooden beams used to span this space are unusually large; the local monks claim they were imported from the nearby region of Kunawar. The apse behind the main shrine hall is almost eight feet square (Plan 1a). The back retaining wall (the western wall) is unusually thick. Upon entering the *'du-khang*, we find ourselves facing a wooden bookcase, which also serves as an altar, and contains the sacred texts (the Kanjur canon and Tanjur commentaries). At the center of this wooden structure is an opening through which one can see the face of the main deity of the chapel, the four-faced image of Sarvavid Vairocana. Along the wide central aisle there are rows of benches where the monks sit, facing inwards to recite the liturgy. At one end of the central aisle, facing this row of benches, is a throne containing a picture of the Dalai Lama. On either side are butter lamps (Fig. 53). Ranged around the walls and attached to them by wooden armatures about four feet above ground level, are thirty-two life-size clay images, each seated on a raised lotus throne. Behind each figure is a round nimbus and halo which is painted and ringed with stucco flames (Fig. 49). The multicolored rays sometimes painted inside the halo seem to represent the supernatural effulgence of the deity.

The thirty-two clay sculptures are symmetrically ordered around the main deity in such a way that the worshipper is placed at the theoretical center of the *maṇḍala*. On each of the long side walls are two slightly larger images. These represent the Buddhas of the four directions. Each Buddha is attended by four Bodhisattvas, two Bodhisattvas to each side, equaling sixteen Bodhisattvas. The Buddhas are distinguished by their slightly larger size and strict frontality. There are eight goddesses of offering. Two are placed at either side of the entry and two are seated on either side of the opening near the altar which leads to the passage leading towards the apse. The *maṇḍala* is also protected by four male guardian deities, two inside the entry and two inside the passage leading to the apse. The life-size sculptural ensemble then forms a completely integrated *maṇḍala* which appears unrelated to the figures in the apse.

Narrative Paintings

The lower portion of the wall is a painted panel adorned with both inscriptions and a continuous narrative frieze. The inscriptions are of several types. On either side of the doorway are various accounts of the founding and repair of the monastery. Some of these have been published by Tucci (1935:III/1) and will be published more completely by the present author in the complete publication on Ta-pho monastery. In addition to these historical inscriptions, there are other inscriptions of a religious nature interspersed among the narrative scenes. These inscriptions have been translated by the Venerable Thartse Khen-po, Rinpoche. Among these writings, he found portions of the *Avataṃsaka-sūtra*. Shorter and longer versions have both been preserved. The practice of inscribing religious texts on monastery walls has a long history in China and Tibet[7].

The pictorial narrative on the north wall depicts the last section of

51. Wall painting, *mgon-khang*, Ta-pho.

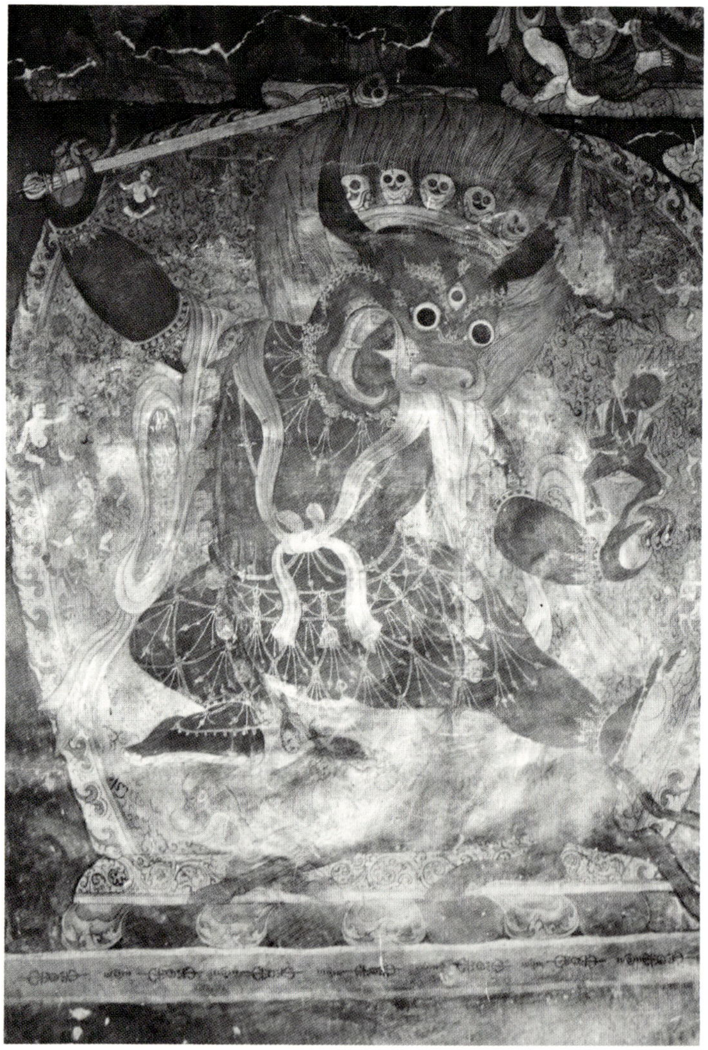

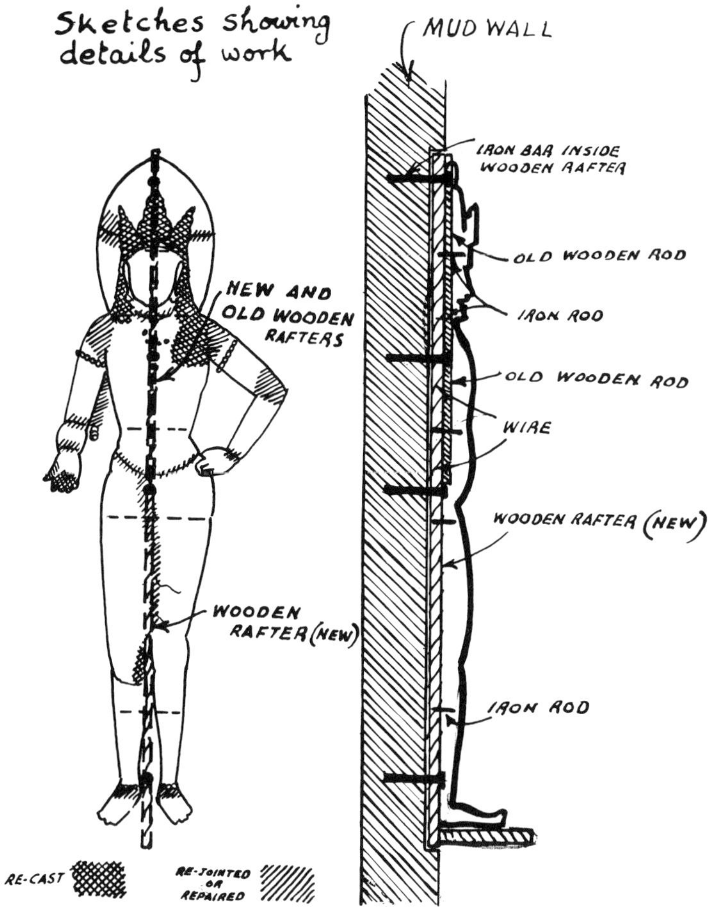

Diagram 1 — Construction and repair of clay sculpture, *'du-khang*, Ta-pho.

the *Gandhavyūha*. The left wall is dedicated to the story of the young Prince Norzang (Sudhana) and his search for enlightenment. The labels with the paintings precisely identify these scenes (Fig. 54, 54a). Located in the same position as these narrative friezes, but on the right wall are scenes from the life of the Buddha and the Avadāna tales (Fig. 55).

Plan 1a — *Du-khang*, Ta-pho monastery.

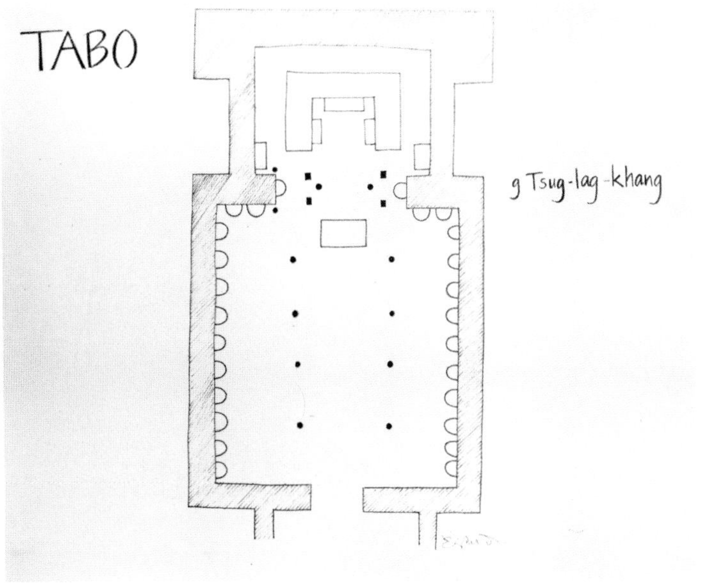

Several of these can be identified. As in other contemporaneous monasteries, some scenes have been taken from the Vessantara-Jātaka while others depict the birth and death of the Buddha (Pls. 105–107).

The depiction of an individual's progress to enlightenment is an ancient theme in Indian art. Scenes from the life of the Buddha Śākyamuni are represented on many early Indian monuments. The story of Sudhana's (Prince Norzang) progress (told in the *Avataṃsaka-sūtra*) is depicted in the eighth-century sculptures on the great *stūpa* at Borbodadur. Images from Luk Monastery in western Tibet show that the traditional themes were still popular in the region in the thirteenth and fourteenth centuries. What is interesting at Ta-pho is the choice of subjects illustrated. We shall return to this theme in our discussion of the philosophical trends depicted in the art of Ta-pho.

The narrative paintings appear to date from the same period as the clay sculptures and the other paintings of divinities on the walls above these sculptures. A comparison of specific details in the devotional paintings, the narrative paintings, and the sculptures reveals that the basic forms are the same—the shapes of the crowns, the garments, the treatment of the torsos. In addition, the details of the secular figures—the clothing, hats, and hairstyles—and also the depictions of architecture and the drawing style are comparable to narrative paintings from eleventh-century Mang-nang Monastery in western Tibet and Iwang Monastery in central Tibet (Tucci 1935–36:IV/3, figs.46–48). The men's clothing—coats with wide lapels, broad sashes, soft black boots with upturned toes, and the wide flat hats depicted in paintings

52. Masks, *mgon-khang*, Ta-pho.

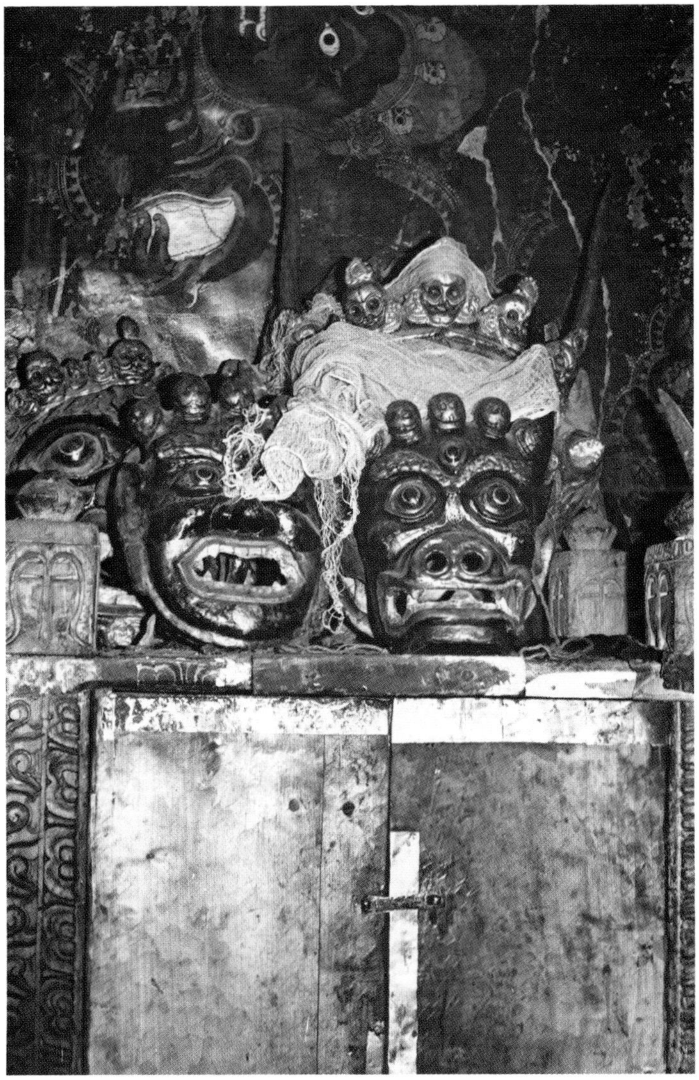

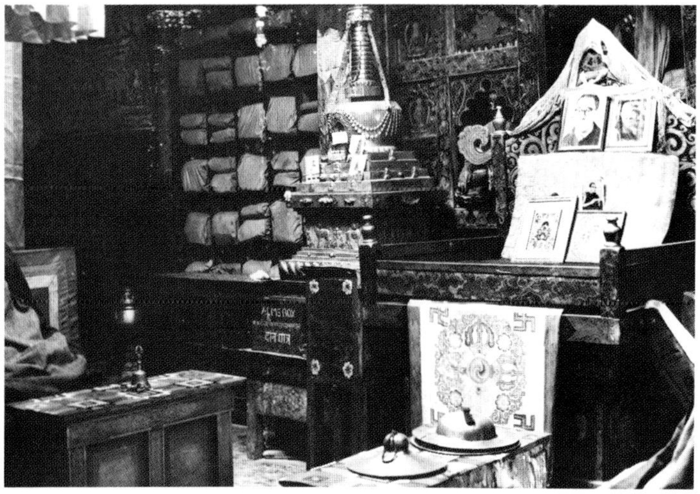

53. *'Du-khang,* Ta-pho.

of the Norzang legend—can also be seen in a leaf from the *Avatamsaka-sūtra* (Pls. 101–102) from T'oling Monastery, West Tibet, ca. eleventh century. These particular details can be related to the costumes still worn today in western Central Asia. Other features of secular dress, such as the large turbans represented in the Sum-tsek Chapel paintings from Alchi, can be identified with royal Tibetan apparel on the basis of the paintings of Tibetan kings preserved in Dunhuang Caves 158 and 159 (Karmay 1977:71–72). The narrative paintings at Ta-pho are extraordinarily important because they document both the history of religion and the history of secular culture, about which so little is known. A detailed study of these paintings and the other works at Tapho is in preparation.[8]

The Apse

The wooden altar screen and bookcase separate the assembly hall from the apse. Behind this altar is a very different pictorial and architectural space. Here a passage allows the circumambulation of the main icon, a four-faced Vairocana, which stands in the middle of the space. The wall of the ambulatory is completely covered with quite late paintings of the Thousand Buddha theme. The fact that no early paintings remain on this wall suggests the possibility that both the wall and the ambulatory passage may be later additions.

In the space between the circumambulatory passage and the main assembly hall stands the extraordinary figure of the white four-faced Vairocana. This image is actually composed of four seated figures (placed back to back), each performing the teaching (*dharmacakra mudrā*). The style of this over-life-size clay figure is identical to that of the other clay figures in the *'du-khang*. There is an elegance in the treatment of the torso; the round, harmonious features of the face; and the proportions of the body parts, which all follow the aesthetic of Kashmiri art in the late ninth and tenth centuries (Pl. 47). The image is seated on a large processional carriage called a *ratha*. It is difficult to understand how this carriage would have been transported into or out of the assembly hall. As I noted earlier, the present entry, which is off-center and reached through a second vestibule, is probably not original. The temple might originally have had another vestibule with large portals. These annual image processions were reported by Xuanzang in his seventh-century account of ceremonies in India and Central Asia. Similar Hindu processionals occur today throughout India.

In order to circumambulate the four-faced Vairocana and complete the *maṇḍala*, the worshipper has to pass by the guardian deities (Fig. 56) and enter a passageway which leads to an apse. At the back of the apse, a Buddha is seated on a throne decorated with two lions, which stands on an elevated platform (Fig. 57). He is attended by four clay Bodhisattvas: Avalokiteśvara and Mahāsthamaprāpta are placed next to the throne; on the lower platform, the two Bodhisattvas are Ksitigarbha and Ākāśagarbha. The Buddha is in the meditation *mudrā* and is painted red. It is difficult to identify this Buddha, but the color and *mudrā* suggest that the figure represents Amitābha; however, the peacock is Amitābha's vehicle, while the lion is associated with Vairocana. The style of the Buddha and the over-life-size standing Bodhisattvas appear somewhat later than the style of the figures in the main *'du-khang*. Certainly, the facial features have been considerably altered and do not have the grace of the earlier sculptures. The bodily proportions, too, are different. The torsos are thinner and flatter, and the hip areas bulge out in a rather pronounced curve which is reminiscent of the thirteenth-century sculptures found in Ladakh. The shape of the Buddha's *mandorlas* is totally different from the shape of the *mandorlas* in the main hall. The position of the Buddha Amitābha and the style of the clay *mandorla* relate to similar features also found in the *'du-khangs* at Alchi and Lamayuru in Ladakh. It is possible that parts of this group were added later, particularly the four standing Bodhisattvas. It is also probable that the Amitābha figure replaced an earlier image of Vairocana to which the lion throne originally belonged. Vairocana can also be depicted in the meditation *mudrā*, but has a white color. It is possible that an image of Vairocana (probably a Sarvavid Vairocana) originally occupied the back wall of the apse and was meant to be the main divinity of the *Vajradhātu-maṇḍala*. The position of the deity would then be analogous to the image of Vairocana

54. Wall painting, *'du-khang* Ta-pho. Sudhana meets Maitreya in the Bodhisattva's palace. He is surrounded by his students. The scene is identified by an inscription which is a summary from the *Gandhavyūha* of the *Avatamsaka-sūtra*.

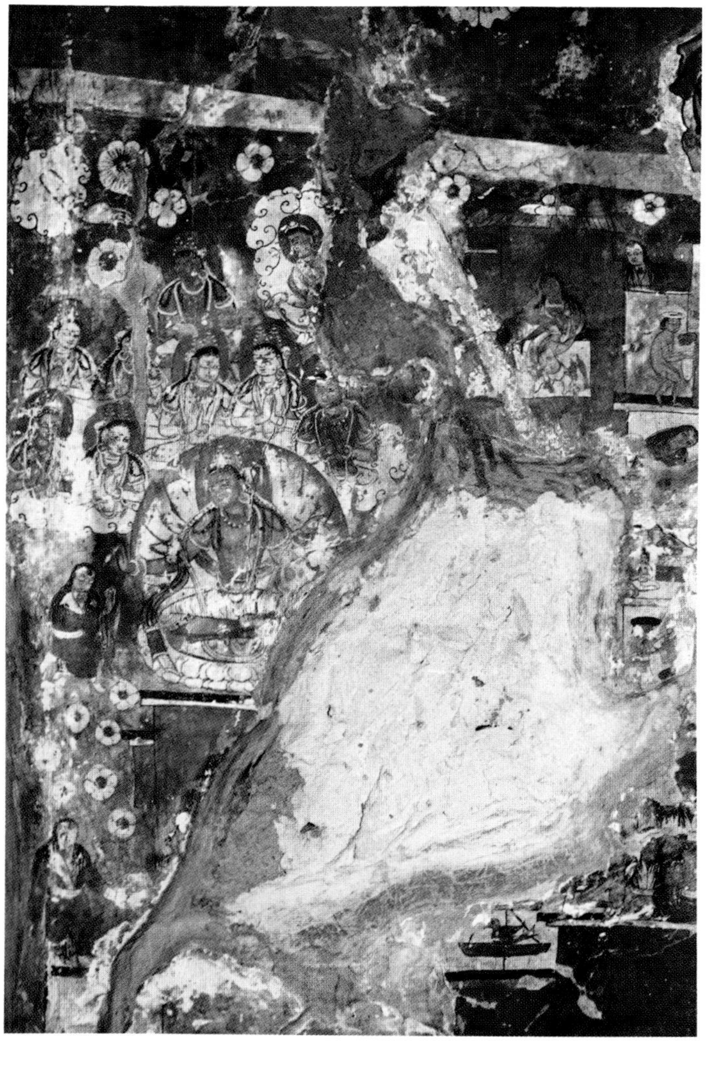

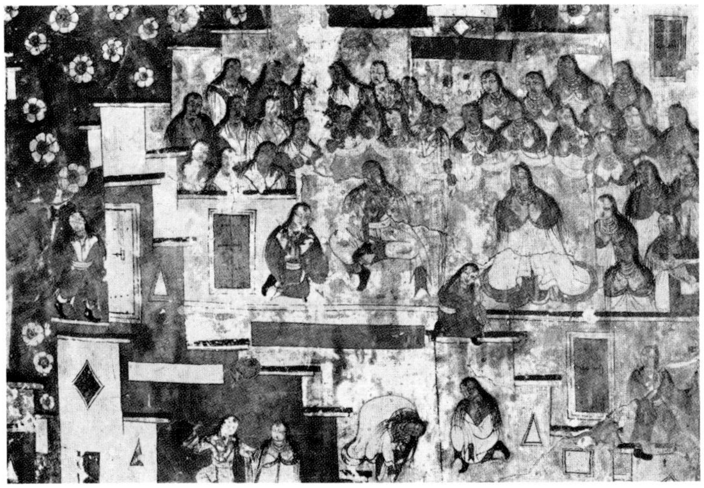

54a. Wall painting, *'du-khang;* legend of Sudhana: Sudhana meets Śrī-Saṃbhava and Srī-mati. According to the inscription, which is a synopsis from the *Gandhavyūha* of the *Avatamsaka-sutra,* Sudhana here meets two of his *kalyanamitra* (good friends), Śrī-Saṃbhava and Śrī-mati. His clasped hands signify that he is requesting teachings. "We have understood the Bodhisattva's path and realized its illusionary nature, so we saw that, in this illusion, everything comes and goes; so, karma and delusions, ignorance, saṃsāra and sentient beings, all these we see as illusions; the dying person and the reborn one, sickness and old age, all sufferings we see as illusions; Arahats, Pratyeka Buddhas and Bodhisattvas, all, we see as having the same illusionary nature. Also, all Buddhas and Bodhisattvas' powerful activities we see as illusionary. But we cannot describe the qualities of this illusion, so you must go to the Southern part of India and there, near the ocean, you can visit Maitreya Bodhisattva and ask Him the directions for the practice of the Bodhisattva's Path, and you will receive all you need to know. If you want to know more, you have to go and visit other teachers . . ." (translated by Thartse Khenpo, Rinpoche).

in the *'du-khang* at Alchi. The present Sarvavid Vairocana originally might not have occupied its present position. This large movable statue is, however, contemporaneous with the *maṇḍala* statues placed against the wall in the main *'du-khang.* It has also been suggested (Snellgrove 1957:186–7) that Amitābha has been placed on a lion throne because he represents a sixth supreme Buddha, known in other systems as Vajradhara or Vajrasattva.

On the north and south walls of the apse, which are definitely part of the original structure, there are paintings of the sixteen supreme Bodhisattvas of the *Vajradhātu-maṇḍala* according to the *STTS.* They are conceived as aspects of Buddhahood arising from Vairocana's mental concentration. At the same time, they are manifestations of the Bodhisattvas named either Samantabhadra, Vajrapāṇi, or Vajradhara (Lokesh Chandra and Snellgrove 1981:25). This recent publication of an edited Tibetan version of the *STTS* should facilitate the correct

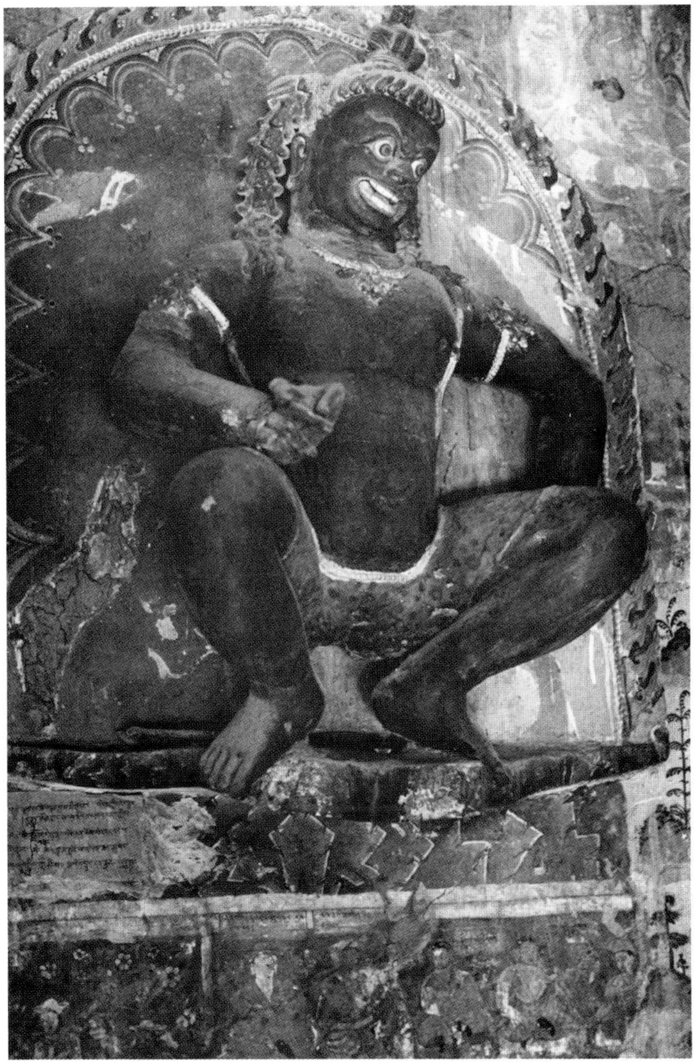

56. Sculpture of guardian statue, *'du-khang,* Ta-pho.

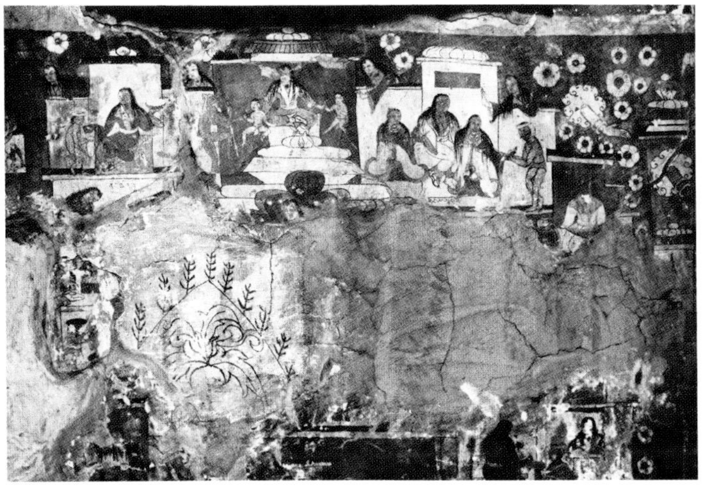

55. Wall painting, Jātaka story, *'du-khang,* Ta-pho: Three scenes from the Vessantara Jātaka. The scenes are identified by Tibetan inscriptions. 1st scene left: Vessantara gives away his money; 2nd scene center: he gives away his children; 3rd scene right: he gives away his wife.

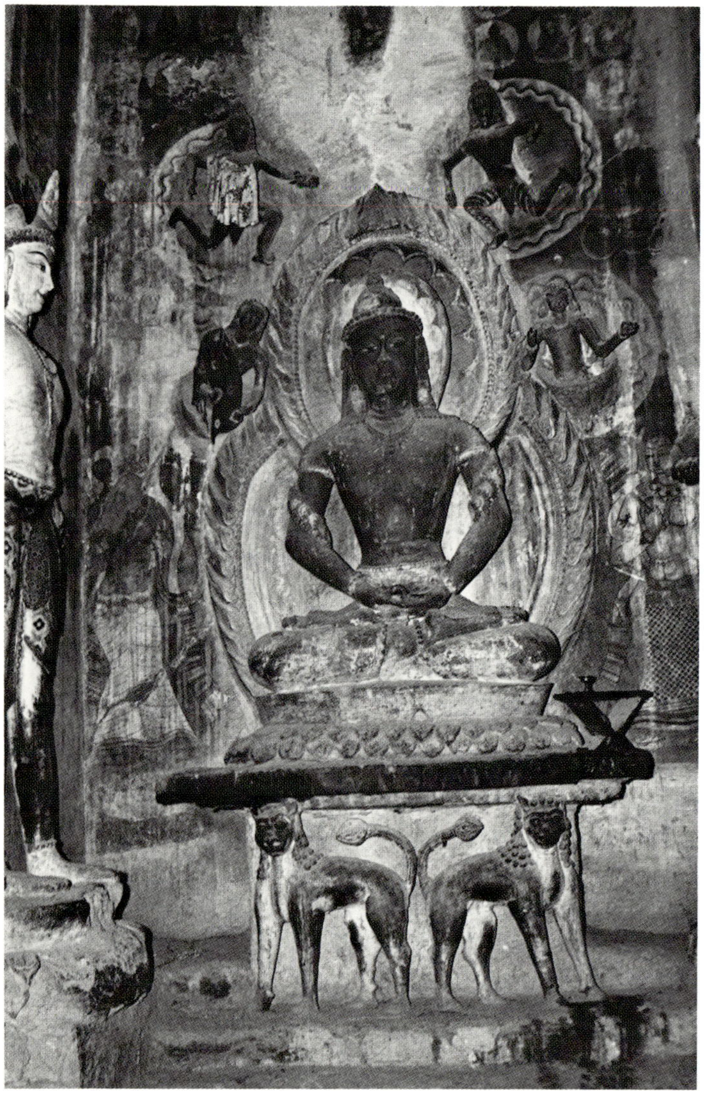

57. Clay sculpture Amitābha, *'du-khang,* Ta-pho.

identification of these extraordinary images whose colors and details have been preserved to an astonishing degree. Only in rare instances can repainting be observed. It seems that the lack of windows and the elevated position of the paintings have protected them from damage by the elements and human contact (Figs. 58,59). All of the Bodhisattvas appear to belong to the *vajra* family because each of them performs the same variant of the *vajra-mudrā* with his right hand. This *mudrā* is peculiar to the early painting of the western Himalayas (Tapho and T'oling; Pl. 102) and Dunhuang (Pls. 66,67) in the ninth through eleventh centuries[9].

The iconographic details in some cases are so unusual that they are now difficult to interpret. For example, one green Bodhisattva, whose right fist is in the *vajra-mudrā,* holds in his left hand a crystalline substance that could be a gem, or possibly, an early form of a *vajra* (Fig. 59). The magnificent dark blue Bodhisattva, whose form and facial features are reminiscent of paintings from Foladi (Fig. 60) in the Hindu Kush, holds at heart-level a crescent on top of a lotus (Fig. 58). This may well be a form of lotus.

The painted Bodhisattvas in the apse must complement the stucco sculptures in the main part of the assembly hall since they were clearly painted at the same time (compare details such as the crown, garments, and torso construction Fig. 41). An explanation for the total complex must await further study of the *yoga-tantras* (Lokesh Chandra and Snellgrove 1981; Skorupski 1981). Tucci was under the impression that the present thirty-three clay images (thirty-two deities plus the central four-faced Vairocana Tucci 1935:III/1,31–36) represented an incomplete, much altered *maṇḍala* from which four images had disappeared. He therefore believed there were originally thirty-seven images arranged according to a scheme similar to the one outlined by Snellgrove in Ch. V, Ill. 2. Tucci identifies the Ta-pho figures on the basis of a text of the Sakya order written several centuries after the Ta-pho *'du-khang* was built. His identifications, based on a system of thirty-seven deities, do not in fact coincide with the figures presently in the *'du-khang.* Tucci attributes the discrepancies to massive repairs and alterations (Tucci 1935:III/1,31–36). There is, however, absolutely no evidence that any statues are missing or have been removed or replaced. Although repairs are visible everywhere, no drastic changes, such as totally altering the position of an image's arm, can be observed. In fact, reference to a Tibetan translation of the *STTS,* a text known to have been used at Ta-pho, is more helpful. Snellgrove has proposed that the four missing goddesses are those located within the inner circle of his diagram (Ill. 2) taken from the *STTS,* viz. Mamākī, Pāṇḍaravāsinī, Locanā, Tārā. Thus, the thirty-three divinities now at Ta-pho could be considered a complete and integrated representation of the *Vajradhātu-maṇḍala* of Sarvavid Vairocana (Lokesh Chandra and Snellgrove 1980).

The style and iconography of the paintings and sculptures in the *'du-khang* at Ta-pho summarize the many cultural influences that converged on the western Himalayas in the late tenth and early eleventh

58. Wall painting blue Bodhisattva, *'du-khang* ambulatory, Ta-pho.

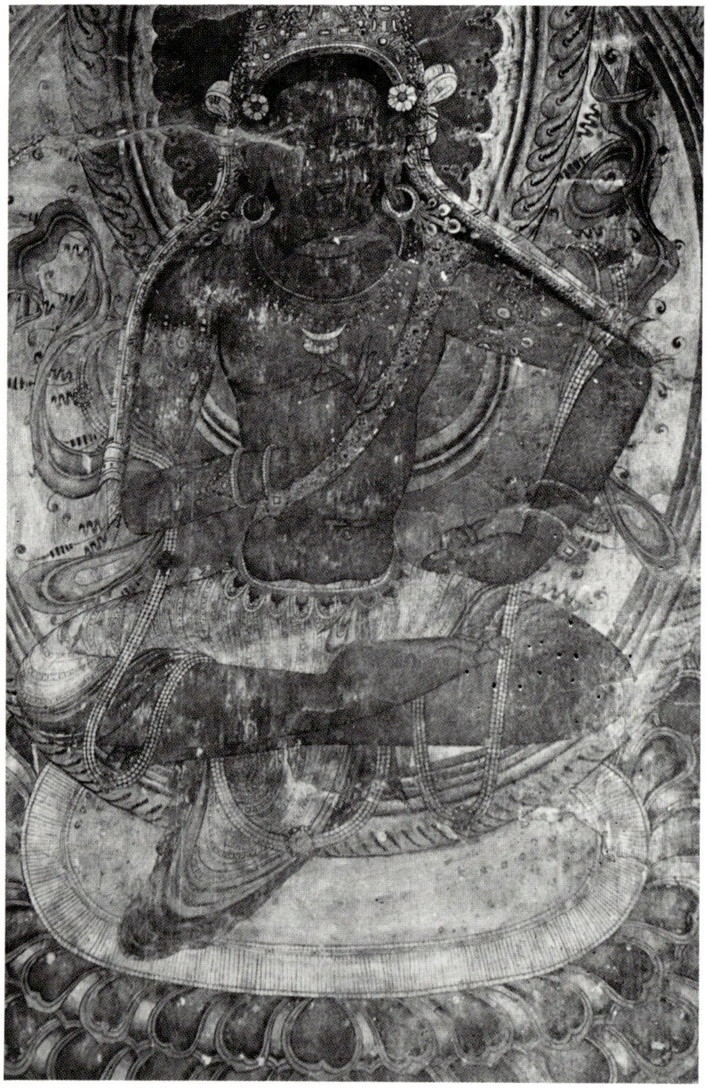

centuries. The large-scale painted clay Bodhisattvas and Buddhas (Pls. 42,48) were made by a technique current in historical northwest India and Central Asia from about the fourth century A.D. Full-scale images such as these still survive in Central Asian cave monasteries where they also originally formed a configuration of devotional images. Likewise, the technique of superimposing clay or stucco forms on a painted ground so that three-dimensional forms merge with two-dimensional ones is used to create an illusionistic environment. This technique was also used in the cave paintings of Bāmiyān and can be seen in Central Asian cave temples such as the ones at Dunhuang. Such motifs as the triple crescent crown containing rosettes; the layered and waved hair; and the simple jewelry consisting of a pearl girdle, a plain rosette on a pearl necklace, and pearl armbands occur both in the art at Ta-pho and in ninth and tenth-century Kashmiri depictions of royal or divine dress (Pl. 30).

At Ta-pho, the raised lotus throne, which consists of a single lotus on a raised pedestal with the folds of the skirt (*dhotī*) flowing over it, gives the impression that the divinity is floating in space. This is precisely the type of lotus throne represented in the Kashmiri sculpture of a six-armed Avalokiteśvara from the British Museum (Pl. 31) and in the famous tenth-century Queen Diddā bronze now in the Śrī Pratāp Singh Museum in Kashmir. This type of throne also appears in the earlier Chinese Buddhist art of Central Asia and may have its prototype in Gandhāran art. In summation, the style and iconographic details of both the painted and sculpted images datable to ca. 1000 A.D. from

59. Wall painting green Bodhisattva, *'du-khang* ambulatory, Ta-pho.

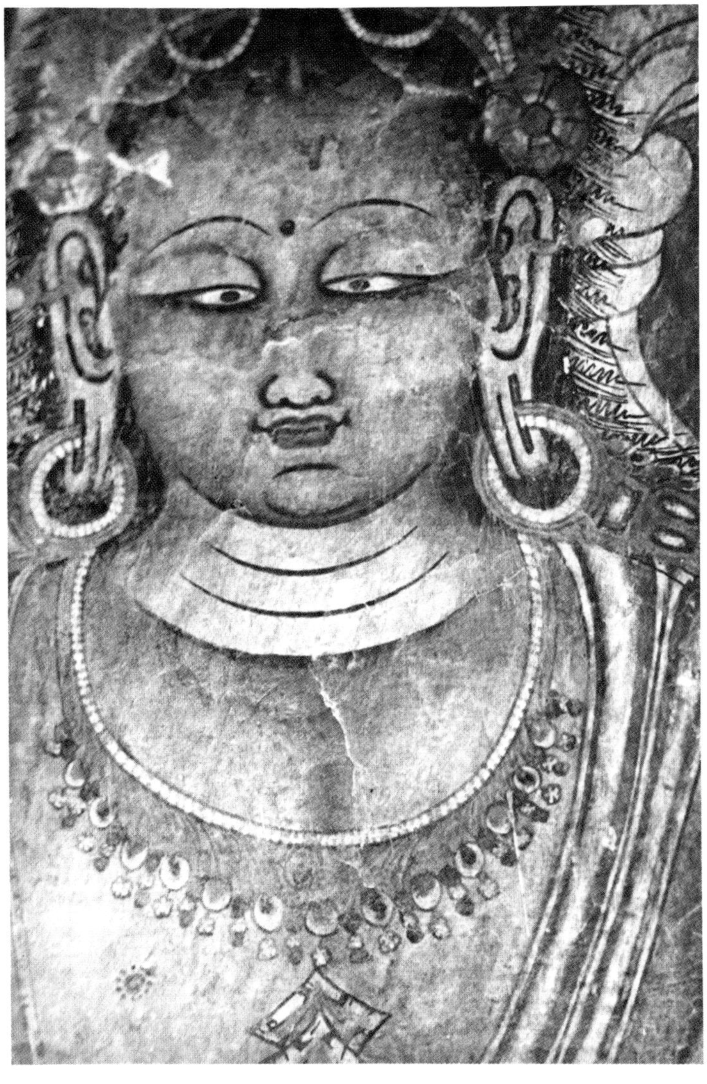

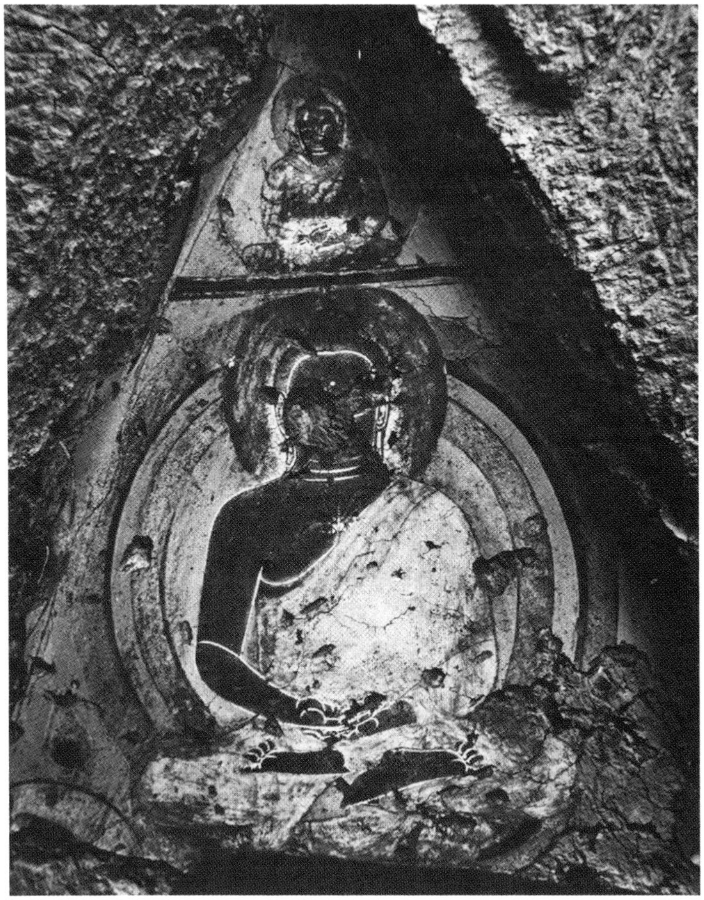

60. Buddha, Foladi, Afghanistan.

the *'du-khang* at Ta-pho derive from the same artistic sources. Thus, the paintings clearly show the influence of both historical northwest India and also, to a lesser degree, Central Asia. In fact, the genesis of the style can be traced to the lost paintings of Kashmir, represented by the Gilgit painted manuscript covers (Figs. 30–33) and eighth to ninth-century wall paintings (the last phase) at Bāmiyān and at Foladi in the Hindu Kush (Fig. 60).

Undoubtedly the most compelling feature of the *'du-khang* lies in the extraordinary fineness and elaboration of each detail, be it the delicately painted scarf of a divinity (Fig. 58) or the splendid articulation of a stucco crown (Fig. 48). The effect is accomplished by the use of fine line, clearly articulated forms, and brilliant primary colors. These same features are found in contemporary manuscript painting (Pls. 101,102). But the most dramatic and original feature of the chapel is its total aesthetic conception. When the practitioner enters into the chapel and moves forward to worship the main image of the four-faced Vairocana, he finds himself in the center of a life-size *Vajradhātu-maṇḍala*. Through meditational practices (outlined in Ch. VII), the worshipper becomes the center of the symbolic universe represented by the *maṇḍala*, and thus is transformed through identification with the deity who is the symbolic center of the universe. Because the scale of the deities is proportional to the worshipper, the ensemble is truly a living *maṇḍala*. No extraneous details disrupt the integrated concept of the cosmic setting inhabited by the deities.

The artistic and psycho-physical functions of the clay sculptures just described occurs in both Central Asia and northwest India. In the fourth and fifth centuries, sculptured images formed an iconic group meant to receive devotional worship. In the seventh century, a *maṇḍala*-like composition, depicted by sculpted images, appears in some caves at Bāmiyān. In effect, the small round chapel decorated with sculpture and paint created a total environment, and the worshipper was the theoretical center of the composition (Klimburg-Sulter in press). The *maṇḍala* is a diagrammatic representation of the universe. An example of an early stage of the conception of the chapel as the cosmic sphere may be seen at Kizil, where paintings of the Tuṣita heaven adorn the upper part of the small cave temples. An example of the next phase in the evolution of this theme is found at Dunhuang, where mural paintings depicted the four paradises. When the worshipper entered the chapel he figuratively entered the cosmic sphere. The ambitious sculpted *maṇḍala* at Ta-pho is the ultimate realization of this theme. Conceptually, it seems to be the animated expression of the pan-Indian idea of the temple as a *maṇḍala*. Likewise, painted *maṇḍalas* in Tibet are symbolic representations of temples (Pls. 125,126).

The Ta-pho sculpted *maṇḍala* may be dated to about 1000 A.D. After this date, architectural clay sculpture is used in a more conventional manner at Ta-pho, Alchi, Lamayuru and other chapels in the Trans-Himalayas (Fig. 21). In the apse at Ta-pho, the Amitābha image is placed against the back wall on a raised platform. At Ta-pho, as at Lamayuru, the Amitābha originally formed the center of an extraordinarily elaborate composition which covered the back wall and used paintings and clay forms to create a cosmic environment. These compositions must also represent the cosmic sphere, a heaven or paradise, presided over by the divinity. Once again the worshipper is separated from the divinity he serves; he stands in awe before the deity and is not part of the cosmic setting. In contrast, the plastic *maṇḍala* at Ta-pho accomplishes a sense of intimacy, in part, through the life-size scale of the images. In the twelfth and thirteenth centuries, clay figures in Ladakh are enlarged and placed on a platform at the back of the chapel (Fig. 21). The distance between the worshipper and the worshipped has been increased by the combined effect of the placement of the image, and by its scale.

This same elaborate concept of a heavenly setting for the deity is seen in paintings from the twelfth and thirteenth centuries (Pl. 108), as well as small portable images (Pls. 86,87) all from the western Himalayas. In these images, as in the earlier three-dimensional architectural configurations and also in the later paintings from Tibet (Pl. 120) the Buddha figure is the center of an elaborate and stylized composition that becomes progressively more abstract.

The origin of these large scale painted and sculpted cosmic environments in the western Himalayas can be identified in the cave temples of Central Asia. But the earliest example which remains of a three-dimensional *maṇḍala*-like composition was in the Hindu Kush (Klimburg-Salter in press). An expanded version of the three-dimensional cosmic environment can be seen in the sculpted *maṇḍala* at Ta-pho. The hieratic scale of the deities, uniform geometric compositions of the painted backgrounds, and the deliberate elimination of pictorial detail contributes to the idealization of the painted and sculpted superhuman forms, as well as the entire supernatural environment. These timeless settings, filled with vivid color and diffused with light, were meant to mirror the divine universe.

In Ta-pho, these sculpted and painted devotional images were complemented by the narrative scenes which were depicted directly underneath the three-dimensional *maṇḍala*. These murals employed the conventions associated with narrative painting in both India and Central Asia. In fact, the use of these two modes of representation together in the same chapel can be found earlier in the eighth-century wall paintings of Dunhuang and some of the larger banners, also from Dunhuang (Pls. 61,68). In the narrative paintings from Ta-pho, as in the narrative paintings at Dunhuang, all of the figures are small in scale and have a natural relationship to each other and to the landscape. In addition, we find that, to a certain degree, the narrative paintings are characterized by the use of genre details and three-dimensional perspective. These techniques are not used in the devotional paintings on the upper part of the wall. In the narrative paintings of the western Himalayan monasteries (Fig. 54), as in the Buddhist narrative paintings of Central Asia and India, motifs deriving from the secular arts, and particularly the courtly world, are liberally interspersed with Buddhist themes. In the narrative paintings of Ta-pho, the Bodhisattvas inhabit the opulent courts of contemporary palaces (Fig. 54). This association between the Bodhisattva and the courtly life is extravagantly expressed in the wall paintings of the Sum-tsek Chapel at Alchi (Fig. 46). The narrative panels at Alchi occupy the same position and serve the same function as those found in Ta-pho. At Alchi, however, separate vignettes also have been isolated from narrative scenes and are used as decorative motifs. These genre scenes, which often appear on the robes worn by divinities (Fig. 21), frequently depict secular figures in Tibetan and Central Asian dress who enjoy a life of luxury and refinement.

The stylistic differences between the devotional paintings in the *'du-khang* at Ta-pho and the didactic or narrative scenes should not be considered an indication of different dates of execution. Small details, such as the treatment of the hair, the crown, and the garments of the divine figures, show that all the works (with the exception of small areas that were repainted later) were created at the same time as part of a single conception. The different styles merely reflect the different function of these two kinds of paintings. In fact, in mediaeval Buddhist art from historical northwest India and Asia there was always a distinction between the styles used for devotional and narrative paintings (Klimburg-Salter in press). These two modes are also found together in the devotional *t'angkas* from the western Himalayas (Pl. 112) as well as later narrative murals (Pl. 106–108).

One might say that these two types of art—devotional and narrative—were actually addressed to the two different groups of people who used the temple. The devotional paintings and sculptures depict the *Vajradhātu-maṇḍala* according to the *Sarva-tathāgata-tattva-saṃgraha (STTS)* of the *yoga-tantras*. The meditational practices and ritual observances associated with these images were known only to the initiate who had received the teachings orally from his tantric master (see explanation of Vajrayāna ritual in Ch. VII and a description of this class of literature in Ch. V). The majority of Buddhists were more concerned with the simpler devotional practices.

The narrative paintings found in the same assembly hall were based on both earlier texts such as the *Avadānas* and a portion of the Mahāyāna *sūtras*, the *Avataṃsaka* literary corpus. The latter part of the *Avataṃsaka* contains the *Gandhavyūha* from which these narrative panels derive. It is interesting to note that Vairocana is the central deity in both the *Avataṃsaka-sūtra* and the *Sarva-tathāgata-tattva-saṃgraha*. Images depicting the Vairocana of the *Avataṃsaka-sūtra* have survived in the art of Central Asia. Some, for example, were found at Khotan (Williams 1973).

Furthermore, we know that the *Avataṃsaka-sūtra* and the other important class of *sūtras*, known as the *Prajñāpāramitā*, were taught in all the early monasteries founded by Rinchen Zangpo. For example, we are told that in the second quarter of the eleventh century commentaries on *Prajñāpāramitā* were written at Ta-pho. This class of text was important to the Kadampa sect which was founded during the eleventh century, and was later associated with this group of monasteries. A recent study has identified in the early Vajrayāna art from Indonesia the complementary symbolic function of the Norzang (Sudhana) legend of the *Ghandhayūha* and the *Vajradhātu-maṇḍala* of the *STTS* (Lokesh Chandra 1981:21–31).

The presence of these two types of images in the main assembly hall at Ta-pho reflects the position of the Buddhist monastery and Buddhism at that time. As we pointed out earlier, the small size of these early monasteries suggests that the actual monastic community must have been quite small. The people in the surrounding area who supported the monastery probably followed Buddhism and other more ancient indigenous practices. Most of these individuals would not have been initiated into the *tantras*. According to Tibetan scholars the *Mahayāna* has two divisions—the *Prajñaparamitra* and the tantric method (*vajrayāna*). Tsoṅ-kha-pa calls these divisions cause and effect. The *vajrayāna* is seen as including the necessary and preliminary teachings of the *prajñaparamita* (see Trungpa, Rinpoche Ch. VII). The second tantric division, which involves more complex and arduous practices, necessitates special instruction and initiation into specific teachings (Wayman 1973:4). This path would necessarily be followed by fewer people. These two divisions of the *Mahayāna* are clearly expressed in the *'du-khang* at Ta-pho.

ALCHI

The *'du-khang* at Ta-pho is now a valuable historical treasure because of its completeness, but it was neither unique, nor the most important monument in the western Himalayas. Important temples from this period remain in Tibet. Some of them, such as Mang-nang and T'oling, were studied by Tucci in the nineteen thirties. Their present condition is unknown, but Chinese archaeologists are beginning to study them (Ye Xinshen 1981).

Their easy accessibility makes the monasteries of Ladakh and Zangskar significant sites for the study of the monastic art of the western Trans-Himalaya. Recent studies on these monuments by Snellgrove and Skorupski (1978, 1980), and the critical editions of two fundamental Tibetan texts (Lokesh Chandra and Snellgrove 1980; Skorupski 1981) will promote art historical research. The earlier phase is best represented in temples at Sumda (Snellgrove and Skorupski 1980:61–69), Lamayuru, and, in particular, the *'du-khang* and Sum-tsek at Alchi, (Kobayashi 1980). In addition there are some remains at Mang-gyu (idem 22) and Phugtal (idem 1980:49–53). The art of the twelfth and thirteenth centuries is best preserved at the Lha-khang Soma and Lotsawa Lha-khang at Alchi (idem 1977:64–80).

In general, these early temples, like those in Ta-pho, were small, built of mud bricks and timber (see Sengupta) on a rectangular plan, and sometimes equipped with a pillared wooden porch. The altar, containing the main cult image, stands clear of the back wall so that the visitor can circumambulate the icon, keeping his right shoulder towards the image. In some places, as at Ta-pho, there is a passage around an inner chamber which is used for this ritual circumambulation (Plan 1).

This simple form of architecture is present all over Tibet and the western Trans-Himalaya (cf.Khosla 1979), and was the forerunner of the great monastic complexes of the later periods (Tucci 1973: 91ff.). From the outside these crumbling mud structures are often undistinguished, an exception being the Sum-tsek at Alchi (Fig. 20a) which still retains its original porch. Inside the temples, however, the vividly colored murals, and the painted and gilded life-size statues convey the impression of paradise.

The *'du-khang*, as the assembly hall, is the heart of the monastic community, and was usually built first. The *'du-khang* at Alchi dates to about the mid-eleventh century, founded by the wealthy aristocrat sKaldan Shes-rab (Snellgrove and Skorupski 1977:30). The simple, almost square building is similar to the *'du-khang* at Ta-pho. It measures 7.5 by 7.9 meters (Khosla 1979:59), and is divided by fluted columns into three bays. The main divinity, as in other early temples associated with Rinchen Zangpo, is a four-faced Vairocana placed against the back wall; he is seated on a throne and surrounded by an elaborate clay arcade. The corresponding arcade framing the Amitābha image at Ta-pho (Fig. 57) may originally have been of a similar kind. To either side of the Vairocana image are placed the Four Buddhas. In addition, there are six well-preserved *maṇḍalas* dating from the founding period, covering three walls, the fourth wall containing the Vairocana image. They portray different cycles of divinities associated with Sarvavid Vairocana (Snellgrove and Skorupski 1977:34–45, fig. 17,18). Such painted *maṇḍalas* replaced the sculptural one in the assembly hall at Ta-pho. Here the life-sized *maṇḍala* is complemented by painted rows of Bodhisattvas and Buddhas who represent the principle divinities of the different cycles related to Sarvavid Vairocana.

The style of these devotional paintings at Alchi appears connected with both northwest India and Central Asia, if compared with the Gilgit manuscript covers (Fig. 33) and the paintings in "Himalayan style" in Dunhuang (e.g., Pl. 62). As at Ta-pho, the secular figures found in the narrative scenes suggest a relationship to Central Asia (ibid.: figs. 45–47), particularly with regard to customs and costumes. One of the most interesting of the courtly scenes is the cup-drinking ceremony depicted in the Alchi *'du-khang* (ibid.: pl. XVIII). This ceremony was popular among the Turkic peoples throughout Central Asia, where it symbolized an oath of allegiance to the ruler (Esin 1967). It is represented in the Buddhist art of Bāmiyān (Klimburg-Salter in press: Fig. 28), and it also frequently appears in the early Islamic art of the Iranian-speaking world. Early Islamic pictorial arts from Iran or Turkestan may assist us in understanding the origin of these scenes in Alchi.

The most interesting building at Alchi is the Sum-tsek (three-tiered) temple whose extraordinarily well-preserved paintings constitute one of the major monuments of mediaeval art in Asia. The present efforts of the Archaeological Survey of India to conserve and protect this monument deserve international encouragement and support. Due to the complexity of the temple it is difficult to summarize, and the reader is referred to published studies of the paintings and inscriptions (Snellgrove and Skorupski 1977:45–64) and the architecture (Khosla 1979: 56–63).

There are three other mediaeval temples within the extensive Alchi complex (Plan 2): the Lha-khang Soma, Lotsawa Lha-khang, and the Manjusri Lha-khang, all of which contain important art treasures. Combined with the artistic evidence available from the *'du-khang* and the Sum-tsek, as well as the *'du-khang* and later temples at Ta-pho, there is sufficient material for the study of the stylistic development of the arts of the western Trans-Himalaya from the beginning of the eleventh to the sixteenth centuries. However, such a study would also need to be combined with a reevaluation of the arts of Gu-ge, the center of the kings of western Tibet (Tucci: 1932-41).

These major monuments have not been studied since Tucci's original research. The early monasteries such as Mang-nang and T'oling are contemporaneous with Ta-pho and provide indispensable evidence for the study of the early monastic art of the Trans-Himalaya. By the twelfth century the foreign influences were integrated into distinctive regional styles. The style of the murals in the Lha-khang Soma, Alchi can also be identified in painted scrolls and sculpture from Ladakh. Quite different styles are found during this period in the art from monasteries in west Tibet such as Man-nang and Luk (Tucci: fig. 155) and in the monastic art from Tsang (e.g., Tucci 1973: fig. 159, 160) such as from Iwang, Sumada and Nesar.

LATER MONASTIC ART: THE FIFTEENTH TO SEVENTEENTH CENTURIES

In the thirteenth century several important events took place which affected not only the form and content of Trans-Himalayan Buddhism, but Tibetan society as a whole. In the region south of Tibet, Muslim armies from Afghanistan and historical northwest India succeeded in conquering all of northern India. This led to the final destruction of Buddhism in the land of its birth. In consequence, the traditional interaction with the more cosmopolitan culture of India through monastic contacts came to an end; and Tibet not only became a refuge for Indian Buddhists, but also a center of missionary activity.

Another important event was the Mongol conquest of all of Central Asia and much of China. In the mid-thirteenth century, the Sakya (*Sa-skya*) lamas formed a peculiar relationship with the Mongol khāns which was formalized towards the end of the thirteenth century. This relationship is known as *yon-mchod*, "patron and priest." Under this arrangement, the Sakya patriarch provided the khāns with religious counsel in return for political patronage. From this time until 1368, the successive heads of the Sakya order held enormous political power. Branches of the Kagyud-pa (*bka'-brgyud-pa*) order successfully contested the supremacy of the Sakya order in the fourteenth century. From the fifteenth century on, the Gelug-pa order became progressively more important and in 1642 the Dalai Lama, head of this order, was installed in Lhasa as the virtual ruler of Tibet.

The relatively small monasteries founded prior to the fourteenth century traditionally concentrated on achieving educational and cultural hegemony. Now they expanded their political and economic foundations, thanks to the active patronage of local aristocratic families, and entered into bitter feuds in their fight for supremacy. A new class of monastic warriors emerged, monasteries increased in size and were built, fortress-like, on impregnable hilltops (Figs. 7,7a). In time, the abbots of the main religious orders came to replace the hereditary feudal nobility as the regional political authorities.

This economic and political expansion of monastic centers was

Plan 2 — Alchi monastic complex.

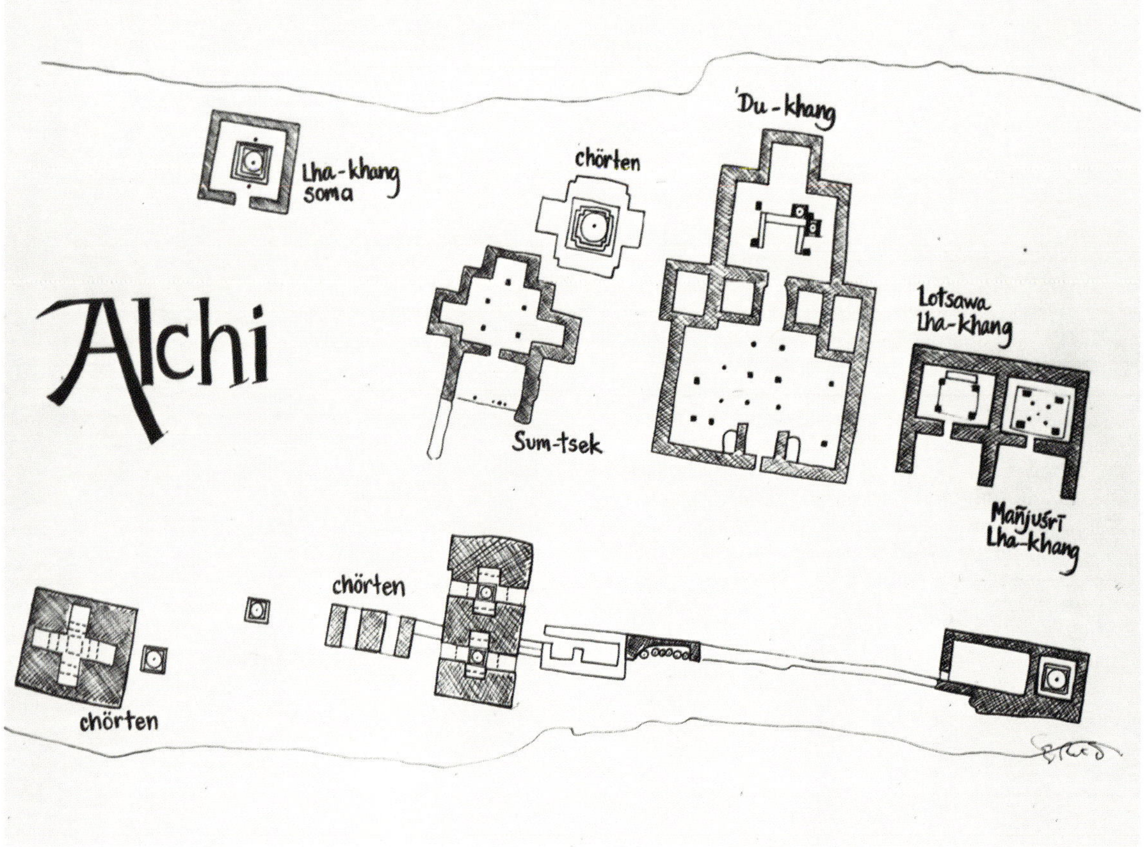

accompanied by creative literary and artistic activity. In the thirteenth century, the official Tibetan canon (Kanjur) was closed, but philosophical inquiry continued and important religious and secular treatises were written. The main sects had already developed their own doctrinal and liturgical traditions and these were pursued vigorously in their respective major centers. Masters of all the schools were mutually respected and there was significant interaction among them. Doctrinal differences did, of course, cause some conflicts, but these were never as violent as disputes occasioned by the desire for political power. The flourishing state of the arts at this time can be attributed to a high level of intellectual activity and, perhaps more importantly, to the increased patronage of the land-owning aristocracy. The additional wealth was in part used for the embellishment of monasteries and the production of a significant body of religious art and literature.

Tibetan Buddhist sects are distinguished principally by different monastic traditions and variations in doctrine and liturgy. Each of these sects was headed by a high lama and had its headquarters in one of the great monasteries, each of which was associated with a number of regional monasteries. The changing fortunes of the different monastic orders naturally affected the monasteries of the western Trans-Himalaya. Some of the old monasteries such as Alchi and Ta-pho came under Ge-lug-pa control. Politically, however, Ladakh retained its independence from Lhasa. Under the great Ladakhi king Senge Namgyal (ca. 1570–1642) Ladakh controlled territory as far as the border of Tsang in west-central Tibet. The king of Tsang was the most important power in Central Tibet until the establishment of the fifth Dalai Lama in Lhasa in 1642 (Snellgrove and Skorupski 1977: XII). The late fifteenth to the early seventeenth century was an active period of artistic production in Ladakh, Gu-ge, and Tsang, and it is interesting to compare a few examples of the art from the major monastic centers of these adjacent regions.

As I have said in Chapter I, two main artistic currents merged in Tibetan art: one came from northeast India, Nepal, and—later—China; the other, from northwest India, particularly Kashmir and Central Asia. This second current of artistic influence affected the art of the western Himalayas, the area which has been the focus of this study. I have chosen to concentrate on the early, lesser known examples of western Himalayan art that survive in India today, in the monasteries of Ladakh, Spiti, and Lahul. It is interesting to note briefly the influence of this early art on the mature art of western Tibet created during the fifteenth to seventeenth centuries, and to compare the regional styles of this later monastic art. In this study, both the art of western Tibet (Gu-ge) and the art of west central Tibet (Tsang) are represented by the well-documented paintings obtained in local monasteries by Professor Tucci (Pls. 120,121,123). As we shall see, the art from Tsang differs from the art of western Tibet in numerous ways.

The art patronized by the kings of western Tibet had distinct chronological phases. The first phase can be clearly related to the art of Kashmir (Pls. 81,89), Central Asia (Pl. 94), and Himachal Pradesh (Pl. 96) from the eighth to the eleventh centuries. This can be seen in the eleventh-century page from the *Avataṃsaka-sūtra* (Pls. 101,102) found by Tucci at T'oling monastery, and the eleventh-century sculptures of Kālacakra (Plate 99) and Uṣṇiṣāvija (Pl. 97), attributable to Spiti. By the twelfth century, a distinctive western Himalayan style can be identified in the murals in Ladakhi monasteries and in individual sculptures (Pl. 82) and paintings (Pls. 108–112). Some of the latter works had previously been attributed to Nepalese artists (Pal 1975 and 1978). However, comparison with Ladakhi murals and architectural sculpture leaves no doubt that there is a distinctive western Himalayan style (Pl.112) which, nonetheless, also shares certain artistic features with the contemporaneous art of Nepal.

Features of this western Himalayan style prevalent in the eleventh to thirteenth centuries survive in the western Himalayan art produced between the fifteenth and seventeenth centuries. Tucci has identified a "Kashmiri school" of painting which continues in West Tibet (Pl. 121) in the sixteenth century. In this later art, in both Ladakh and Gu-ge, the heads of the Buddha figures tend to be somewhat shovel-shaped (Pl. 120); they become rounder by the seventeenth century, but always remain flat. This flatness is frequently punctuated by an inverted widow's peak and gently arched brows (Pl. 121). The attendant figures have similarly shaped heads, and their long bodies with attenuated torsos twist slightly at the waist. These characteristics—the long body and ribless torso—are found in Ladakh in the eleventh and twelfth centuries and in art from Karakhoto (Pl. 108. The earliest examples of this figure style are found in the clay sculpture from Fondukistan in Afghanistan and Kucha in Central Asia (Pls. 51,52).

For the most part, the compositions in the western Tibetan style are less crowded than the paintings from the Tsang region. In the earlier phase (eleventh to thirteenth centuries) of western Himalayan art, backgrounds tend to be red, as is also the case in Nepalese painting. In Gu-ge art from the fifteenth to seventeenth centuries, the backgrounds are usually dark blue (Pl. 121). It is also interesting to note the consistent treatment of certain motifs, such as Śākyamuni's throne, in the thirteenth (Pl. 108) and sixteenth centuries (Pl. 121).

Although the doctrinal sources for the art from Gu-ge, Ladakh, and Tsang are essentially the same and the socioeconomic systems are also similar, the long political independence of the kingdoms in the western Himalayas and traditional trade connections with Kashmir and Central Asia contributed to the formation of distinctive artistic styles. These differences in composition, color, and individual motifs can be appreciated if one compares a painting in the style of Tsaparang Monastery in western Tibet (Pl. 122) with a painting from Ngor Monastery in Tsang (Pl. 125). When Tsang and Gu-ge paintings are compared, one can see that the red tones in Tsang paintings tend to be blood-red or orange-red; similar reds are also seen in Nepalese art. The figures and the floral decorations have lyrical, circular forms which also suggest Nepalese influence. Between the fourteenth and seventeenth centuries, we also notice the influence of Chinese art (Pl. 126); this can be seen, for example, in the treatment of landscape motifs and cloud forms.

From the fifteenth century on, the various influences from India, Nepal, and China were integrated into a truly Tibetan art. The differences we have been discussing between the paintings from Gu-ge, Ladakh, and Tsang help us to identify regional styles. Tucci notes that "the inspiration of various origins which had produced the Tibetan schools of painting and had given them rules and a direction, slowly led to a new style: this contains them all, though transfigured by the Tibetan people's artistic sensibility, which has now matured and become well defined" (1949:I,280).

SUMMARY

A brief analysis of the stylistic characteristics of the art of the western Trans-Himalaya allowed us to define five regional artistic schools. However, there are also significant features relating these regional schools, which allow us to distinguish seven chronological phases throughout the western Himalayas. These chronological phases are identified not only by their style but also by changes in iconographic motifs, and in patronage groups. These phases can be summarized as follows:

1. *Ca. 700-1,000 A.D.* A period of foreign influences, of cross-cultural contact and intensive cultural change; the steady cultural Tibetanization of the western Trans-Himalayan region, Kashmiri influence predominates in the arts (Pl. 89) but Chinese Central Asian influence can also be noticed (Pls. 83,88,94). Little remains from this period in India prior to the end of the tenth century, but evidence for the art is reflected in the Esoteric art of Central Asia, particularly Dunhuang (Pls. 54,58,59,61,62,63,66,67,68,69,70).

2. *Ca. 1,000 A.D.* The earliest surviving monastic foundations in the western Trans-Himalaya date from this period; e.g., Ta-pho in Spiti, Sumda in Zangskar and T'oling, and Mang-nang in Gu-ge (Pls. 85,92). The debt to artists from Kashmir and Himachal Pradesh is especially clear but influences from Central Asia can still be detected.

3. *Eleventh and twelfth centuries* The most complete monuments surviving from this period are in Ladakh, particularly in Alchi; the Sumtsek and the *'du-khang* as well as the old temple at Lama-yuru. Painting continues in the Kashmiri tradition (Pls. 101,102). In architectural decoration, cycles of divinities related to the *Yoga-tantras* predominate but a great variety of tantric divinities are represented in diverse media (Pls. 95–99). Frequently their iconography differs slightly from the textual sources that are presently known to us.

4. *Twelfth to thirteenth centuries* The Lha-khang Soma and the Lotsawa La-khang temples at Alchi provide important evidence for this artistic period in the western Trans-Himalayas. This style contains archaicizing tendencies (Pls. 58,90). Other styles derived from different sources continue to be important in western Tibetan monasteries. This is the first period from which a significant number of painted scrolls have survived in India (Pls. 108–112).

5. *Fourteenth century* A period of political-economic changes in which the expansion and consolidation of monastic institutions is a dominant factor. Earlier artistic styles continue (Pls. 86,87, and 103–107). From this period onwards a large corpus of materials is available for the study of the diverse Tibetan philosophical and contemplative traditions (Pls. 115, 100).

6. *Fifteenth and sixteenth centuries* A particularly active artistic period in the western Himalayas. By this time a truly "Tibetan" style had emerged, but regional artistic schools patronized by the great monasteries characterize the art of this period in Tsang (Pl. 125), Ladakh (Pl. 119), and Gu-ge (Pl. 122).

7. *Seventeenth and eighteenth centuries* A new style emerged, combining elements of the earlier regional styles (Smith 1970). This style (Pl. 128) characterized by a new figure style, Chinese landscape elements, and a palette including intense pinks and light greens, became associated with the Lhasa or Central Tibetan style, which remains popular in contemporary Tibetan art.

Although the formal features of the art changed over the centuries, the iconographic components remained remarkably consistent. Above all, the essential function of the art never deviated from its central purpose, to serve as an aid in the quest for enlightenment.

Notes

---

1. Rock inscriptions in the upper Indus Valley testify to the presence of Tibetan troops in Ladakh, stationed along these routes (Snellgrove and Skorupski 1980:162ff.). The personal names in these inscriptions show affinities with Tibetan names appearing in documents from Dunhuang, which date to the period of the second Tibetan occupation of the site (ca. 760–840). The cultural Tibetanization of Ladakh is usually believed to have begun in the second half of the ninth century, but the military occupation may easily have started this process at least a century earlier.
2. Evidence for Buddhist art prior to the tenth century comes mostly from rock sculpture (Figs. 4,5), which testifies to the Indian and particularly Kashmiri background of western Himalayan Buddhist art. However, several wall paintings inside monasteries as well as literary sources also suggest artistic influences from Central Asia. Tibetan literary sources have noted the presence of Khotanese artists in Tibet at different times. Tucci has suggested stylistic influences from centers as diverse as Khotan, Bäzälik, and Pendzhikent (Tucci 1973:182ff.) while Snellgrove has drawn attention to the donor figures in Alchi whose dress may reflect Central Asian influence. There was probably a period of close contacts between the western Trans-Himalaya and Central Asia when Tibet controlled much of both areas, and Central Asian influences may have reached central Tibet through Ladakh and Gu-ge. Needed are more detailed studies that would help to establish more precisely the artistic interaction between the two regions.
3. In his biography it is related that Rinchen Zangpo commissioned a life-sized bronze statue in Káshmír and transported it by cart to Go-khar in Kha-tse. He wished this to be "an exceptional memorial" to his father (Snellgrove and Skorupski 1980:92).
4. Except for rock engravings (Figs. 2,3,6,6a) and inscriptions, little is known about the Buddhist art of the more remote areas of India's inner Asian frontier, such as Baltistan. It is probable that the art reflected influences from Central Asia (Pl. 5), at least through the ninth century, although Kashmiri influence predominated. Later, until its Islamization in the fourteenth century, Baltistan was influenced by the art of Ladakh (Fig. 2).
5. A four-armed Avalokiteśvara image from Chamba, ca. eleventh century (Tucci 1973:fig. 154), preserves the metropolitan style of Kashmir as represented by the British Museum Avalokiteśvara (Pl. 31), which could have served as the model for the Chamba image. Certain modifications in the representation of the Chamba Avaloketeśvara occur in later images from the western Himalayas (Pl. 95): color of the metal, horseshoe-shaped mandorla,

additional jewelry, knotted garment on the chest, and the donor figures.

6. Tucci has frequently drawn attention to the influence of Central Asian art on the early Buddhist art of Tibet (e.g., Tucci 1973:140 ff.). However, it is usually difficult to be precise about points of contact and direct influence. "This early period of its history, when Tibet was open to all kinds of cultural influences from Central Asia, was clearly the most formative and creative of all the various periods into which, for convenience, we are dividing Tibetan history from the seventh to the twentieth century. Yet because of its distance in time and the comparative paucity of relevant documentation, it is the one of which we can write with least precision. At the same time there can be no doubt that the most extraordinary 'cultural connections' came about." (Snellgrove and Richardson 1968:110).
7. The complete transcription of Tu-pho *Avatamsakasutra* from the *'du-khang* murals is available from the Trans-Himalayan project, University of California at Los Angeles.
8. The author is presently preparing a detailed comparative analysis of the art of Ta-pho Monastery. This publication is part of the interdisciplinary Trans-Himalayan Project at the University of California at Los Angeles.
9. Unpublished M.A. thesis, University of California at Los Angeles, 1982, by Chandra Reedy, *The Function of Mudrās at rTha-pho Monastery*.

A NOTE ON ARCHAEOLOGICAL ACTIVITY IN THE WESTERN TRANS-HIMALAYA

The Archaeological Survey of India (ASI) has a long history of involvement in the exploration of the Trans-Himalayan region. It was under their auspices that Dr. A.H. Francke, a Moravian missionary, conducted the first scientific survey of the Buddhist monasteries there in 1909. Recently, the plan for the preservation of Ta-pho monastery, Spiti Valley, was implemented. This program was begun while Śri M.N. Deshpande was Director General of Archaeology and R. Sengupta Chief of the Dept. of Conservation. When the project was first surveyed the present road to Ta-pho did not exist. Even now, the isolation, altitude, scarcity of supplies, and extreme climate severely test the ingenuity of the Survey teams working there.[1] Recent developments in Ladakh have greatly facilitated travel and research there, including the activities of the ASI now under the Director Generalship of Dr. Debela Mitra. Among other projects, ASI is surveying and conserving the monastery at Alchi. The registration and preservation of monuments are also continuing under the auspices of the State Government of Kashmir and Jammu. Of course, renewed interest from scholars and tourists is inevitably accompanied by exploitation as well as exploration of these mediaeval treasures. The continuing challenge is to conserve the monuments for the future while also insuring their integrity and accessibility to visitors and residents alike. The following note indicates the nature of the conservation work now being conducted in these monasteries. Further, the structural analysis of the monuments which precedes the actual conservation work enables us to understand the original techniques of manufacture.

Note

1. I would especially like to acknowledge the ASI team working at Ta-pho in 1978 for their assistance in this study: R. Veeraraghavan, Satish Gupta, J.S. Bisht, Mohan Lal Gupta, Mela Ram Koundal.

CONSERVATION WORK AT TA-PHO MONASTERY
by R. Sengupta

Gönpas at Ta-pho

The Kinnaur and Lahul-Sipti area falls within the Alpine-Himalayan seismic belt. Therefore, occurrences of earthquakes in that area are common; between 1902 and 1975, there were twenty-two shocks of magnitude varying from 5.0 to 7.0 on the Richter Scale. To cope with the frequent seismic disturbances, local people have devised suitable methods of construction. The houses are mostly of adobe, with appropriately spaced wooden bracings. A similar concept was applied to the construction of earthen sculpture.

During the earthquake of January 19, 1975, there was much damage done to houses in the Spiti Valley. The *gön-pas* (monasteries) suffered similarly, and considerable damage occurred to the earthen sculptures of Buddhist deities and to the mural paintings within the monasteries. Most of the deities are placed on wooden brackets resting on walls giving an impression of their hovering in the sky around the central figure of the Buddha (Fig. 57).

In the *'du-khang,* damage to the idols revealed the technique of construction of the clay figures (Fig. 42; Diagram 1). In addition to the wooden armature which forms the rudimentary framework, there are horizontal and vertical bracings—their number, spacing and direction varies according to the size and posture of the figure. The standing figures rest on the ground, held in position with wooden pegs which are driven through the back of the figure into the supporting backwall. The brackets and other supports are generally covered with clay and painted to remain inconspicuous. Since the idols and paintings are all inside the gönpas they are fairly well-protected. The damage they suffered was mainly due to earthquake shocks and seepage of water from rain and snow-melt. A study of these features helps a restorer to understand the mechanism of decay and damage, and to evolve remedial measures which one hopes would offer resistance to the phenomenal earthquake shocks.

For the preservation of the objects within the *gönpas* it is most essential to make the roof and walls water–resistant. Earthquake shocks of less intensity sometimes cause cracks in the roof, especially at the junction between side-walls and terrace, if the structure is not provided with wooden planks as ties inside the mud-walls. Wooden planks were used in the original mud-walls, during construction of the *gönpas* at different levels. They are made to meet at the corners where wooden pins, nailed from the top, put them in position. These planks and the concealed vertical post, placed at intervals, make a framework and help to absorb oscillation of the structure during an earthquake. The roof is also supported by wood beams on which planks are spread to carry a thick cushion of clay.

In the course of restoration of the damaged *gönpas,* layers of alkathene sheets were spread in a layer of clay. The clay was laid on top with a slope. Care was taken to make the sheets run into the side-walls to prevent any seepage through the junction. Alkathene sheets were used because of their workability, their effectiveness as water-repellent layers, and for their ease of transport. The use of alkathene sheets in an ancient structure amounts to an introduction of a foreign element, but the "Venice Charter" permits use of foreign material as long as it does not clash with the structure in volume, shape, mass or color. In the case of the Ta-pho *gönpas* the sheets remain concealed beneath the layers of clay on the roof, invisible to visitors.

From the experience gathered at Ta-pho, and the study of local ancient constructional methods which are still practiced and followed in the restoration work, it is clear that wooden bracings used in the thickness of adobe walls help in protecting houses in an earthquake-prone area. The use of wooden bracings or tie-beams in walls has withstood the test of time in Afghanistan and Central Asia as well. A similar system of wooden braces accounts for the longevity of the clay sculptures some of which date to the early eleventh century.

While restoring the fifteenth-century Timurid mosque, Khwaja Parsa, in Balkh, Afghanistan, I observed the use of wooden logs inside the brick walls at varying levels. One can still see them in the derelict structure of the gateway to the enclosure.

Catalogue Entries

Plates: 78—127

Pl. 78
Head of a Divinity
Sandstone
Himachal Pradesh
eighth-ninth century
H. 26 cm.
Lent by Marie Hélène and Guy Weill

The round serene face is richly bedecked with a heavy jeweled crown and large circular earrings. The hair, parted in the middle, forms, tight curls along the brow, a fashion found on female figures in the temple of Avantiśvārman in Kashmir. A well-worn crescent is inscribed on the forehead. Crescents, which are worn as hair ornaments by Śiva, are also a prominent motif in Hephtalite and post-Hephtalite period crowns from Afghanistan to Kashmir. A group of Hindu sculptures of the Gupta and Śāhī period from northern India and Afghanistan have the crescent (sometimes with another form drawn within the crescent) inscribed on their foreheads. One of the most unusual of these Śāhī images is the silver rhyton (ca. 700 A.D.) with Durgā's head having a gilt crescent inscribed on her forehead (Carter 1979:315). Also the head of the Mahiṣāsuramardinī from Tepe Sardār, Ghaznī has a tiny crescent hung from a chain which lies on her forehead. The style of our stone head may be compared to that of an image of the goddess seated on a lion in the Himachal State Musejm, Simla, which is believed to come from one of the Hindu temples at Masrur. Our piece may be somewhat later, however, and may have come from one of several largely unstudied stone temples in Himachal Pradesh (Ohri 1973:116–141).

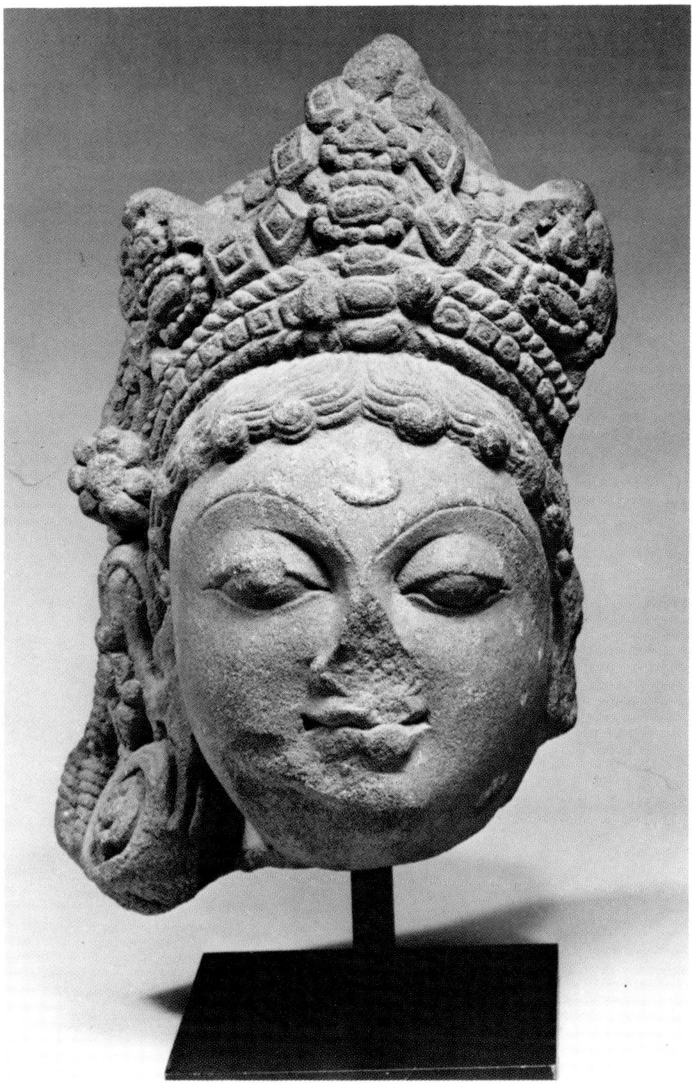

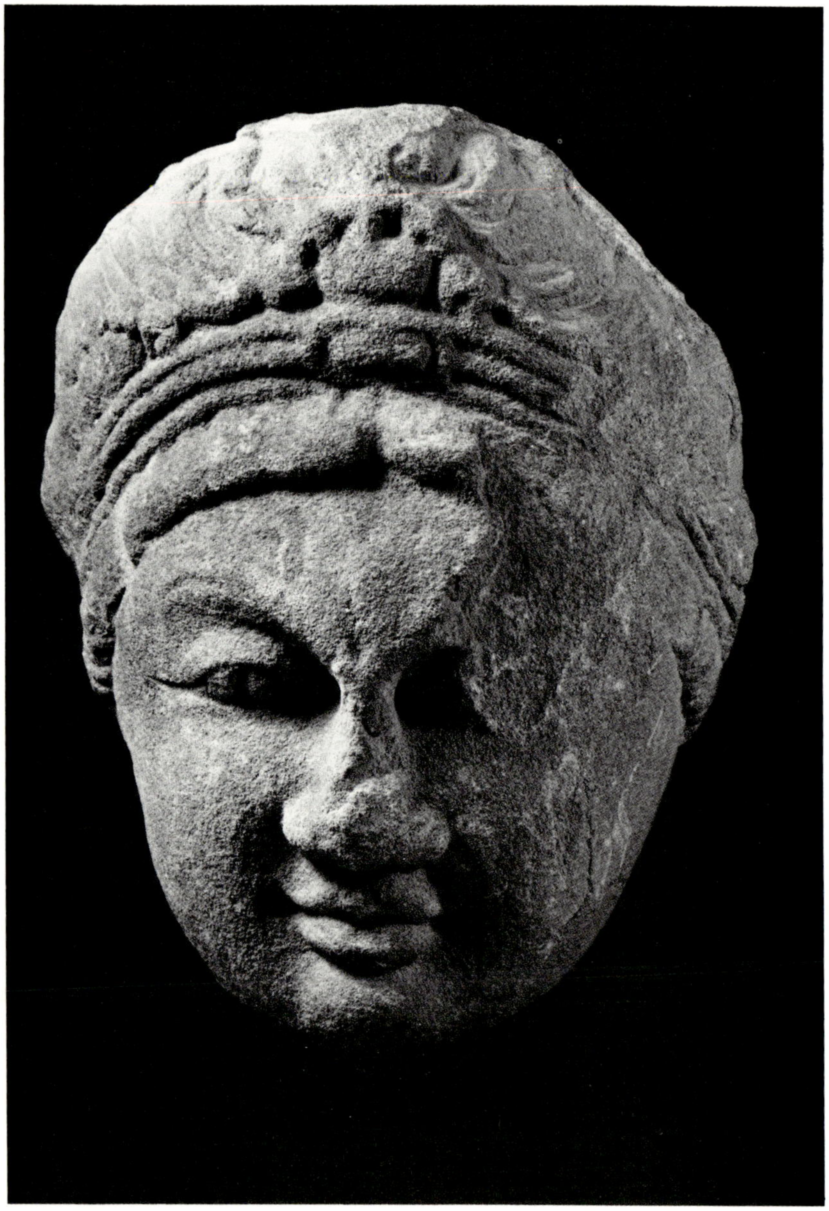

Pl. 79
Head of a God
Sandstone
Himachal Pradesh/Masrur, Kangra
Eighth century H. 30 × 23 cm
Lent by Mr. and Mrs. Walter Eisenberg

This divinity's round face with gently curving upturned mouth and eyes, and wide, flat nose is quite comparable to a sculpture of Śiva (his central face) in the Himachal State Museum, Simla (Ohri 1975:183). This stone sculpture came from one of the nine rock-cut Hindu temples of Masrur (Kangra district) which have been dated to about the eighth century (*Archaeological Survey of India* 1912–1913,1915–1916). The sculptures which continue the late-Gupta style of northern India also have a strong affinity to Kashmiri sculpture of the Kārākota period. An analysis of the late Gupta architectural sculpture of Himachal Pradesh helps us to understand the relationship between eighth-century Kashmiri art and Gupta art of northern India.

Pl. 80
Chörten
Brass
West Tibet
Thirteenth century
H. 34.3 cm. *Chörten* base 16.8 cm diameter.
Spire base 8.9 cm diameter
The Newark Museum. (81.23)

This small reliquary *stūpa* from Tibet provides a considerable amount of historical information thanks to the meticulous "archaeological" recording and scientific analysis of the *stūpa* and its contents by Dr. Hatt, its previous owner. If such analysis (Hatt 1980) were carried out on other art objects, art historians could develop a corpus of "benchmark" pieces which would make possible the establishment of a relative chronology for Himalayan art. Radio-carbon testing of the barley grains contained inside the *stūpa* gave a reading of A.D. 1230 (±65 years) (Hatt 1980:176). A thirteenth century date has also been confirmed by an analysis of the two drawings (Figs. 58 and 59) retrieved from the *stūpa*. A comparison of Figs. 40 and 40a with Pl. 109 is particularly interesting. In addition to the similar style of the three figures, the helmet-like crowns (Hatt 1980:204–205) also resemble one another, and may be considered a later variant of the helmet-crown in the Dunhuang painting (Pl. 68). Through examination and metallurgical analysis, the fabrication, construction, assembly and alloy were determined. (Hatt 1980:211–219). It would seem that the *stūpa* was made "of fairly pure copper, possibly with some iron content, which was alloyed with zinc by the calamine process" (p. 214). This information can be integrated with the results obtained from other analysis on Indo-Tibetan bronzes (von Schroeder 1981, Werner 1970; 1972) so that eventually the history of Indo-Tibetan metallurgy and the production of so-called Indo-Tibetan "bronze" sculptures can be understood.

Previously published: (Hatt 1980).

Metal content: Copper 70–75%; Tin 0.1%; Zinc 20.2–25.3%; Iron 1.2–1.3%.

Pl. 81
Seated Buddha
Bronze
Western Himalayas
Tenth-eleventh century
H. 20.6 × 16.9 cm × 10.5 cm
Navin Kumar, Inc.

The Buddha figure sits in the meditative posture, his right hand in the earth-touching *mudrā*. This elegant image is a study in fine detail and smoothly flowing lines. The folds are depicted as incised lines; strips of inlaid copper accent the edge of the robe, mouth and fingernails. This piece is clearly influenced by northeast Indian art of the ninth and tenth centuries. (e.g., Snellgrove 1978:fig. 213).

(See Color Plate 81)

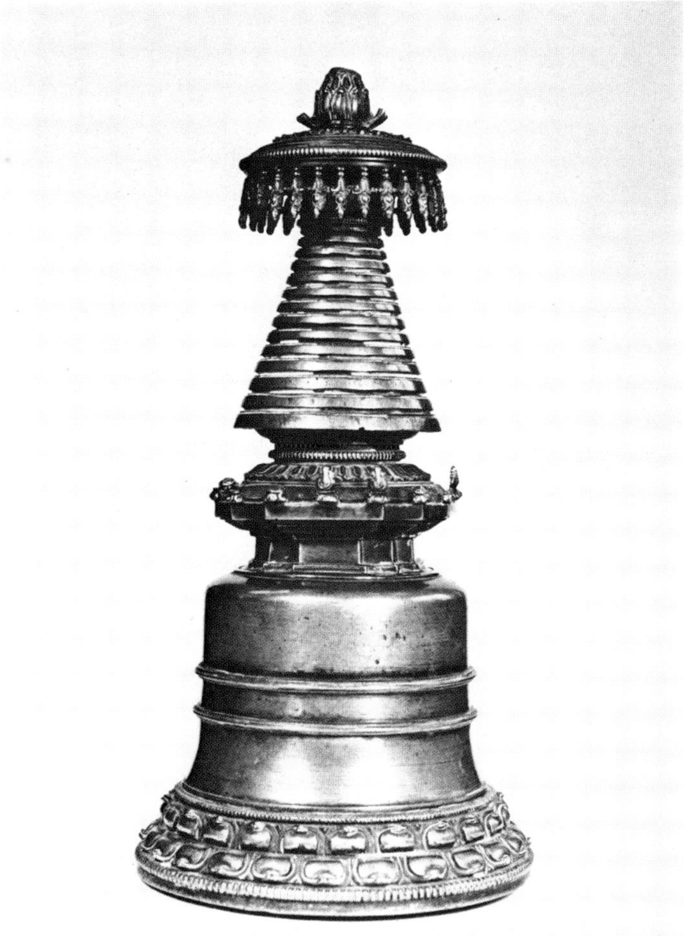

Pl. 82
Buddha
Bronze
Western Himalayas, perhaps Ladakh
Twelfth-thirteenth century
H. 28.1 cm
Kreitman Gallery

Both the style of the Buddha figure and the lotus throne permit attribution of this image to the western Himalayas in the twelfth through thirteenth centuries. Comparison to murals in the Lhakhang Soma (New Temple) in Alchi Ladakh (Snellgrove and Skorupski 1977:64–76) and (Figs. 14, 17, 26) suggest that Ladakh is the region of manufacture. The broad, shovel-shaped head, the tight snail-shaped curls and the extra knob atop the *uṣṇīṣa* appear in these murals as well as in the portable scroll painting (Pl. 108) from the western Himalayas. This style can be traced westward to Baltistan, where it is found in a rock engraving of a standing Buddha.

Metal Content:

Buddha Figure: Copper 86.148; Zinc 13.290; Iron 0.304; Lead 0.196; Tin 0.060; Antimony 0.004; Silver 0.003; Arsenic 0.001; Bismuth 0.0003; Barium 0.0003; Manganese 0.0003; Gold 0.000009.

Base: Copper 59.384; Zinc 30.240; Lead 5.933; Iron 2.758; Tin 1.633; Silver 0.031; Manganese 0.008; Antimony 0.003; Barium 0.003; Arsenic 0.003; Gold 0.00008.

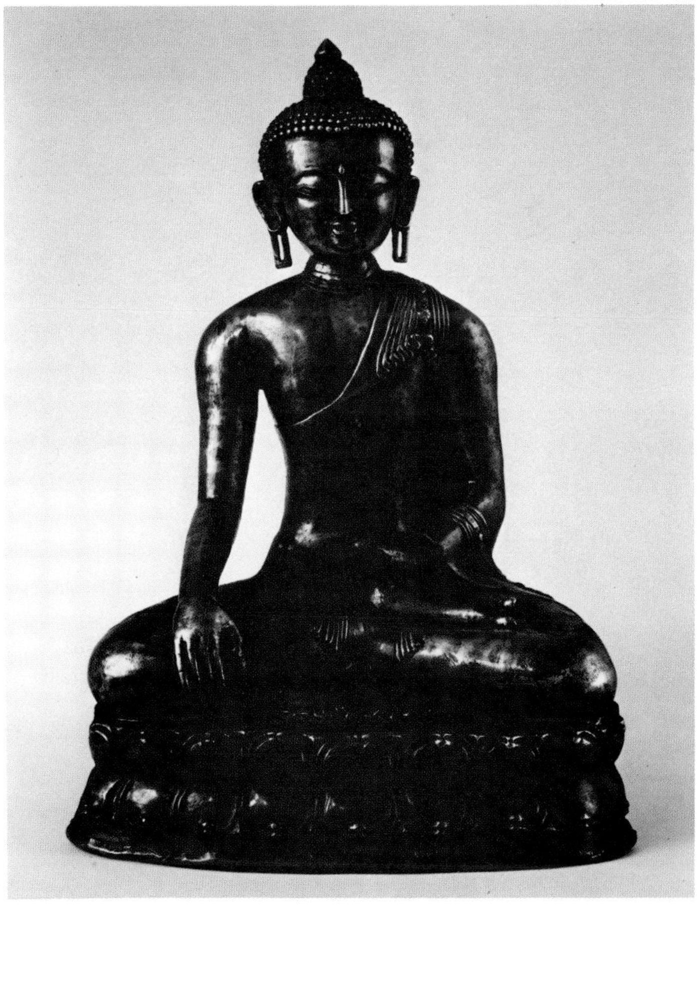

Pl. 83
Amoghasiddhi
Brass
Ladakh or northern Pakistan
Ca. tenth century
H. 34.3 cm
Pacific Asia Museum, Pasadena
Promised gift of Mr. and Mrs. Robert King

This Buddha wears a crown, with monastic gown, necklace, earrings, bracelets and armbands. The addition of royal finery to the monastic dress suggests that this image represents one of the Five Buddhas (or Five Jinas or Tathāgata). An exact identification is difficult since the "gesture of charity" exhibited by this figure is usually associated with Ratnasaṃbhava, whose vehicle is a horse (Pl. 109). Here five birds, holding garlands or a snake in their beaks, are found in the throne. The mythical bird, Garuḍa, is associated with Amonghasiddhi, but he usually presents the "do not fear" gesture (*abhaya-mudrā*). However, an image of Amoghasiddhi with his left hand in the charity *mudrā* is known in Central Asia (Gansu) (Getty 1974:42). The place of manufacture of this image is also problematic. Although the motif of several animals supporting a compound throne is found in northern Pakistan circa ninth century (Pl. 11), the height of the throne, the long, flat, slender figure and the stylized shape of the crown-ties seen here rather suggest the western Trans-Himalayas.

Metal content: Copper 65.668%; Tin 28.373%; Lead .01%; Zinc .35%; Bismuth .0005%; Gold .00005%; Antimony .017%; Silver .016%; Indium .314%; Selenium .0004%; Arsenic .059%; Nickel .256%; Iron 4.792%; Manganese .0001%; Chromium .0004%; Calcium .108%; Potassium .032%.

Pl. 84
Ratnasaṃbhava
Bronze
West Tibet
Thirteenth-fourteenth century
H. 39 cm
Navin Kumar Gallery

The crowned figure wearing Bodhisattva garments can be identified as Ratnasaṃbhava by the "gesture of charity," as well as by the mode of representation. As with all meditating Buddhas, the image is frontal, symmetrical and immobile; the eyes half-closed in meditation, a serene expression on its face. The elaborate crown, the scarf which forms a stiff arch around the shoulders, the triangular-shaped jewelry, and particularly the elongated torso with the rather long, slender stomach flowing into the waist and upper torso in an hourglass shape, are all features shared by other Buddhas attributed to fourteenth century western Tibet (von Schroeder 1981:pls. 35D and 35G).

(See Color Plate Frontispiece)

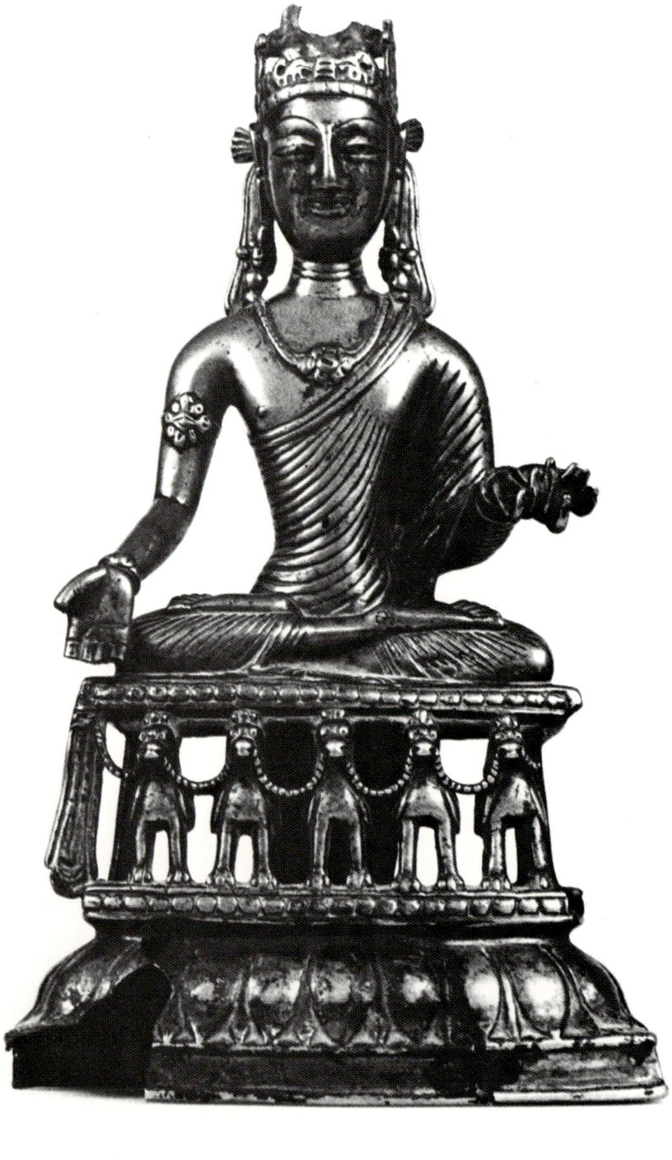

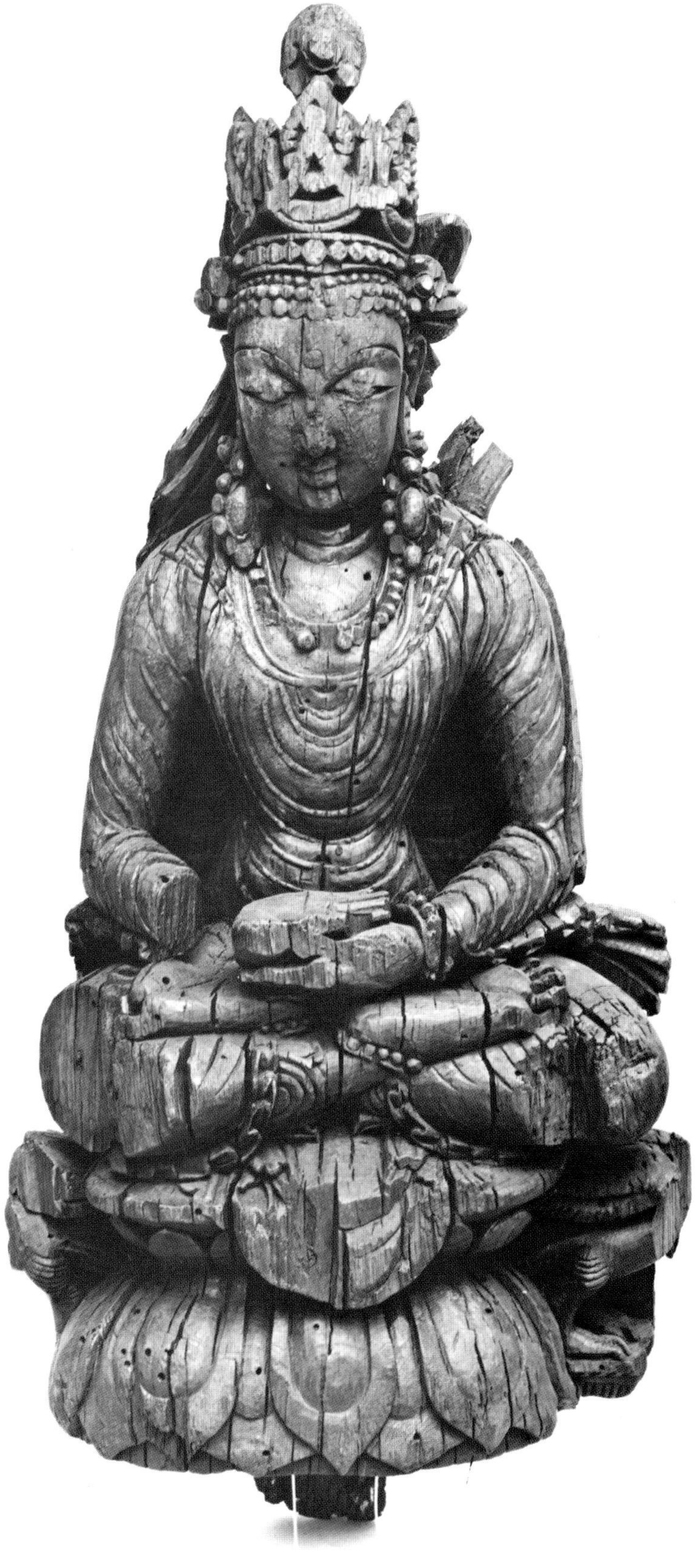

Pl. 85
Amitābha
Wood
Lahul, Kyelong Monastery
Ca. tenth century
H. 60 × W. 29 × D. 13 cm with dowel
Trustees of the British Museum, London. Given by Mrs. H. G. Beasley. (1954.2.22.1.)

This extremely important sculpture is reported to have come from the Kyelong Monastery in Lahul. Since this piece must have originally been part of the architectural decoration of a monastery, it provides important evidence for both Kashmiri and Central Asian artistic influence in the western Himalayas. Comparison of the figure style and drapery, particularly with Kashmiri ivories, suggests a date in the tenth century. The Buddha's crown and jewels, combined with monastic dress, the meditation *mudrā*, and what appear to be the vestiges of peacocks on either side of the lotus base suggest an identification of this figure as Amitābha.

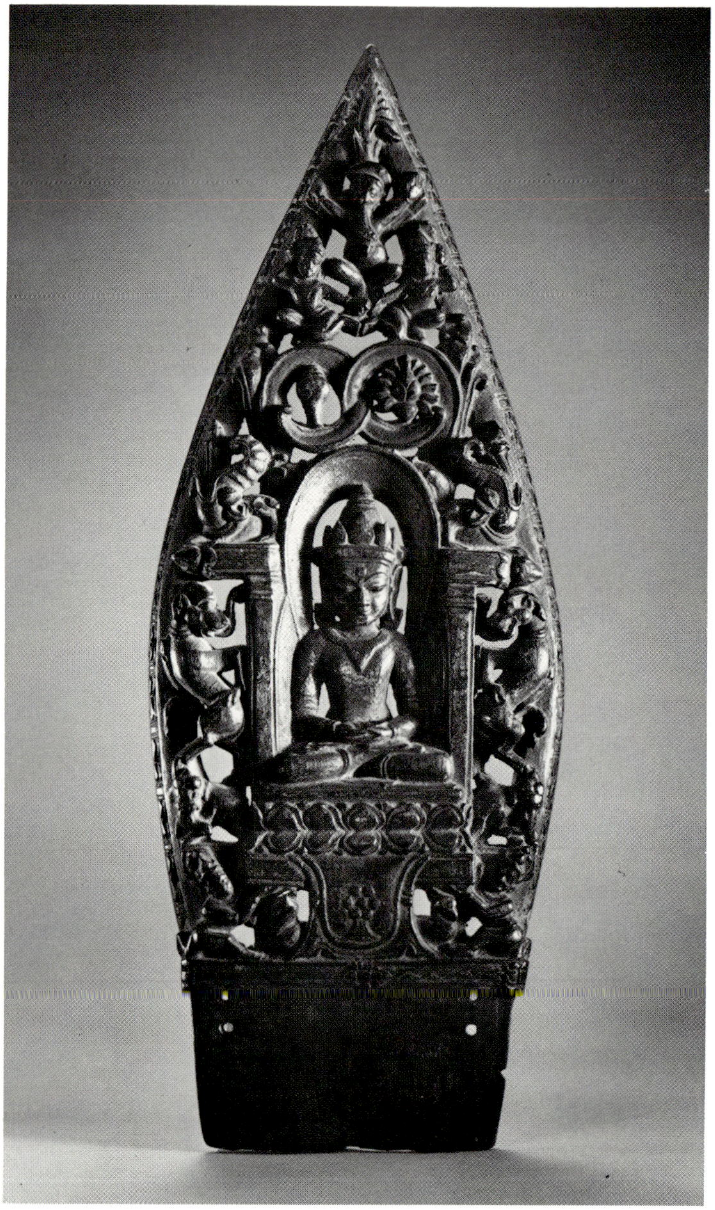

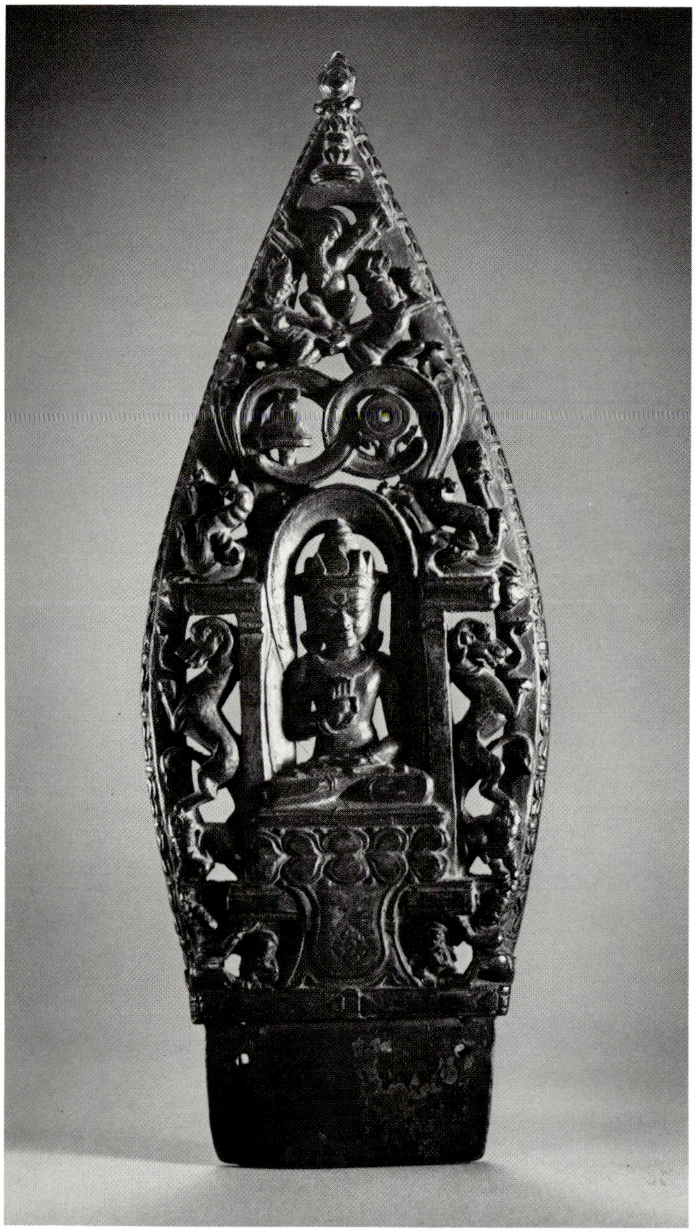

Pl. 86
Wood Crown
Wood covered with lacquer
Tibet
Thirteenth-fourteenth century
H. 31.7 × 12.7 cm
Los Angeles County Museum of Art. Gift of Dr. and Mrs. P. Pal. M.79.151.1

Pl. 87
Wood Crown
Tibet
Thirteenth-fourteenth century
H. 12.5 × 5 cm
Los Angeles County Museum of Art.
M.79.151.2.

These two pieces originally must have been part of a set of five, composing a crown. Such crowns, painted and gilded, may adorn large-sized Buddha sculptures in Himalayan monasteries. The Buddha in Pl. 86 holds his right hand in the "do not fear" gesture and hence may be identified as Amoghasiddhi; the Buddha Amitābha in Pl. 87 sits in meditation with his hands in his lap. The shape of the lotus throne and textile overhang, as well as the lion and *makara* supports, are found also in the painting in Pl. 108, and may ultimately derive from northeast Indian art. Early examples of these forms also appear in Vairocana's throne in the tenth-century painting from Dunhuang (Pl. 68). The style of these carved wooden pieces suggests a slightly earlier date than that given for the western Tibetan wood sculpture in the Victoria and Albert Museum, which is attributed to the fourteenth century (Lowry 1973:43).

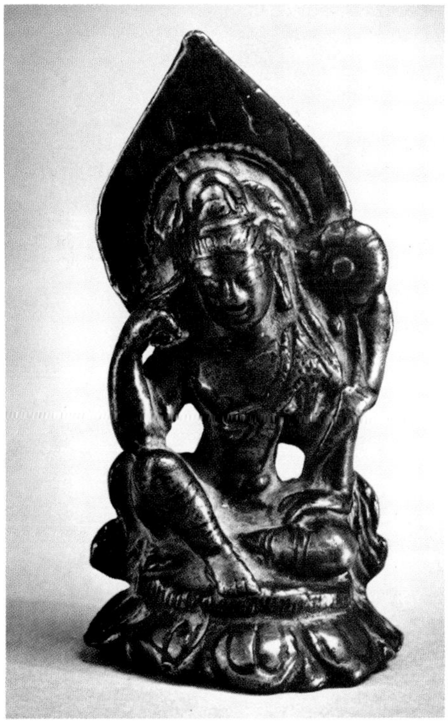

Pl. 88
Avalokiteśvara
Copper with traces of gilt
Western Himalayas or Kashmir
Eighth century
H. 8.2 × W. 4.5 × D. 2.8 cm
Los Angeles County Musum of Art. Nasli and Alice Heeramaneck Collection, Museum Associates Purchase. M.72.53.5.

Although previously attributed to Kashmir (Pal 1975:236, and Pal 1967–68), the shallow single lotus base with incised petals suggests the western Himalayas as a possible place of manufacture. (See von Schroeder 1981:27). Although this piece is conceptually close to the Rockefeller Avalokiteśvara (Pl. 28) attributed to Kashmir, eighth century, the style of the latter is quite different. The right elbow resting on the raised right knee and the pensive leaning against raised fingers is a gesture found infrequently in the Himalayas and historical northwest India. The aureola, tied scarf, and facial features can all be related to Chinese Central Asian art of ca. sixth century (Pal 1975b:236).

Previously published: (Pal 1967:45, pl. XIII.9; Pal 1975b:no.94).

Pl. 89
Avalokiteśvara
Bronze
West Tibet (Kashmir style) or Western Himalayas
Tenth-eleventh century
H. 19.05 × W. 8.25 × D. 7.62 cm
Navin Kumar Gallery

The style of this standing Bodhisattva holding an exceptionally large lotus contains elements which relate this image both to Kashmir and the western Himalayas. So few bronzes from this region and period can be firmly attributed that it is often difficult to delimit specific iconographic or stylistic characteristics. Various motifs, such as the single lotus base, fleshy face and nipples surrounded by a circle of dots, are more frequently found in the western Himalayas (Fig. 39 Ta-pho). The exaggerated delineation of the upper torso and the large side rosettes of the crown are found in images from both regions during the eleventh–twelfth centuries. (See for example, a Padmapāṇi in the Brooklyn Museum 78.256.4 anonymous gift attributed to Kashmir, von Schroeder 1981:126).

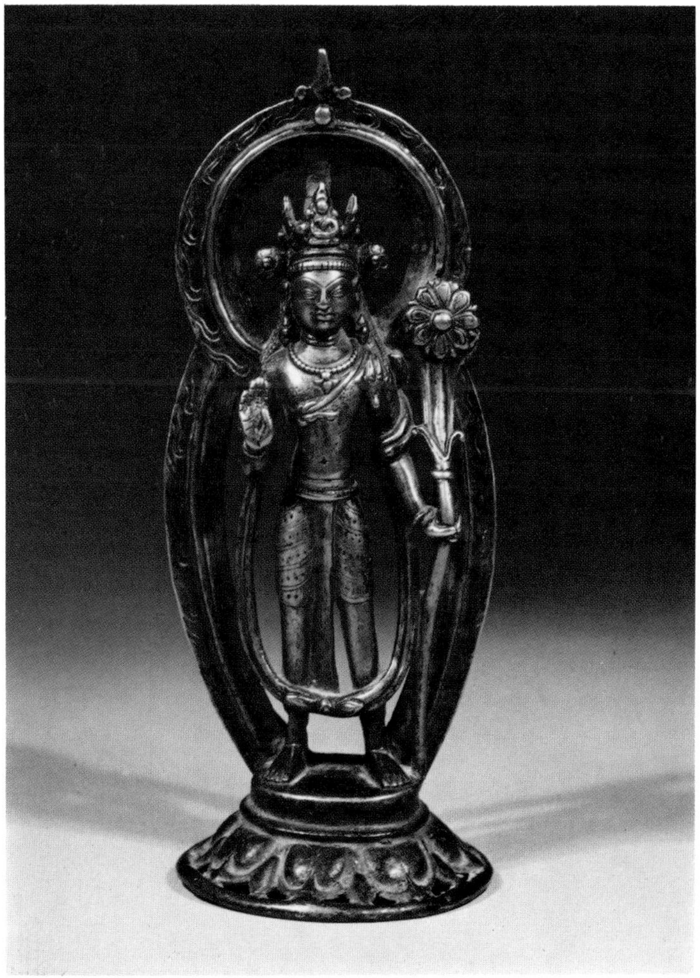

Pl. 90
Standing Mañjuśrī on Lion Throne
Brass
Western Himalayas
Eleventh-twelfth century
H. 12.4 × W. 6 × D. 6 cm
The Trustees of the British Museum, London. (1905.5.19.15.)

This small Mañjuśrī standing on a lion base was found inside a bronze sculpture of a lama when it was acquired in 1905 by the British Museum. The sculpture, said to have been purchased at the Tsechen Monastery in Tibet, belongs to a group of small figures: most depict Mañjuśrī and have bases cast separately of a different and darker alloy than the sculpture itself. These pieces have a somewhat awkward style such as straight legs, large head, sketchy irregular facial features. These same characteristics are found in eighth century Khotanese painting. They also show a rather summary treatment of the surface details. Similar stylistic features can be seen in a group of paintings considered in the "Tibetan-style" (Pl. 58). (See the examples pictured in von Schroeder 1981:176–177.)

Previously published: (von Schroeder 1981:176–177, fig.32F).

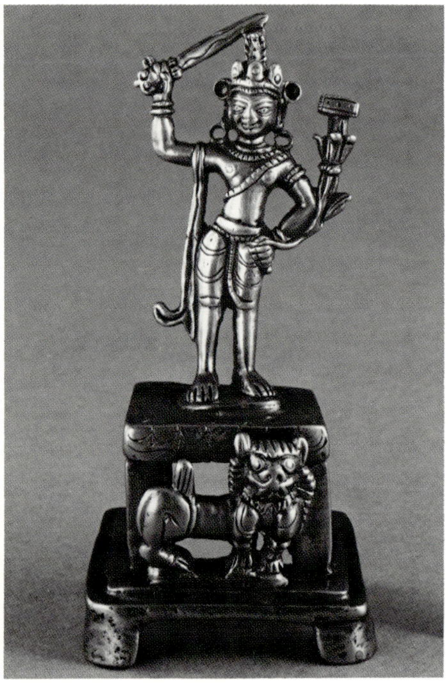

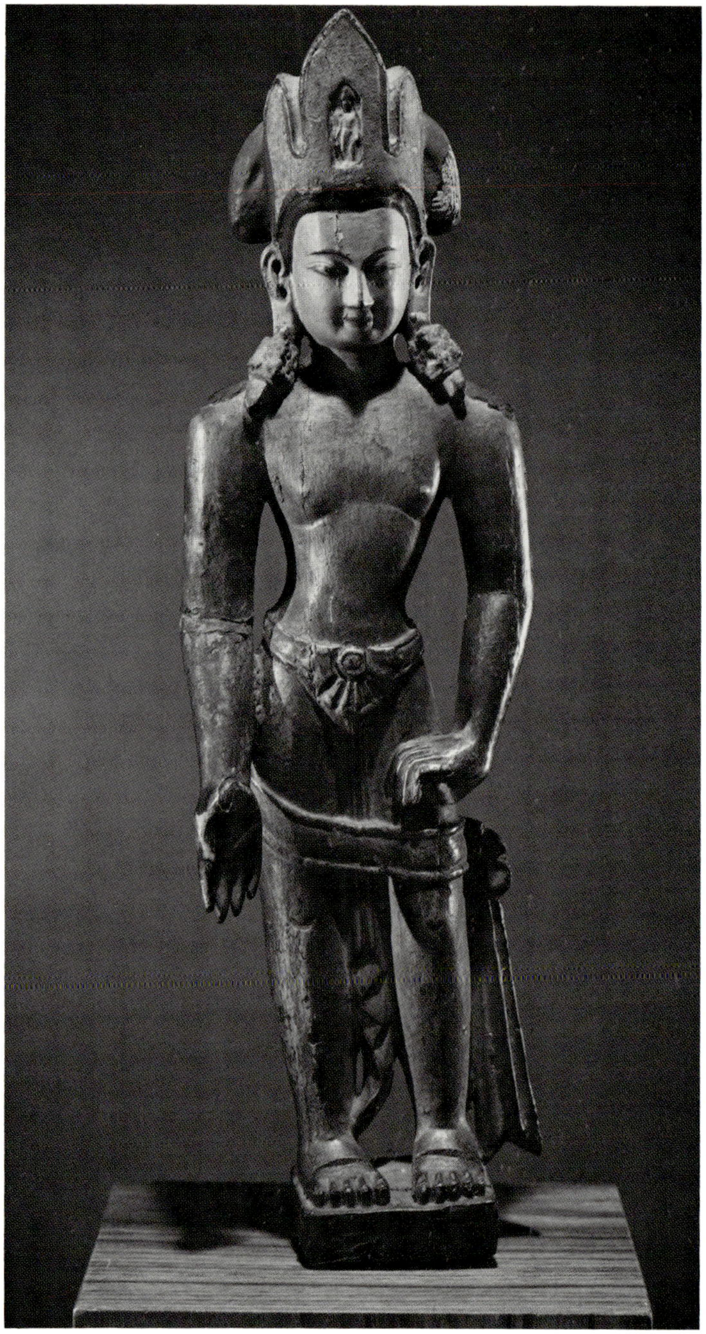

Pl. 91
Bodhisattva
Painted and gilded wood
West Tibet
Ca. thirteenth century
H. 33 cm
Los Angeles County Museum of Art, Museum Purchase, Unrestricted Acquisitions Fund. M.75.67.

This Bodhisattva, standing with his right hand in *abhaya-mudrā*, has wide shoulders, heavy crown and short, thick legs which give the figure a very solid appearance. A quite similar figure is placed in the crown. A wooden painted and gilded Bodhisattva related to this example has also been attributed to Nepal (Kramrisch 1964:73). Figures with short legs and heavy proportions similar to those of this image are found in the twelfth and thirteenth century wall paintings of the Lhakhang Soma (New Chapel) at Alchi monastery in Ladakh. However, the styles of dress, jewelry and crowns of the figures in the Lhakang Soma murals are quite different from that of our figure.

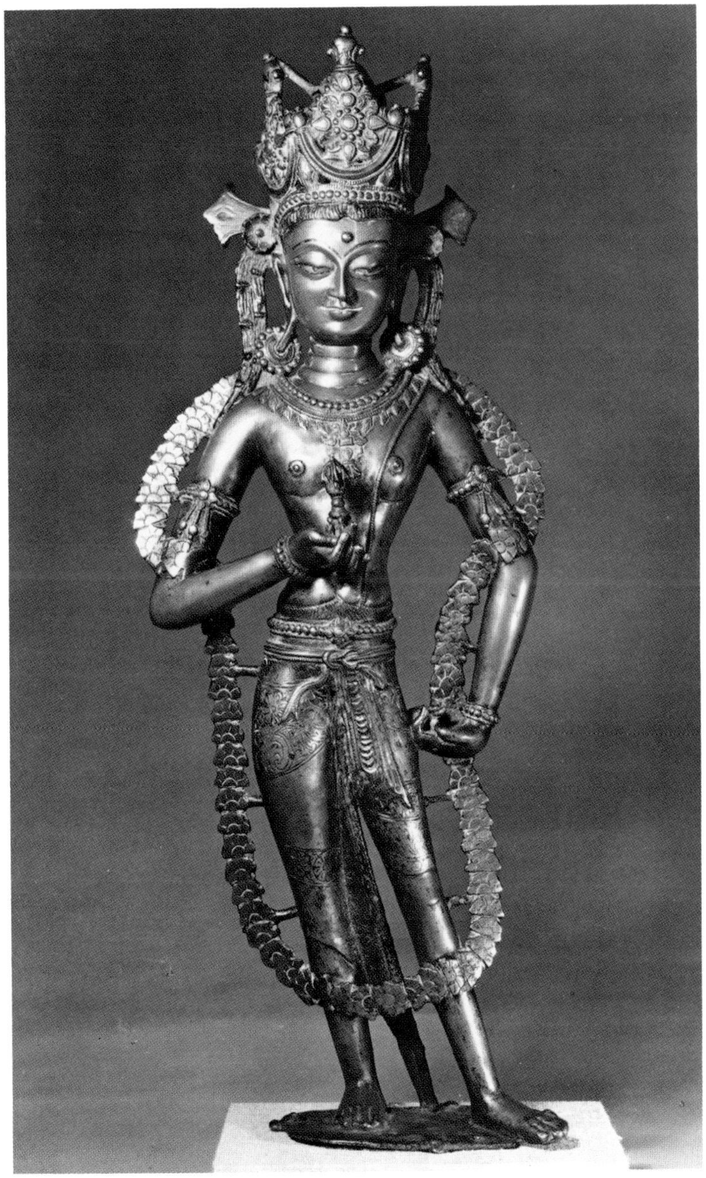

Pl. 92
Bodhisattva Vajrapāṇi
Brass
Western Trans-Himalayas
Eleventh-twelfth century
H. 69.3 cm
Musée Guimet, Paris. (MA 3546.)

The style of this large standing image suggests that it was made in the western Himalayas between the eleventh and twelfth centuries, when the influence of Kashmiri art and artists was widespread. A comparison with the Rockefeller Bodhisattva (Pl. 30) demonstrates the transformation of Kashmiri elements in western Himalayan art. The sensuously modeled body of the Kashmiri image is replaced by a long and exceedingly slender figure. The over-large head and crown may have been an attempt to adjust the proportions of the image after it was placed on a high monastic altar. The elaborate crown with side rosettes and the richly patterned *dhotī* which leaves one knee exposed are also found in the clay sculptures from Ta-pho (Fig.42), and in a large bronze sculpture photographed by Tucci in T'oling monastery, West Tibet. (Tucci 1973:Fig 27). The madra is characteristic of Western Trans-Himalayan art.

Previously published: (Pal 1969:no.6; Béguin 1974:333–334, fig.1–3; Pal 1975b:no.98; Musée Guimet 1977:no.40; Musée Guimet 1979:12, fig.8; von Schroeder 1981:131, fig.22E).

Pl. 93
Mañjuśrī with Inscription
Bronze
Central or Southwest Tibet
Thirteenth century
H. 45.72 × 25.40 cm
Navin Kumar Gallery

Tibetan Inscription on both legs of image. Translation: Hey, through the support of the gentlemen, Mr. Tibuthrikyab, who has great faith in Buddhism and the learned lady, Mrs. Nyang-mo Sher-cam, this statue of Mañjuśrī was molded by the great artist Zhalbo-Lhaso and offered to the Guru Tampa-can who is identical to Buddha. By this merit, may we reach Enlightenment. Namo Mañjuśrī.

This lovely image of Mañjuśrī, inlaid with turquoise stone, wears an elaborate five-part crown composed of large rosettes and streamers which curl upward from flowers at the side of the crown. He holds a flower in his left hand together with a book, and thus can be identified as Mañjuśrī. The jeweled belt and simple beaded necklaces are frequently found in seated images of this period from western Tibet (von Schroeder 1981: pls. 35C to 35G). The red and blue paint is a later addition. There is a Tibetan inscription written on the thighs of the statue. Since inscriptions usually appear on the base of the statue, this would appear to be a later addition. The inscription has been translated by the Venerable Thartse Khenpo, Rinpoche (New York, 1981). The lady's name may indicate that she lived in the small Tibetan principality of Nyang in the thirteenth century and/or fourteenth century.

(See Color Plate 93)

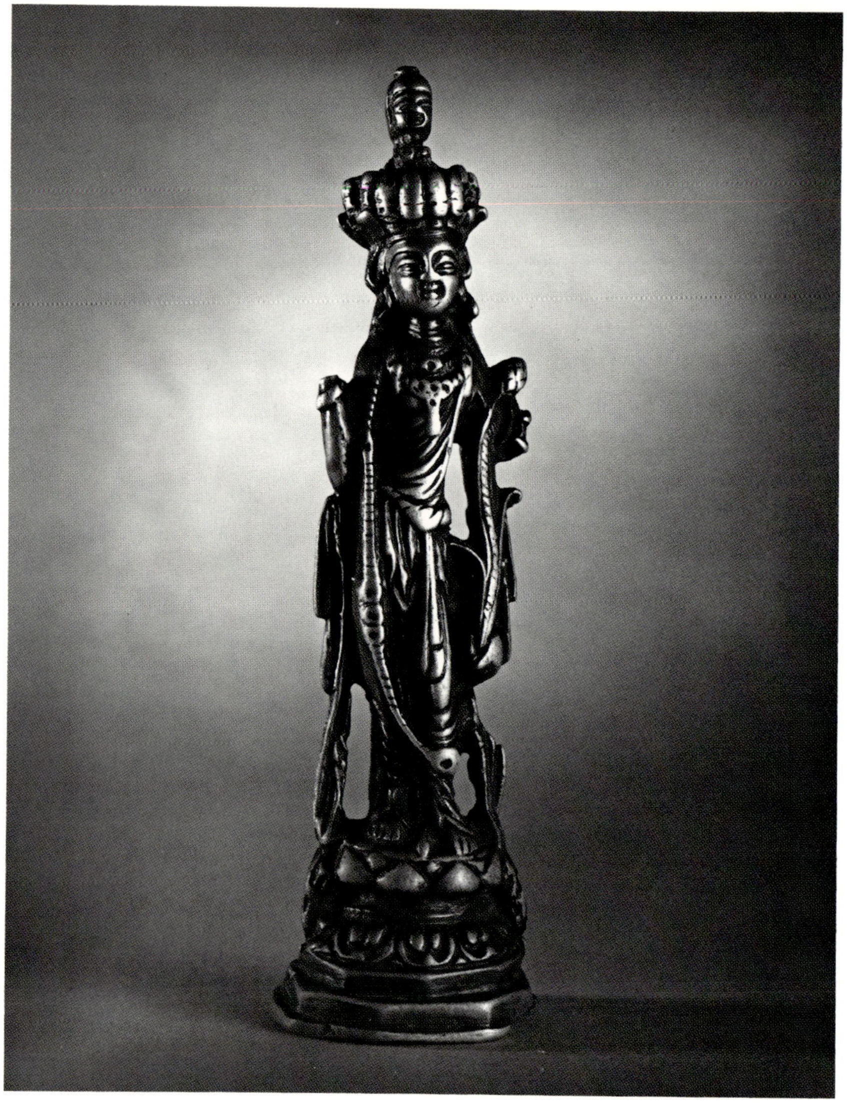

Pl. 94
Eleven-headed Avalokiteśvara
Brass
Tibet
Ca. eighth century
H. 15.24 cm
Neil Kreitman

Made wretched by the sunken state of humanity, the Bodhisattva Avalokiteśvara momentarily gave way to his grief; whereupon, his head burst and splintered into fragments. These were restored by Amitābha to permit the Compassionate One to watch in all directions. Thus does legend explain this specialized form of Avalokiteśvara.

Perhaps the earliest known reference to this form of the Bodhisattva occurs in a Sanskrit work entitled *Avalokiteśvara-Ekādaśamukha-nāma-dhāranī,* found in Gilgit and datable to about the sixth century (Dutt 1939:I, 42). Prior to this twentieth-century discovery, *sūtras* referring to the Eleven-Faced Avalokiteśvara were known only from Chinese and Tibetan texts. Four Chinese translations dating from the mid-sixth to late-eighth centuries are known, and fragments of those by Yaśogupta (651–677 A.D. Taishō 1070) and Xuanzang (655 A.D. Taishō 1071) have been found at Dunhuang.

The earliest example of the Eleven-faced Avalokiteśvara is in a rock-cut *vihāra* at Kanheri, *ca.* sixth century (Satō Ryūken 1960:43). Elsewhere, images of this form with eleven heads and two or four arms are found in China; in the Turfan region of Central Asia; at Dunhuang; and in Japan, and date from the seventh to tenth centuries. The Kashmiri image (Pl. 32) of circa tenth century belongs with the latest images of this group.

The provenance of this unusual bronze is unknown. The Eleven-faced, Two-armed Avalokiteśvara stands on a multi-level pedestal with octagonal base and two tiers of lotus leaves. The right lower arm and hand are missing. The torso, draperies, and pedestal appear to be almost a direct copy of a small (14-1/4 cm. high) Chinese bronze Bodhisattva datable to the Sui Dynasty (581–618 A.D. Matsubara Saburō 1966:I, pl. 223). Unlike the Chinese image, however, this Bodhisattva holds a lotus stalk and pod in its left hand, while its head carries eight small, badly worn faces in a semicircle. This wreath of faces is crowned by one larger head, presumably Amitābha. Only one other Chinese image with a similar semicircular arrangement of heads is known: a Tang Dynasty stone sculpture from Sichuan (Ōmura

1915–1930:II, pl. 764). Such an arrangement, however, is frequently found in Japan, where images of the Eleven-faced Avalokiteśvara enjoyed considerable popularity from the eighth century on. The figure is completely unfinished on the back, save for the presence of a lug at shoulder level (designed to hold a *mandorla*) and one additional face in the center of the main image's head.

No Chinese image of the Eleven-faced Avalokiteśvara can be dated with certainty to a period earlier than the Tang Dynasty (618–906 A.D.) (Lee and Ho 1959). Technical considerations—the absence of gilding and the unfinished back—as well as stylistic anomalies, strongly suggest that the image is not of Chinese manufacture. However, the fact that it is copied in part from a Chinese bronze statue, and the fact that, with the exception of the sculpture in the Kanheri Caves, all known early images of the Eleven-faced Avalokiteśvara appear in China or in regions influenced by Chinese culture (e.g., Turfan, Japan), lead us to seek a provenance within the sphere of Chinese influence.

Summary treatment of the backs of bronze images is characteristic of Tibetan craftsmanship (Pal 1978:179; John Huntington, personal communication, December 1981). The Tibetan scholar Bu-ston (1290–1364) records that an image of the Eleven-faced Avalokiteśvara was first introduced to Tibet in the seventh century by King Sroṅ-btsan-sgam-po (Obermiller 1932:II, 184). John Huntington has further noted the existence of Tibetan copies (unlike this image, however, of nearly pure copper) of Chinese images that were duplicated with apparent disregard for the historical validity of the style (personal communication, Dec., 1981). It is possible that this unusual image was made in Tibet, copied in part from a small Sui Dynasty bronze, but altered to suit prevailing iconographic interests. Although based on an earlier image, the deeply incised drapery folds suggest a later date, perhaps late eighth or early ninth century, or even later.

Audrey Spiro

Metal content: Copper 43.303%; Tin .561%; Lead 6.119%; Zinc 39.983%; Bismuth .003%; Barium .0009%; Cesium .007%; Iodine .002%; Antimony .003%; Silver .001%; Indium .001%; Selenium .002%; Strontium .0005%; Rubidium .0006%; Bromine .0002%; Arsenic .039%; Nickel .037%; Cobalt .023%; Iron 9.48%; Manganese .003%; Titanium .003%; Calcium .214%; Potassium .217%.

Pl. 95
Eleven-headed Avalokiteśvara, or Unidentified Bön Deity
Bronze. Inscription on pedestal.
Western Trans-Himalaya
Eleventh-twelfth century
H. 29.2 cm
Los Angeles County Museum of Art. Gift of Mr. and Mrs. Harry Kahn. (M.78.40)

The eleven-headed deity sits on a double lotus supported by a high podium. The podium contains a dancing small figure and two rather crudely depicted lions. The large *mandorla* and halo are decorated by incised flame designs, two heavenly creatures and topped by a large *stūpa* with sun and moon symbols on top. There is an inscription in Tibetan letters which runs along the top part of the pedestal. There are several unusual features about this image which in part, demonstrate relationships to Central Asia. In Dunhuang, the six-armed seated version of Avalokiteśvara, often, as here, has one hand offering the *vitarka-mudrā* (see description of Pl. 70). Also in Dunhuang, representations of the deity hold sun and moon discs, and here they crown the *stūpa*. (Pal:1982:17–18).

The inscription, which has not yet been successfully interpreted, may contain a Tibetan reference to the Mongol Buddhist title *hutuktu*. According to this interpretation, the inscription may contain the name of a non-Tibetan donor, Hu-t'og Trir Hyag, and also a place of manufacture. Another interpretation suggests that this may, in fact, be a Bön deity whose name is included in the inscription (The Ven. Thartse Khenpo, Rinpoche, Los Angeles, 1981). Although the fact that this image has seven ferocious heads, instead of the one ferocious head usually found in Himalayan images, might support the Bön hypothesis, Pal (1982) has recently demonstrated that this feature occurs in other Buddhist bronzes as well. In fact Avalokiteśvara with seven ferocious heads is only one of several variant forms representing the eleven-headed Avalokiteśvara.

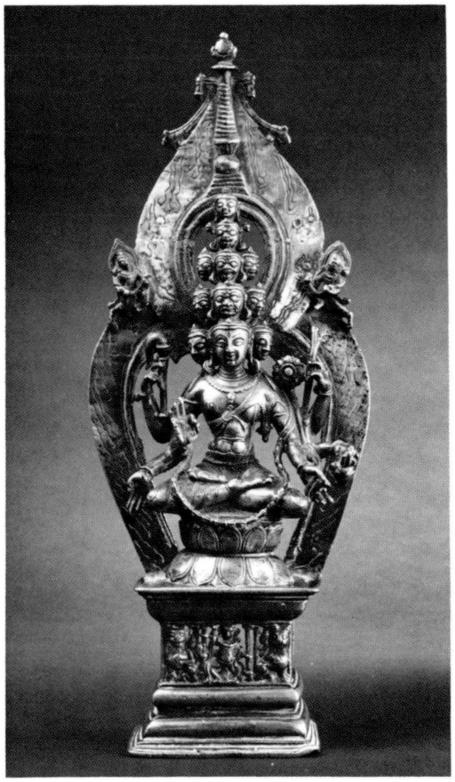

Pl. 97
Uṣṇīṣavijayā
Bronze
Spiti
Tenth-eleventh century
H. 18.4 cmPrivate collection

In Himalayan art, the goddess Uṣṇīṣavijayā is frequently depicted sitting inside a *stūpa* (Kramrisch 1964:Pls 93 and 97). This three-headed, eight-armed goddess, who is often represented in mural paintings in the western Trans-Himalaya, may also be understood as sitting within a "descent from heaven" type *stūpa* (see fig. 9). The tiered pedestal, in fact, represents the base of such *stūpas* and is found in monumental *stūpas* as well. The lotus on the pedestal may be analogous to the dome of the *stūpa* and the tiers above the goddess's halo may have held umbrellas (see Pls. 80 and 95).

The style of this image may be related to the sculptures attributable to both Kashmir and the western Himalayas of the tenth and eleventh centuries. It also has been suggested that the patron may have been one of the Śāhī rulers of northern Pakistan. (Pal 1975:186). Prior to the tenth century the *uṣniṣavijaya dhārāni* was important in China and Japan (Chou-Yi-Liang 1944:322–3).

Previously published: (Pal 1975b:no.70; von Schroeder 1981:148–149, fig.26C).

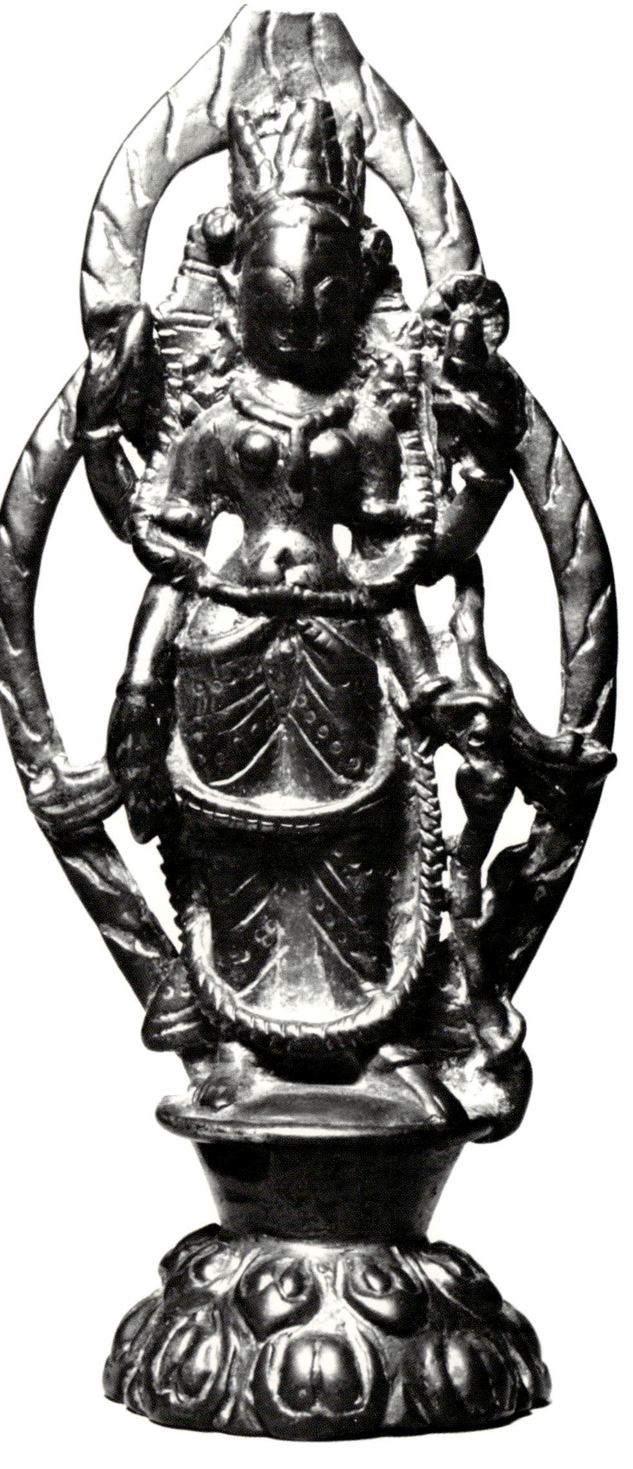

Pl. 96
Dhanadā-Tārā
Brass
Himachal Pradesh
Ninth-tenth century
H. 11.5 cm
Professor Samuel Eilenberg

This small, four-armed image of Dhanadā Tārā, although badly worn, displays the essential stylistic and iconographic features associated with Himachal Pradesh sculptures from the tenth to eleventh centuries: the painted halo, the vesica, and decorative pattern of stylized flames. The three-pointed, straight-sided crown with long side-streamers, as well as the skin-tight bodice exposing the rounded belly, are frequently found in the contemporaneous art of the region, and also in the slightly earlier art from Central Asia and Kashmir. According to the *Sādhanamālā* (Bhattacharyya 1968:231), the four-armed goddess should ride an animal, which is not the case here. This image also diverges from the text with regard to the symbols held—the lower left hand does not seem to hold a book, as is customary, although the other hands do hold the lotus, rosary, and give the charity *(varada)* mudrā as prescribed. See related sculptures now in the Robert H. Ellsworth collection (Pal 1975b:180–184).

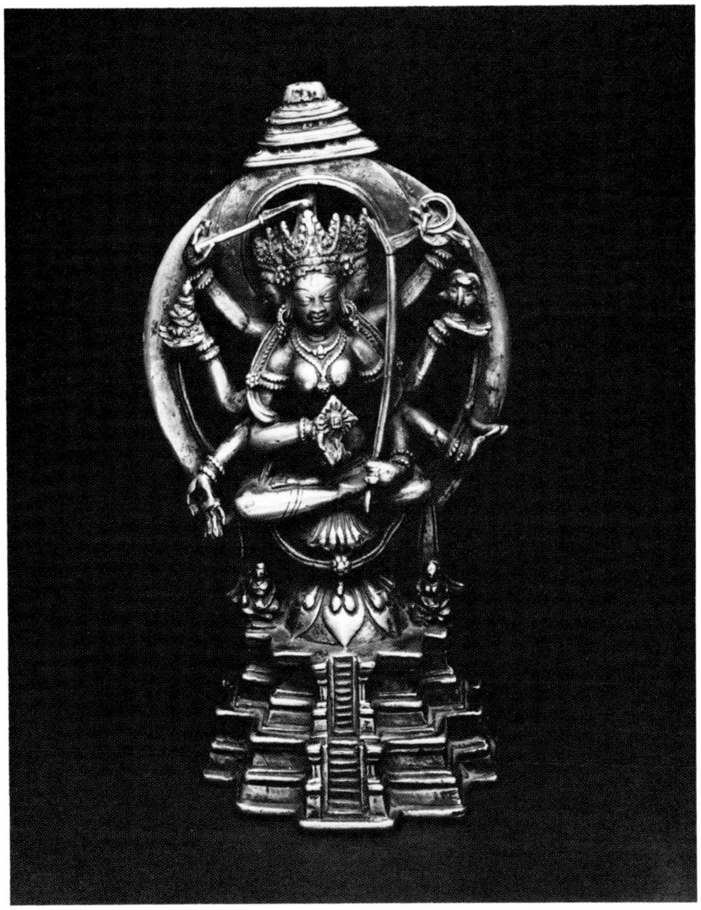

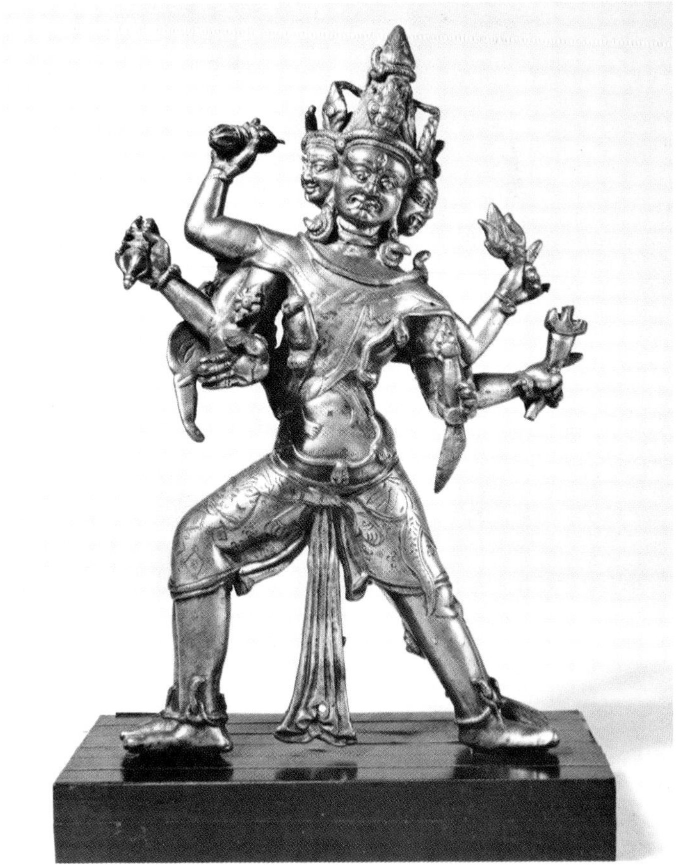

Pl. 98
Vajrakīla
Brass
Western Trans-Himalaya
Eleventh century
H. 27.4 cm
Collection The Newark Museum. Gift of Mr. and Mrs. Jack Zimmerman in honor of Eleanor Olson. (70.27.)

This iconographic form, also known as *Dorje phurba*, exemplifies the tendency in Himalayan art to deify liturgical instruments or ritual formulas. (Tucci 1949 Vol. 2 p.588). This example corresponds for the most part to textual descriptions except for the lack of a consort, a phenomenon frequently noted in the art of northwest India and the western Himalayas (tenth through twelfth centuries). This image has three heads (two fierce and one benign) and six arms which hold a nine-pronged *vajra*, a five-pronged *vajra*, a trident (broken) and a *kīla*. He wears human, tiger and elephant skins and is decorated with snakes. For a related image in the Los Angeles County Museum of Art (M.70.1.6) see Musée Guimet 1977:no.198.

Previously published: (Musée Guimet 1977:183–184, fig.199; Reynolds 1978:no.198).

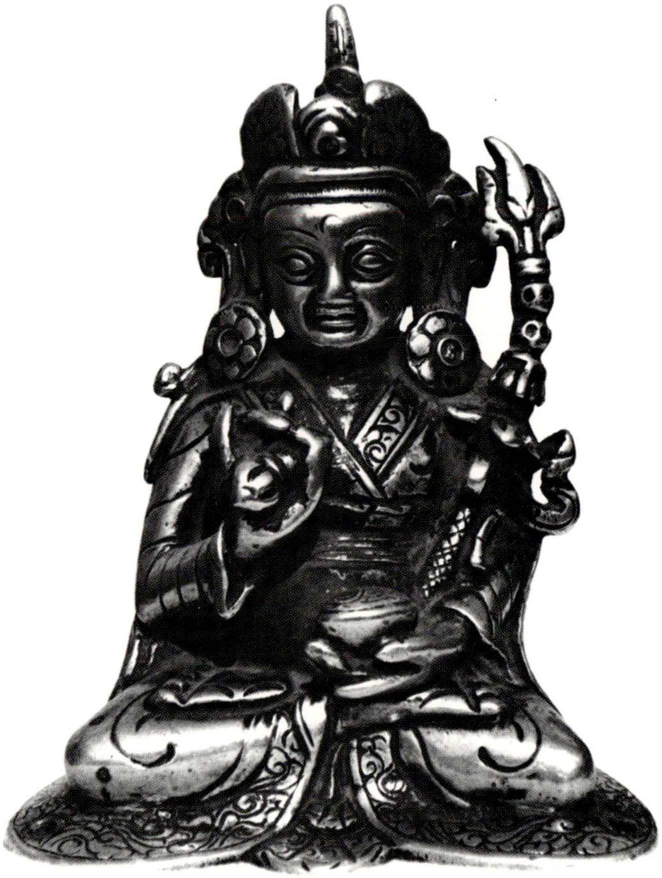

Pl. 99
Kālacakra and Consort
Brass
(Spiti/Guge?) Western Himalayas
Ca. eleventh century
H. 21.6 × 17.5 cm
Collection of The Newark Museum (76.27)

This extraordinary complex image has been tentatively identified as the earliest known representation of Kālacakra in India. As the cult is said to have developed somewhere in the western Himalayas or Central Asia in ca. the tenth century or earlier, an iconographic form of this divinity in the western Himalayas would not be surprising (Pal 1975:176). Although it is still debated when and where this cult originated we do know that the teachings were important during the "second diffusion of Buddhism." Given the early stage of the cult, it would also not be surprising that this image would differ iconographically in some respects from later representations of the deity (Pl. 126). The figure of Kālacakra has four heads, twelve arms and twenty-four hands (each arm dividing into two hands). The principal pair of hands, which embrace his consort, also holds a thunderbolt (*vajra*) and bell (*ghaṇṭā*). Most of the other hands are holding weapons. The female divinity has four heads and eight arms. Four unidentified figures, two male and two female, are being crushed under the weight of the divine couple.

Previously published: (Pal 1975b:fig.65; von Schroeder 1981:fig.27E).

Pl. 100
Padmasaṃbhava
Bronze
West Tibet
Fourteenth century
H. 13 cm
Navin Kumar Gallery

This sculpture of Padmasaṃbhava (Guru Rinpoche) depicts the great "Master" seated in the lotus or diamond seat with a *vajra* in the right hand, a *patra* in the left, and his staff (or *khaṭvāṅga*) held against his left shoulder. His cap ends in a peak or half-*vajra* and its lapels are turned up. The large earrings and cap are inlaid with turquoise. The flowing robe crosses and ties just under the left arm and has an incised floral border. Although our figure is more elegantly proportioned, its vacant gaze and broad, expressive face resembles the portrait of a lama in a private collection in Germany. (Uhlig and von Schroeder 1976:25).

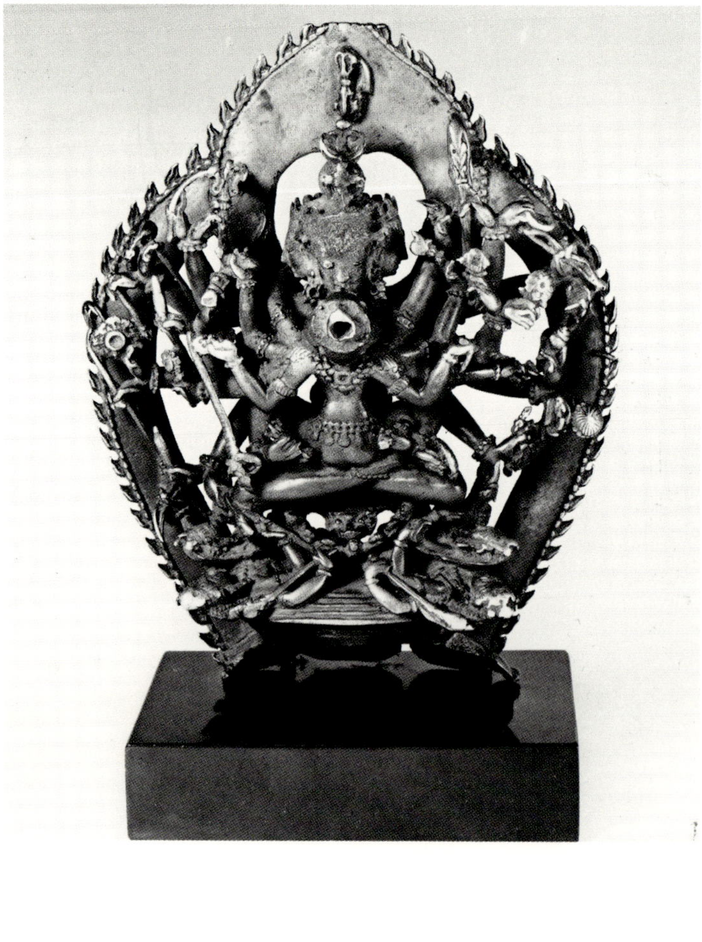

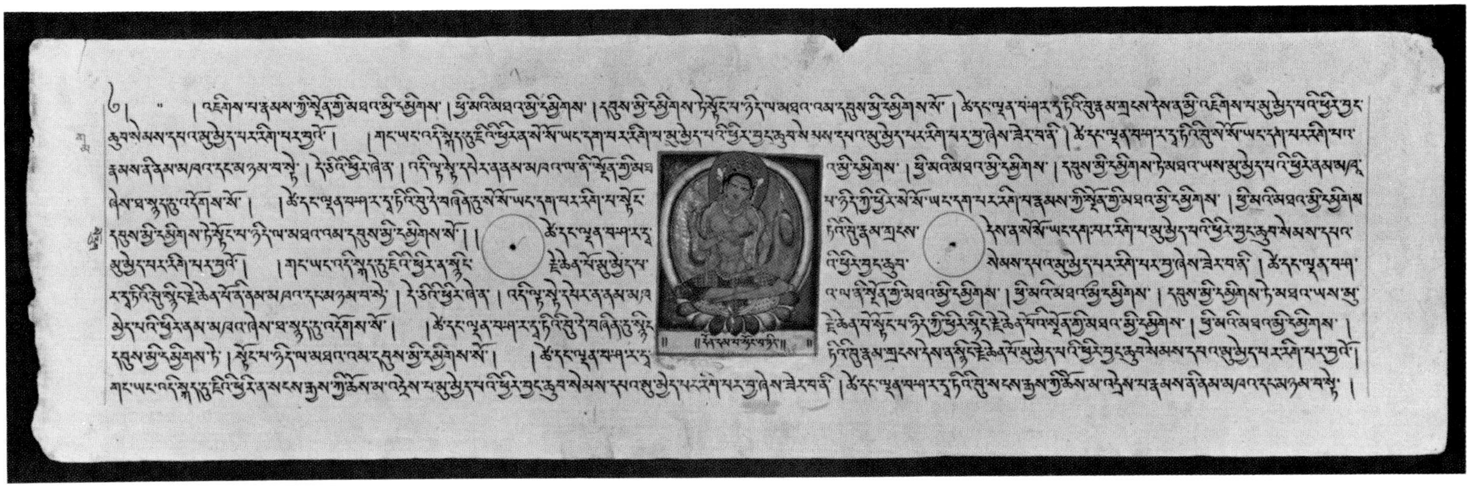

Pl. 101
Prajñāpāramitā Manuscript, p. 56
Ink, colors, gold on paper
T'oling
Eleventh century
H. 19 × 66.4 cm
Los Angeles County Museum of Art. Nasli and Alice Heeramaneck Collection; Museum Associates Purchase (M.81.90.14.)

Pl. 102
***Prajñāpāramitā* Manuscript, p. 36 of Vol. "gam"**
Ink, colors, gold on paper
T'oling
Eleventh century
H. 17.8 × 66.4 cm
Los Angeles County Museum of Art. Nasli and Alice Heeramaneck Collection; Museum Associates Purchase (M.81.90.6).

The twelve leaves in the Los Angeles County Museum of Art come from at least three, or perhaps, four different manuscripts. These manuscript pages vary slightly in size but are all written in black ink and illuminated with color and gold. Some panels are covered with a resinous varnish or lacquer.

The seated six-armed figure of Prajñāpāramitā (most examples have two or four arms) wears a crown composed of three triangular plaques, an ornament at the left side of her crown describes an arabesque shape and is silhouetted against the goddess' elaborate coiffure, heavy gold earrings, and armbands. The tight bodice accentuating the goddess' attenuated torso and narrow waist terminates in two thin triangular projections that reach toward the elaborate jeweled girdle and emphasize the navel.

These manuscript pages were purchased by Tucci in T'oling Monastery, Gu-ge (western Tibet). The style of the figure as well as the costume details may be related to eleventh-century painting from Alchi in Ladakh, Ta-pho in Spiti and sculpture from Himachal Pradesh (Pl. 96), in India. In the eleventh century, these regions were ruled by "the kings of Western Tibet." The arts of the tenth and eleventh century reflect Kashmiri cultural influence. Tucci has long maintained that the influence of northwest Indian art, particularly from Kashmir, provided one of the common threads which related the art of the western Himalaya from the eleventh to thirteenth century.

In the frieze below Prajñāpāramitā are seen two pairs of devotees at either side of an altar. Also represented are two conch shells, bowls containing water, incense and a *torma* offering (butter sculpture). At the center of the altar, a round dish, shown in aerial perspective, holds cakes of rice shaped in a *maṇḍala*.

On the left side of the frieze is a novitiate monk with shoulder-length braids who wears a short, flowing cape and upturned Tibetan black boots. Next to him is a shaven-headed monk who wears a patchwork robe and black boots. The two secular figures wear slim-fitting robes with broad triangular collar flaps. Their wide-brimmed hats seem to float behind them, which may be the artist's device to suggest recession into space. Both figures offer lotus blossoms to Prajñāpāramitā.

Of interest for the history of art is the similarity between the figures at the bottom of the page and those in the Nor-bzang narrative in the *'du-khang* at Ta-pho (Fig. 34). On this page has been written "just as Nor-bzang (Nor-bzangs) attained the highest stage (of Bodhisattvahood) may I and all beings, without exception, move in the *prajñāpāramitā* (perfection of wisdom). . . ." This page appears to be p. 56 containing a concluding prayer of the *Ārya-dhvajaketu-praṇidhāna-rāja*, which appears to have been part of a *Prajñāpāramitā* text.
Elsie Ritchie

Pl. 102 is page 36 of volume "gam." Because of the slightly different size of the page, it appears to have belonged to a different manuscript. This page also appears to be part of a *Prajñāpāramitā* text. In the center of the leaf is an image representing a personification of one of the forms of emptiness (śūnyatā).

Previously published: (Le Coq 1922–1933:I, pl.32,35; Tucci 1949:II,273–274, III, pl.C; Pal 1969:no.92; Huntington 1972:pl.LVIII; Musée Guimet 1977:no.49.

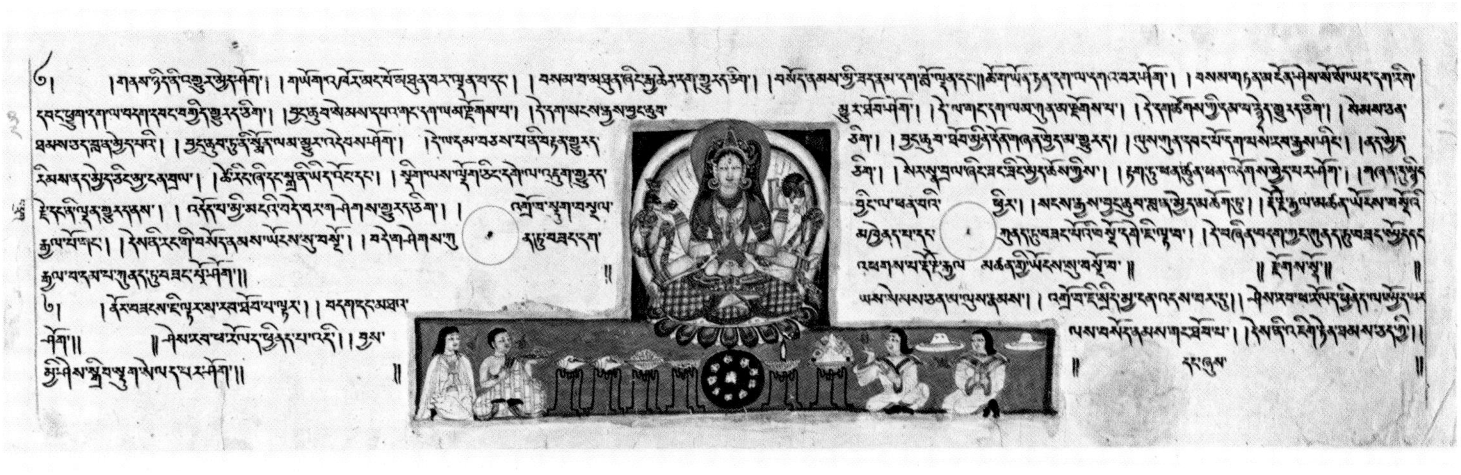

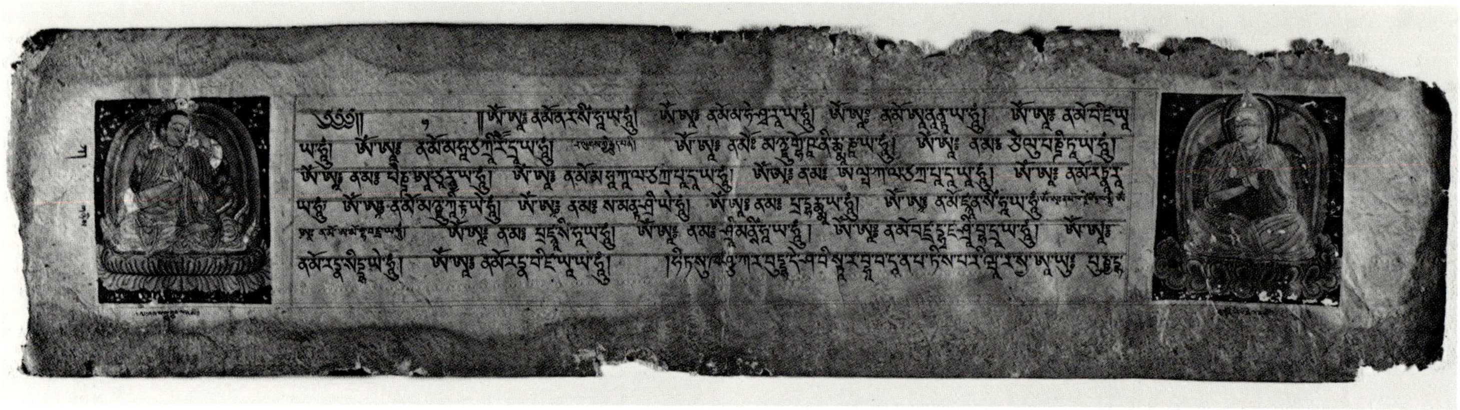

Pl. 103
Kālacakra-tantra Manuscript
Opaque watercolor on paper
West Tibet
Fourteenth century
H. 14.3 × 63.7 cm
Los Angeles County Museum of Art. Louis and Erma Zalk Foundation. (M81.9.1 and 2.)

Pl. 103a

These pages appear to have been written by the same hand and may be part of the same manuscript which contains a Tibetan transcription of the Sanskrit text of the *Kālacakra-tantra.* Both pages are marked side "a" of p. 2. If they do belong to the same manuscript this is either an error or may be explained by the fact that each page belongs to a different section of the text. On Pl. 103a there is a small square on each side of the page, in which a teacher is represented. Nāgārjuna is seated with a protective hood consisting of five snakes (*nāga*); the other personage is Rinchen 'Grub-pa, Bu-ston (1290–1364). The text on this page gives the lineage of transmission of the *Kālacakra-tantra* according to the tradition of Rwa Lotsawa (see *Blue Annals:*Vol.2; p.756). The last name given is that of Rin-chen rNam-rGyal-ba, successor to Bu-ston in the Bu-lugs subsect of the Sakya-pa. Therefore, this text was probably written during the lifetime of Rin-chen rNam-rGyal-ba in the fourteenth century (see also Dharbyey 1975).

Pl.103b

The blue *yab-yum* figure is Guhya Samāja with his consort; the red figure is the deity Yamāntaka with his consort. This page contains the beginning of the liturgy in which the deities are described.

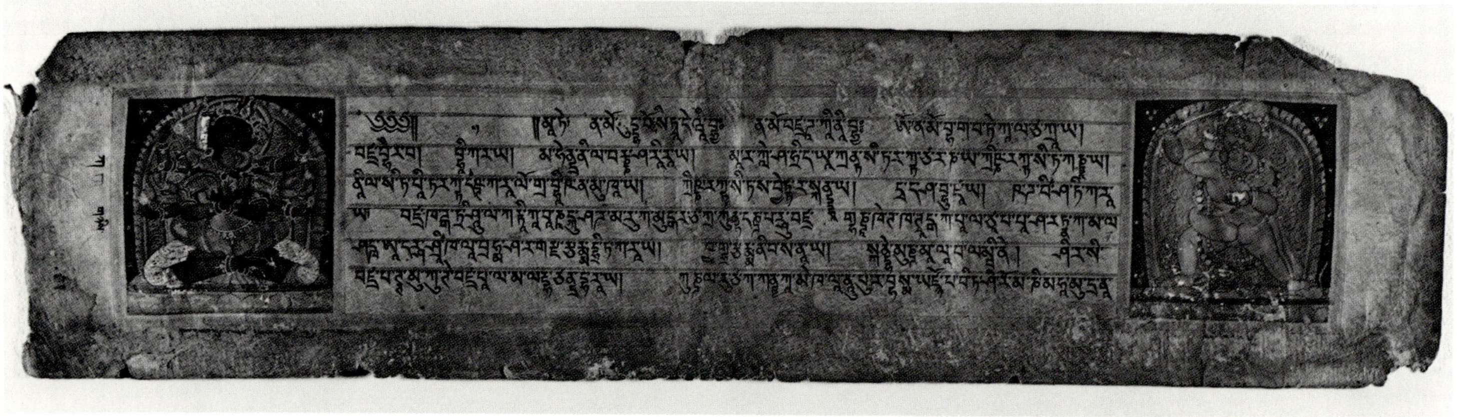

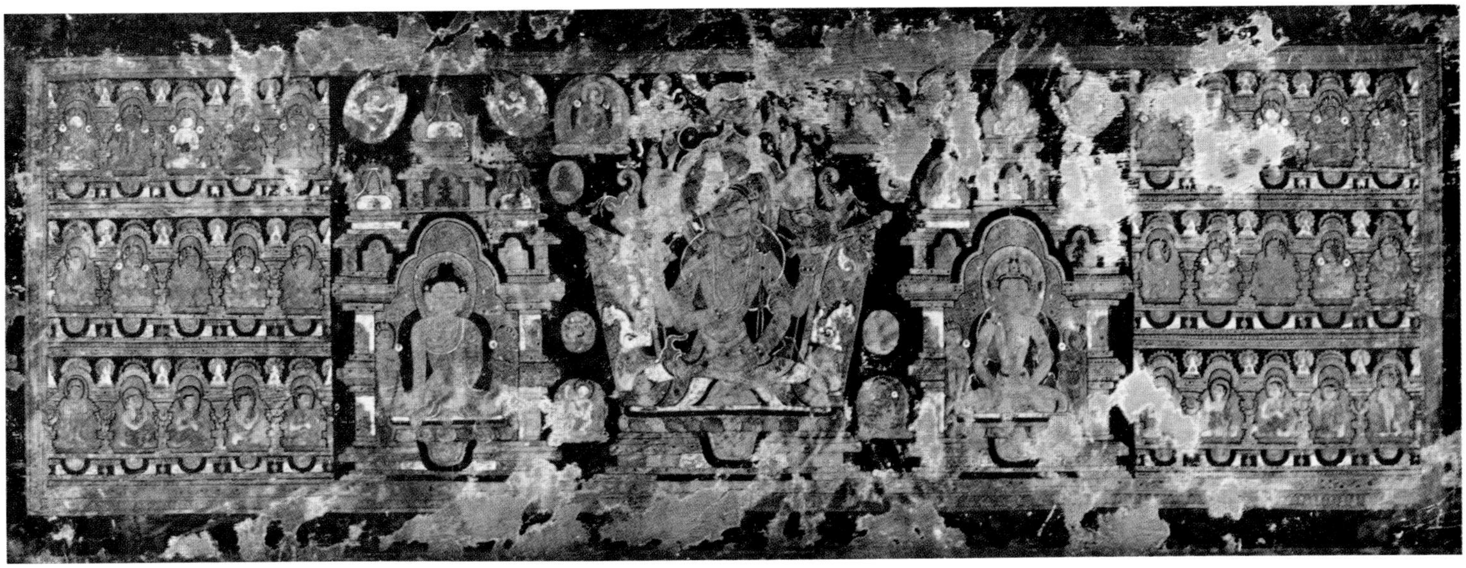

Pl. 104
Vajradhara Manuscript Cover
Carved and painted wood
West Tibet
Fourteenth century
H. 24.8 × W. 68.5 × D. 3.2 cm
Los Angeles County Museum of Art. Nasli and Alice Heeramaneck Collection, Museum Associates Purchase. M.71.1.48.

The red-orange figure of Vajradhara sits enthroned between two Buddhas also seated on lotus thrones. The tiered thrones of gold, orange and blue are silhouetted against the dark blue background. To either side are three rows of five figures each. Each figure is placed in an arcade as if seated in a balcony. The figures represent lamas, teachers and divinities. Grouped at the top and around the central figure are more figures representing similar themes. The four small circles, two to either side of Vajradhara, are goddesses Locanā, Māmaki, Panduravāsini and Tara. The long slender figure style may be compared to the mural painting from Luk monastery. Other details such as the fashion in which Śākyamuni's robe is draped and the small flowers over his ears relate to the painting of Vairocana from Po Monastery, Himachal Pradesh (Pl.108).

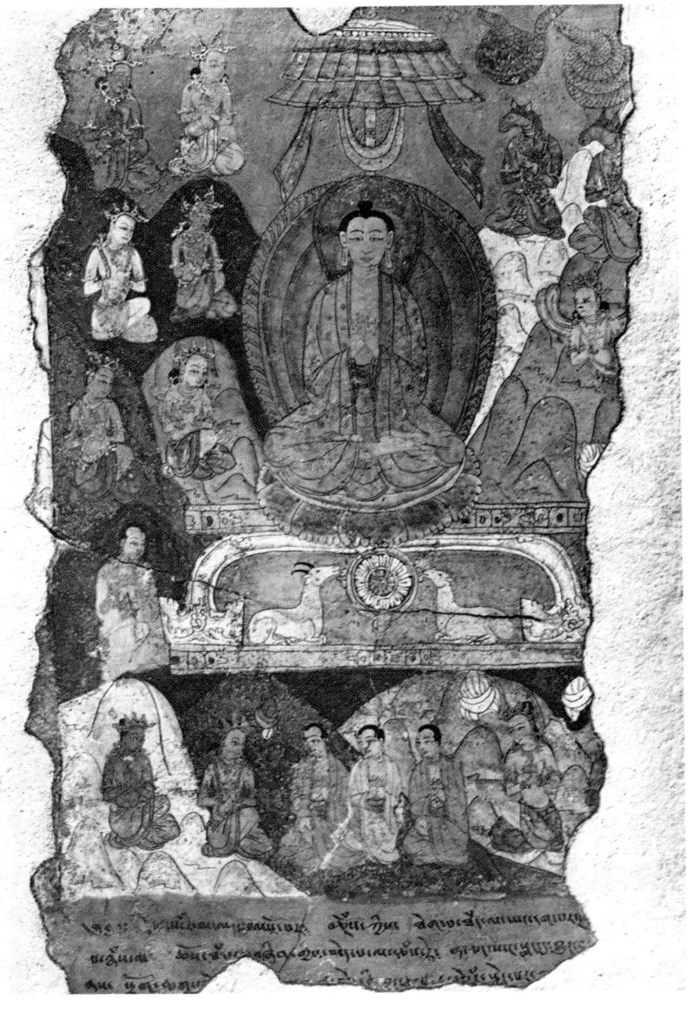

Pl. 105
Fragment of Wall Painting
Luk Monastery
West Tibet
Fourteenth century
H. 49 × W. 29 cm
Instituto Italiano per il Medio e Estremo Oriente, Rome (389)

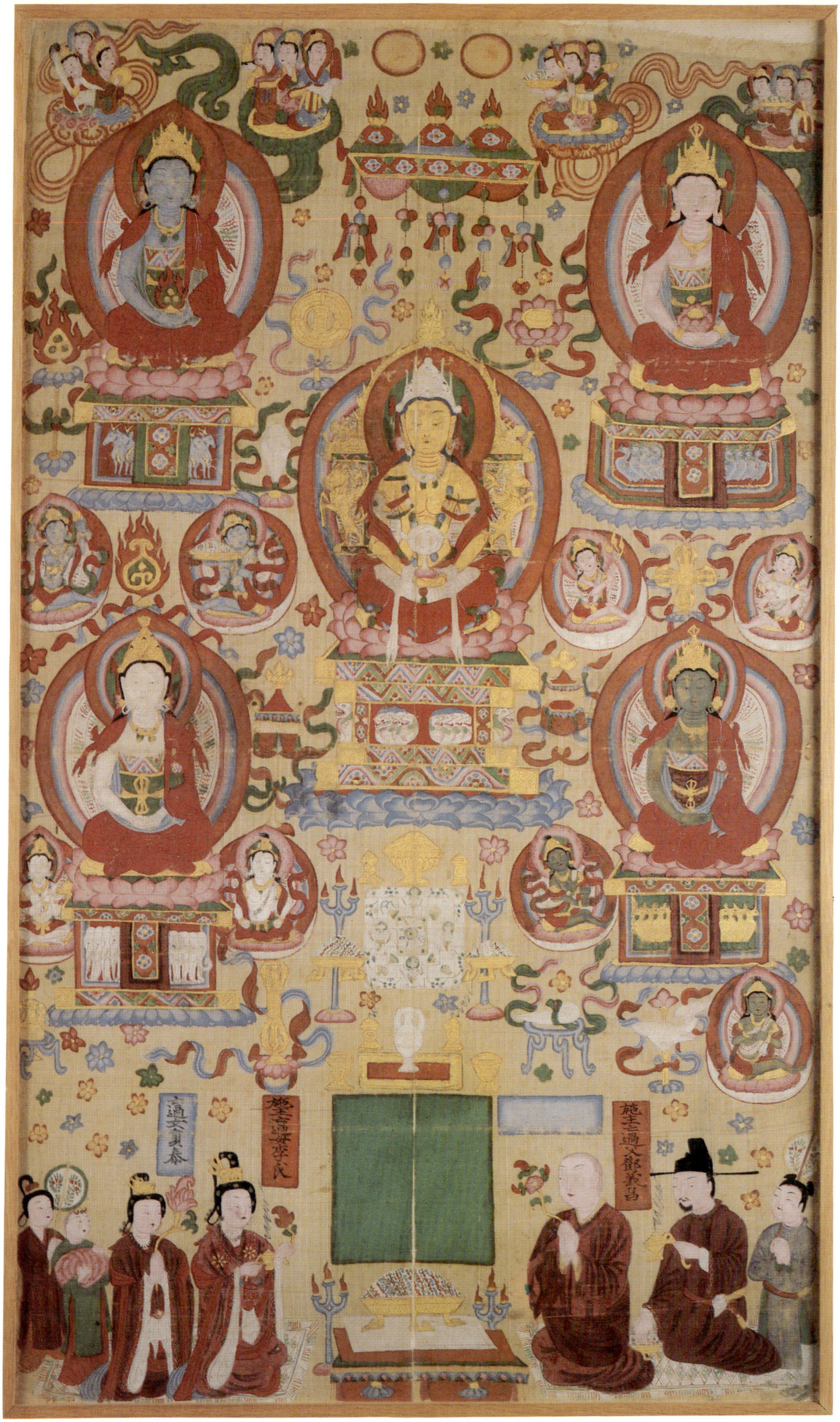

Pl. 68

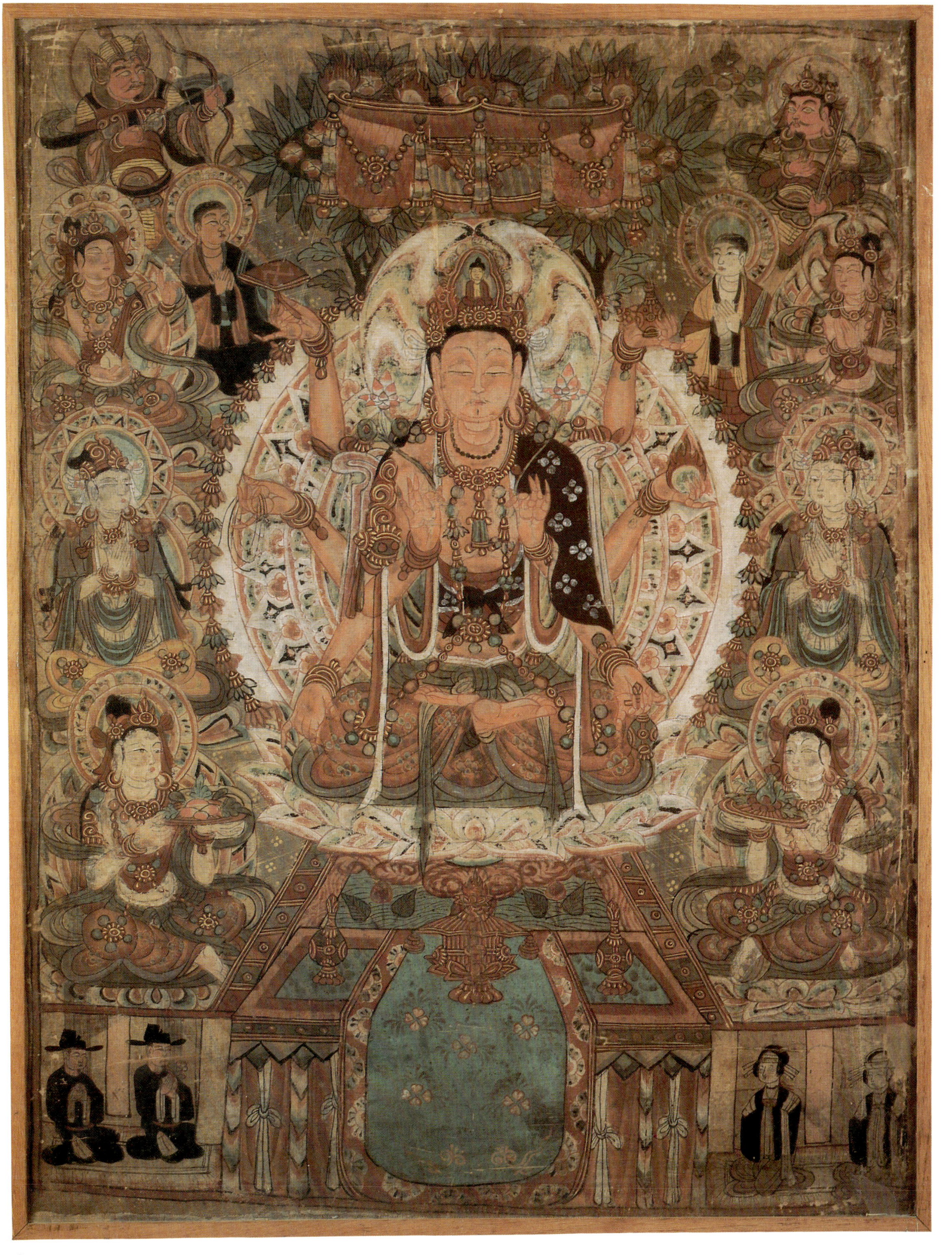

Pl. 70

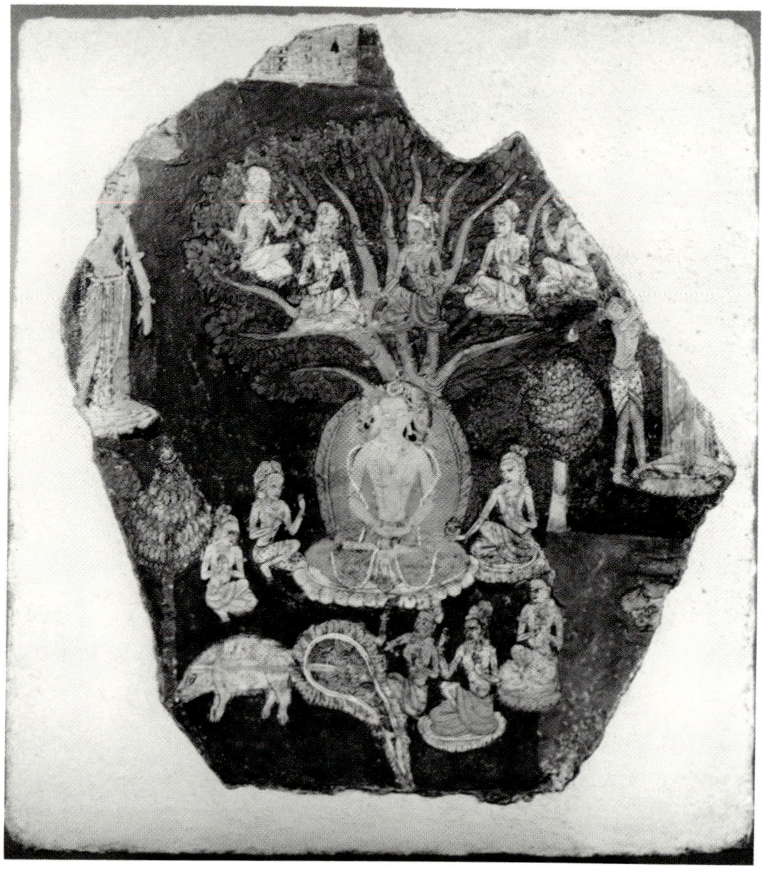

Pl. 106
Fragment of Wall Painting
Luk Monastery
West Tibet
Fourteenth century
H. 31 × W. 28 cm
Instituto Italiano per il Medio e Estremo Oriente, Rome (392)

(See Color Plate 106)

Pl. 108
Vairocana
Painting on cloth
Spiti, Po Monastery, Himachal Pradesh
Thirteenth century
H. 64.77 × 55.88 cm
University of Michigan Museum of Anthropology. (17461)

This *t'ang-ka* (painted scroll from Po monastery) was purchased by Dr. Walter Koelz in 1934 and is part of the Koelz collection at the Museum of Anthropology, University of Michigan, one of the few documented art collections obtained from Ladakh and Himachal Pradesh (Copeland 1980). The Vairocana figure sits on a lotus throne supported by lions and attended by two Bodhisattvas. He is surrounded by rows of meditating Buddhas displaying different *mudrās*. The bottom row contains the *dikpālas*; the second row from the bottom contains the four guardians, *lokapālas*. The background of the painting is blue; the *mandorlas* and many of the monastic gowns are bright red. The Buddhas are painted in white, blue, red and yellow. Both the figure style and the individual motifs, such as the elongated *mandorlas*, are comparable to thirteenth century mural paintings from the Western Himalayas.

Previously published: (Copeland 1980:no.K584, figs.70–71)

(See Color Plate 108)

Pl. 107
Fragment of Wall Painting
Luk Monastery
West Tibet
Fourteenth century
H. 35 × W. 25 cm
Instituto Italiano per il Medio e Estremo Oriente, Rome (391)

These mural fragments were obtained by Prof. Tucci in Luk monastery in West Tibet. Mural paintings containing narrative scenes were often placed on the same wall with devotional paintings. The compositions tend to be rather more spacious than in devotional paintings and thus the scenes are more easily read (Fig. 54). These scenes appear to represent Pl. 105, Śākyamuni preaching the first sermon in the deer park; Pl. 106, unidentified narrative scene from the life of the Buddha; Pl. 107, Śākyamuni and *the attack of the māras*.

It is difficult to date these paintings because of the continuous use of this style over several centuries. (See also Tucci 1932–41:III/pt.2, pls. CXXV–CXXXIV). These murals have been attributed to the eleventh-twelfth century (Olshack 1973:49) and the fifteenth-sixteenth century (Musée Guimet 1977:94). Comparison to Pl. 108, as well as to later examples of this same style which appear in the upper part of a devotional *t'ang-ka* published by Tucci (1949:III, pls.16), suggests a date in the fourteenth century but this is by no means certain.

Pl. 105—Previously published: (Tucci 1967:17, pl.1; Pal 1969:34, fig.10; Musée Guimet 1977:fig.52).

Pl. 106—Previously published: (Musée Guimet 1977,fig.51).

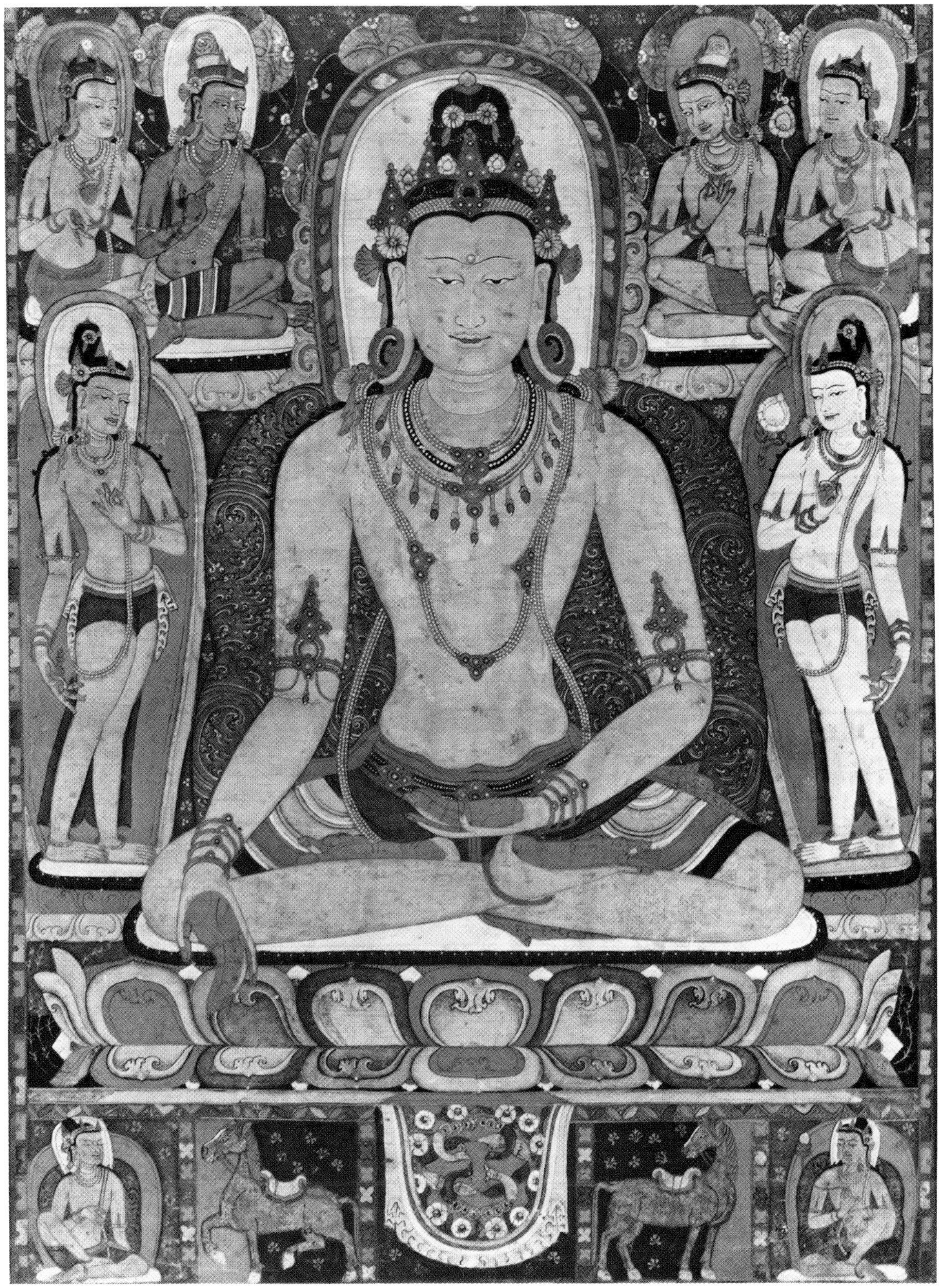

Pl. 109
Buddha Ratnasaṃbhava
Paint on Cotton
Western Trans-Himalaya
Twelfth century
H. 92.7 × 68.3 cm
Los Angeles County Museum of Art
Nasli and Alice Heeramaneck Collection
(M.78.9.2)

Ratnasaṃbhava is surrounded by the eight Bodhisattvas. The composition, figure style, and individual motifs, such as the scroll pattern on the back of the throne, can also be identified in mural paintings of the Lhakhang Soma temple at Alchi Monastery in Ladakh (Fig. 17). The color scheme as well as individual motifs, such as the elongated halo, are also found earlier in Central Asian paintings. Although this painting has been associated with Nepal (Tucci 1949:II,331 and II pl.E; Museum of Fine Arts, Boston 1966:110), More recent scholarship recognizes that this style found in Nepal, Central Asia, and the western Himalayas must derive from a common Indian antecedent (Musée Guimet 1977:75). The drawing found inside the Hatt Stūpa (Pl. 80 and figs. 40 and 40a) is stylistically related to this painting and also to Pls. 111 and 112, which share the curious border motif of alternating blue and red U-shaped forms bordered on yellow (see Pal 1969:49 for a related painting).

Previously published: (Tucci 1949:II,331 and III pl.E; Museum of Fine Arts, Boston 1966:122; Pal 1969:49,131; Pal 1972:fig.4; Los Angeles County Museum of Art 1975:no.21; Musée Guimet 1977:no.20; Snellgrove 1978:no.266).

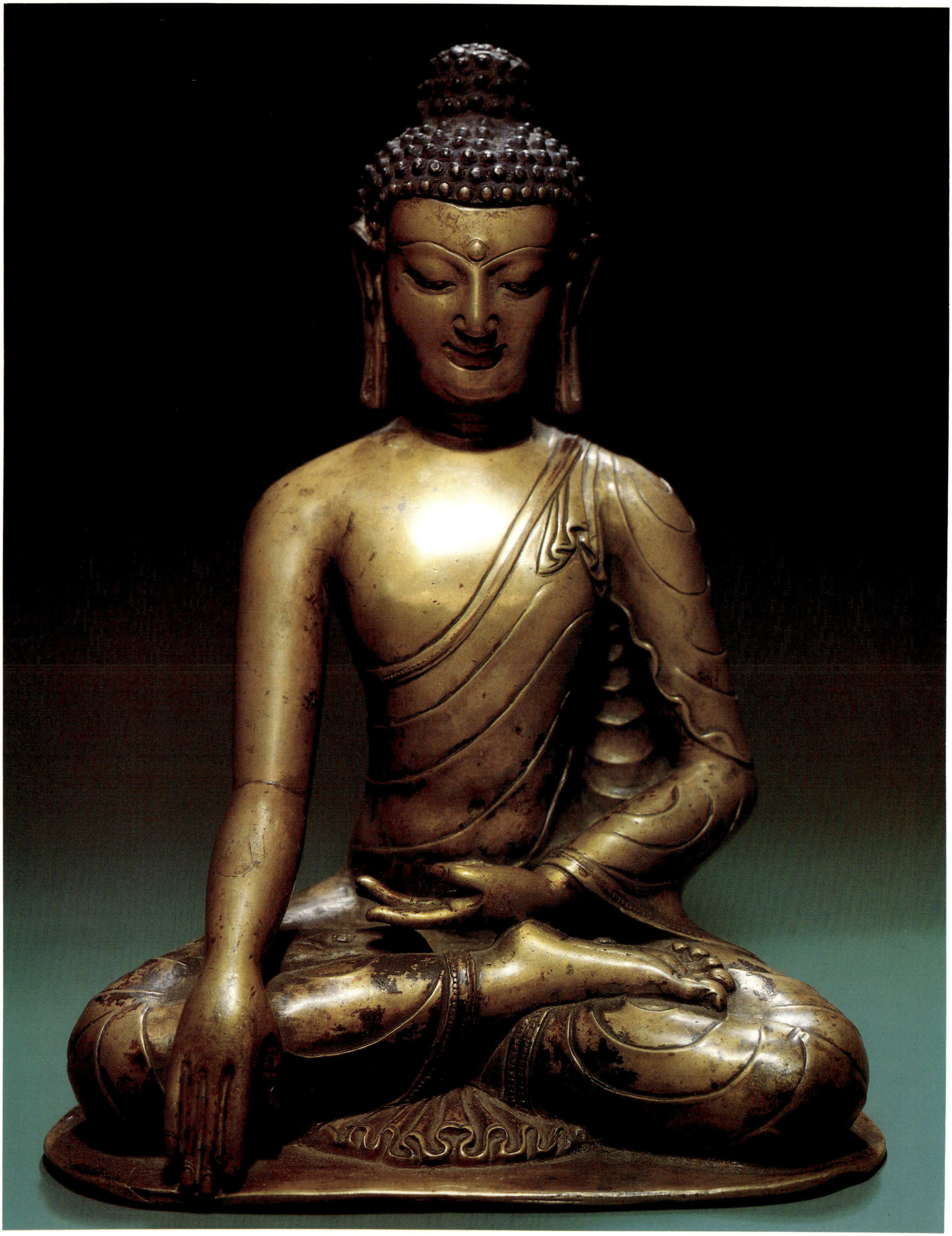

Pl. 81

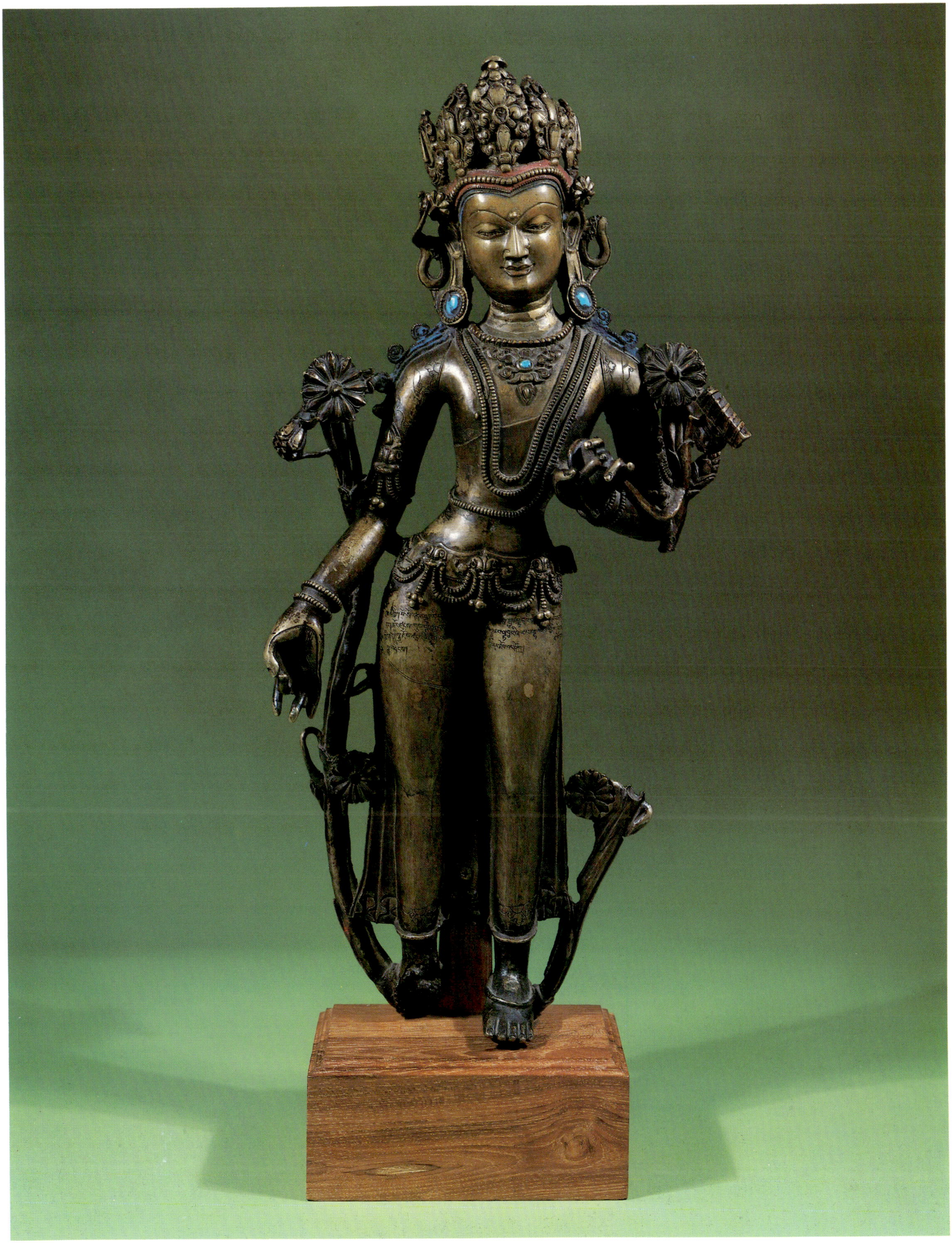

Pl. 93

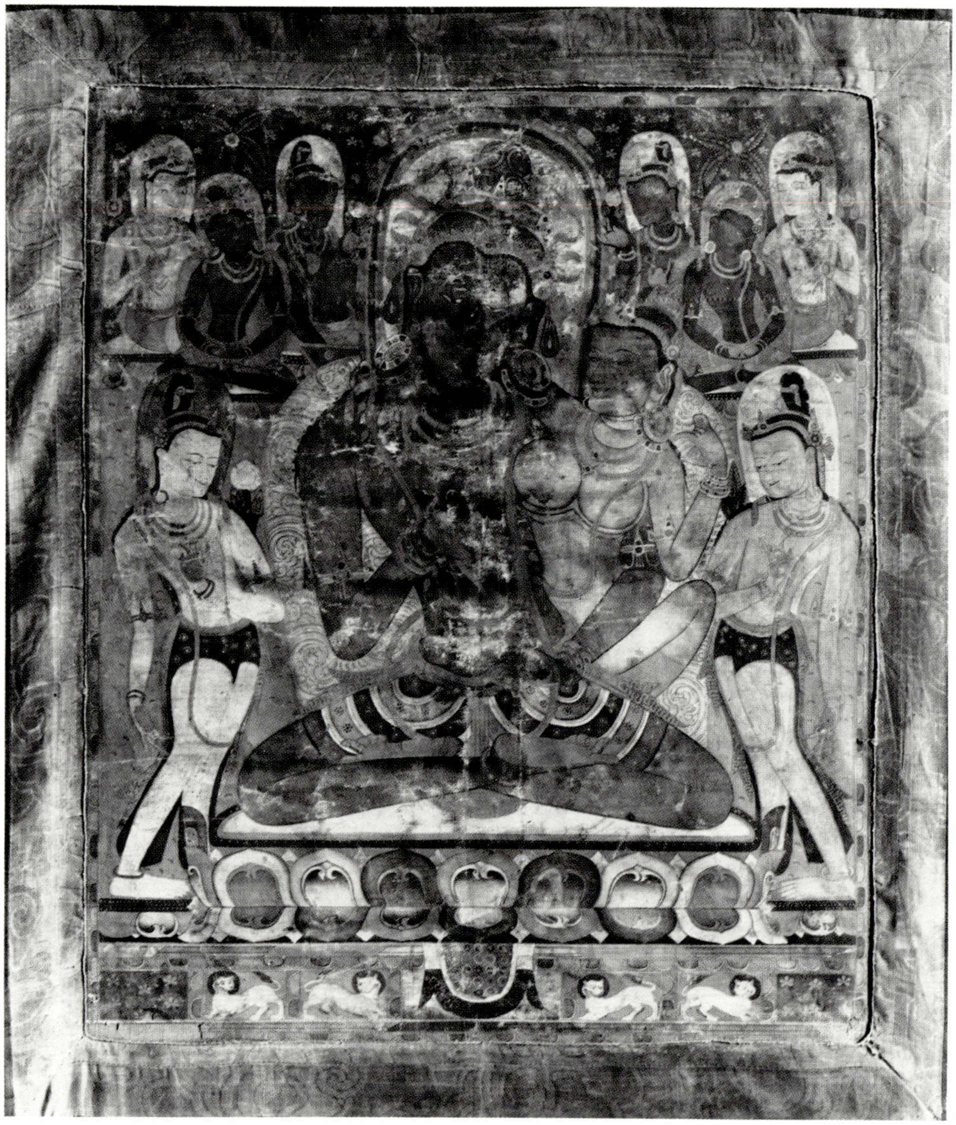

Pl. 110
Vajrasattva and Consort
Paint on cotton
Western Trans-Himalaya
Late twelfth century
H. 62 × 52 cm
Musée Guimet, Paris
Gift of Benedetti, 1952 (MA 1089)

The subject of this important painting is Vajrasattva with his consort seated on a lion throne and surrounded by the eight Bodhisattvas, a popular theme in both Central Asia (Pl. 54) and the Himalayas (Pl. 110). This painting was originally published by Tucci, who concluded that this ancient *t'ang-ka* was the product of a Nepalese tradition in Tibet. In numerous succeeding studies, its historical importance has been reaffirmed, and it is now attributed to the mid-thirteenth century (Musée Guimet 1977:75) and the western Himalayas. The figure style of the Bodhisattvas, the details of the dress and jewelry, and the treatment of the throne—particularly the lotus petal—permit a relative chronology: Pl. 109 may be slightly earlier than this plate; Pls. 111 and 112 somewhat later; and Pl. 108 slightly later still. These scroll paintings might be more firmly dated when future studies clarify the dates of the western Himalayan monastic murals (Figs. 17, 45) and the Kharakhoto paintings which form a stylistic group together with the *t'ang-kas* exhibited here.

Previously published: (Tucci 1949:II, p.331, no.3: III, pls.1,F; Huntington 1968:48; Musée Guimet 1977:no.21, pl.10; Monod, Inde, Khmer and Champa 1966:238–239)

Pl. 111
Saṃvara and Prajñā
Paint on cotton
Western Trans-Himalaya
Late thirteenth century
H. 43 × W. 27 cm (without frame)
Anonymous, Courtesy of Doris Wiener (exhibited only in Washington, D.C.) Gallery

This extraordinarily dramatic painting employs many of the stylistic motifs found in the slightly earlier paintings in Pls. 110 and 111: the helmet-crown of Saṃvara, the shape of the lotus throne, the figure style and the color scheme. The entire group (Pls. 108–112) uses a dark blue background and deep red as the dominant color. These two hues, along with accents of blue, green and yellow (together with white) are the five colors associated with the Five Buddha families. The simple rendition of Saṃvara and his consort, each having only one head and two arms, serves to emphasize the diagonal placement of the main divinities. The Saṃvara cycle is important throughout the Himalayas, and the clay sculptures of this divinity at Tsaparang are particularly impressive (see Tucci 1932–41:III,17).

(See Color Plate 111)

Pl. 112
Vajravārāhī (the Adamantine Sow)
Paint on cotton
Western Trans-Himalaya
Late thirteenth century
H. 82.87 × 60 cm
Anonymous loan

Inscription on reverse side: The *mantra* of Tārā: Oṃ Tāre Tuttāre Ture Svāhā: The enlightened one has declared, "Patience is the supreme penance; patience is truly the highest liberation."

This painting is stylistically and iconographically related to the painting of Śaṃvara and consort (Pl. 111). In addition to the features already mentioned in the discussion of Pls. 110 and 111, the similarity of the compositions is quite striking. Both paintings isolate the central divinity in a shallow arcade. Each painting has two rows of figures in separate arcades at the top and one row on the bottom. The dancing figure of Vajravārāhī, a form of the goddess Vajrayoginī with a sow's head protruding from the left side of her head, is accompanied by six goddesses. The central arcade is framed by the ten cemeteries which are treated as small narrative scenes, each separated by a curving strip of water. Compare this composition to the circular arrangement of the cemeteries in Pls. 125 and 139. A similar framing effect is accomplished in Pl. 111 by a vine stalk which frames a row of personages. A similar composition is also used in a painting from Karakhoto (Musée Guimet 1977:no. 23). Both Vajravārāhī and her consort are represented in paintings from Karakhoto now in the Hermitage Museum (Musée Guimet 1977:28,29). For additional discussions on the liturgy, see deMallmann 1969; Meisezahl 1967.)

Previously published: (Fogg Art Museum 1974:no.138; Pal 1975a:no.46; Pal 1978b:II, fig.203).

(See Color Plate 112)

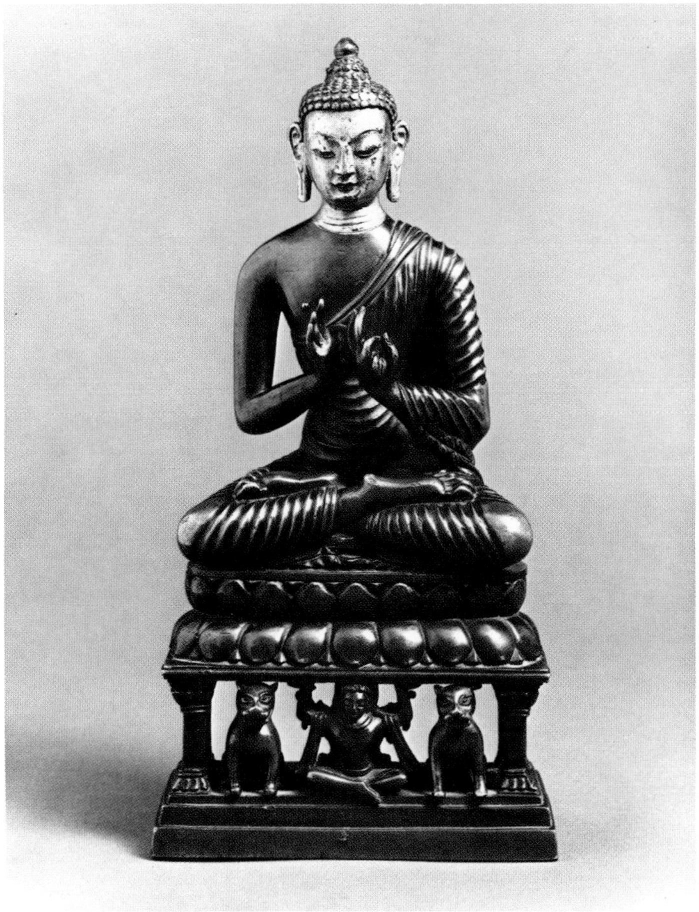

Pl. 113
Vairocana
Bronze
Western Trans-Himalaya
Fifteenth century
H. 22.5 × W. 11.4 × D. 5.4 cm
Michael Phillips

This lustrous, brown-toned Vairocana image, whose face is painted in "cold gold," is identified by his "teaching *mudrā*" and the lion throne. This Tibetan image copies a type of Kashmiri Buddha which is known from several examples. The hairstyle, the monastic robe falling in symmetrical U-shaped folds, and the throne supported by two dwarf pillars, two frontal lions and a seated figure at the center are all found in the Los Angeles County Museum of Art Kashmiri bronze (Snellgrove 1978:pl.257) and the Fatehpur bronze (*Archaeological Survey of India Report* 1904–1905:107–109).

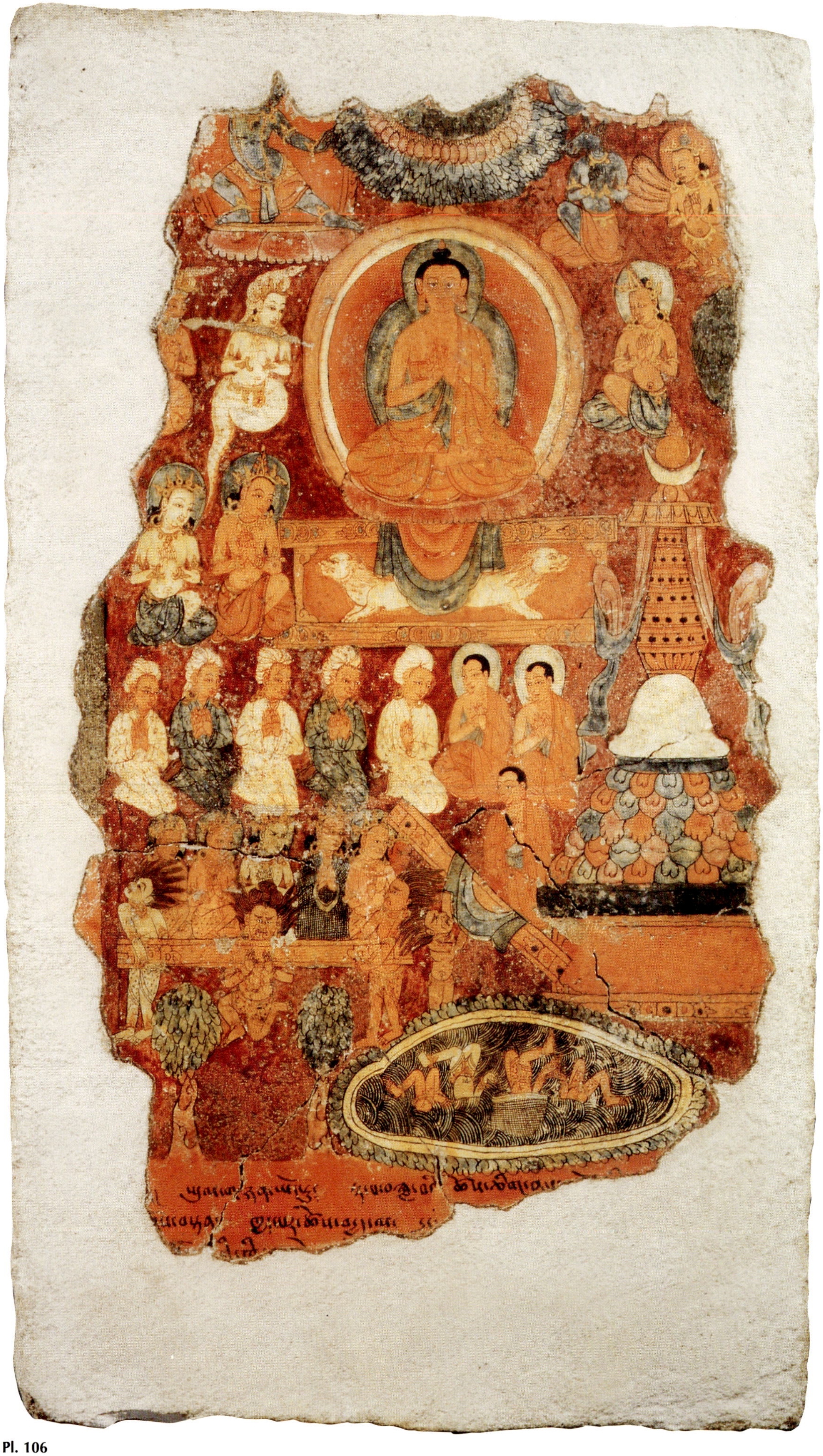

Pl. 106

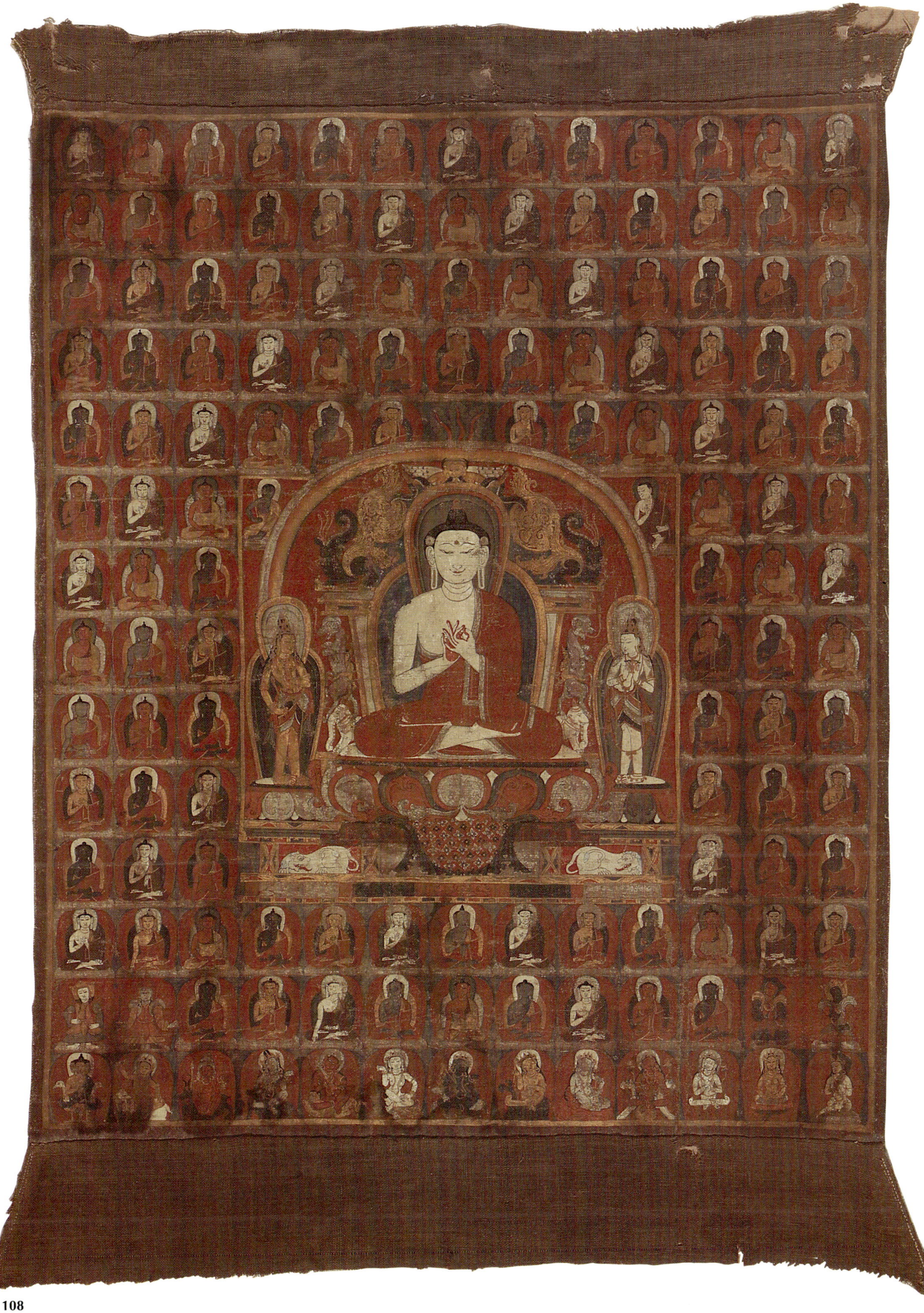

Pl. 108

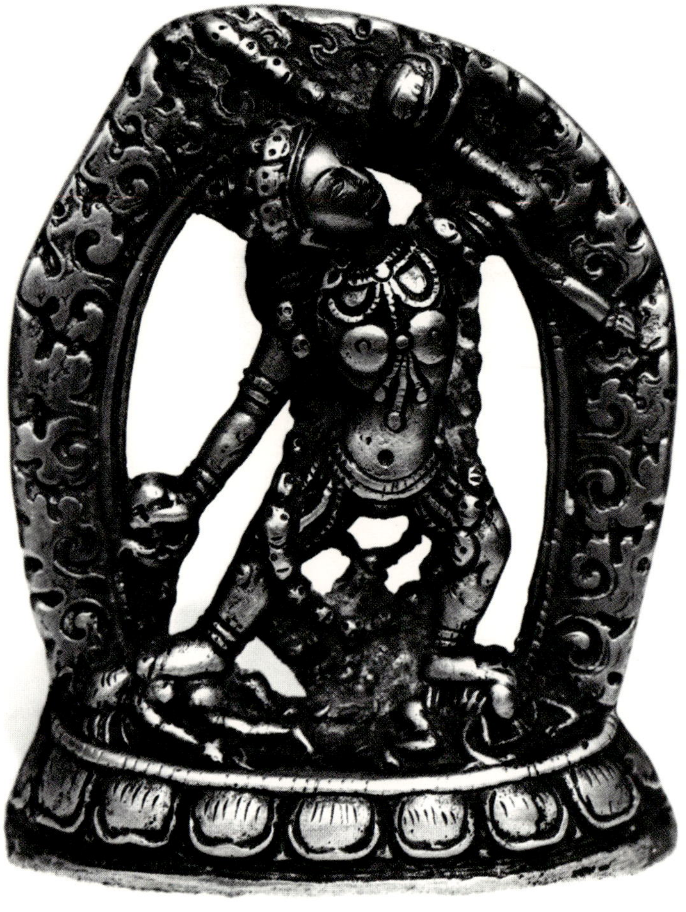

Pl. 114
Vajrayoginī
Bronze. Tibetan inscription on pedestal.
West Tibet or Tibet
Fourteenth century
H. 12.06 cm
Navin Kumar
(Inscription: oṃ maṇi padme hūṃ hrī)

This small image represents the goddess Vajrayoginī according to the tradition found in the Sakya liturgy. At the back of the base is a *mantra* of Avalokiteśvara which appears to be a later addition. Except for the posture, the essential iconography is that of the Kagyud tradition, which is explained in Chapter VII. Stylistic features of this image are found in both western Tibetan and Nepalese art of this period.

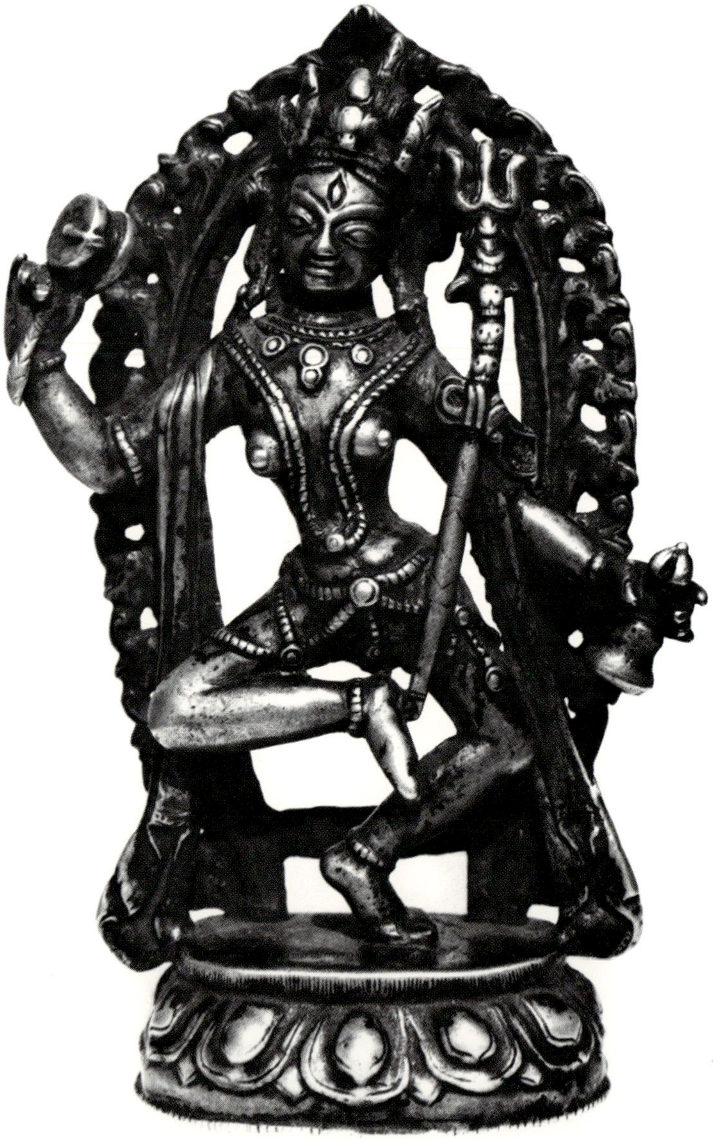

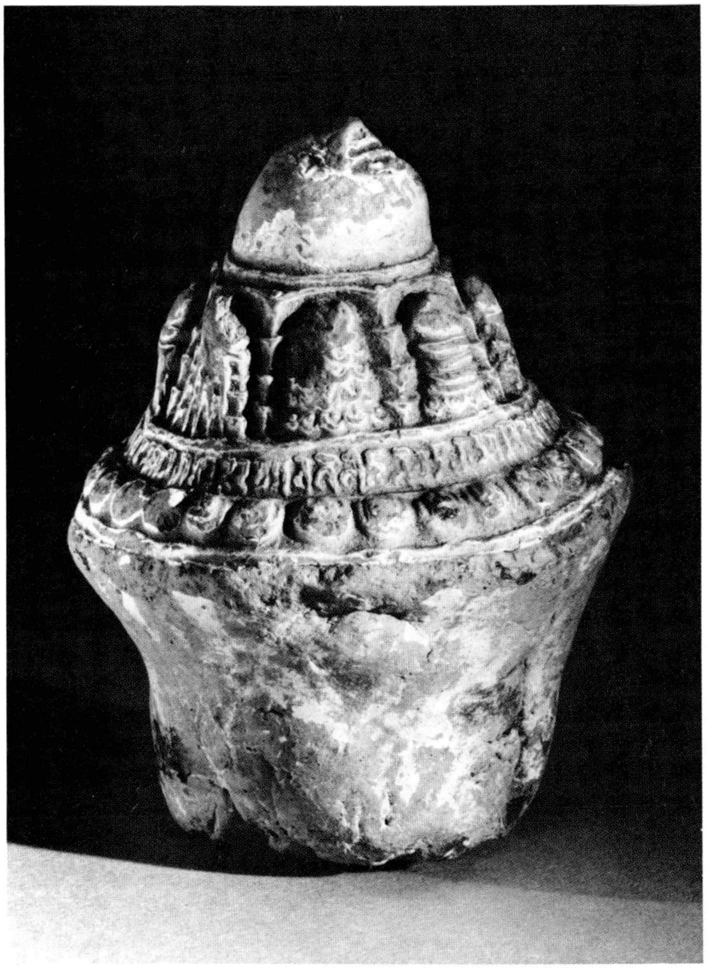

Pl. 116
Stūpa *ts'a ts'a*
Clay
Ladakh
Date undetermined
H. 8 × 6 × 6 cm
Museum für Völkerkunde, Vienna (38269)

Pl. 117
***Ts'a-ts'a* Śākyamuni with Attendants**
Clay
Ladakh
Date undetermined
H. 4.5 × 1 cm
Museum für Völkerkunde, Vienna (38278)
(Śākyamuni in *bhūmisparṣamudrā*; attendant figures may be the disciples Śāriputra and Maudgalyāyana)

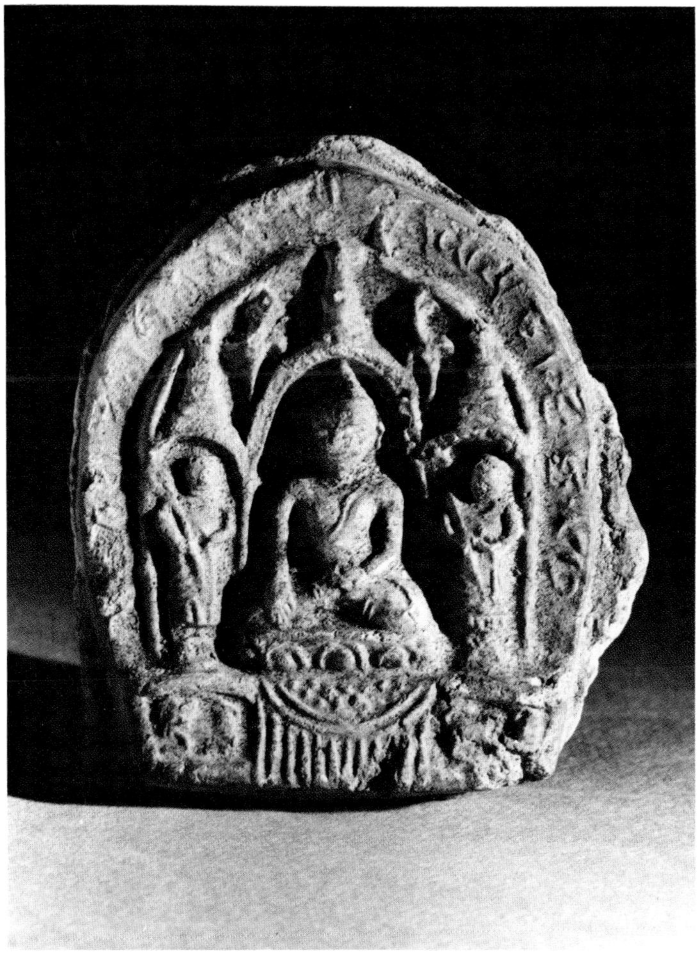

Pl. 115
Ma-chik Drönma
Bronze. Tibetan inscription on pedestal.
West Tibet or Tibet
Fourteenth century
H. 7.94 cm
Navin Kumar

Inscription: Salutations to the one mother, good fortune to the patrons.

One of the few females to have become renowned as a great teacher, Ma-gcig bslab-kyi sGrön-ma (1055–1149) was one of the chief disciples of Dam-pa Saṅs-rgyas, founder of the Źi-byed-pa sect. As a female teacher, she carries the attributes of *Yoginī*—*damaru*, bell, and *triśula*—and she dances against a rainbow of flames. This representation follows the Nying-ma tradition. This concept is also found in Śaivite images. Ma-chik Drönma propagated the teachings known as the *gCod* doctrine in West Tibet. This psychologically and physically demanding system associated itself with (often) bizarre practices. Those practices which have survived appear to have been absorbed into the Nying-ma and Kagyud teachings (Tucci 1980:39, 87–93).

(Inscription read by Thartse Khenpo, Rinpoche, Los Angeles 1981)

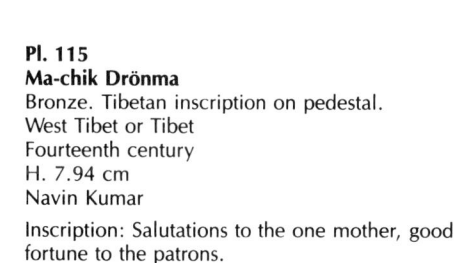

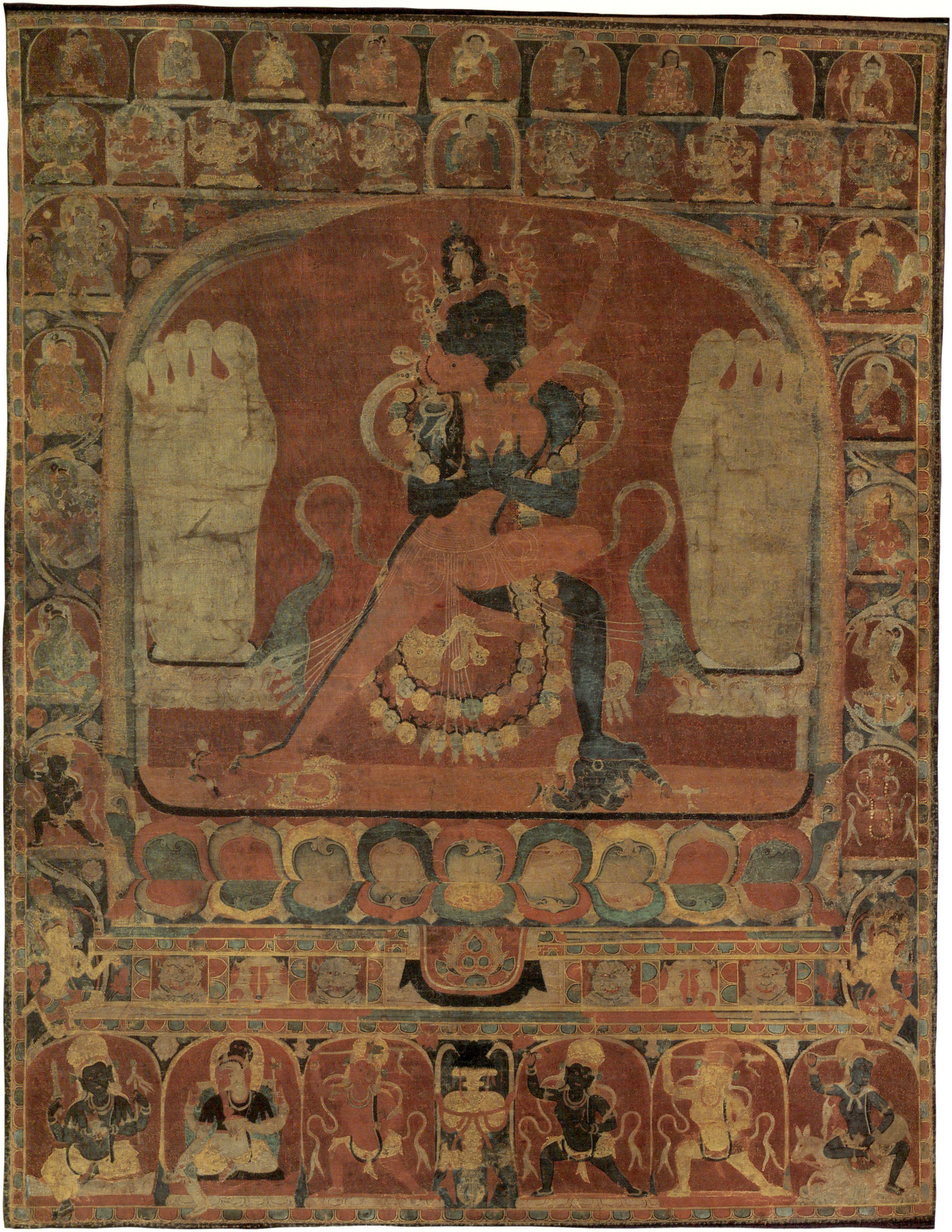

Pl. 111

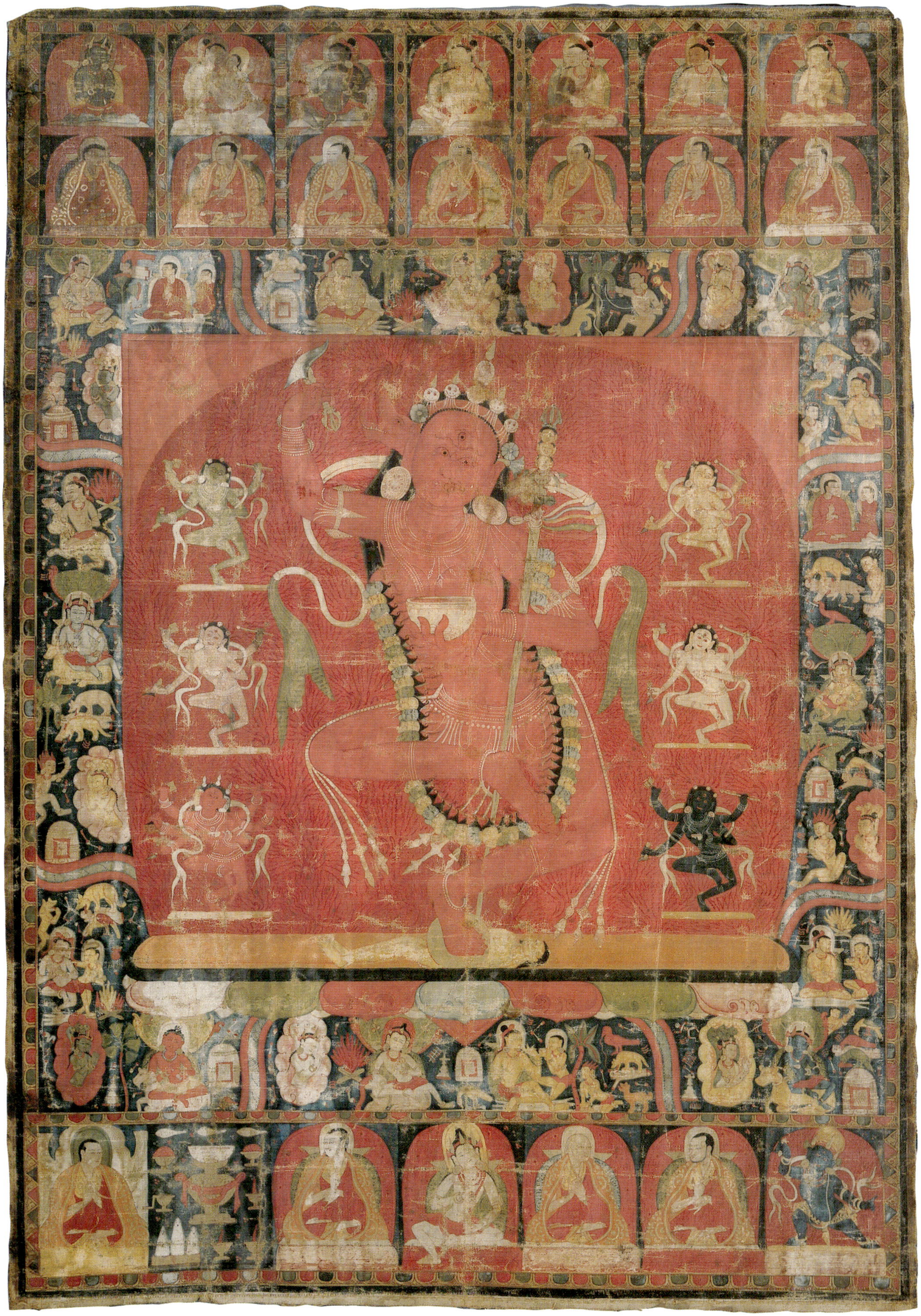

Pl. 112

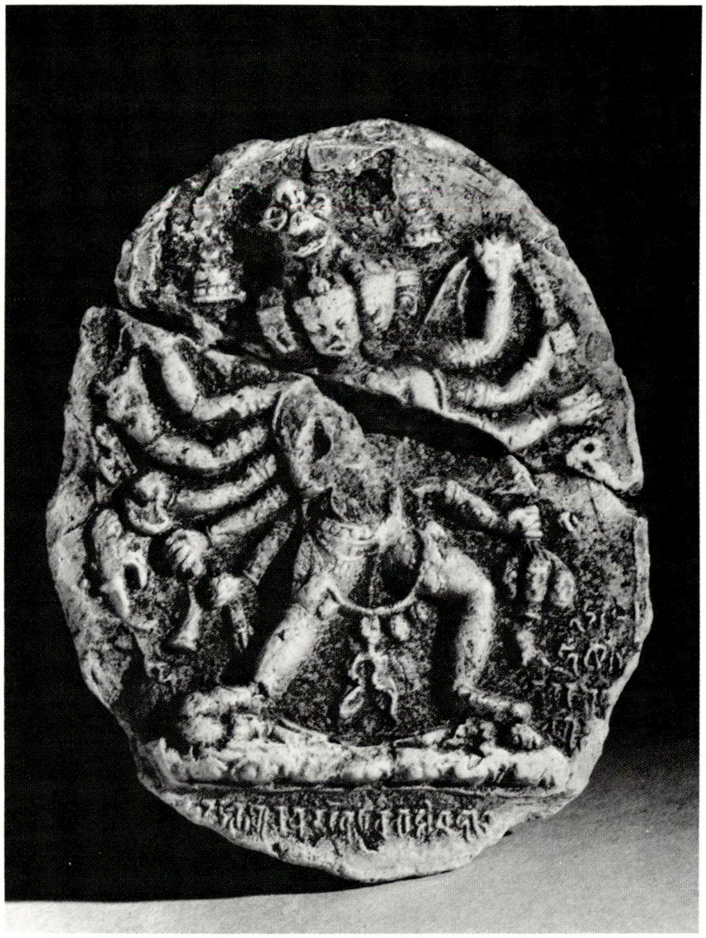

Pl. 118
***Ts'a ts'a* Cakraśaṃvara**
Clay
Ladakh
Date undetermined
H. 8 × 6.5 × 2 cm
Museum für Völkerkunde, Vienna (38272)

These votive clay offerings were collected by Dr. Troll in 1888–89 in either Ladakh or Baltistan. Dr. Troll's expedition took him from Central Asia to the western Himalayas via Yoktan, Khotan, and Leh, eventually ending his journey at Śrīnagar. *Ts'a-ts'a* have been found in Afghanistan dating from the eighth to ninth centuries and are still found throughout the Himalayas. Since clay images were inexpensive and easy to produce, clay plaques, usually depicting *stūpas* or tantric divinities, were made in great numbers and sold to pilgrims who used them as votive offerings. In some cases, the ashes of a deceased abbot or other esteemed person, or other sacred substances, were mixed with clay and molded into a *ts'a-ts'a*. These could also be gilded or painted.

Pl. 119
Buddha
Paint on cloth
Ladakh (Lamayuru), Western Trans-Himalaya
Fifteenth century
H. 161.29 × 99 cm (unframed)
Navin Kumar, Inc.

The Buddha sits serenely centered in a spacious, uncluttered environment, his left hand in the earth-touching gesture. As with earlier paintings from the western Himalayas, the background is blue, although here the blue is somewhat lighter than was customary earlier. The shape of the face and the style of the gown is also different from earlier periods (Pl. 108) and can be compared to paintings acquired in Lamayuru Monastery, Ladakh (Copeland 1980:73). The round shape of the combined *mandorla* and aureola is also seen in earlier West Tibet painting (Tucci 1949: III, pl. 24). An upturned lotus with a simple lion throne and rug overhang is a later elaboration of an earlier motif. The elaborate overlapping flame-like forms of the border are also found in the fifteenth century paintings from this region. Large-scale images were frequently painted on cloth on monastery walls.

(See Color Plate 119)

Pl. 120
Buddha
Paint on cloth
West Tibet
Fifteenth century
H. 0.97 × 0.90 cm
Museo Nazionale d'Arte Orientale, Rome.

This painting was acquired by Professor Tucci in western Tibet (ancient Gu-ge) in the 1930s and belongs to the significant group of paintings which, together with murals, assist us in defining Tibetan regional schools of painting. This ancient theme of a Buddha surrounded by myriads of meditating Buddhas decorates the walls of earlier Buddhist chapels in Central Asia, India, and the Himalayas, and also appears in *t'ang-kas* (Pl. 108). As in the earlier *t'ang-kas* from western Tibet (Pl. 108–112), the background here is blue, and red is used throughout the painting. This painting uses motifs well-known in Gu-ge painting, such as the elaborate lotus throne with different tendrils curving to frame individual vignettes but here the ornamental character of the throne completely overwhelms any structural logic, so that the Buddha is framed by groups of eight lamas, *stūpas*, and Buddhas. Tucci has identified this scene as representing the heaven of our present age, the *bhadra-kalpa* (1949:II,359–360).

Previously published: (Tucci 1949:II,359–360; III,pl.29; Tucci 1973:illus.208; Musée Guimet 1977:no.58).

(See Color Plate 120)

Pl. 121
Śākyamuni
Paint on cloth
Luk Monastery, West Tibet
Sixteenth century
H. 0.63 × 0.52 cm
Museo Nazional d'Arte Orientale, Rome

Acquired by Tucci in Luk village in western Tibet. Buddha Śākyamuni sits in the earth-touching gesture. The throne has a stepped, almost geometric shape which supports six *stūpas*. The slightly horseshoe-shaped *mandorlas* and elongated figures retain the stylistic preferences seen in the earlier mural fragments also acquired by Tucci in the same locale (Pls. 105–107). The blue background appears again, but here it is strewn with small red flowers, and the various tones of red have a more orange cast. The Buddha's face with a widow's peak and the shaded folds of the garments are found in sixteenth-century wall paintings at Ta-pho and the so-called "white temple" at Tsaparang. The figure style and decorative elements prompted Tucci to class this painting with his "Kashmiri" style.

Previously published: (Tucci 1973:illus.208; Musée Guimet 1977:fig.58)

(See Color Plate 121)

Pl. 122
Lokeśvara, Tsaparang Style
Painting on cloth
West Tibet
Fourteenth-fifteenth century
H. 91.5 × 66 cm (unframed)
Navin Kumar, Inc.

Although the eleven-headed, thousand-armed Avalokiteśvara was not popular in India (see Pl. 94), it was well-known in Central Asia, China, Japan and in the Himalayas. This image appears frequently in architectural sculpture and mural paintings in the monasteries of the western Himalayas. Comparison of this painting with both painted scrolls and murals establishes a relationship to the Tsaparang style. In addition, the lamas wearing yellow caps and the figure of Tsong-kha-pa confirm that this painting was associated with Gelug-pa patronage, probably in the fifteenth century.

An eleven-headed, thousand-armed Avalokiteśvara stands on a lotus, its multiple heads and body encased by a *prabhāmandorla*. A miniature landscape occupies the base. Subsidiary figures and a ritual scene fill out the lower sides. Apotheosized lamas and other minor deities appear across the top of the painting. While there is a marked frontality and an informal but powerful symmetry, the curvilinear element emerges as a result of the repetition of parabolic curves, spiral and ogee shapes. An engaging play of shapes occurs in the likening of the tip of the lion's tail to a flower bud, and a lotus petal to a cloud. A parallel sense of luxury can be found in mural paintings from the western Himalayan monasteries such as Alchi and Tsaparang. The background of the composition is blue, but the predominant color is a cinnabar red, complemented by a dark bluish-green. A subtle cream hue colors much of the face, body and multiple arms, which also show traces of white.

The central image has a rather broad flat face with a widow's peak. A slight attempt at modeling is revealed by the still-visible socket of the right eye. The long earlobes indicate aristocratic birth. The expression is bland and rather detached. In contrast, the adjunct figures have a sweet, engaging look often associated with Nepalese work.

The relatively simple fall of the central figure's scarf contrasts with the elaborate curves, bows, and flourishes associated with the drapery found in later works. The use of a two-sided fabric, such as that in the shawl ends, also occurs in Ta-pho textiles.

The Kumar painting's clear connection to the Gu-ge region can be readily seen in the similarity of the treatment of the lotus and spiral forms, and in the facial type. One painting from sixteenth-century Tsaparang (Gu-ge region) suggests a close parallel but shows the earlier date of our painting: (1) an architectural element usually noted in later works is found in the corner; (2) there is a flattening and schematization of the lotus; and (3) slightly more overlap in the decor.
Cheryl Snell

Previously published: (Pal 1982).

(See Color Plate 122)

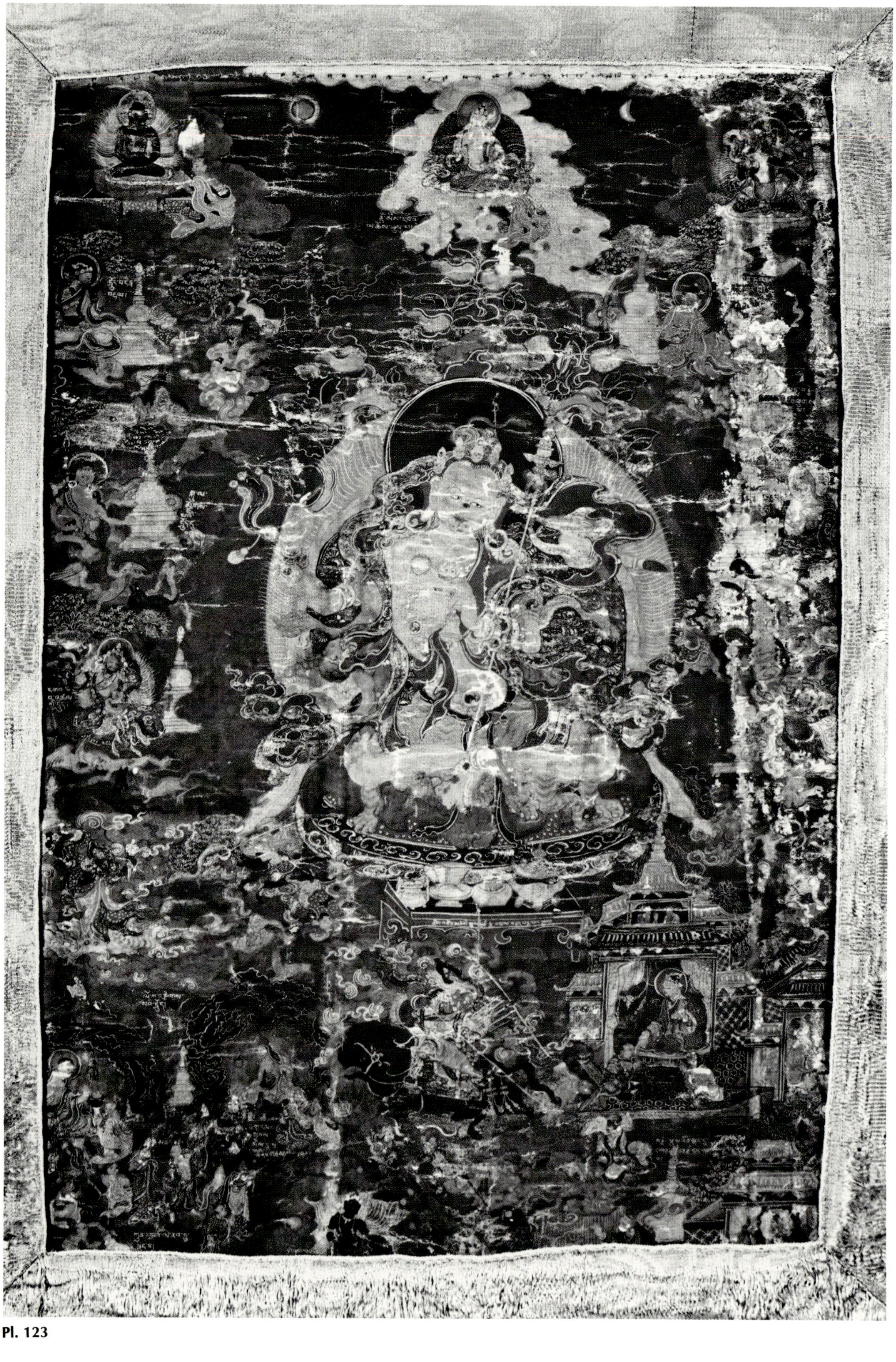

Pl. 123

Pl. 123
Padmasambhava
Paint on cloth
Tibet
Seventeenth century
H. 41 × 23 cm
Museo Nazionale d'Arte Orientale, Rome. (No.916/749).

This painting was originally part of a series of twelve dedicated to the eight aspects of Padmasaṃbhava (Guru Rinpoche). Six paintings from this set were acquired by Tucci, who has discussed both the paintings and the textual sources for the iconography at length (1949:II,540–547), as well as the importance of "Guru Rinpoche" (precious teacher) for Tibetan and particularly Nying-ma tradition (1949:I,109–115). According to an inscription on the back, the set was commissioned by Kunga Namgyal, a merchant in K'ar in Tibet; the name of the lama who consecrated the *t'ang-kas* is given as Pad ma'i miṅ can. The form of Padmasaṃbhava represented in this *t'ang-ka* is Rig-dzin mchog-sprul-pa'i-bskal-bzang Pad-ma dbang-phyug. In the upper part of the painting, from left to right, is Samantabhadra (blue), Vajrasattva (white), and another aspect of Padmasaṃbhava with his consort. The use of stylized Chinese motifs, and the freer composition distinguishes this painting from the earlier western Tibetan school (Pls. 120,121).

Pl. 124
Guardian Deity
Paint on cloth
Ladakh
Sixteenth century
H. 117 × 95.3 cm
Navin Kumar

The bright blue background of the painting is repeated in the deeper blue skin of the main and two subsidiary deities, as well as in the lotus petals; shades of red, and pink-red are used throughout. The figure is encircled by a halo of stylized flames surrounding six crows. The deity carries a sword in his right hand and a mongoose spitting jewels in his left. The mongoose is an attribute of Vaiśravaṇa, King of the North, and also of Jambhala, god of wealth. The deity wears a cape which appears to be made of peacock feathers, soft felt boots, and a five-part jeweled crown. A similar figure appears in the lower left hand corner of a Kālacakra *t'ang-ka* and is considered to belong to a composite style which integrates styles associated with both the Sakya and Nying-ma orders. A figure with a similar style and iconography, but without the mongoose, is painted in the *mgon-khang* at Phyang monastery in Ladakh.

(See Color Plate 124)

Pl. 125
Maṇḍala of Kurukullā
Paint on cloth
Ngor Monastery, Tsang, Tibet
Sixteenth century
H. 73.5 × 85 cm
Jerry Solomon, Los Angeles

The goddess takes many forms and is worshipped throughout India under many names. Although several devotional paintings dedicated to the goddess are known (Pl. 112) from the earlier period of western Himalayan art, the true *maṇḍala*-palace schemes are known only in mural painting (Fig. 22). The traditional *maṇḍala*-palace scheme (see descriptions accompanying Pls. 61–64; 73), were painted on paper and cloth in Dunhuang in the ninth and tenth centuries, and must also have existed in the western Himalayas. The Dunhuang diagram of the *maṇḍala* of Uṣṇīṣavijayā (Pl. 73), a popular goddess in the western Himalayas (Pl. 97), is particularly interesting in this regard. This sixteenth century *tang'ka* of a *maṇḍala* dedicated to the tantric goddess Kurukullā demonstrates one variant of the fully-developed *maṇḍala*-palace scheme (Burway 1978). Here the goddess is red, she is of the family of Amitābha and is often identified with the red Tārā. In this example, the goddess Kurukullā dances at the center of a red lotus surrounded by the four goddesses Vajrayoginī (at the top), then Vajraḍākinī, Vajrā, and Gaurī. In the top row the divinities and great teachers of the Śakya lineage, including Abhayakāragupta, who wrote the text illustrated by this *maṇḍala* are represented. This painting is a remarkable example of the sixteenth-century Ngor school of painting. The color scheme and dark blue background strewn with flowers also occurs in other Śakya paintings (Pl. 120), and earlier in western Himalayan art (Pl. 109).

Previously published: (Galerie Robert Buraway 1978, *Peintures du Monastere de Nor.*)

(See Color Plate 125)

Pl. 126
Kālacakra Maṇḍala
Paint on cloth
Tibet
Sixteenth century
H. 71 × W. 81 cm
Navin Kumar, Inc.

The complex iconography of this *maṇḍala* is clarified to some degree by the use of an extremely fine line and clear luminous colors. The *Kālacakra-tantra* became important in about the tenth century. It was taught in the great Buddhist monasteries in northeast India and propagated by teachers in the western Himalayas during the "second diffusion" of Buddhism. There is an extremely sophisticated cosmology (Kālacakra means "wheel of time") which is part of this text, and its teachings continue to be revered in Tibet, particularly among the Gelugpa. Kālacakra, the main deity of this *maṇḍala* according to the *Niṣpannayogāvāli*, is blue, has four heads, twenty-four arms, and dances with his consort in the *ālīḍha* posture. His consort is yellow. There are five rows of deities—*yab-yum* figures, goddesses, and guardian deities—whose colors correspond to the Buddha Family which rules the section of the *maṇḍala* in which they reside. It was commissioned by one of the Sakya subsects, perhaps Bu-lug-pa. Neither the eight pandits or four monks depicted at the top of the painting nor some of the deities are easily recognizable. (For additional reading see Dhagyag 1977.)

(See Color Plate 126)

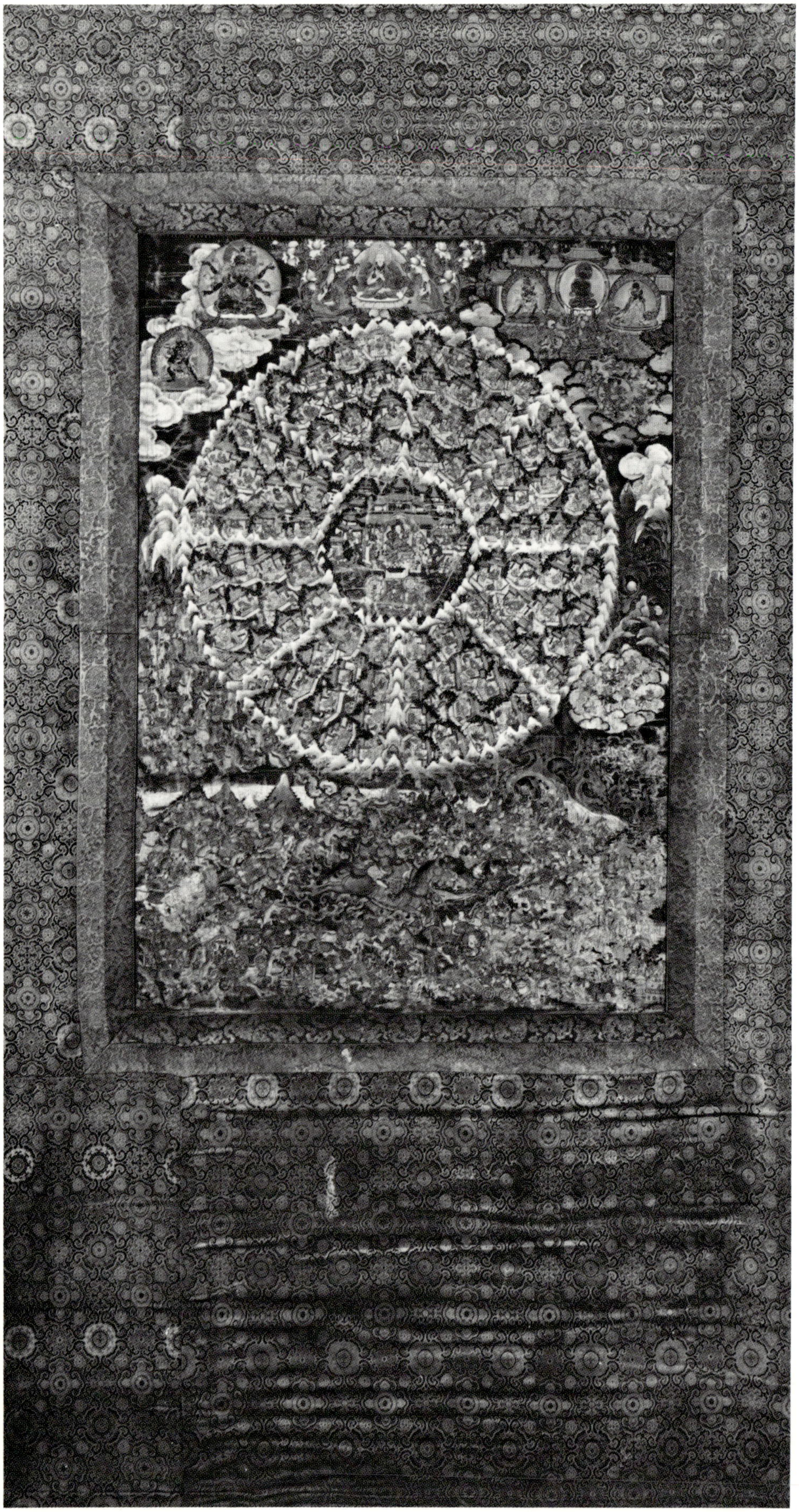

Pl. 127
The Kingdom of Shambhala
Paint on cloth
Tibet
Seventeenth-eighteenth century
H. 60 × 83.5 cm
Österreichisches Museum für Angewandte Kunst, Vienna
(32 315 mal. 164)

The theme of the Kingdom of Shambhala has a long and complex tradition which encompasses several regional variations. The legend of Shambhala is associated with the Kālacakra tradition (see Pls. 99,126). The mythic country of Shambhala is usually placed somewhere in the north, generally in Central Asia, and is sometimes suggested to be Khotan. Although called a *maṇḍala*, this representation has quite a different structure, as Tucci has pointed out (Tucci 1949:I,598–599). The upper two-thirds of the painting is occupied by an eight-part circle symbolizing the Kingdom of Shambhala as an eight-part lotus, each section (lotus leaf) containing twelve palaces, thereby equaling the ninety-six kingdoms. At the center is the capital, Kālapa, ruled over by the Rigs-ldan kings. Their association with the Kālacakra tradition is demonstrated by the presence of three of Rigs-ldan kings in the upper right-hand corner of Pl. 126. Painted at the top (center) of the painting is Tsong-kha-pa with a lama on either side; various deities are arranged around him, including Vajradhara and Yamāntaka. The Kingdom is protected by snow-covered mountains and the sacred river "Sita" (which some have identified with the Tarim River) runs beneath. At the bottom of the painting, a fierce battle rages between the Rigs-ldan Dragpo 'khorlo-can, his general Hamumanda, and the Muslim armies (the *Kla-klo*). According to one tradition, the success of Drag-po 'khorlo-can restores the Buddhist law—thus, a parallel can be seen with the traditions associated with Kalkī, an avatar of Viṣṇu. The various meditative teachings associated with Shambhala as well as the regional folk traditions have been studied by numerous scholars. [See related *t'ang-kas* in Musée Guimet (MA 1041; MG 24416); formerly Tucci collection (Tucci 1949:II,178); American Museum of Natural History, New York (70.2.870); Völkerkundemuseum der Universität Zürich (NR 13090); private collection, New Yorkc.)] For additional reading see Lokesh Chandra and Raghu Vira 1961–1972:20,260–262; Fux 1969; Birnbaum 1979; Béguine 1981:54–56; Hummel 1958.

Previously published: (Fux 1969).

See Color Plate 127

(d) Epilogue:

Vajrayāna Ritual and Art, A Contemporary Example

Although Buddhism disappeared in India, the land of its birth, its traditions and essential principles were preserved in Tibet. We have briefly surveyed the events that brought Buddhist monks, artists and ideas to the Himalayas, where they greatly enriched monasteries built to perpetuate the faith. But the law of impermanence, a fundamental Buddhist precept, admits no exceptions. Today these monasteries too are empty and once again Buddhist monks have travelled to India along the same routes which, seven hundred ago, had brought Buddhist refugees to the Himalayas. The cumulative effects of this history can be seen in the contemporary practice of Vajrayanā. An example, is the Tibetan ritual associated with the goddess Vajrayoginī. Both the altar assembled here (Pls. 128–140) and the ritual associated with it (Ch. VII.) further demonstrate the preservation of these traditions in America.

TIBETAN BUDDHISM IN EXILE

At certain times in its history, Buddhism has spread to new cultures with remarkable speed. In each of these cases, a force—either positive or negative—impelled Buddhist monks to leave their homeland. When Buddhism initially spread to Central Asia, China, and Tibet, missionaries were attracted by opportunity or invitation; economic conditions also encouraged the establishment of the new institutions. At other times, political and military hostility forced Buddhist monks into exile. The Muslim conquest of Afghanistan and western Central Asia in the eighth and ninth centuries forced monks to take refuge in the safer valleys of historical northwest India and the western Himalayas. The destruction of Buddhist monasteries in Tibet in the ninth century encouraged the foundation of new monasteries in the western Himalayas in the tenth century. In the twelfth and thirteenth centuries, the Muslim conquest of northeast India drove Indian Buddhists to Tibet and Nepal; since 1959, the Chinese occupation of Tibet has caused the reestablishment of Buddhist institutions in Nepal and India.

As we have noted, when Buddhism first came to Tibet it was embraced by only a small number of people; indeed the first monasteries had only a handful of monks (see Chapters V. and VIa). The story of the rebel Śākyamuni who renounced his home, class, and caste was enacted many times over as converts to the new philosophy in Tibet or Central Asia set themselves against the traditions of their fathers. When we consider the cultural transformation of Buddhism and most particularly the evolution of the esoteric systems, it is the image of the individualist, as well as the nonconformist which comes to mind. Of course, the monk could maintain his opposition to society's norms only so long as he remained outside society's establishments, including monastic institutions. Once Buddhism became a social institution with vested economic interests, the monk's role as social critic was severely restricted, and eventually eliminated.

As Buddhism was established in its various homelands, the socially critical attitude advanced by Śākyamuni changed drastically (Ch. VIa) and conventional Buddhist institutions received the support of established rulers and played a number of important roles in society. The members of these Buddhist orders possessed considerable social status and, as in all religious systems, many were more dedicated to worldly matters than to advanced meditative and intellectual teachings. The Mahayāna school has always encouraged the participation of laymen, and it was through their support that monastic communities survived. In the feudal periods the interlocking interests of the lay and monastic communities took on expanded economic and political dimensions, which sometimes obscured the spiritual role of the monastic community.

In response to this drastically different social function of Buddhism, new viewpoints and practices developed. One example is the meditative disciplines associated with Shambhala literature (Pl. 127). These disciplines relate Buddhist philosophical principles to secular (even military) life. Through the application of methods and perceptions derived from Vajrayāna psychology, the practitioner of these disciplines learns to transmute potentially negative or destructive situations into productive ones. The Shambhala teachings are only one example of

Vajrayāna practices which allow the layman, even someone with an apparently non-Buddhist occupation (such as a military man), to follow the Buddhist *dharma*. This is perhaps the most creative example of Buddhist involvement in secular life.

The long distance which Buddhism had traveled from the ascetic ideals and simplicity preached by Śākyamuni is well-illustrated by a seventeenth-century painting of Padmasaṃbhava. Here the image of the *yogī*, the ascetic character of earlier literature, or the divinized patriarch (Pl. 100) is replaced by a worldly teacher dressed in brocades and enthroned in a luxuriant paradise. But this is only one of the aspects of Padmasaṃbhava, as it is only one of the ideals of later Tibetan Buddhism. As we mentioned earlier (Chapter VIa), Padmasaṃbhava is best known as a *siddha*, a holy man. This tradition originated in the Indian *siddha* schools from which the special Tibetan technique of Yoga also derived. In reading the stories of the lives of the eighty-four *siddhas* and the descriptions of their frequently anarchistic behavior, one is reminded of the early conflict between Buddhism and established social tradition. The bizarre character depicted in the legends of the magician-saint Padmasaṃbhava may well represent an ascetic tradition prevalent in northwest India of about the eighth century A.D. In Vajrayāna, the respect accorded unconventional Buddhist practices is found in later centuries as well. The poet Milarepa (*Mi-la ras-pa*) began his life by practicing black magic, endured incredible trials in order to study *dharma* with his teacher Mar-pa (the Kagyud patriarch, d. 1098), then spent the rest of his life meditating in a cave, eating green nettles, and composing songs which are still sung in Tibet. Another example of an extreme individualist is the female saint Machik Drönma (*Ma-gcig bslab-kyi-sgron-ma,* 1055–1145; Pl. 115), who founded a special branch of the *gcod* tradition. The teachings of this school are quite distinct from the major sects. They are based on the Prajñāpāramitā tradition, but also show the influence of ancient Tibetan and shamanist practices. The use by *gcod* practitioners of demonic forces and macabre rituals clearly demonstrated their disdain for society and its conventions (Tucci 1980:87–92).

An ascetic is bound to reject a materialist society. The necessity of formulating an independent and critical attitude toward one's society was one of the essential lessons taught through the example of the life of the Buddha Śākyamuni. This perception persists in other monastic systems, such as Christianity. In a talk on "Marxism and Monasticism," the Capuchin monk, Thomas Merton, compared the monk and the socialist revolutionary and pointed out that each is "essentially someone who takes up a critical attitude toward the contemporary world and its structures." (quoted in Fields 1981:300). The difference is that the Marxist seeks to change economic structures, while the monk seeks to change psychological structures. But it is always difficult for an individual to maintain a socially critical attitude from within a community. As in all organized religious systems, the self-perpetuating interests of the institution frequently took precedence over spiritual functions. I noted earlier that these different trends always existed in Tibetan Buddhism—the conventional practice of Buddhism being tied to monastic establishments and official patronage while the more unconventional, individualist practitioners eschewed both.

It is perhaps too early for a sociological study of Buddhist converts in North America and Europe, but such a study might find that the spread of Buddhist sects in the West is connected with the bourgeois alienation found throughout Western urban centers. Western converts are likely to come from the urban bourgeoisie. Both their relative economic stability and their taste for exoticism enables these twentieth-century converts, like the new converts of the eighth or tenth century, to support new Buddhist institutions and accept foreign and somewhat socially critical ideas (Fields 1981).

This sense of alienation and conflict with existing social norms has attracted Westerners to other Asian cults besides Buddhism, as well as to new Christian movements. One indication of the link between the phenomenon of western involvement in these cults and social discontent is the curious fact that many of these western converts had previously been involved in political activism. While today these practitioners are often seen by their peers as attempting to "escape from life," there are others who are drawn to Buddhism for exactly the opposite reason. The principal technique of Buddhism, meditation, is now being sought by an educated elite in both the East and West as a means of successfully coping with urban stress and thereby acquiring material advantages. As we have seen, when Buddhism travelled beyond the confines of the Hindu-Buddhist societies of India, aspects of both its belief structures and institutions adapted to the varying social and economic circumstances. Similarly today, various forms of Buddhism, Mahayāna, and Theravadin are adapting to new social environments far beyond their traditional cultural settings. One can presume that the gap between doctrine (as recorded in scriptures) and actual beliefs and practices (which incorporates non- and pre-Buddhist elements) continues today in Western and traditional Eastern societies as it had in mediaeval Himalayan societies.[1]

Another limited but historically interesting phenomenon that deserves study is the recent interest in Buddhism in India. This fascinating process, which preceded the Tibetan refugee movement, involves for the most part conversion to schools of Buddhism other than Vajrayāna. The small number of converts appear to come from different regions. The majority belong to the Harijan (untouchable) caste, while some belong to the intelligentsia. This movement is generally said to have begun in 1891 with the founding of the Mahā Bodhi Society of India, which since then has actively propagated Buddhism in the land of its birth. The single most dramatic event occurred in 1966 when Dr. B.R. Ambedkar, the Harijan leader, announced that he and a half million of his followers had converted to Buddhism. This new phase of Buddhism in India is so recent that it is not yet possible to understand its true impact on Indian society, nor the effect of this experience on the various Buddhist institutions in different parts of India. But it would seem that once again, Indian Buddhism is playing a role in the expression of social protest.

The majority of Tibetan refugees and new converts is concentrated in northern India, the area where Buddhism flourished a millennium ago. This relocation of Buddhism back across the Himalayas is not really surprising for, as Staal pointed out in the third chapter, "most features of Tibetan Buddhism were originally Indian." Furthermore, as we have seen in Chapter VIa, there has always been a fluid and creative interaction between Buddhism and Hinduism. From one point of view, it is possible to see this new phase of Buddhism in India as the latest stage in the continuous exchange of peoples and ideas across the Himalayas. It is undoubtedly in part because of this appreciation of the Indian roots of Vajrayanā that the Indian government has substantially assisted the Tibetans in preserving their culture. One important example is the government-sponsored college of Buddhist studies near Leh. Its ambitious goal is to train Buddhists of all sects, who for decades have been cut off from the Tibetan institutions of higher learning that had nurtured Ladahki Buddhism for centuries. (Ch. III).

Seen from an historical perspective, the revival of Buddhism in twentieth-century India and the transplantation to America is simply a new phase in the old process of transmission and revitalization. Once again, the migration of teachers and Buddhism has been motivated either by adverse political circumstances (as in the case of Tibetan Buddhism) or favorable circumstances (as in the case of Japanese or Southeast Asian Buddhism). Not surprisingly, the re-creation of Buddhist institutions has been facilitated by access to economic resources.

I use the term re-creation to refer to the inevitable need to translate and interpret Buddhist texts for each new culture. The subtle transformation of Buddhism that occurred as texts were translated, commented on, and retranslated has been referred to several times in this study. We have also noted that differences in language and cultural perspective inevitably result in change and confusion. The translations of Buddhist texts into the Iranian and Altaic languages found in Central Asia provide fascinating evidence of this process of adaptation and transformation. Strickmann has examined this process in China (Ch. IV). Xuanzang tells us that it was his concern about the authenticity of the texts Chinese Buddhists had received that prompted him to travel to India to search for Sanskrit originals. Today, many centuries later, Buddhists are still arguing over whether Chinese, Japanese, or Tibetan texts convey the "original" meanings of the *sūtras* or *tantras*. As we have seen, in China the importance of "authentic Indian textual sources" was openly espoused, while the usefulness of Chinese adaptations of Indian Buddhism was tacitly acknowledged (Ch. IV).

TIBETAN BUDDHISM IN THE WEST

Since the nineteenth century, Buddhist texts have been translated from a variety of Asian languages into western languages. Because of the inaccessibility of Tibetan Buddhist teachers and their texts, translations from Tibetan Buddhist sources were relatively limited until the 1950s. Today, Tibetan Buddhist teachers themselves are collaborating on the translation of Tibetan texts so that entire rituals can now be performed in English.[2] Future scholarship will undoubtedly analyze how English translations of Asian Buddhist literature have unintentionally distorted the original meaning of these works.

A parallel phenomenon is the admission of Westerners into Asian Buddhist orders. This process has been occurring since the previous century, but it seems to have become increasingly popular in recent years because affluence and air travel have made it easier for Western Buddhists to travel to Asian monasteries. It is presumed that in many cases these new monks will return to participate in the establishment of American Buddhist institutions, such as Vajrayāna centers.

The study of Vajrayāna became popular in the West only after Tibetan refugees began arriving in the 1960s. Since that time, interest in Vajrayāna has increased sufficiently to suggest that some Tibetans consider the United States as a new center for the practice of Vajrayāna Buddhism. In the summer of 1981, the Dalai Lama, spritual and temporal leader of the Tibetan people and the head of the Yellow Hat reform sect called the Ge-lug-pa, performed the entire Kālahakra (Pl. 126) initiation (including the explanatory teachings) in Deer Park, Wisconsin. This ceremony was rarely performed even in Tibet. According to tradition a Dalai Lama is only supposed to perform it three times in his life, but the present Dalai Lama has already performed this ceremony more often.

In the fall of the same year, the sixteenth Gyal-wa Karmapa, then terminally ill, chose to return to the United States. He had taught in America on three earlier occasions and considered this country fertile ground for the teaching of Buddhism. Some ten days after his arrival, he died in Zion, Illinois. It was the first time any high incarnate lama (believed by Tibetans to be "living Buddhas") had died outside Asia. The lineage of the Karmapas was committed to the active propagation of the teachings of the Kagyu lineage and, for this reason, many of the earlier Karmapas had traveled incessantly throughout Tibet, Mongolia, and eastern China. The extensive travels of the sixteenth Karmapa (including his visits to America) were seen by his followers as a continuation of this responsibility.

This contemporary phase of missionary work is a continuation of the historical process that was responsible for the spread of Tibetan Buddhism in the Indian Himalayas, China, and Mongolia. The Karma Kayud continues to operate monasteries in India, the Himalayan states, and Europe; and an incarnate lama (tulku) of the order, Chogÿam Trungpa, Rinpoche, former abbot of a group of monasteries in Kham (eastern Tibet), has been teaching and establishing monasteries in the West for almost two decades. In Chapter VII, he translates from the traditional Kagyud liturgy on Vajrayoginī and provides his own explanation (derived from traditional commentaries) of this practice as it relates to, and is understood by, contemporary Westerners. He provides a bridge between the past and the present. All the Tibetan orders are similarly attempting to perpetuate their traditions through teaching, the establishment of contemplative centers, and the translation of their texts into western languages.

In addition to the Gelug-pa and Kargyupa orders, the heads of the other major communities also live in exile and have established centers in North America as well as in many other countries. The Nying-ma-pa (rñin-ma-pa) is the oldest of the orders and traces its lineage to the eighth century and Padmasaṃbhava (Pl. 100). His Holiness, Dudjom Rinpoche, is the head of this order. He lives in Kathmandu, Nepal. Following the tradition of the yogis, he wears his hair long and is a married layman. The hereditary head of the Sakya-pa order (Sa-skya-pa), His Holiness Sakya Trizin is descended from the noble Khoṅ family, which in 1073 founded Sakya monastery, the seat of this order until 1959. Today, his main monastery is in Dehra Dun, India. One of the major sub-monasteries of this order, Ngor Evam (founded in 1429), was a major cultural center (Pl. 125). It was destroyed after the Chinese occupation of Tibet in 1959. One of the last abbots of Ngor, Thartse Khen-po Rinpoche, has taught in the United States, Europe, and Japan and has contributed to this study.

Most of the monasteries in Tibet are now closed; but the lamas educated in those monasteries, considered the "lineage holders" of these traditions by their followers, are now scattered throughout the world. Today, they continue the missionary traditions of their respective orders, and preach the *dharma* just as the wandering monks of India did more than two thousand years ago. This missionary activity has always been facilitated by the ease with which Buddhism can be adapted to different ideas and lifestyles. In contrast to several other religious systems, Buddhism has neither a racial nor an ethnic bias. Buddhist philosophy (the more sophisticated insist Buddhism is not a religion; see Ch. III) is often easily grasped by Westerners attracted to a nonmaterialist viewpoint. There are, of course, many reasons for the impact of eastern philosophical systems on many leading intellectual and artistic figures in the West, but an examination of this interesting phenomenon would take us far beyond the confines of this study. It is only necessary to note here that what we are actually dealing with is a process of cross-cultural interaction. Many monks are naturally affected by their exposure to western philosophical traditions as well. Equally important, many Eastern Buddhists have been profoundly affected by western materialist doctrines such as Marxism. Many Tibetan intellectuals, after coming to the West, have openly discussed the weaknesses that had existed in Tibetan Feudal society prior to 1959. These discussions inevitably lead to a critical examination of the history of Buddhism, its methods and goals.

Vajrayāna is distinguished from earlier forms of Buddhism by its complex ritual and associated imagery. The goal of most Vajrayāna rituals is to achieve power over oneself and the various "forces" of the phenomenal world, then ultimately to transcend the limitations of both. Given this grandeur of purpose it is remarkable that the iconograhy associated with specific rituals has remained so consistent in the various countries where they were performed. The strict preservation of the iconographic details was important to the ultimate success of the ritual. In this context it is of some interest to consider Buddhist imagery as it is used in ritual practice (Chs. V and VII).

The demands for objective accuracy in the ritual over subjective, artistic interpretation has meant that the iconography has remained essentially the same for almost one thousand years. Naturally, these practices did not survive as discrete entities, but rather as part of the entire ritual and philosophical system of contemporary Tibetan Buddhism. The focus of these ritual practices is an altar, represented here by the Vajrayoginī altar (Ill. 4).

One of the most striking examples of this phenomenon is the survival of the cult of the female divinity, Vajrayoginī, who, according to legend contained in the liturgy, originated in Uḍḍiyāna, northern Pakistan, where the worship of female spirits and divinities is particularly popular. The cult of this goddess is found throughout the Himalayas (Pls. 112,114,125,128), and is now even observed in the West by those who practice the traditional Tibetan ritual in English.

The image and the liturgy—*mudrā*, *mantra* and visualization, combined with the distinctive music—remain similar to those used hundreds of years ago. But the nature of the individual experience is more elusive. The Tibetans believe that the liturgy transforms the nature of consciousness, so that through meditation and devotional practice, one may ultimately attain "enlightened mind" (*bodhi*). In this sense, therefore, the contemporary Buddhist is descended from the worshipper in ancient Uḍḍiyāna who devoutly called forth the image of Vajrayoginī in the hope that the goddess would assist him or her in the quest for enlightenment.

Notes

---

1. Among the anthropological studies analyzing this phenomenon in traditional Buddhist societies of Southeast Asia see Melford E. Spiro, *Buddhism and society, a great tradition and its Burmese vicissitudes* Berkeley, 1970; and Sherry B. Ortner, *Sherppas through their Rituals*. Cambridge, 1978.
2. The liturgy (*sādhana*) for Vajrayoginī quoted in Chapter VII was translated by the Nālandā translation committee in Boulder, Colorado under the direction of the Vajrācārya, Chōgyam Trungpa, Rinpoche. This English text has been used in Colorado since 1977 in the Kagyud-pa performance of the Vajrayoginī ritual.

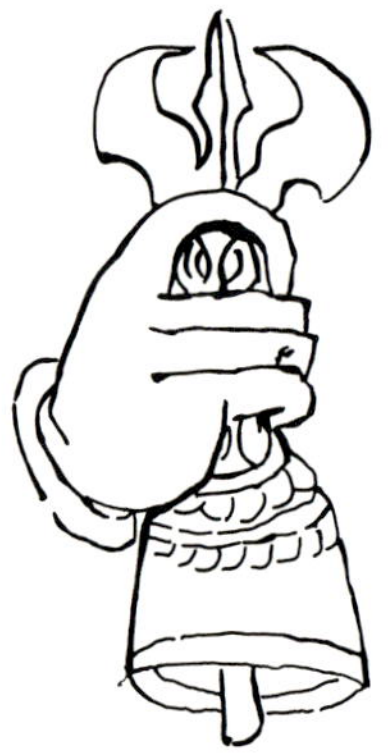

Catalogue Entries

Plates: 128-140

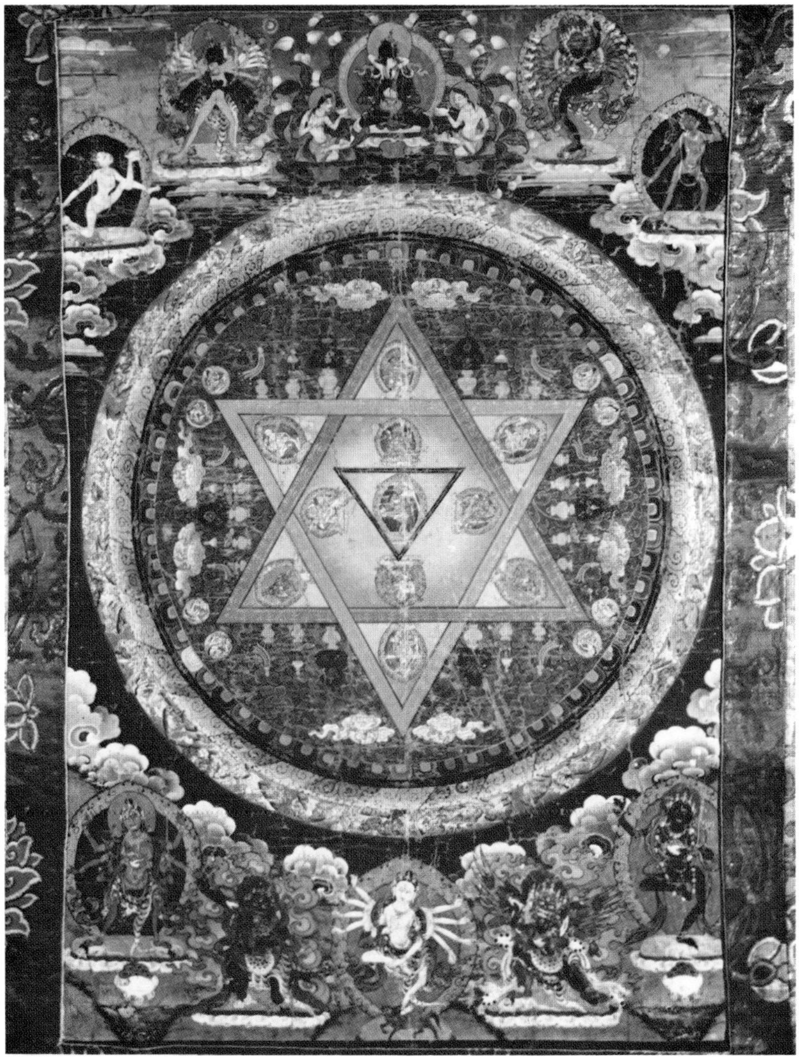

Pl. 128
Vajrayoginī
Paint on cloth
Tibet
Seventh century
H. 66.04 × 43.81 cm
Doris Weiner Gallery, New York
Previously published: (Doris Weiner Gallery 1974)

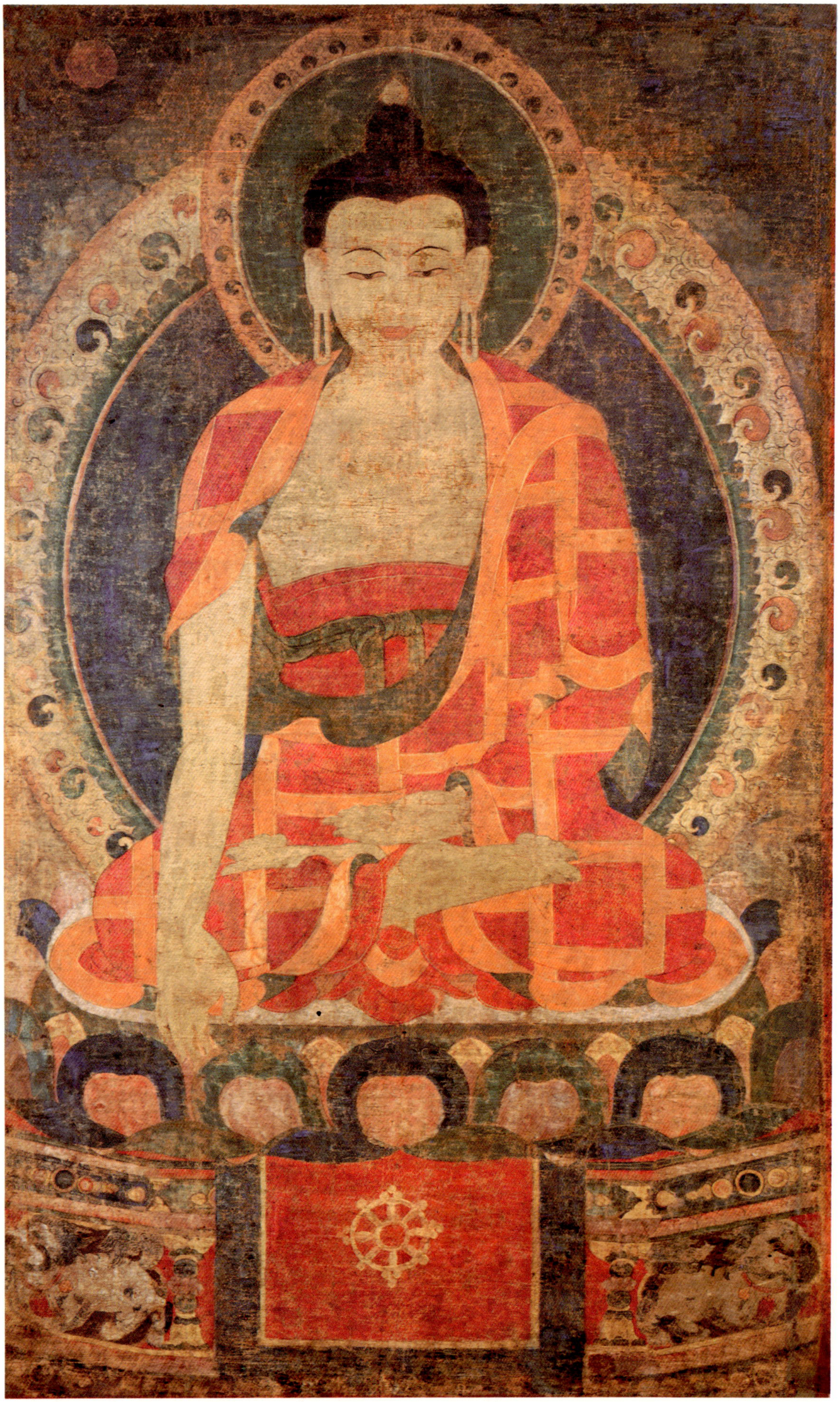

Pl. 119

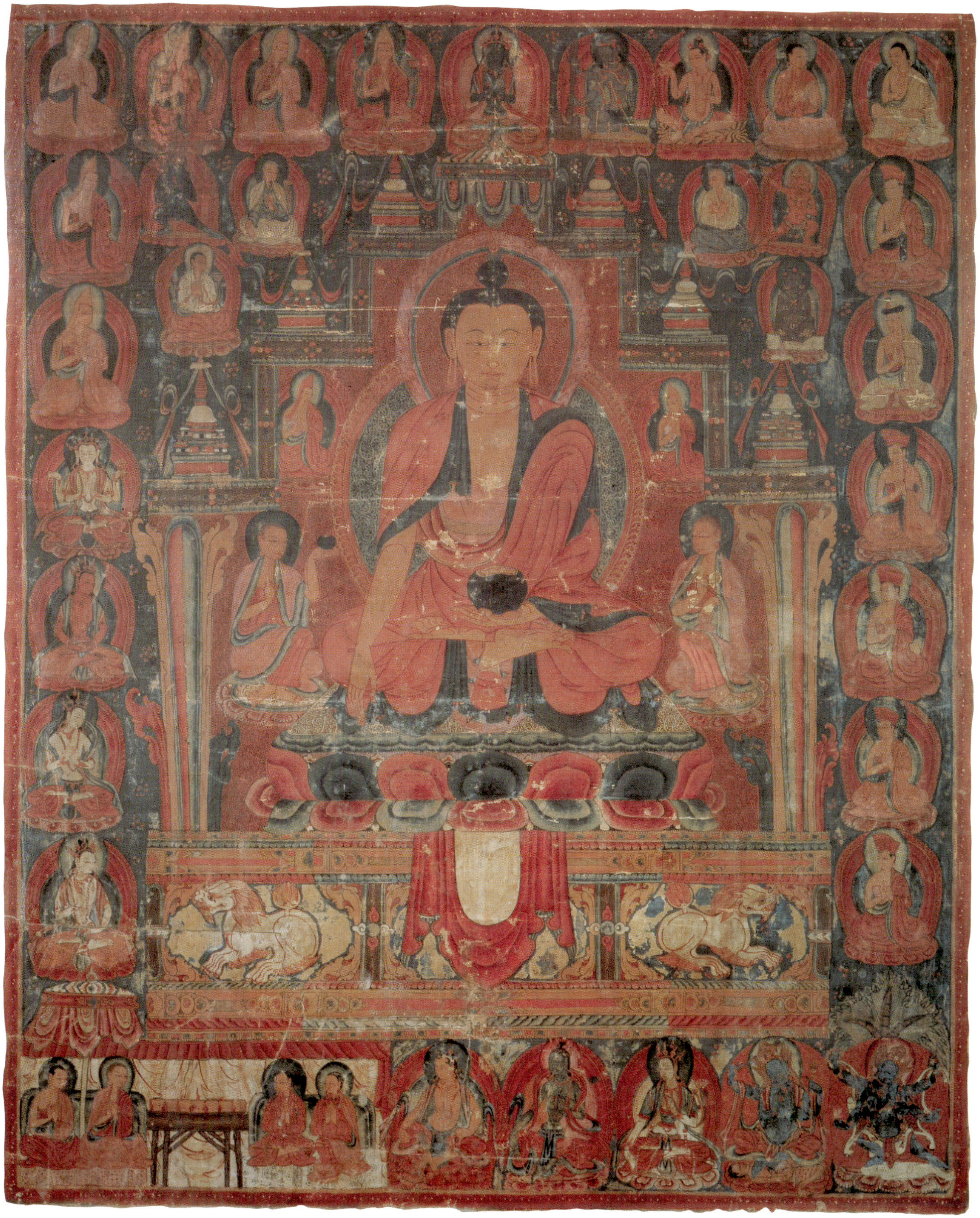

Pl. 120

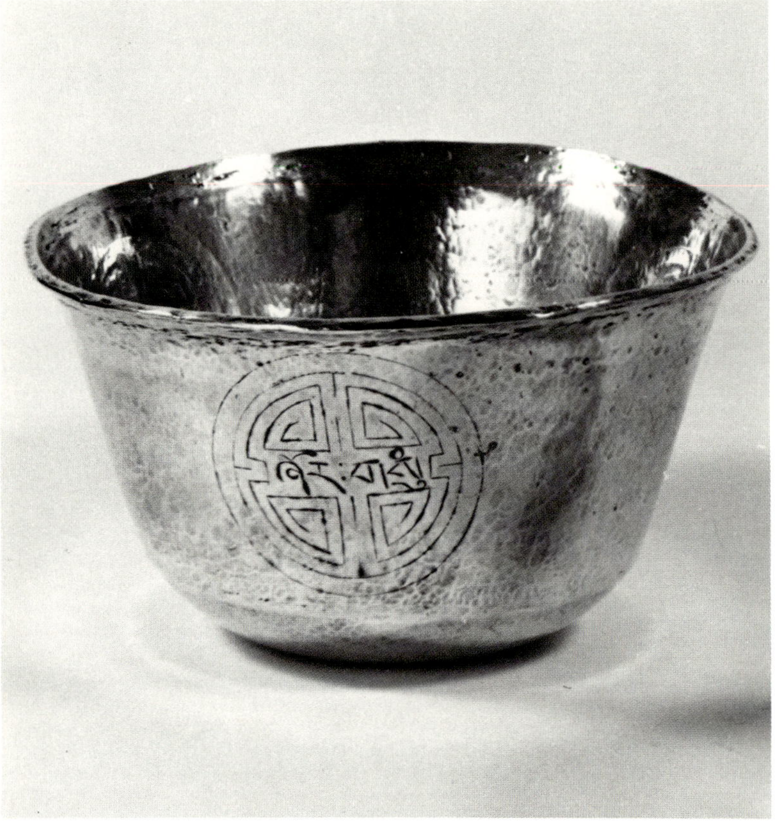

Pl. 129
Offering Bowl
Silver
Tibet
Nineteenth century or earlier
H. 16.5 × 18.4 cm
The Newark Museum
(#320.316–78, #324-5-6-7)

Pl. 130
Wall Hangings
Brocade. Applique: cut and sewn silk brocade, cord and floss on cotton backing stiffened with cardboard filling. Streamers formed of cut and sewn chevrons with silk floss tassel, some added watercolor tints.
Materials of Chinese manufacture; painting, cutting and stitching done in Tibet. Reportedly from a monastery in Lhasa.
Eighteenth-nineteenth centuries

L. 350.84 cm. each
Collection of the Newark Museum. 74.125 A–B

Used to decorate pillars in Tibetan Buddhist chanting hall or altar.

Previously published: (Reynolds 1978:no.136).

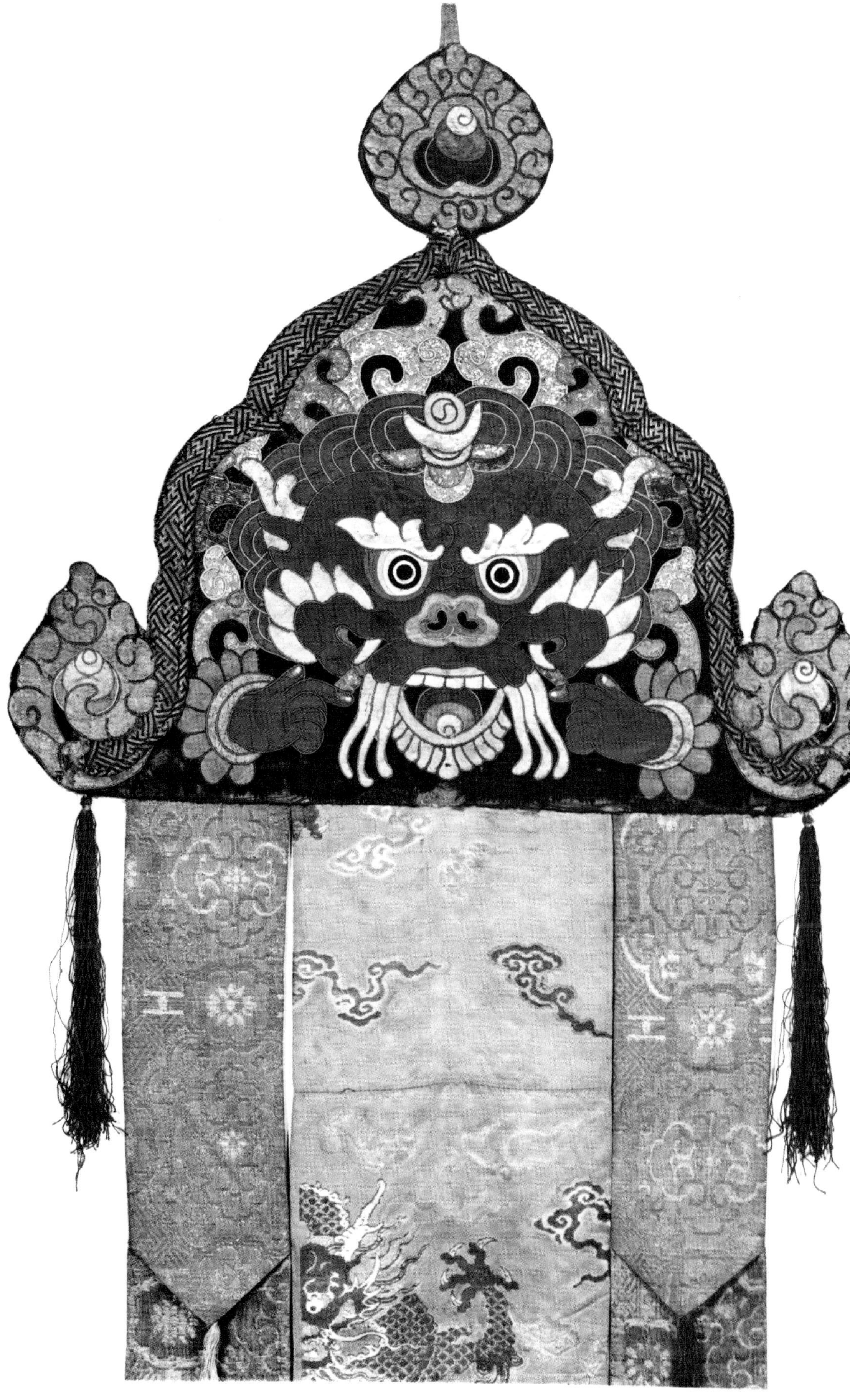

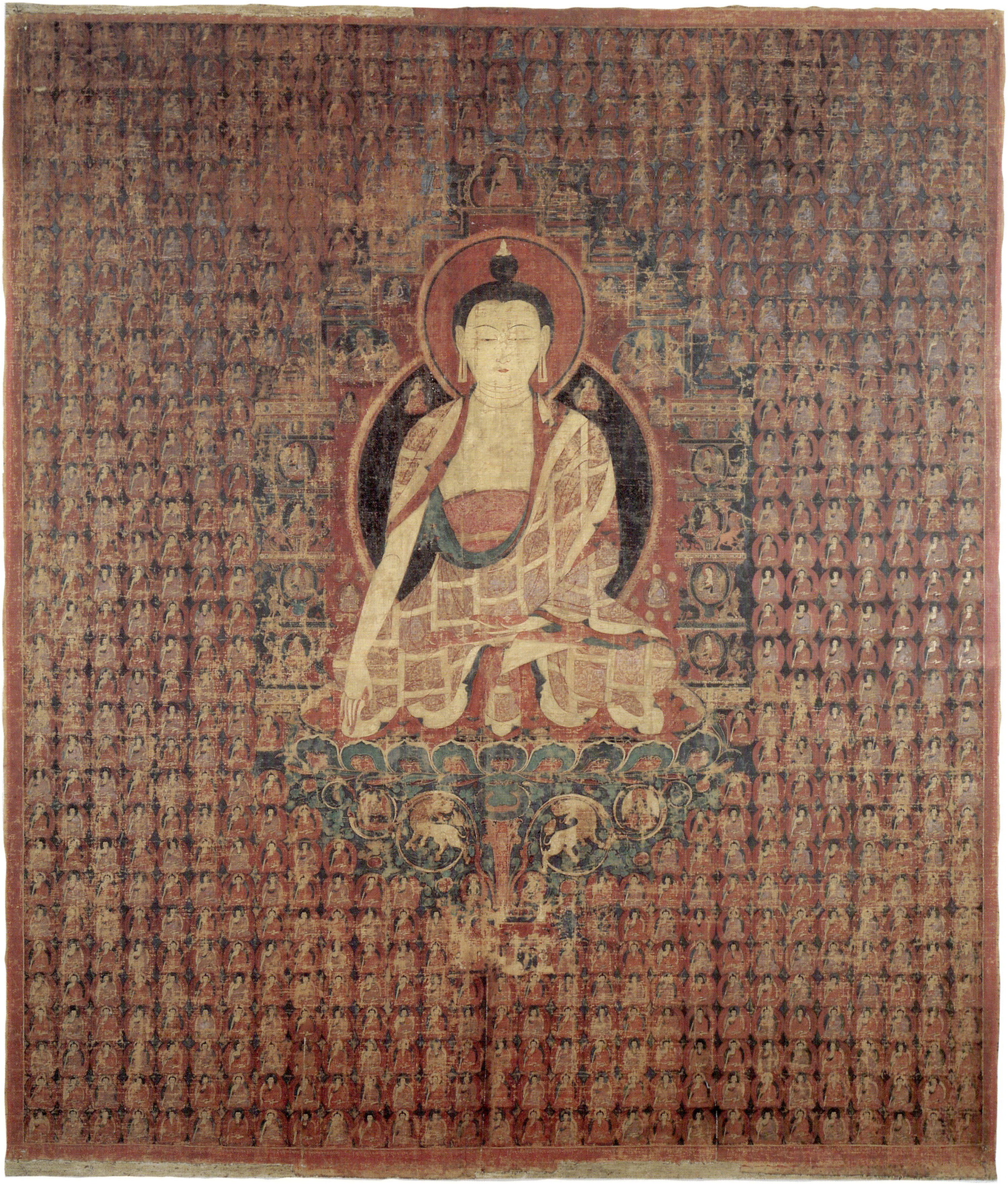

Pl. 121

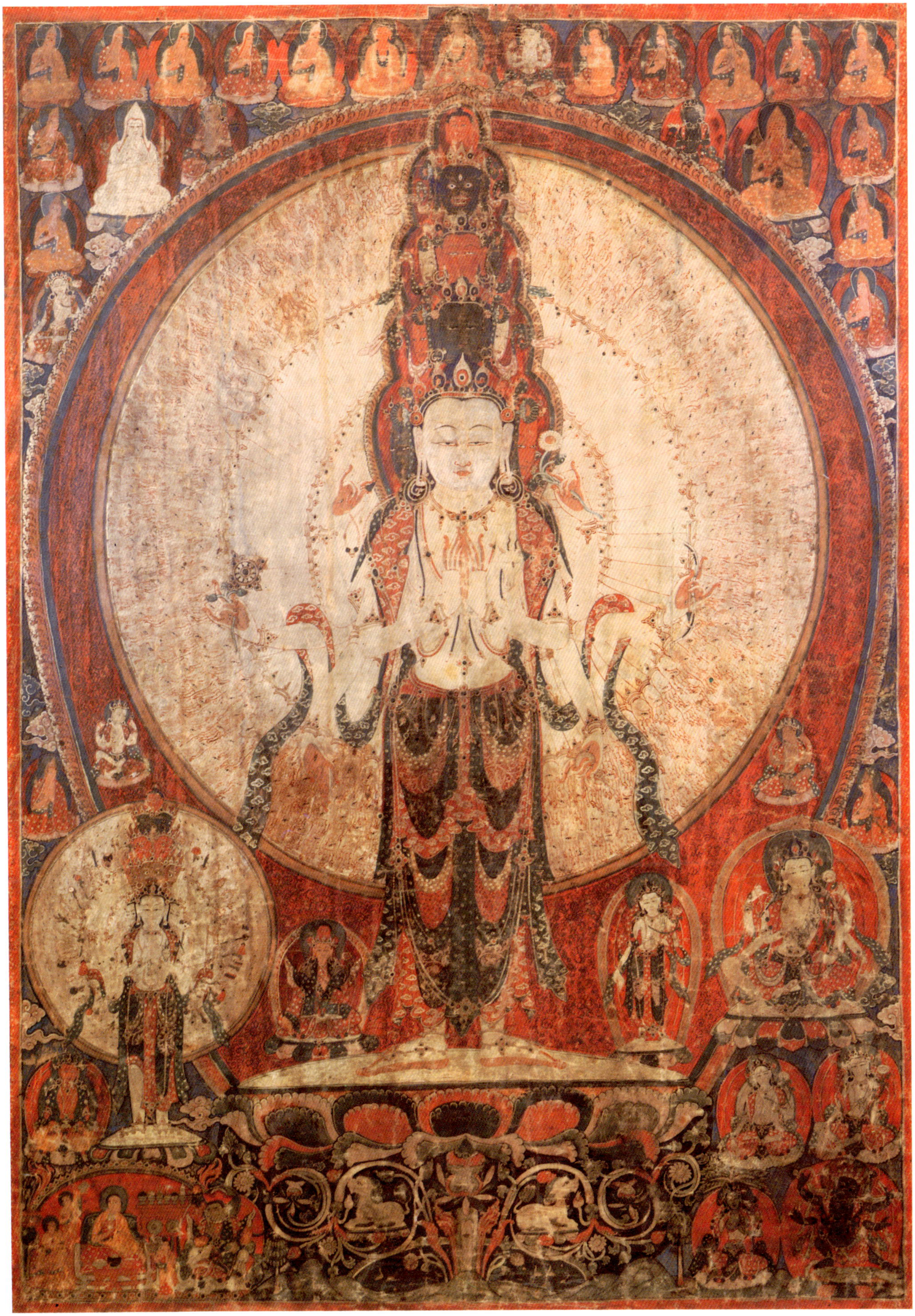

Pl. 122

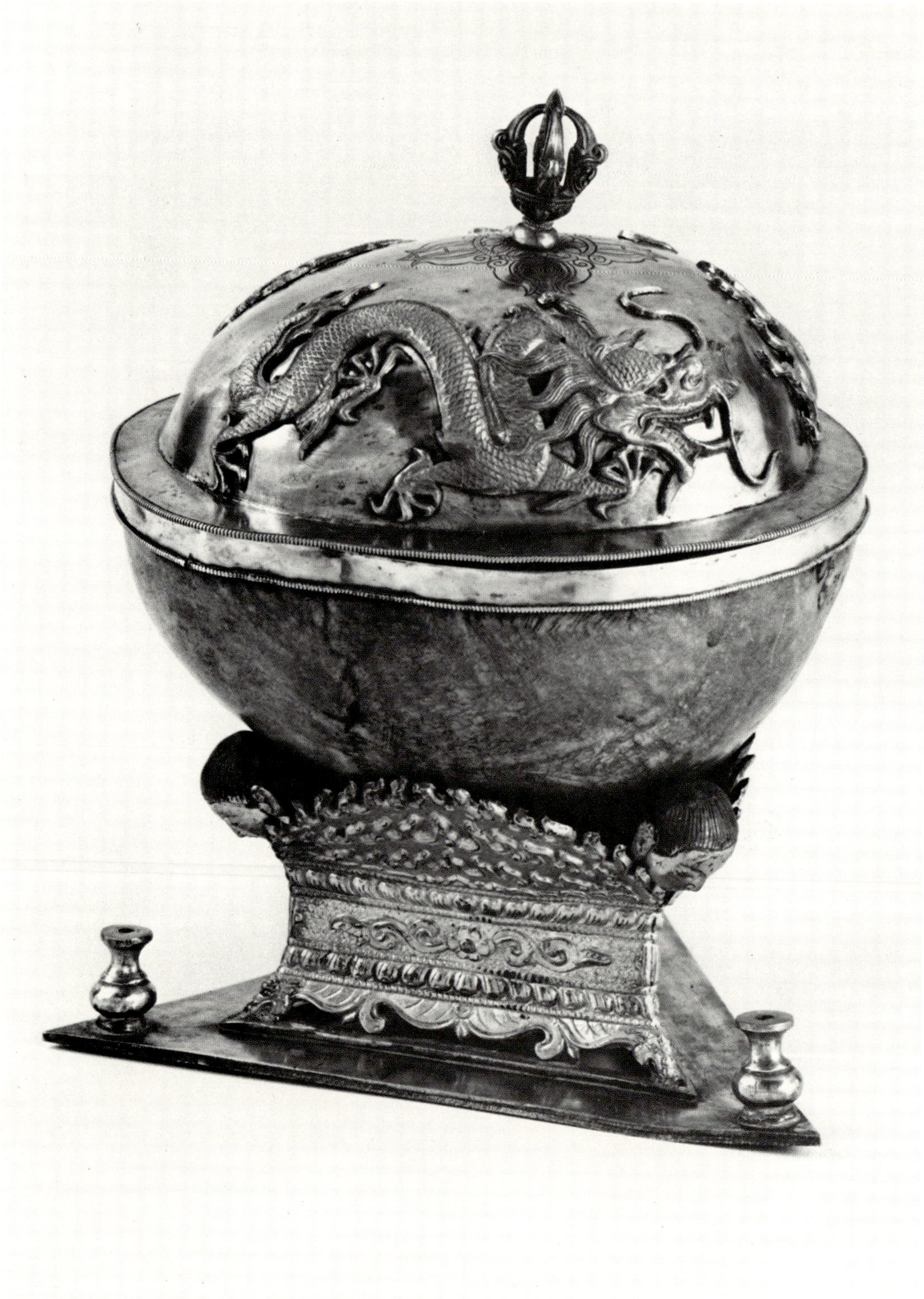

Pl. 131
Skull Cup with Stand and Lid
Human skull lined with copper, silver trim; copper lid with gilt appliqué; gilt copper stand.
Tibet, possibly of Newar workmanship
Nineteenth century or earlier
H. 21.5 cm
Collection of the Newark Museum. 62.103.

Used in ceremonies involving the fierce deities.

Previously published: (Newark Museum 1950–1971:V,34,pl.19).

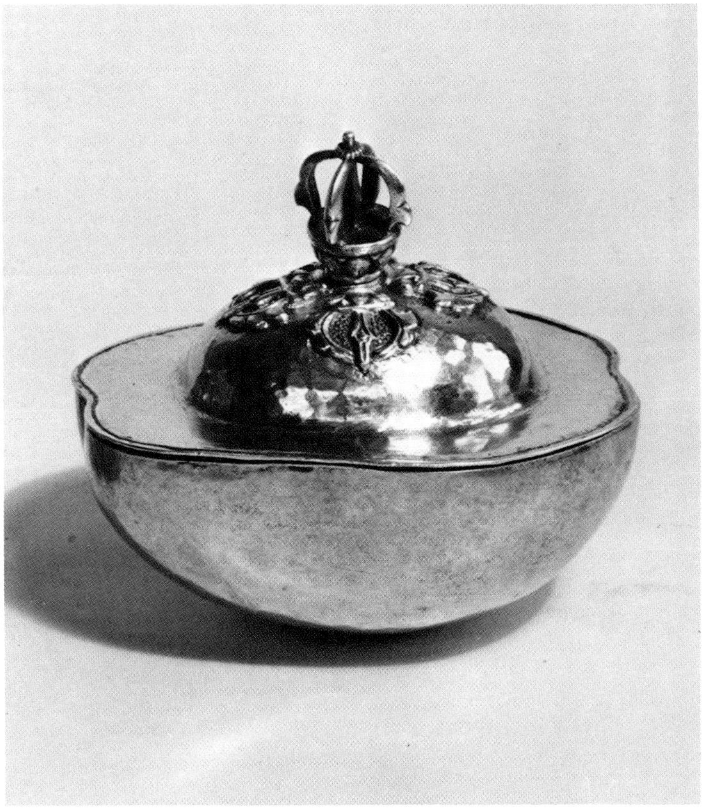

Pl. 132
Skull-shaped Cup with Cover
Cast and hammered silver
Eastern Tibet
Nineteenth century or earlier
H. 7.62 cm
Collection of the Newark Museum. 11.669

Used in ceremonies involving the fierce deities. Obtained by Dr. Shelton in Sichuan, East Tibet, probably from Batang monastery.

Previously published: (Newark Museum 1950–1971:V,50; Reynolds 1978:no.132).

Pl. 133
Offering Bowl
Hammered brass (bell metal)
Eastern Tibet
Nineteenth century
Range: 12.7–20 cm
Collection of the Newark Museum. 20.366 A–G; 20.365 A–F. Obtained by Dr. Shelton from Batang monastery.

Previously published: (Newark Museum 1950–1971:II,46–47).

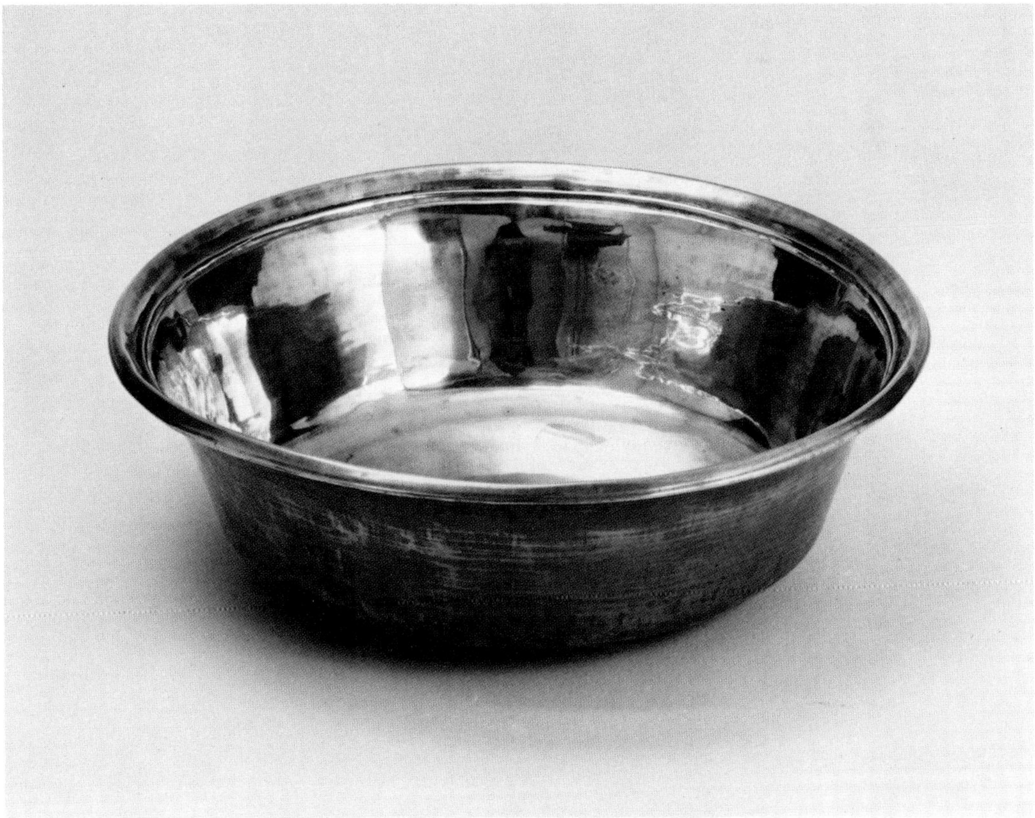

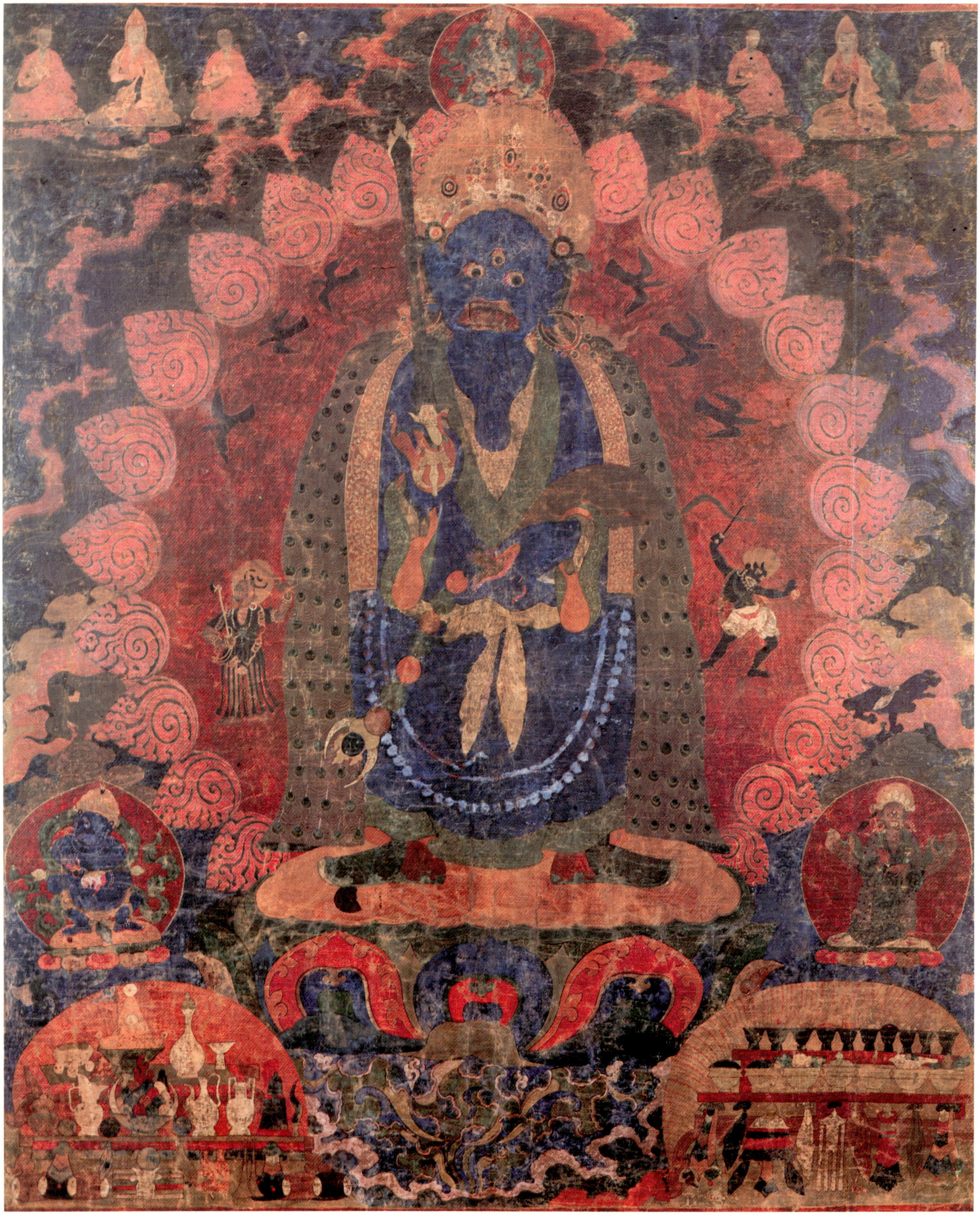

Pl. 124

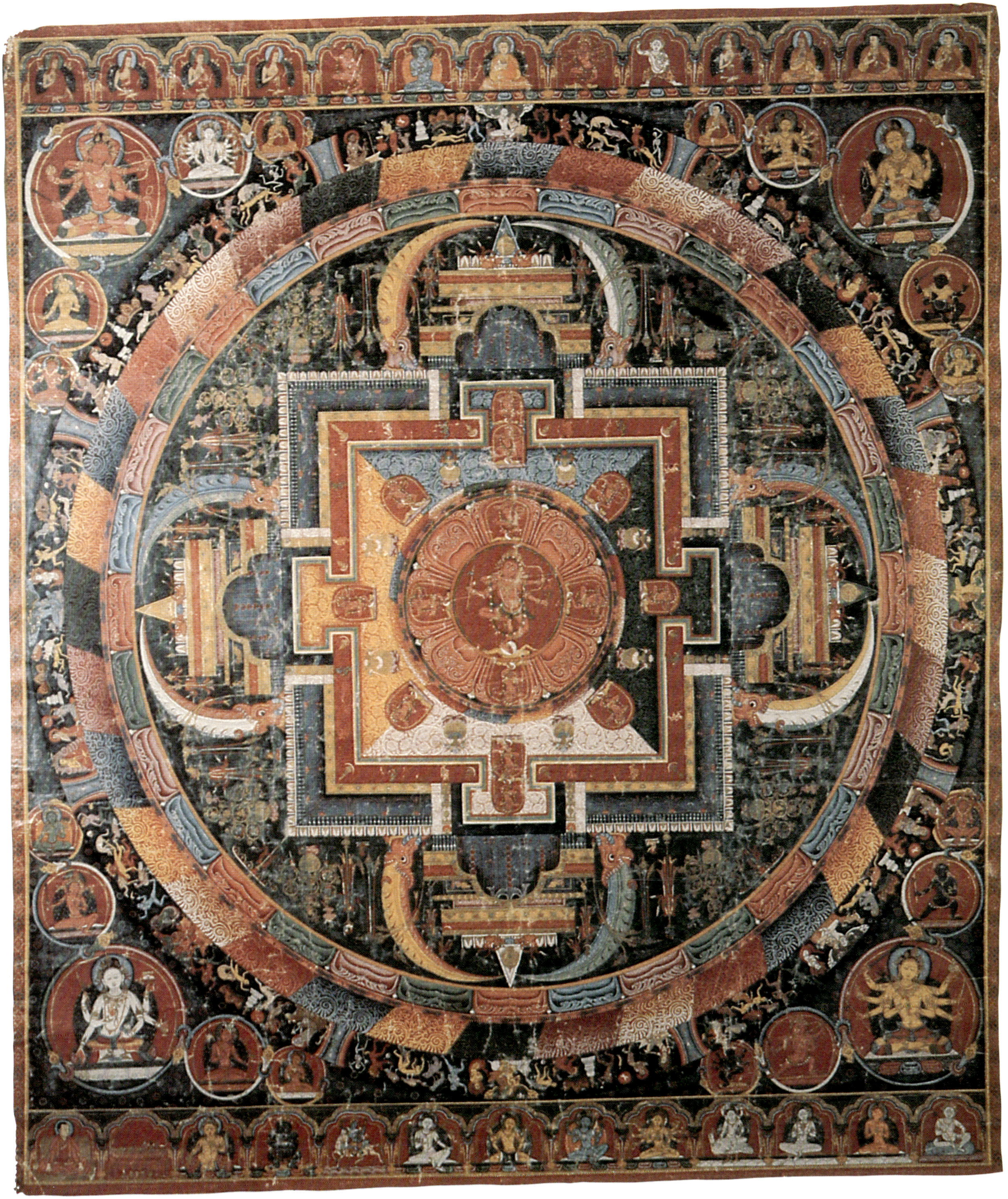

Pl. 125

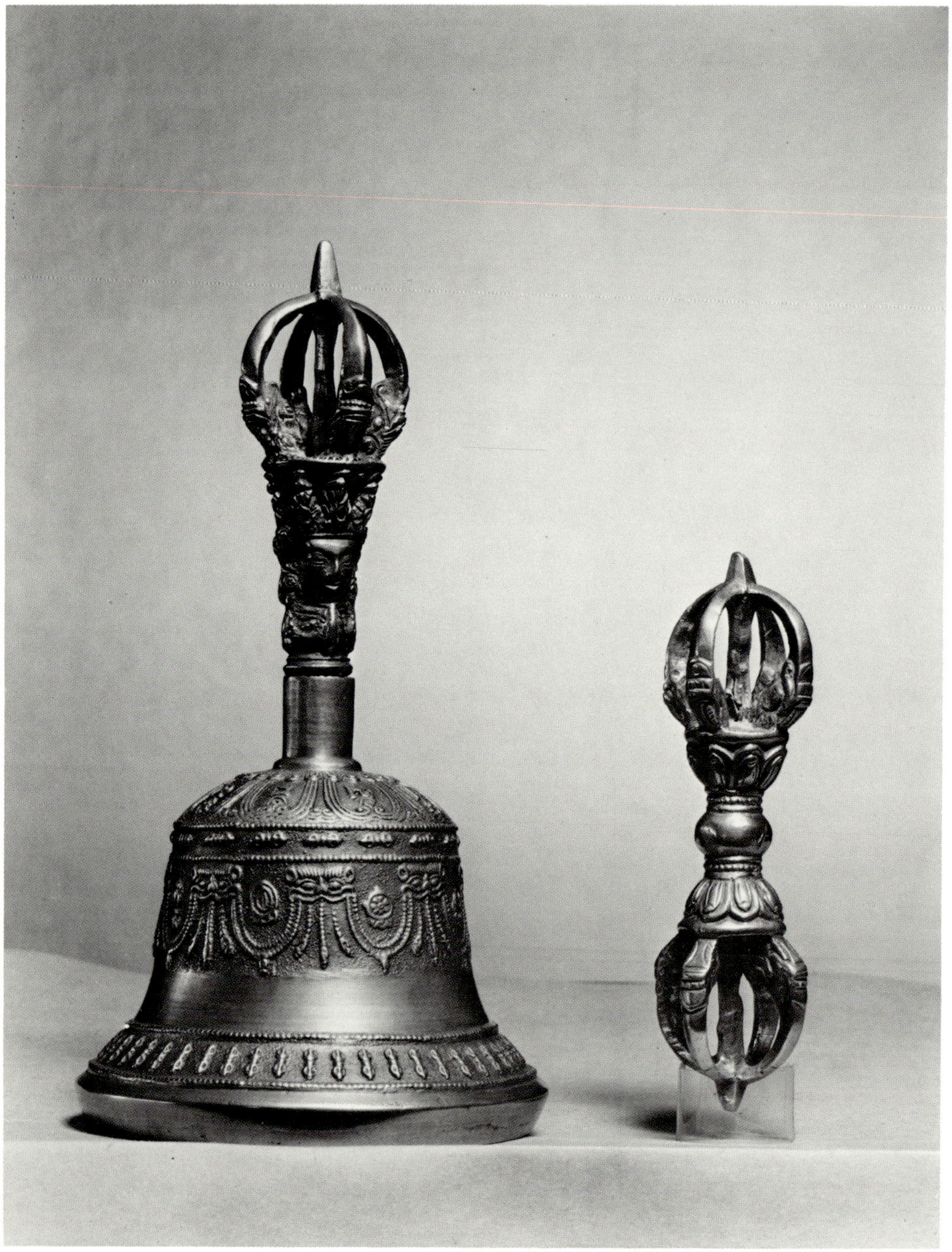

Pl. 134
Bell and rDor-je
Bell: hollow cast brass (bell metal) with solid cast brass handle; cast brass handle attached with leather. Eight Tibetan syllables in cast relief on shoulder: lam, bam, mam, tsum, pam, bhrim, tam, nam(?); interior syllables: Om Āḥ Hūm. rDor-je: solid cast brass.
Tibet
Nineteenth century
Bell: H. 18.1 cm; rDor-je: H. 11.4 cm
Collection of the Newark Museum. 20.398–9. Obtained by Dr. Shelton from Batang monastery.

Previously published: (Newark Museum 1950–1971:II,35–36).

Pl. 135
Butter Lamps
Hammered silver
Eastern Tibet
Nineteenth century or earlier
H. Range 10.5–18.2 cm
Collection of the Newark Collection. 20.341, 346, 348 A–B, 349.

Previously published: (Newark Museum 1950–1971:II,39; Musée Guimet 1977:no.364; Reynolds 1978:no.124).

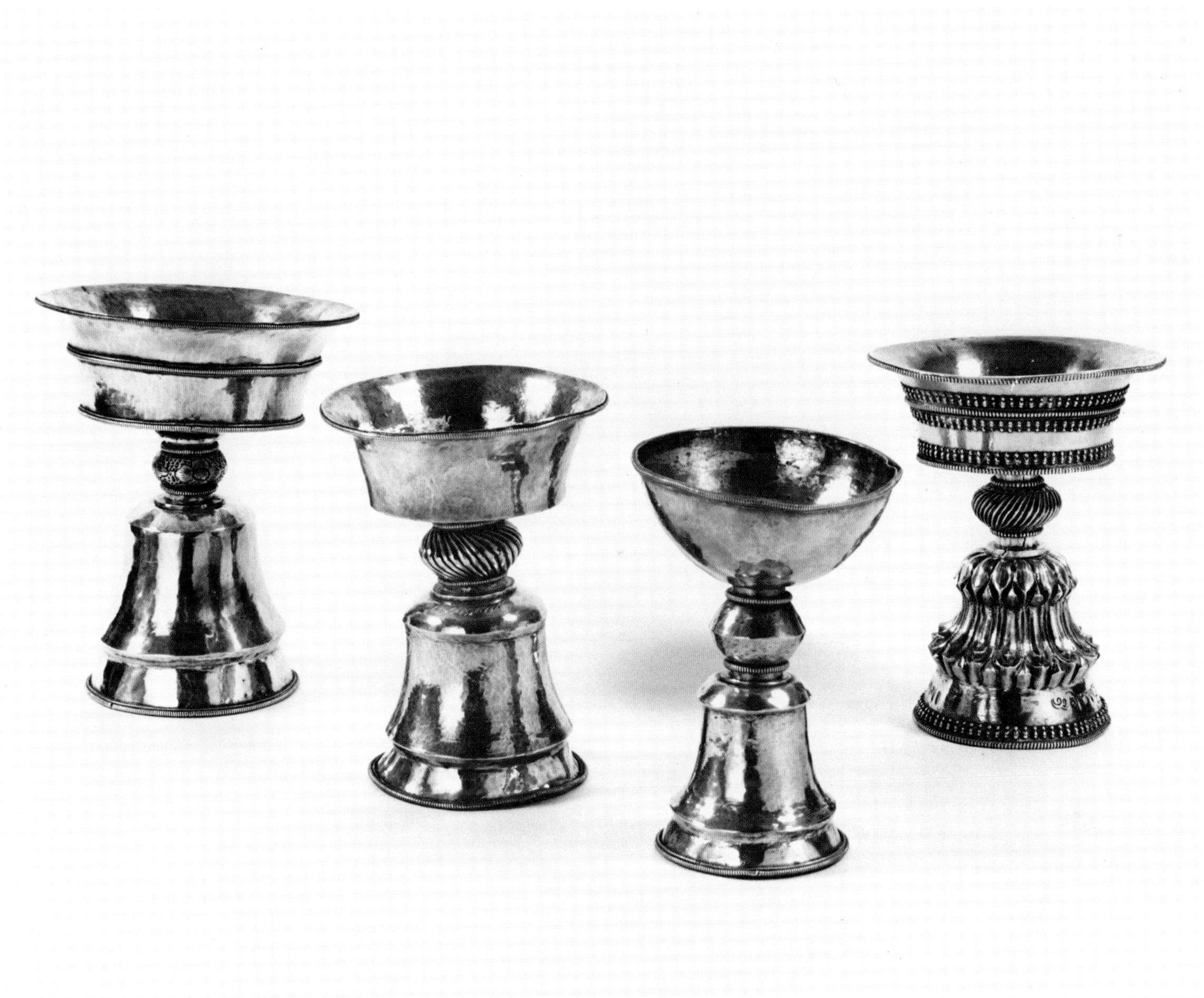

Pl. 135

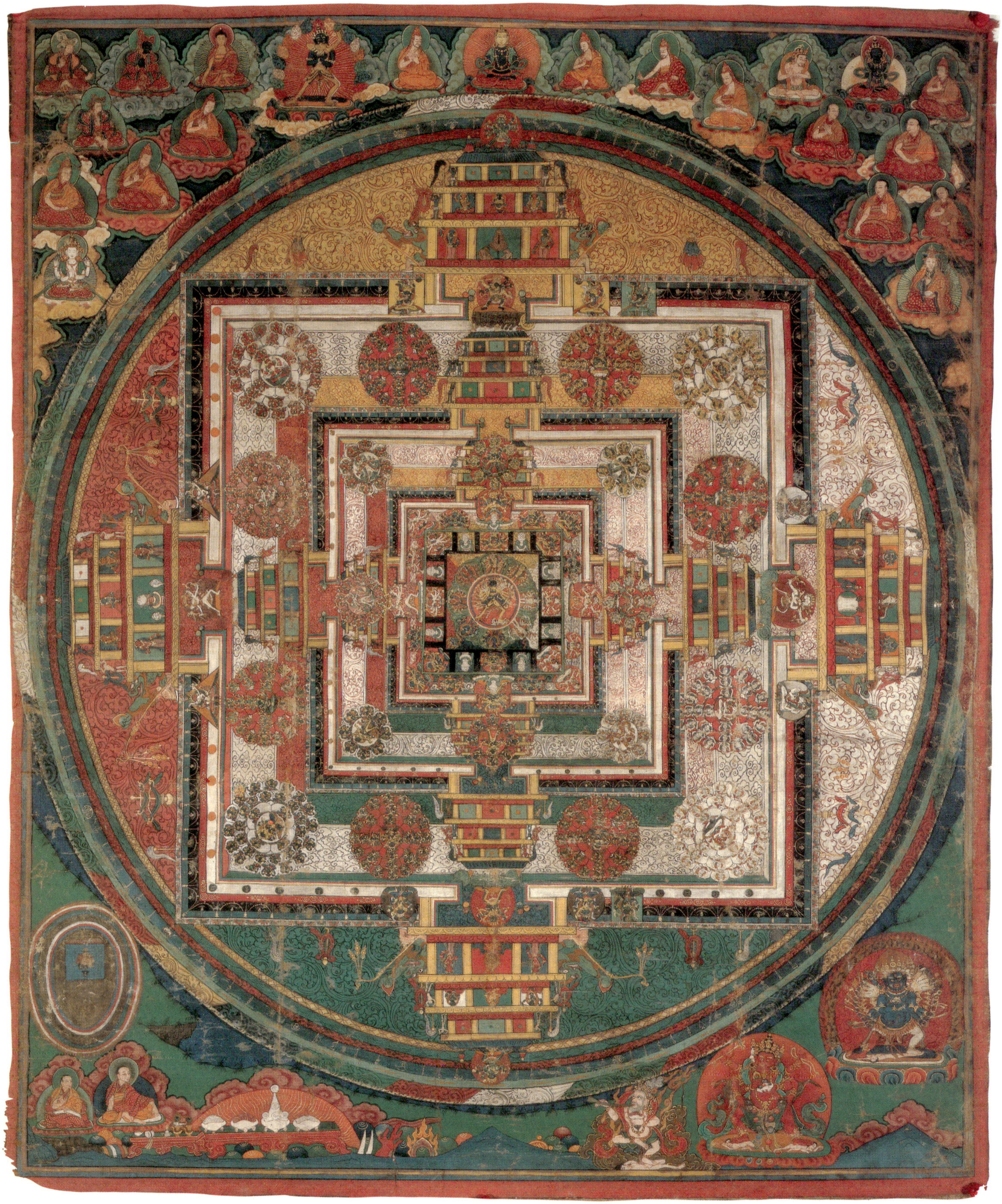

Pl. 126

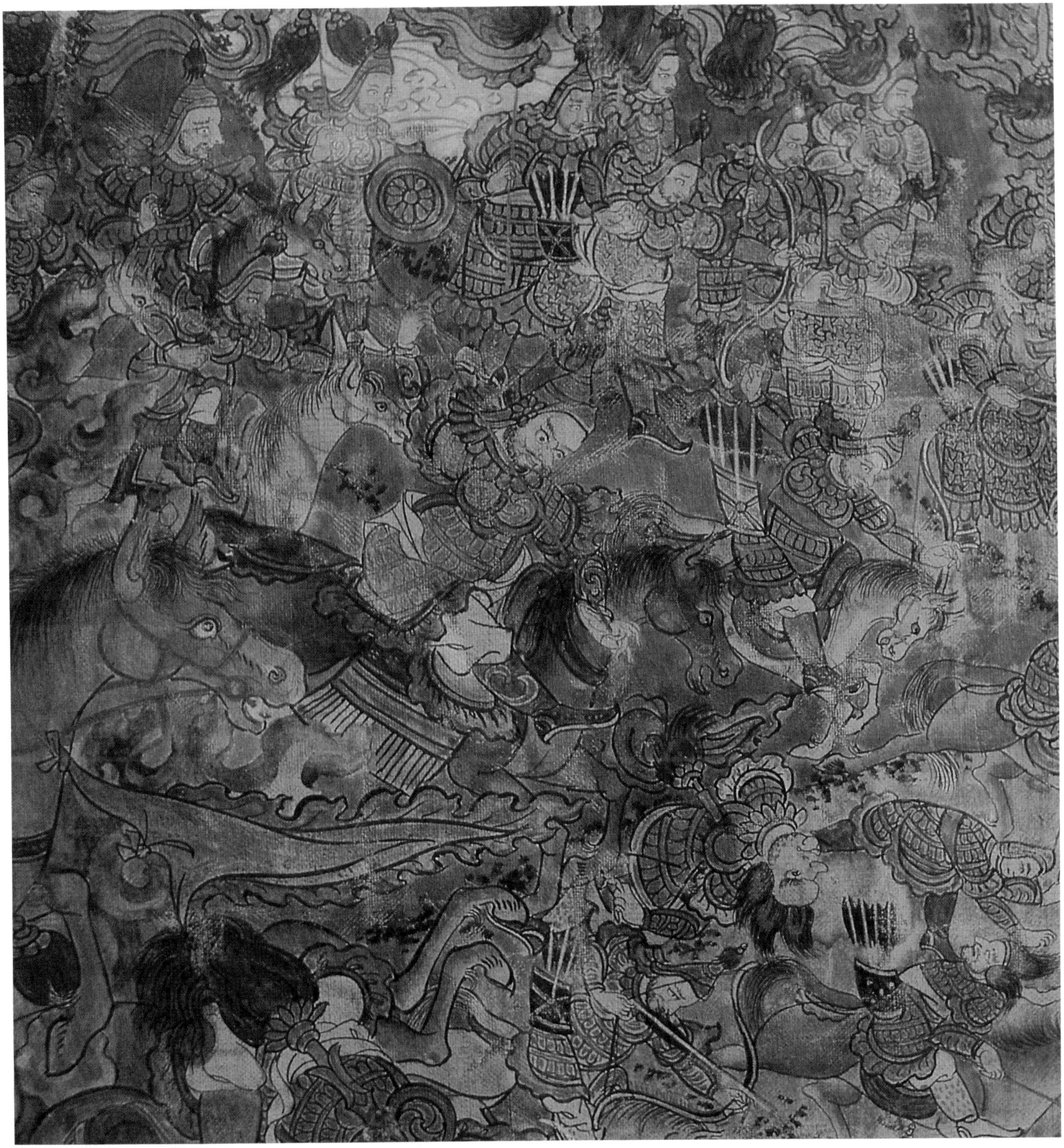

Pl. 127

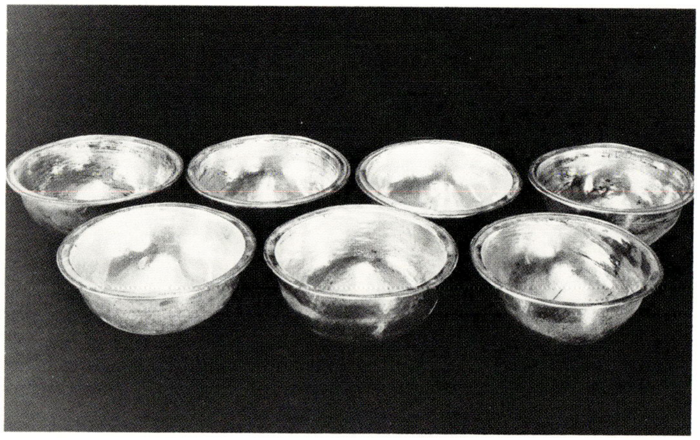

Pl. 136
Set of Seven Offering Bowls
Silver
Tibet
Twentieth century (?)
D. 6 × 17 cm
Field Museum of Natural History, Chicago.
12478 A–G.

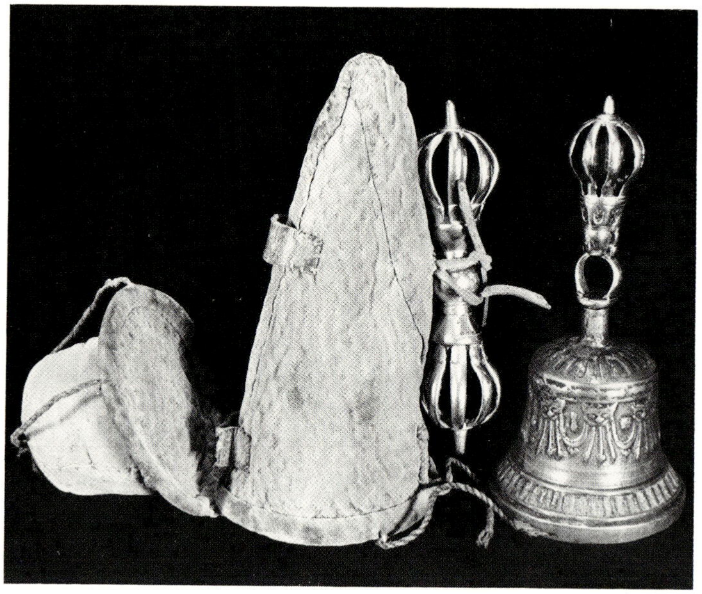

Pl. 138
Bell and rDor-je with Carrying Case
Brass, cotton, wool and leather
Tibet
Twentieth century
Bell: H. 17.5 × D. 8.7 cm
rDorje: H. 15 × D. 3.7 cm
Case: H. 21 × D. 10.2
Field Museum of Natural History, Chicago.
235354 A–C.

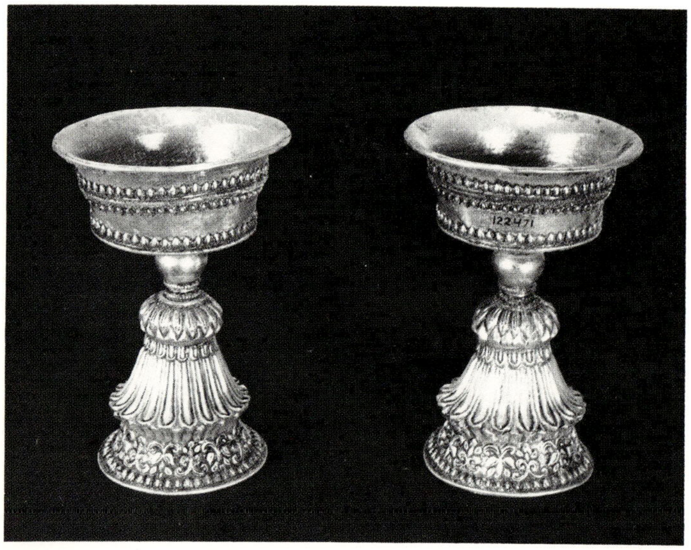

Pl. 137
Set of Two Butter Lamps
Silver
Tibet
Twentieth century (?)
D. 14 × 9.7 cm
Field Museum of Natural History, Chicago.
122472, 122471.

Pl. 139
Altar Table: Vajrayoginī Maṇḍala
Constructed and painted wood
Tibet
Twentieth century
H. 10.79 × 22.86 × 22.86 cm
Navin Kumar, Inc.

Sādhana of the Glorious Coemergent Mother Vajrayoginī—Liturgical Music

Tibetan monastic ritual is a dramatic and complex combination of several elements (image, words, music, hand gestures) with profound symbolic and psychological dimensions which are intended to create particular states of mind. The performance of the ritual lasts many hours, even days. Tibetan liturgical music is an integral part of the Buddhist ritual. In Tibetan religious ceremonies, recitation of the scriptures alternates with instrumental sections. After one portion of a chant is completed, the instrumentalists play until the next part of the chant begins. In contrast to the reserved style of the chant, the instrumental section is dynamic and textually complex.

The master of chant *(dbu-mdzad)* uses the neumatic musical score *(dbyaṅs-yig) in conducting the chant section. The musical score, which is written in notational signs or symbols, indicates the direction of the chant's melody and also contains specific directions to the instrumentalists.*

The Tibetan style of chanting which is normally in unison, although sometimes polyphonic, is often performed in extraordinarily low tones, about an octave below the normal bass range, and can involve the audible projection of the overtone series. There are three main styles of chanting—the sustained chant, the hymn of melodic chant, and the recitative parlando. The primary tonal center of the chant section may be the same as the instrumental section but with a different scale or mode. The tonal center of the two sections, however, may be different. The melody of the chant section is most often confined to the range of an interval of a third and rarely exceeds a fifth or a minor sixth. It usually consists of three or four pitches. The religious texts are rhymeless and frequently are chanted in stanzas of four lines of uneven numbers of syllables, seven and nine being the most common. Typically, a nine-syllable line occurs in a ten-beat measure, the last beat being a rest, and a seven-syllable line in eight-beat measure.

The instrumental section is completely separate from the chant section and is performed exclusively on wind and percussive instruments. There are eight essential instruments employed in the monastic ensemble—four wind and four percussion. The wind instrumentalists play in pairs. Tibetan musicians have developed the ability to breathe circularly. By constantly inhaling air through the nose and storing the air in puffed cheeks, the airflow through the instrument is constant and enables musicians to play a tone continuously without stopping to breathe.

A full orchestra consists of as many as fourteen instruments—two conches, two shawms, two short trumpets, two long trumpets, a hand-bell, a hand-drum, two drums and two pairs of cymbals. The Vajrayoginī Sādhana uses all the instruments of the Tibetan orchestra except the shorter trumpets (*rkaṇ-glin*). The melody of the shawm, embellished with microtones and frequent glides, accompanied by the drone and variations of the other wind instruments, and combined with the percussion, offers a sound which is unusually rich and complex, and highly unique.

The version of the *Vajrayoginī Sādhana* was composed by the Sixth Karmapa, Thongwa Dönden, and recorded at Rumtek Monastery in Sikkim, India in February 1982 by Elizabeth Ann Goldblatt. The full ceremony is available from the UCLA Archives. It lasts approximately eight hours and has been edited by Chögyam Trungpa, Rinpoche, and Elizabeth Ann Goldblatt for use in the exhibition *The Silk Route and the Diamond Path: Esoteric Buddhist Art on the Trade Routes of the Trans-Himalayan Region.*

Elizabeth Ann Goldblatt

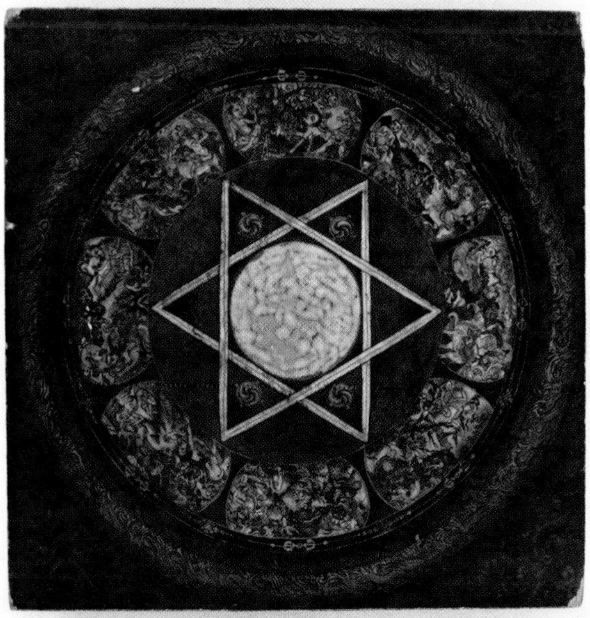

Pl. 140
Chopper
Copper
Tibet
Early nineteenth century
H. 15.2 × D. 15.2 cm
Doris Weiner Gallery, New York

VII

Sacred Outlook:

The Vajrayoginī Shrine and Practice

Chögyam Trungpa, Rinpoche

Vajrayāna, the tantric teaching of the Buddha, contains tremendous magic and power. Its magic lies in its ability to transform confusion and neurosis into awakened mind and to reveal the ordinary everyday world as a sacred realm. Its power is that of unerring insight into the true nature of phenomena and seeing through the ego and its deceptions.

According to the tantric tradition, the Vajrayāna is regarded as the complete teaching of the Buddha. It is considered to be the path of complete discipline, complete surrender, and complete liberation. It is important to realize, however, how firmly grounded the Vajrayāna is in the basic teachings of the Sūtrayāna, the teachings of egolessness and compassion.

Frequently, the exceptional strength and efficacy of Vajrayāna are misunderstood as a promise of instant enlightenment. But one cannot become enlightened overnight; in fact, it is highly deceptive and even dangerous to think in such a way. Without exception, the Buddhist teachings point to the erroneous belief in a self, or ego, as the cause of suffering and the obstacle to liberation. All of the great teachers of the past practiced the preliminary meditative disciplines diligently before becoming students of the Vajrayāna. Without this basic training and practice of meditation, there is no ground to work with Vajrayāna at all.

The Vajrayoginī principle, as it has been experienced, understood and transmitted by the *gurus* of the Karma Kagyu (*karma bka'-brgyud*) lineage of Tibet, to which I belong, is part of the Vajrayāna tradition. I feel very honored to have the opportunity to explain the Vajrayoginī principle and the shrine connected with Vajrayoginī practice. At the same time, I have a responsibility to the lineage, as well as to those who view this exhibit, to introduce Vajrayoginī properly.

EGOLESSNESS AND COMPASSION

A brief discussion of fundamental Buddhism and Mahāyāna is necessary so that it will be clearly understood, in the discussion of Vajrayoginī, that Vajrayoginī is not perceived as an external deity or force. This is sometimes rather difficult for Westerners to understand because of the Judeo-Christian belief in God. Buddhism is a nontheistic religion; there is no belief in an external savior. Nontheism is synonymous with the realization of egolessness, which is first discovered from the practices of *śamatha* and *vipaśyanā* meditation. In *śamatha* meditation, one works with breath and posture as expressions of one's state of being. Assuming a dignified and upright posture and identifying with the breath as it goes out, one begins to make friends with oneself in a fundamental sense. When thoughts arise, they are not treated as enemies, but they are included in the practice and labeled simply as "thinking." *Śamatha*, or *shiné* (*źi-gnas*) in Tibetan, means "dwelling in a state of peace." From *śamatha* practice one begins to see the simplicity of one's original state of mind and to see how confusion, speed, and aggression are generated by ignoring the peacefulness of one's being. This is the first experience of egolessness, in which one realizes the transparency of fixed ideas about oneself and the illusoriness of what one thinks of as "I" or "me."

With further practice, one begins to lose the reference point of one's self-consciousness, and one experiences the environment of practice and the world without bringing everything back to the narrow viewpoint of "I." One begins to be interested in "that," rather than purely being interested in "this." The development of perception that is penetrating and precise without reference to "myself" is called *vipaśyanā*, or *lhak-t'ong* (*lhag-mthoṅ*) in Tibetan, which means "clear seeing." The technique of *vipaśyanā* does not differ from *śamatha*; rather, *vipaśyanā* grows out of the continued application of *śamatha* practice. The "clear seeing" or "insight" of *vipaśyanā* sees that phenomena have no more of a solid existence than oneself, so that one begins to realize the egolessness of "other." One also begins to see the suffering that is caused in the world from clinging to erroneous conceptions about self and phenomena. One perceives that philosophical, psychological, and religious ideas of eternity and external liberation are myths created by ego-mind. So, in *vipaśyanā* practice, egolessness is the recognition of fundamental aloneness, the nontheistic realization that one cannot look for help outside of oneself.

Altogether the ground of Buddhist practice is called the path of "individual liberation," which is *prātimokṣa* in Sanskrit and *so-sor t'arpa* (*so-sor-thar-pa*) in Tibetan. By practicing the disciplines of *śamatha* and *vipaśyanā*, both in meditation and throughout one's life, one can actually liberate oneself from personal confusion and neurosis and one can free oneself from causing harm to oneself and others. One becomes inspired to commit oneself fully to this path by taking refuge in the Buddha (as the example of a human being who attained enlightenment by renouncing external help and working with his own mind), in the *dharma* (the teachings of egolessness that can be heard and experienced), and in the *saṅgha* (the community of practitioners who follow the path of the Buddha by practicing as he did). One realizes that in this spinning world of confused existence one has had the rare good fortune to encounter the true path of liberation.

The Mahāyāna or the "great vehicle" goes beyond the inspiration of individual liberation. On the whole, the Mahāyāna approach is basically one of working for the benefit of others with whatever the world presents; therefore, it is an endless journey. As one embarks on this journey without destination, one's preconceptions begin to fall away. This experience of nonreference point, which initially could be just a momentary flash in one's mind, is the first glimpse of *śūnyatā*. *Śūnya* means "empty," and "*tā*" makes it "emptiness." According to tradition, *śūnyatā* is empty of I, empty of other, absolutely empty. This experience of emptiness is realizing that there is no "I" as actor; no action; and no "other" to be acted upon.

Śūnyatā is not the nihilistic idea of nothingness, or voidness. It is the complete absence of grasping and fixation (*gzuṅ-ba daṅ 'dzin-pa*), complete egolessness of subject and object. It is therefore the absence of separation between self and other.

The experience of *śūnyatā* provides tremendous room and tremendous vision. There is room because one sees that there is no obstacle to going out, to expanding. And there is vision because there is no separation between oneself and one's experience. One can perceive things clearly, as they are, without filters of any kind. This unbiased perception is called *prajñā*, or "discriminating awareness." It is the sharpness of the perception of *śūnyatā* and the knowledge that comes from that perception.

In fact, *prajñā* literally means "superior" or "best knowledge." The highest knowledge that one can have is the knowledge of egoless insight, which begins as the experience of *vipaśyanā* and matures in the Mahāyāna into *prajñā*. The discriminating awareness of *prajñā* sees that "I" and "others" are not separate; and therefore, that the enlightenment of oneself and the enlightenment of others cannot be separated.

In this way, the perception of *śūnyatā* makes one more wakeful and compassionate altogether. One feels immense interest in others and immense caring for others, whose suffering is not different from one's own. This is the beginning of the Mahāyāna practice of exchanging oneself for others (*bdag-gzhan brje-ba*).

The notion of exchange means giving whatever assistance is needed—extending kindness, sanity, and love to other people. In exchange, one is willing to take on others' pain and confusion and hypocrisy. One is willing to take the blame for any problems that might come up, not because one wishes to be a martyr, but because one feels that there is an infinite reservoir of goodness and sanity to share. At the Mahāyāna level, egolessness is expanded into the path of selfless action which goes completely beyond ego-clinging. It is this surrendering of ego, which we shall discuss later, that makes it possible to enter the Vajrayāna path.

VAJRA NATURE AND THE YI-DAM PRINCIPLE

When one lets go of grasping and fixation completely, one is able to rest in the intrinsic goodness of one's mind, and one regards whatever discursive thoughts that arise—passion, aggression, delusion, or any conflicting emotions—as merely ripples in the pond of mind. Out of that, one begins to realize that there is a greater vision beyond grasping and fixation. That vision is very firm and definite. It is not definite in the style of ego, but it is like the sun, which shines all the time. If one flies in an airplane above the clouds, one realizes that the sun is always

shining even when it is cloudy and rainy below. In an analogous fashion, when one ceases to hold on to one's identity, one's ego, one begins to see that the nonexistence of ego is a powerful, real, and indestructible state of being. One realizes that, like the sun, it is a continuous situation that does not wax or wane.

This state of being is called *vajra nature*. *Vajra*, or *dorje* (*rdo-rje*) in Tibetan, means "indestructible," or "having the qualities of a diamond." *Vajra* nature is the tough, immovable quality of egolessness which is the basis for the Vajrayāna path. The term *Vajrayāna* itself means the "vehicle of indestructibility," the "*vajra* vehicle." The Vajrayāna is also called the *tantrayāna*, or the tantric vehicle. *Tantra*, or *gyud* (*rgyud*) in Tibetan, means "continuity" or "thread." *Vajra* nature is the continuity of egolessness, the continuity of wakefulness, which, like the sun, is brilliant and all-pervasive.

The deities of the Vajrayāna are the embodiments of *vajra* nature. Important for the practice of Vajrayāna are the deities called *yi-dams*. The best translation for *yi-dam* that I have found is "personal deity." Actually, *yi-dam* is a shortened form of the phrase *yid-kyi dam-ts'ik* (*yid-kyi-dam-tshig*), which means "sacred bondage of your mind." *Yid* means "mind," *kyi* means "of," and *dam-ts'ik* means "sacred word" or "sacred bondage." *Dam-ts'ik*, which in Sanskrit is *samaya*, will become important in the later discussion of the tantric *samayas*, or sacred commitments. "Mind" refers to *vajra* nature, the basic sanity and wakefulness of our being, freed from ego-clinging. The *yi-dam* is the manifestation of this enlightened mind, and the *yi-dam* is what connects, or binds, the practitioner to that enlightened sanity within himself or herself. So the *yi-dam*, according to the tantric understanding, is a nontheistic deity who embodies one's innate *vajra* nature rather than any form of external help.

There are many thousands of tantric deities, but in the Karma Kagyu lineage, Vajrayoginī is a particularly important *yi-dam*. When a student has completed the preliminary Vajrayāna practices, called the *ngöndro* (*sṅon-'gro*), he receives *abhiṣeka*, or empowerment, to begin *yi-dam* practice, which is identifying with a personal deity as the embodiment of his innate wakefulness or *vajra* nature. In the Karma Kagyu tradition, the Vajrayoginī *abhiṣeka* is the first empowerment that a practitioner receives and Vajrayoginī is the first *yi-dam* given to a student. In order to understand the Vajrayoginī principle in any depth, a discussion of the stages of Vajrayāna practice through which a student is introduced to the *yi-dam* is necessary.

DEVOTION

In the Buddhist tradition, relating to a teacher is not hero worship; one appreciates the teacher as an example of living *dharma*. Upon entering the Buddhist path, the practitioner respects the teacher as a wise man or an elder. The teacher in the Mahāyāna is called the *kalyāṇamitra* or "spiritual friend"—a friend in the sense that he is willing to share one's life completely and to walk with one on the path. He is truly the example of the Mahāyāna practice of exchanging self for others.

At the Vajrayāna level, one begins with faith (*dad-pa*) in the teachings and the teacher, because one has already experienced the truth and the workability of the teachings for oneself. Then, with the discovery of *vajra* nature, faith begins to develop into devotion, which is *mögü* (*mos-gus*) in Tibetan. *Mö* means "longing," and *gü* means "respect." One develops tremendous respect for the teacher and a longing for what he can impart because one sees that he is the embodiment of *vajra* nature, the embodiment of wakeful mind. At this level, the teacher becomes the *guru*. He is the *vajra* master, the one who has mastered *vajra* truth, indestructible truth, and who can transmit that *vajra* power to others. However, the Vajrayāna can be extremely destructive if one is not properly prepared to receive these teachings. Therefore, in order to practice Vajrayāna, one must have a relationship with a *vajra* master, who completely understands the practitioner and the practice and knows how to bring the two together.

One's relationship with the *vajra* master involves surrendering oneself to the teacher as the final expression of egolessness. This allows one to develop fully the threefold *vajra* nature: *vajra* body, *vajra* speech, and *vajra* mind. The maturation of devotion into complete surrendering is called *lote-lingkyur* (*blo-gtad ling-bskyur*) in Tibetan. *Lote* means "trust," *ling* means "completely," and *kyur* means "abandoning" or "letting go." So *lote-lingkyur* means to trust completely and to let go, to abandon one's ego completely. Without such surrender, there is no way to give up the last vestiges of ego, nor could the teacher introduce the *yi-dam*, the essence of egolessness. In fact, without such devotion to the teacher, one might attempt to use the Vajrayāna teachings to rebuild the fortress of ego.

NGÖNDRO

In order to develop proper devotion and surrender, a student of the Vajrayāna begins with the practice of the *ngöndro*, the foundation practices that are preliminaries to receiving *abhiṣeka*. *Ngön* means "before," and *dro* means "going." In the Karma Kagyu lineage, there are five practices that make up the *ngöndro*: prostrations, the recitation of the refuge vow, the Vajrasattva *mantra* practice, the *maṇḍala* offering, and the practice of *guru-yoga*. These are called "The Extraordinary Foundations."

Ngöndro is the means of connecting oneself with the wisdom of the *guru* and of the lineage to which he belongs. In prostrations, as the starting point, one is humbling oneself and expressing one's gratitude for the example of the *vajra* master and the lineage forefathers. The student visualizes the *gurus* of the lineage, including his or her own *guru* in the form of the primordial Buddha. Over the course of many practice sessions, the practitioner prostrates to the lineage 108,000 times while reciting the refuge vow 108,000 times. In that way, the student reaffirms the commitment to the basic path of discipline and renunciation at the same time that he or she expresses surrender to the Vajrayāna teachings and to the *vajra* master. Through this practice, one catches one's first glimpse of the lineage.

Mantra practice leads to a closer experience of the lineage wisdom. It allows one to work directly with obstacles and psychological obscuration and to realize that defilements are temporary and can be overcome. Vajrasattva, literally the "*vajra* being," is visualized as a youthful white prince who is both the essence of *vajra* wisdom and the wisdom body of one's *guru*. In contrast, the practitioner visualizes his own body filled with impurities of all kinds: physical, mental, and emotional. While reciting the *mantra* of Vajrasattva 108,000 times, one visualizes that one's body is slowly cleansed of these impurities by the action of Vajrasattva. By the end of a practice period, the student visualizes himself or herself as possessing the same pure nature as Vajrasattva. The point of *mantra* practice, therefore, is to recognize one's own inherent purity.

In *maṇḍala* practice, one gives oneself and one's world as an offering to the lineage. The student offers 108,000 *maṇḍalas* made from heaps of saffron-scented rice mixed with jewels and other precious substances. While constructing the *maṇḍala*, one visualizes the world and everything in it, all its wealth and beauty and myriad sense perceptions, as an offering to the *gurus* and Buddhas visualized before oneself. One's sense of pure being should also be included in the offering and given up. This is called giving up the giver. When one gives up so completely, there is no one left to watch what is being given, no one to appreciate how generous one is being. The more one surrenders in this way, the more richness one develops. There is never a problem of running out of things to offer. Just the fact of one's human life is an immensely rich situation to offer to the lineage.

Having completed the *maṇḍala* offerings one also practices *guru-yoga* as a part of *ngöndro*. *Guru-yoga* is like actually meeting the *guru* face-to-face for the first time. *Guru-yoga* is the first opportunity to receive the *adhiṣṭhāna*, or the blessings, of the *guru*'s wisdom.

In *guru-yoga*, one begins to realize the nondual nature of devotion: that there is no separation between the lineage and oneself and that, in fact, the *vajra* being of the *guru* is a reflection of one's own innate nature. In this way, the practice of *ngöndro*, culminating in *guru-yoga*, helps to overcome one's theistic notions about the teacher or the Vajrayāna itself. One realizes that the lineage is not an entity outside of oneself: one is not worshipping the teacher or his ancestors as gods. Rather, one is connecting with *vajra* sanity, which is so powerful *because* of its nonexistence, its utter egolessness.

SACRED OUTLOOK

When one begins to mix one's mind with the energy of the lineage, one is not trying to protect oneself from the world by becoming devoted to the teacher. In fact, devotion brings one closer to one's experience, to one's world. As a result of the practice of *ngöndro*, one feels a greater sense of warmth and gentleness in oneself. Because of that, one can relax and take a fresh look at the phenomenal world. One finds that life can be an easy, natural process. Because there is no need to struggle, one starts to experience "goodness" everywhere—a tremendous sense of freedom and sacredness is everything one experiences.

When one experiences this self-existing sacredness, one realizes that the only way to abide continuously in this state of freedom is to enter completely into the *guru's* world, because such freedom is the blessing of the *guru*. It is the *guru* who has presented the practice that leads to the experience of freedom, and it is the *guru* who manifests the epitome of this freedom. In fact, one begins to see that the self-existing sacredness of the world is simultaneously an expression of the *guru*. This experience is known as "sacred outlook," or *dag-nang (dag-snaṅ)* in Tibetan. *Dag-nang* literally means "pure perception." The idea of purity here is the absence of imprisonment. Sacred outlook is perceiving the world and oneself as intrinsically good and unconditionally free.

THE FIVE BUDDHA FAMILIES

Developing sacred outlook makes possible a further step into the *vajra* world. When one experiences the self-existing sacredness of reality, the Vajrayāna iconography begins to make sense: it begins to make sense to picture the world as a sacred realm, the *maṇḍala* of enlightened mind. From the viewpoint of sacred outlook, the phenomenal world is seen in terms of five styles of energy: *buddha, vajra, padma, ratna,* and *karma*. Oneself and the people one meets, the seasons, the elements—all aspects of the phenomenal world—are made up of one or more of these families.

The Buddha family or families associated with a person describe that person's intrinsic perspective or stance in the world. The Buddha family principles can have either a neurotic or an enlightened expression. The particular neurosis associated with a Buddha family is transmuted into its wisdom or enlightened form by the taming process of *śamatha-vipaśyanā* meditation, the Mahāyāna training in compassion, and particularly by the development of sacred outlook in the Vajrayāna. In their neurotic expression, the Buddha families are styles of imprisonment. In their enlightened expression, they are the styles or manifestations of *vajra* freedom.

In tantric iconography, the Buddha families make up a *maṇḍala* with *buddha* in the center, and *vajra, ratna, padma,* and *karma* in the four cardinal points. The basic quality of *buddha* energy is spaciousness. The confused manifestation of this spacious quality is ignorance, which in this case is avoiding vivid or unpleasant experience. When *buddha* energy is transmuted, it becomes the wisdom of all-encompassing space. *Buddha* is associated with the color white and is symbolized by a wheel, which represents this all-encompassing, open, nature.

Vajra is in the east of the *maṇḍala* and is represented by the color blue. The symbol of *vajra* is the *vajra* scepter, or *dorje*, whose five prongs pierce the neurosis of ego-mind. The *vajra* scepter is like a thunderbolt, electric and powerful. *Vajra* energy is precise and direct. It is the ability to view situations from all possible perspectives and to accurately perceive the details of experience and the larger frameworks in which things take place. The neurotic expression of *vajra* energy is aggression and intellectual fixation. When the intellectual accuracy of *vajra* is transmuted into its enlightened form, it becomes mirror-like wisdom. *Vajra* is associated with the element of water. Its neurotic expression, anger, is like clouded, turbulent water; its wisdom aspect is like the clear reflection of a still pond.

The *ratna* family, in the south, is represented by the color yellow. The symbol of the *ratna* family is a jewel. *Ratna* energy is the expression of richness. It is like autumn when fruits and grains are ripe and farmers celebrate the harvest. *Ratna* is associated with the element of earth, which expresses its solidity and fertility. The neurotic style of *ratna* is envy or hunger, wanting everything and trying to engulf everything. Its enlightened expression is the wisdom of equanimity, because *ratna* accommodates all experiences and brings out their innate richness. When it is freed from hunger, *ratna* becomes an expression of powerful expansiveness.

In the west is the *padma* family, which is associated with the color red. The symbol of *padma* is the lotus, a beautiful, delicate flower that blooms in the mud. *Padma* is the basic energy of passion or seduction. Its neurotic aspect is grasping or clinging, the confused expression of passion. When passion is freed from fixation on the object of its desire, it becomes discriminating-awareness wisdom, appreciation of every aspect and detail of experience. *Padma* is associated with the element of fire. In the confused state, like fire, passion does not distinguish among the things it grasps, burns, and destroys. In its enlightened expression, the heat of passion becomes the warmth of compassion.

Karma, the last Buddha family, in the north of the *maṇḍala*, is associated with the color green. The symbol of *karma*, a sword, represents cutting through hesitation and confusion and accomplishing one's goals accurately and thoroughly. *Karma* is the wisdom of all-accomplishing action in its enlightened manifestation. The neurotic expression of *karma* energy is resentment and excessive speed. *Karma* neurosis would like to create a uniform world and resents any sloppiness or inefficiency. When *karma* is freed from neurosis, it becomes accurate and energetic without resentment or pettiness. *Karma* is associated with the element of wind, which represents this forceful and energetic quality of action.

Perceiving the energies of the Buddha families in people and in situations, one sees that confusion is workable and can be transformed into the expression of sacred outlook. The student must reach this understanding before the teacher can introduce the tantric deities or *yi-dams*. Every *yi-dam* "belongs" to a Buddha family and is a "ruler" of the wisdom aspect of that family. The Buddha family principles provide a link between ordinary saṃsāric experience and the brilliance and loftiness of the *yi-dams'* world. From an understanding of the Buddha family principles, one can appreciate the tantric deities as the embodiments of the energies of the sacred world and as a means of identifying oneself with that sacredness. With that understanding one can receive *abhiṣeka*, or empowerment; one is ready to be introduced to Vajrayoginī who is described in the *sādhana* as "the wrathful wild protectress, the wondrous body of desire" (Plate 128).

ABHISEKA

By receiving the *abhiṣeka* of Vajrayoginī, the student enters the *maṇḍala* of Vajrayoginī. Through this process, Vajrayoginī becomes the student's *yi-dam*, the embodiment of one's basic being or basic state of mind. *Abhiṣeka* literally means "anointment" or "confirmation." The Tibetan *wangkur* (*dbang-skur*) means "empowerment." The principle of empowerment is the meeting of the minds of the student and *vajra* master, which is the product of devotion. Because the student is able to open fully to the teacher, the teacher is able to communicate directly the power and wakefulness of the Vajrayāna through the formal ceremony of *abhiṣeka*. In reviewing the history of the Vajrayoginī transmission in the Karma Kagyu lineage, the directness of this communication becomes apparent.

The Vajrayoginī-sādhana in the Karma Kagyu Lineage

The *abhiṣeka* of Vajrayoginī is an ancient ceremony which is part of the *Vajrayoginī-sādhana*, the manual and liturgy of Vajrayoginī practice. There are many *sādhanas* of Vajrayoginī, including those according to Saraha, Nāgārjuna, Luyipa, Jalandhara, and Śavarī. In the Karma Kagyu tradition, one practices the *sādhana* of Vajrayoginī according to the Indian *siddha*, Tilopa, the forefather of the Kagyu lineage.

According to the spiritual biographies (*rnam-par-thar-pa*), after studying the Basic Buddhist teachings for many years, Tilopa (998–1069) traveled to Uḍḍiyāna, the home of the *ḍākinīs*, or female *yi-*

dams, to seek Vajrayāna transmission. He gained entrance to the palace of the *ḍākinīs* and received direct instruction there from Vajrayoginī herself, who manifested to him as the great queen of the *ḍākinīs*. It may be rather perplexing to speak of encountering Vajrayoginī in anthropomorphic form, when she is discussed throughout this article as the essence of egolessness. However, this account of Tilopa's meeting is the traditional story of his encounter with the direct energy and power of Vajrayoginī.

Nāropa (1016–1100), who received the oral transmission of the Vajrayoginī practice from Tilopa, was a great scholar at Nālandā University. Following a visit from a *ḍākinī*, who appeared to him as an ugly old hag, he realized that he had not grasped the inner meaning of the teachings, and he set out to find his *guru*. After encountering many obstacles, Nāropa found Tilopa dressed in beggar's rags, eating fish heads by the side of a lake. In spite of this external appearance, Nāropa at once recognized his *guru*. He remained with him for many years and underwent numerous trials before receiving final empowerment as the holder of his lineage. From Nāropa, the oral tradition of the Vajrayoginī practice passed to Marpa (1012–1097), the first Tibetan holder of the lineage. Marpa made three journeys from Tibet to India to receive instruction from Nāropa. It is said that, on his third visit to India, Marpa met Vajrayoginī in the form of a young maiden. Taking a crystal hooked knife, she slashed open her belly and Marpa saw in her belly the *maṇḍala* of Vajrayoginī, surrounded by a spinning *mantra* wheel. At that moment, he had a realization of Vajrayoginī as the Coemergent Mother, a principle that will be discussed later. This realization was included in the oral transmission of Vajrayoginī that has been passed down to the present day.

Marpa gave the oral instructions for the Vajrayoginī practice to the renowned *yogin* Milarepa (1040–1123); he in turn transmitted them to Gampopa (1079–1153), a great scholar and practitioner who established the monastic order of the Kagyu. Chief among Gampopa's many disciples were the founders of the four great and the eight lesser schools of the Kagyu tradition. The Karma Kagyu is one of the four great schools. It was founded by Tusum Khyenpa (1110–1193), the first Karmapa and a foremost disciple of Gampopa. Tusum Khyenpa handed down the oral transmission of the *Vajrayoginī-sādhana* to Drogön Rechenpa (1088–1158); from him it was passed to Pomdrakpa, who transmitted it to the second Karmapa, Karma Pakshi (1206–1283). Karma Pakshi passed the Vajrayoginī transmission to Ugyenpa (1230–1309), by whom it was given to Rangjung Dorje (1284–1339), the third Karmapa (Fig. 62). It was Rangjung Dorje, the third Karmapa, who composed the written form of the *sādhana* of Vajrayoginī according to Tilopa and the oral instructions of Marpa, which is still practiced today. It is this *sādhana* that is the basis for this discussion of the Vajrayoginī principle.

The first Trungpa was a student of the *siddha*, Trungmase (fifteenth century), who was a close disciple of the fifth Karmapa, Teshin Shekpa (1384–1415). When Nāropa transmitted the teachings of Vajrayoginī to Marpa, he told him that these teachings should be kept as a transmission from one teacher to one student for thirteen generations, and then they could be propagated to others. This transmission is called *chik gyud* (*gcig brgyud*), the "single lineage" or "single thread" transmission. Because of this, the Kagyu lineage is frequently called the "Hearing Lineage" (*sñan brgyud*). Trungmase received the complete teachings on Vajrayoginī, Cakraśaṃvara and the Four-Armed Mahākāla, and these became a special transmission (*bka'-babs*) that he was to hold. Trungmase, belonging to the thirteenth generation, became the first *guru* to transmit this particular lineage of *mahāmudrā* teachings to more than a single *dharma* successor, and in fact he taught it widely. The first Trungpa, Kunga Gyaltsen, was one of Trungmase's disciples who received this transmission. I, myself, the eleventh Trungpa Tulku, received the Vajrayoginī transmission from Rolpe Dorje, the regent abbot of Surmang and one of my main tutors.

Since 1970, when I arrived in America, I have been working to plant the Buddhadharma, and particularly the Vajrayāna teachings, in this American soil. Beginning in 1977 and every year since then, those of my students who have completed their preliminary Vajrayāna practices, as well as extensive training in the basic meditative disciplines, have received the *abhiṣeka* of Vajrayoginī. There are now more than three hundred sādhakas (or practitioners of the *sādhana*) in our community (Fig. 63) and many other western students are studying with Tibetan teachers and practicing various Vajrayāna *sādhanas*. So the Vajrayoginī *abhiṣeka* and *sādhana* are not purely part of Tibetan history; they have a place in the history of Buddhism in America as well (Fig. 61).

The Ceremony of Abhiṣeka

The *abhiṣeka* of Vajrayoginī belongs to the highest of the four orders of *tantra*: *anuttara-yoga*. *Anuttara* means "highest" or "unsurpassed," unequaled. *Anuttara-tantra* can be subdivided into three parts: mother, father, and nondual. The Karma Kagyu lineage particularly emphasizes the teachings of the mother *tantra*, to which Vajrayoginī belongs.

Mother *tantra* stresses devotion as the starting point for Vajrayāna practice. Therefore, the key point in receiving the *abhiṣeka* of Vajrayoginī is to have one-pointed devotion to the teacher. By receiving *abhiṣeka*, one is being introduced to the freedom of the *vajra* world. In the *abhiṣeka*, the *vajra* master manifests as the essence of this freedom, which is the essence of Vajrayoginī. He therefore represents the *yi-dam* as well as the teacher in human form. Thus, in receiving *abhiṣeka*, it is essential to understand that the *yi-dam* and the *guru* are not separate.

In the tradition of *anuttara-tantra*, the student receives a four-fold *abhiṣeka*. The entire ceremony is called an *abhiṣeka*, and each of the four parts is also called an *abhiṣeka*, because they are each a particular empowerment. The four *abhiṣekas* are all connected with experiencing the phenomenal world as a sacred *maṇḍala*.

Before receiving the first *abhiṣeka*, the student reaffirms the refuge vow, and the *bodhisattva* vow, the Mahāyānist vow of compassion. In receiving *abhiṣeka*, the attitude of the student must be one of loving kindness for all beings and sincere desire to benefit others. The student then takes a vow called the *samaya* vow, which binds the teacher, the student and the *yi-dam* together. As part of this oath, the student vows that he will not reveal his Vajrayāna experience to others who are not included in the *maṇḍala* of Vajrayoginī. The student then drinks what is known as the *samaya*-oath water from a conch shell on the shrine, to seal this vow. It is said that if the student violates this oath the water will become molten iron. It will burn the student from within and he will die on the spot. On the other hand, if the student keeps his vow and discipline, the oath water will act to propagate the student's sanity and experience of the glory, brilliance, and dignity of the *vajra* world. The notion of *samaya* will be discussed in greater detail after the discussion of the *abhiṣeka* itself.

After taking the samaya oath, the student receives the first *abhiṣeka*, the *abhiṣeka* of the vase (*kalaśābhiṣeka*), also known as the water *abhiṣeka*). Symbolically, the *abhiṣeka* of the vase is the coronation of the student as a prince or princess, a would-be king or queen of the *maṇḍala*. It signifies the student's graduation from the ordinary world into the world of continuity, the *tantric* world.

The *abhiṣeka* of the vase has five parts, each of which is also called an *abhiṣeka*. The first *abhiṣeka* of the vase is also called the *abhiṣeka* of the vase, or jar. The student is given water to drink from a vase on the shrine called the *tsobum* (*gtso-bum*). The *tsobum* is the principal *abhiṣeka* vase and is used to empower the student. In the text of the *abhiṣeka* it says:

> *Just as when the Buddha was born*
> *The devas bathed him.*
> *Just so, with pure divine water*
> *You are empowered.*[1]

The symbolism of receiving the water from the *tsobum* in the first *abhiṣeka* of the vase is psychological cleansing as well as empowerment. Before ascending his throne, the young prince or princess must bathe and put on fresh clothes. The five *abhiṣekas* of the vase are connected with the five buddha families. The *abhiṣeka* of the vase is connected with the *vajra* family, and the student is also presented with

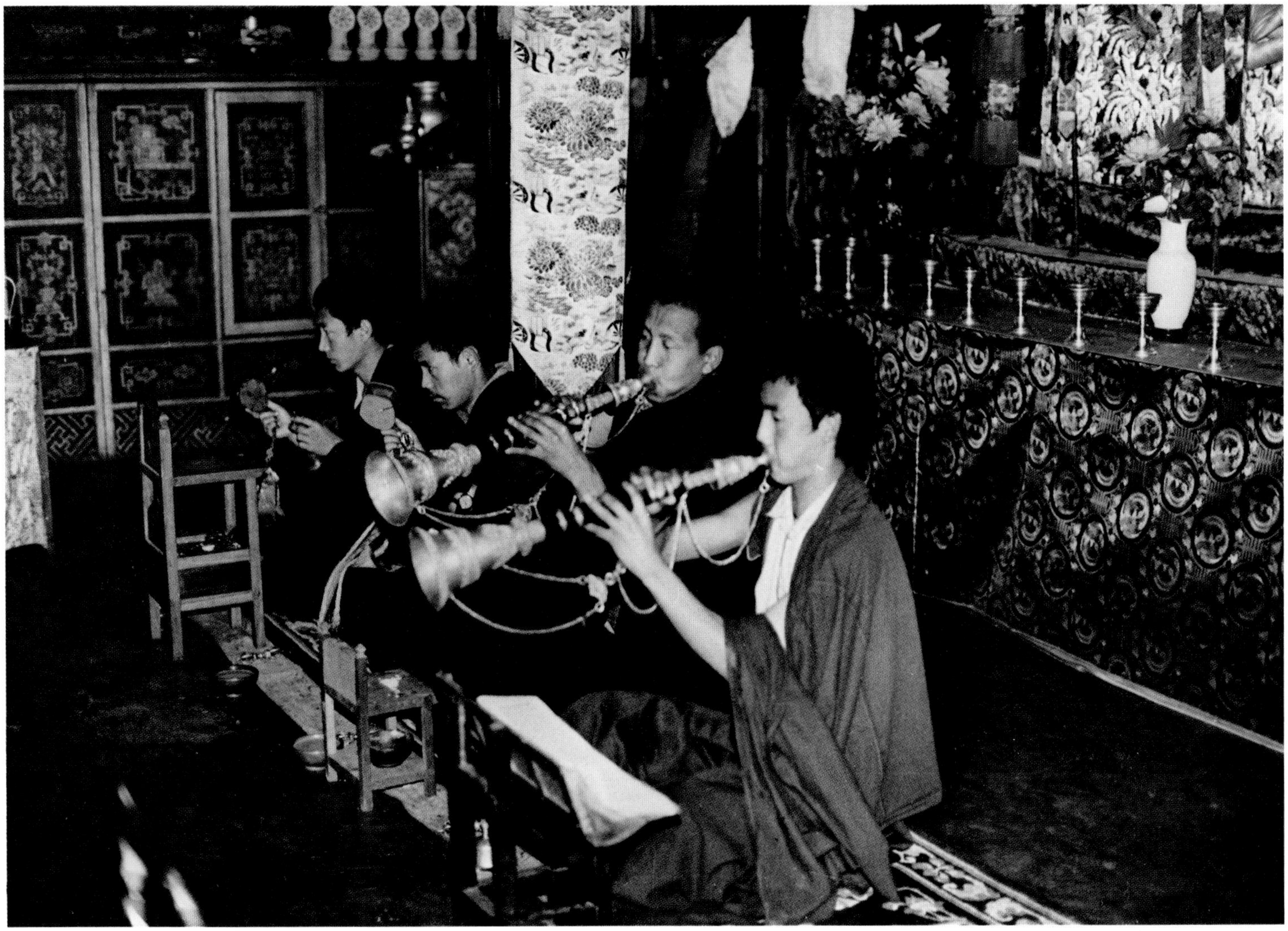

61. Performance of *Vajrayoginī Sādhana,*
Rumtek Monastery, Sikkim.

a five-pointed *vajra* scepter, symbolizing his ability to transmute aggression into mirror-like wisdom.

The second *abhiṣeka* of the vase is the crown *abhiṣeka*. The student is presented with a crown inlaid with five jewels representing the wisdom of the five buddha families. The practitioner is crowned as a confident and accomplished student worthy of taking his or her place in the *maṇḍala* of Vajrayoginī. The crown *abhiṣeka* is connected with the *ratna* family, and the student is also presented with a jewel, the symbol of the *ratna* wisdom of equanimity. There is a sense of being enriched, a feeling of openness and generosity, and a sensation of being able to overcome any sense of threat or poverty.

In the third *abhiṣeka*, the *abhiṣeka* of the *vajra*, the student is presented with a nine-pronged *vajra* scepter, or *dorje*. The *vajra* is the symbol of indestructibility and of complete skillfulness in working with the phenomenal world. So in receiving the *vajra* the student is presented with the means to overcome obstacles and to propagate *vajra* sanity. The *abhiṣeka* of the *vajra* is related to the *padma* family. Although the *vajra* is both a powerful scepter and a deadly weapon, its power comes from generating and extending compassion, warmth and generosity. The student is also presented with a lotus, the symbol of the *padma* family, signifying the ability to transmute the grasping quality of desire into discriminating awareness wisdom.

The *abhiṣeka* of the *ghaṇṭā*, or bell, is the fourth *abhiṣeka* of the vase. Presenting the student with the *ghaṇṭā* signifies that he or she is not only concerned with personal realization but is also willing to proclaim the teachings for the benefit of others. The piercing sound of the *ghaṇṭā* signifies that the *vajra* proclamation of truth is unobstructed. The *abhiṣeka* of the *ghaṇṭā* is connected with the *karma* family. The student is presented with a sword, the symbol of the *karma* family, signifying the wisdom of all-accomplishing action which conquers neurotic speed and jealousy.

The final *abhiṣeka* of the vase is the *abhiṣeka* of name. In this *abhiṣeka*, the *vajra* master rings a *ghaṇṭā* with a *vajra* attached to it above the student's head. When the bell rings, the student is given a tantric name, which is a secret name. This name is not publicized like an ordinary name, but when the practitioner needs to use his power to wake someone up, he says his own *vajra* name, his secret name, as a reminder of *vajra* nature. The giving of the secret name also signifies the final act in the coronation of the tantric prince or princess. Because of merit accumulated through practice and devotion to the teacher, the student deserves to change his name from a common name to the name of a would-be king, a potential master of the *maṇḍala*, a *tathāgata*.

The *abhiṣeka* of name is connected with the *buddha* family. There is a sense of complete spaciousness and openness that comes when one takes one's place in the *vajra-maṇḍala*. In the *abhiṣeka* of Vajrayoginī, the student is presented at this point, as part of the *abhiṣeka* of name, with the hooked knife, which Vajrayoginī holds in her right hand. At this point, the student is introduced to the chief deity of the *maṇḍala* and to her buddha-like quality, which is the wisdom of all-

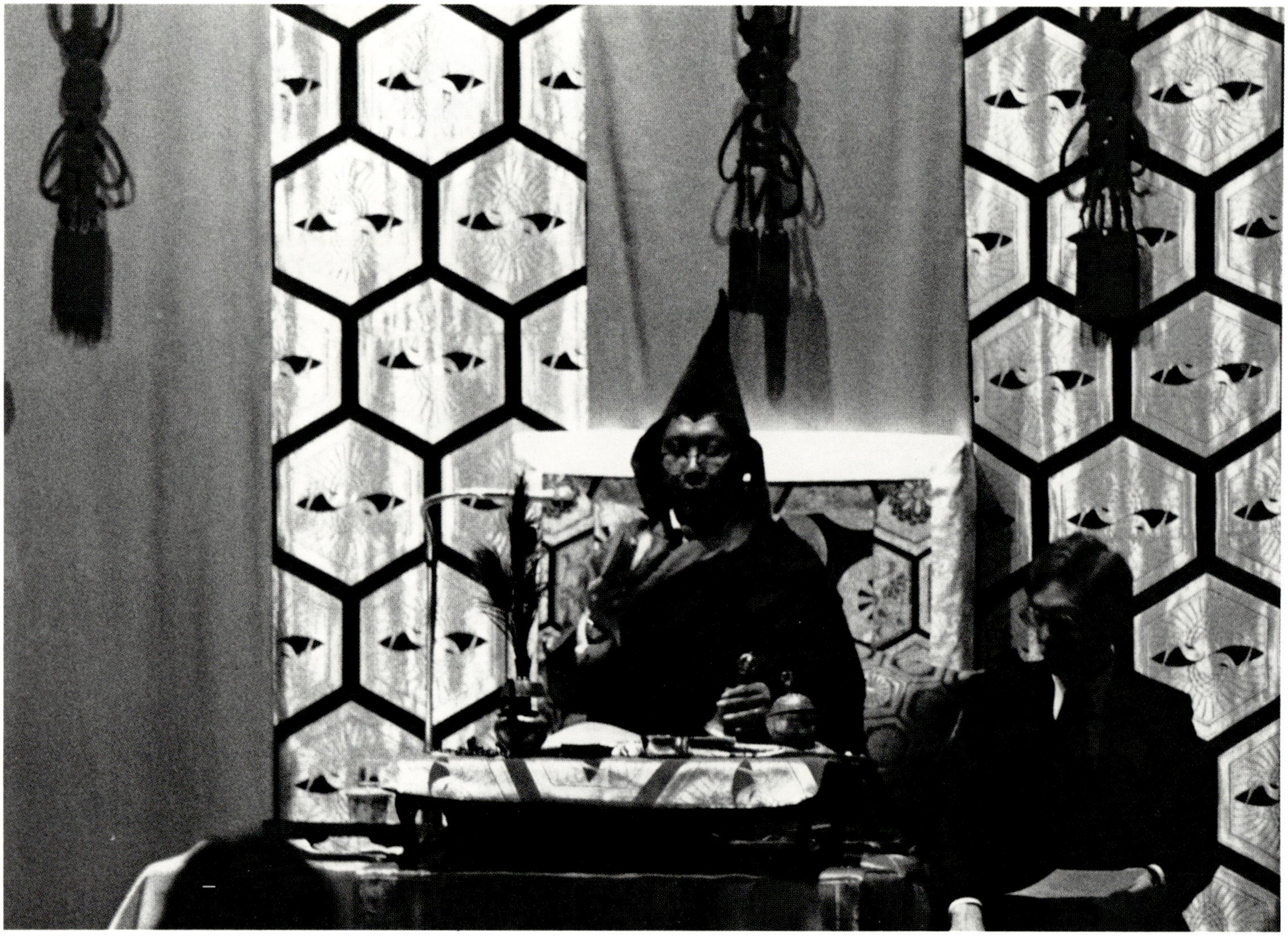

62. Chögyam Trungpa, Rinpoche, performing the initiation of Vajrayoginī.

encompassing space. Although Vajrayoginī is red in color, symbolizing her feminine quality of warmth and passion, her basic quality is definitely that of the *buddha* family.

Having received the complete *abhiṣeka* of the vase, there is a sense of significant psychological progress and psychological change. At that point, the *vajra* master is able to confer the remaining three *abhiṣekas*. We cannot go into too much detail about these aspects of the ceremony. But in brief, the second *abhiṣeka* is known as the secret *abhiṣeka* (*guhyābhiṣeka*). By drinking *amṛta*, a mixture of liquor and other substances, from the skull cup on the shrine, the mind of the student merges with the mind of the teacher and the mind of the *yi-dam*, so that the boundary line between confusion and wakefulness begins to dissolve. In the third *abhiṣeka*, the *prajñā-jñāna-abhiṣeka* of knowledge and wisdom, the student begins to experience joy, *mahāsukha*—uniting with the world. This is sometimes called the union of bliss and emptiness, which signifies greater openness and greater vision taking place.

The fourth *abhiṣeka* (*caturthābhiṣeka*) is known as the *abhiṣeka* of suchness. The student experiences that he does not have to dwell on the past, present or future. He could just wake himself up on the spot. The student's mind is opened into the ultimate notion of sacred outlook, in which there is nobody to flash sacred outlook. There is just a sense of the doer and the doing dissolving into one, which is a sense of basic shock: the possibilities of conventional mind are dissolving into nothing.

SAMAYA

The principle of *samaya*, or sacred bondage, becomes extremely important when a student has taken *abhiṣeka*. The meaning of the word *yi-dam* as the "*samaya* of your mind" was discussed earlier. When one receives empowerment to practice the *sādhana* of Vajrayoginī, one takes on that *samaya* or bondage. One binds oneself to indestructible wakefulness. One commits oneself fully to maintaining sacred outlook throughout one's life. This is done by identifying oneself completely with the *vajra* sanity of the teacher and of Vajrayoginī. One is inseparably bound together with the teacher and the *yi-dam*; and, at this point, one's very being and one's sanity depend on keeping up this commitment.

This is not to say that if one has one "bad" thought or one trace of confusion that one will be rejected or destroyed. There is still a sense of journey and path that takes place once one has received *abhiṣeka*. In fact, it is said that *samaya* is nearly impossible to keep. It is like a mirror that, no matter how thoroughly it is polished, always collects dust and must be polished again. In taking *abhiṣeka*, one is taught to experience sacred outlook on the spot, which *is samaya*. When obstacles or difficulties arise, they become reminders of sacred outlook rather than purely hindrances. This is called the *samaya* of experiencing everything as sacred in *vajra*-like nature, which has three categories: the *samaya* of body, the *samaya* of speech, and the *samaya* of mind.

The *samaya* of body, or the *samaya* of *mudrā*, is that one's basic phenomenal situation is always regarded as an expression of sacredness. One does not doubt the sacredness of one's world. The *samaya* of speech, or the *samaya* of *mantra*, is that any occurrence, anything that comes up in one's experience, is also regarded as sacred. This could be an internal or an external occurrence, so that any subconscious gossip or emotional upheaval is transformed into sacredness through the *samaya* of speech. The *samaya* of mind, or the *samaya* of *vajra*, is connected with the indestructible wakefulness of the *vajra-maṇḍala*, in this case the *maṇḍala* of Vajrayoginī. Even the hint or possibility of neurosis is unable to enter into one's state of being because the whole world is seen as part of the *maṇḍala* of sacredness that one has entered.

It is interesting that *abhiṣeka* brings both a greater sense of freedom and a greater sense of bondage. The more one develops a sense of openness, letting go, shedding ego, the more one develops a commitment to the world of sanity. So taking *abhiṣeka* and beginning *yi-dam* practice is a very, very serious step. In fact, we should be somewhat frightened of it and, at the same time, we could appreciate it as the most precious opportunity to realize our human birth.

COEMERGENT WISDOM (*LHAN-CIG-SKYES-PA'I-YE-ŚES*)

Fundamentally, the magic of the Vajrayāna tradition is the ability to transform confusion into wisdom on the spot. From the point of view of Vajrayāna, real magic (S.: *siddhi*) is the ability to work with and to tame one's own mind. This is completely different from the usual notion of magic as supernatural power over the universe. As previously mentioned in the discussion of the *samayas* of body, speech, and mind, any potential confusion or neurosis becomes an opportunity to experience sacred outlook. At the beginning of the path of meditation, one works to tame one's mind and to subdue the forces of confusion. In the Mahāyāna, one sees the emptiness of self and phenomena; and out of that, one rouses compassion for beings who do not realize the emptiness, and therefore the freedom, of their nature. In the Vajrayāna, one could actually bring together confusion and enlightenment on one spot, and thereby completely overcome the dualism of *saṃsāra* and *nirvāṇa*.

63. *Vajrayoginī Sādhana* practitioners, Dorje Dzong, Boulder, Colorado.

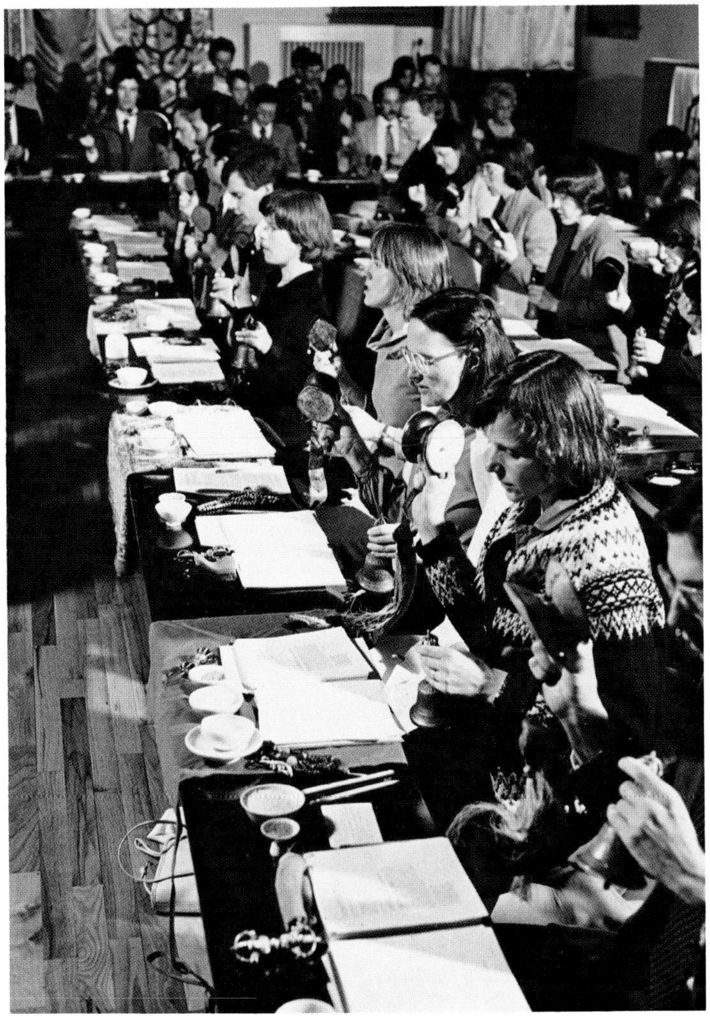

The simultaneous experience of confusion and sanity, or being asleep and awake, is called the realization of co-emergent wisdom (*sahajajñāna*). Any occurrence in one's state of mind, any thought, feeling, or emotion, is both black and white; it is both a statement of confusion and a message of enlightened mind. The confusion is seen so clearly that this clarity itself *is* sacred outlook. Vajrayoginī is called the Coemergent Mother. In fact, the *sādhana* of Vajrayoginī according to Tilopa is entitled *The Sādhana of the Glorious Coemergent Mother Vajrayoginī*.[2] By practicing the *Vajrayoginī-sādhana* and by identifying oneself with the body, speech, and mind of the *yi-dam*, one becomes able to experience the coemergent boundary between confusion and wakefulness. Then one can use confusion itself as a stepping stone for realizing further sanity and further wisdom.

THE SHRINE OF VAJRAYOGINĪ

Some understanding of coemergent wisdom is necessary in order to appreciate the significance of the Vajrayoginī shrine and the ritual objects that are part of it. When one begins to realize the coemergent quality of reality, one recognizes that even a simple object, like a vase or a chair or a table, contains the potential power to spark wakefulness. The same is true for any sense perception or any emotion one may experience. One finds oneself in a world of self-existing messages. Because one is able to "read" the messages of the phenomenal world as statements of sacred outlook, one can properly appreciate the shrine of Vajrayoginī, for the shrine embodies these self-existing messages and communicates them to others. The shrine is not set up for the worship of an external god or force; rather it is designed to focus the messages of sanity and wakefulness that exist in the world, to bring them down into the experience of the practitioner and, in some sense, to amplify their brilliance and power.

The Vajrayāna has sometimes been misinterpreted as a highly symbolic system. For example, one often says that the *vajra* scepter *symbolizes* skillful means or that the *ghaṇṭā symbolizes* wisdom. When it is said that the *vajra* is a symbol of skillful means or of indestructibility, that is true; but, in the genuine Vajrayāna sense, it is not simply that the *vajra* is used to represent or symbolize skillful means because skillful means is too abstract a concept to be dealt with, or shown, directly. The *vajra* scepter *is* skillful means; it actually communicates and transmits skillful action directly if one understands the literalness of the Vajrayāna. For that reason, the shrine of Vajrayoginī and all of the implements on the shrine are themselves regarded as sacred objects.

The shrine that has been constructed for this exhibit is an *abhiṣeka* shrine; that is, it includes all of the objects that are used in conferring the *abhiṣeka* of Vajrayoginī (Ill. 4). A simplified version of this shrine would be used for the daily practice of the *sādhana*.

The painted *maṇḍala* of Vajrayoginī is placed in the center of the shrine. A *maṇḍala* made of colored sand is sometimes used; but in this case it was not possible to construct a sand *maṇḍala*, because of the elaborate preparations needed and the difficulty of transporting it. In fact, traditionally a sand *maṇḍala* is made for a particular ceremony and then destroyed immediately thereafter. Sometimes a *maṇḍala* made of heaps of rice is used, if neither a painted *maṇḍala nor a sand maṇḍala* can be made. The painted *maṇḍala* and the objects above it, which will be discussed next, are regarded as a particular power spot, or focus, of the shrine for magnetizing the energy and blessings of Vajrayoginī, that is, for magnetizing self-existing wakefulness (Pl. 139).

In the center of the painted *maṇḍala* one finds a symbol for the

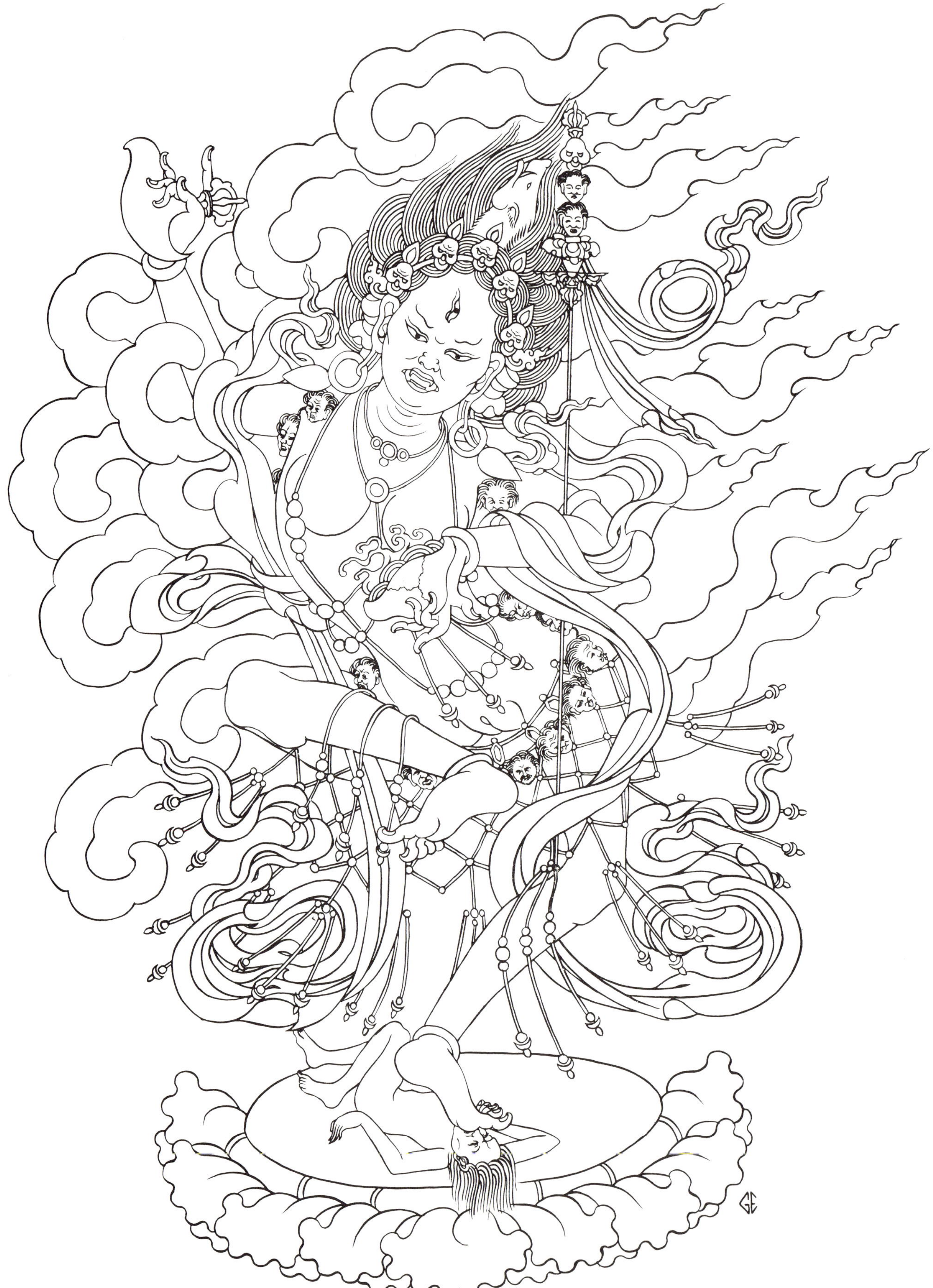

Ill. 3 — Vajrayoginī.

Iconographical Aspect	Symbolic of
a. Hooked knife	a. Cutting neurotic tendencies. Also the weapon of nonthought.
b. Skull cup filled with *amṛita*	b. *Prajñā* and intoxication of extreme beliefs.
c. Staff *(khaṭvāṅga)*	c. Skillful means. The staff is eight-sided, representing the eight-fold Āryan Path taught by the Buddha.
1. Scarf	1. The two folds of the scarf represent the inseparability of Mahāyāna and Vajrayāna.
2. Three skulls	2. The *trikāya* principle: the top head is a skull representing *dharmakāya;* the middle head is of a putrefying corpse representing *saṃbhogakāya;* the bottom head is a freshly severed head representing *nirmāṇakāya.*
d. Sow's head (usually shown over the right ear)	d. Vajra ignorance or nonthought.
e. Hair streaming upwards	e. The wrath of passion. (When Vajrayoginī's hair hangs loosely on her shoulders it is a symbol of compassion. Here the emphasis is more on her wrathful aspect.)
f. Crown of Five skulls	f. The wisdoms of the Five Buddha families.
g. Three eyes	g. Knower of the past, present and future. Also Vajrayoginī's omniscient vision.
h. Wrathful expression, clenching her fangs and biting the lower lip	h. Enraged against the *māras.*
i. Necklace of freshly severed heads	i. The 51 *saṃskāras,* completely purified in nonthought.
j. One face	j. All *dharmas* are of one flavor in *dharmakāya.*
k. Bone ornaments: headdress, earrings, necklace, girdle, anklets and bracelets	k. Perfection of the 5 *pāramitās* of generosity, discipline, patience, exertion, meditation.
l. Two arms	l. Unity of *upāya* and *prajñā.*
m. Left leg bent and right leg raised in dancing posture	m. Not dwelling in extremes of *saṃsāra* or *nirvāṇa.*
n. Corpse seat	n. Death of ego.
o. Sun and moon: disc seats (only the sun is shown)	o. Sun: wisdom Moon: compassion.
p. Lotus seat	p. Spontaneous birth of enlightenment.
q. Vajrayoginī's form: red and blazing with rays of light	q. Enraged against the hordes of *māras* and very wrathful. Also *prajñā-pāramitā.*
NOT SHOWN:	
r. Necklace of red flowers	r. Total nonattachment.

hooked knife (*kartari*) which Vajrayoginī holds in her right hand. This means that the principal *yi-dam*, Vajrayoginī herself, stands at the center of the *maṇḍala*. In the painted *maṇḍala*, the hooked knife is situated in the middle of two crossed triangles, which represent the two "source of *dharmas*" (*chos-'byung*) which are the palace (*mkhar-thabs*) and the seat (*gdan-thabs*) of Vajrayoginī. The "source of *dharmas*" that is Vajrayoginī's palace is actually a three-faced pyramid (trihedron), but it is represented in the painted *maṇḍala* in only two dimensions. The apex of the triangle is an infinitesimal dot that points downward; the mouth of the triangle, in which Vajrayoginī stands, is vast and spacious (Pl. 128, Ill. 4).

The source of *dharmas* arises out of emptiness and has three characteristics: it is unborn, nondwelling, and unceasing. Essentially it is absolute space with a boundary or frame. This represents the coemergent quality of wisdom and confusion arising from the emptiness of space. The source of *dharmas* is sometimes referred to as a channel for *śūnyatā* or as the cosmic cervix. The source of *dharmas* is an abstract form of coemergence while Vajrayoginī is the iconographic or anthropomorphic form of the Coemergent Mother. The shape of the triangle—sharp at the bottom and wide at the top—signifies that every aspect of space can be accommodated at once, microcosm and macrocosm, the most minute situations as well as the most vast.

It is interesting that, in many theistic traditions, the pyramid is a symbol of reaching upward to unite with the godhead. The pinnacle of a pyramid or the apex of a cathedral reaches high into the clouds above. In this case, the source of *dharmas* reaches down, so that pleasure, pain, freedom, and imprisonment all meet at the lowest of the low points of the pyramid. In the nontheistic tradition of Buddhist *tantra*, the triangle reaches down and down into the ground of reality; when one reaches all the way down to the apex of the triangle, one discovers water in that ground, which is known as compassion and as *amṛta*.

In the four cardinal points of the painted *maṇḍala*, surrounding the hooked knife in the center, are the symbols of *vajra, ratna, padma,* and *karma*. Vajrayoginī manifests her basic *buddha* family quality in the central space of the *maṇḍala*. However, the energy of Vajrayoginī creates a complete *maṇḍala* that encompasses, or works with, the energies of all of the Buddha families. Thus, in the iconography of Vajrayoginī, she is surrounded by her retinue: the *vajra ḍākinī* in the east, the *ratna ḍākinī* in the south, the *padma ḍākinī* in the west, and the *karma dākinī* in the north (Pl. 128). This is shown in the painted *maṇḍala* by the symbols of the Buddha families in the four cardinal points: the *vajra* in the east, representing her *buddha-vajra* quality; the jewel in the south, representing her *buddha-ratna* quality; the lotus in the west, representing her *buddha-padma* quality, and the sword in the north, representing her *buddha-karma* quality. The painted *maṇḍala* also depicts coils of joy, which symbolize the *mahāsukha*, the great bliss, that Vajrayoginī confers.

On top of the *maṇḍala* on the shrine is placed the chief *abhiṣeka* vase, the *tsobum*. During the first vase *abhiṣeka*, as discussed earlier, the practitioners are empowered with water from the *tsobum*. Above the painted *maṇḍala* is a tripod on which is placed a skull cup filled with *amṛta*, which is used in conferring the second *abhiṣeka*, the secret *abhiṣeka*. This transmission dissolves the student's mind into the mind of the teacher and the lineage. In general, *amṛta* is the principle of intoxicating extreme beliefs, belief in ego, and dissolving the boundary between confusion and sanity so that coemergence can be realized.

On the skull cup is placed the mirror *maṇḍala* of Vajrayoginī, a mirror coated with red *sindūra* dust, in which is inscribed the *maṇḍala* and *mantra* of Vajrayoginī. The mirror shows that the phenomenal world reflects the wakefulness of Vajrayoginī and that her *maṇḍala* is reflected in the experience of the practitioner. This is the same self-existing message that was discussed earlier. The red *sindūra* dust that covers the mirror represents the cosmic lust and passion of the Coemergent Mother. At this level of practice, passion is no longer regarded as a problem. Freed from grasping, it becomes a force of expansion and communication; it is the expression of "self-luminous compassion" as is said in the *Vajrayoginī-sādhana*.

Surrounding this arrangement of the painted *maṇḍala*, the *abhiṣeka* vase, the skull cup and the mirror are objects connected with the five Buddha families and used in the transmission of the *abhiṣeka* of the vase. Directly in front of the painted *maṇḍala*, in the east, is placed the five-pointed *vajra*, the symbol of the *vajra* family. The symbols of the *buddha* family, the crossed bell and *dorje* and the hooked knife, are also placed here, slightly off to one side. In the south (stage right) are placed the crown and the jewel representing the *ratna* family. In the west (behind the *maṇḍala*) are placed the nine-pointed *vajra* and the lotus, representing the *padma* family. In the north (stage left) are the *ghaṇṭā* and the sword, representing the *karma* family. If the actual objects representing the Buddha families are not available, painted cards (*tsakali*) depicting the objects are placed on the shrine. A second *abhiṣeka* vase, the *lebum* (*las-bum*), is placed in the northeast corner of the shrine. The *lebum* is considered to be the embodiment of the *karma ḍākinī*. At the beginning of the *abhiṣeka*, prior to the *abhiṣeka* of the vase, students drink water from the *lebum* to purify and cleanse themselves; at various points in the ceremony the *vajra* master sprinkles the disciples with water from the *lebum* to signify further purifying and overcoming of psychological obstacles. The conch shell, which holds the oath water of *samaya*, is placed in the front (east) of the shrine between the *vajra* family symbols and offering bowls on the edge of the shrine.

In the southern quadrant of the shrine (stage right) are also placed the *p'agmo tormas* (*phag-mo gtor-ma*) which represent Vajrayoginī and her retinue. *Torma* is a form of bread sculpture made from barley flour, water, alcohol and other ingredients. The *p'agmo tormas* on the shrine are an important means of making offerings to Vajrayoginī, and in doing so, inviting the blessings of the *yi-dam* and of the lineage into the environment of practice. The *tormas* play a central role in the feast offering (*gaṇacakra*), a part of the *Vajrayoginī-sādhana*. The basic idea of the feast offering is to make an offering of all sense perceptions and experience, transforming them into wakefulness rather than expressions of confusion or indulgence.

On the edges of the shrine box are four sets of offering bowls, seven bowls to a set. The seven offerings are: saffron water, flowers, incense, lamps, food, perfumed water, and musical instruments. The offering of saffron water represents cleansing neurotic tendencies and emotional defilements, or *kleśas*, of body, speech, and mind. As is said in the *sādhana*:

> In order to cleanse the *kleśa*-tendencies of sentient beings
> I offer this ablution water for body, speech, and mind.[3]

The offering of flowers represents offering pleasing sense perceptions:

> Flowers pleasing to the victorious ones of all *maṇḍalas*
> Superior, well-formed, celestial varieties.[4]

The offering of incense represents discipline:

> The fragrance of discipline is the best supreme incense.[5]

The offering of lamps represents *prajñā:*

> Burning the poisonous *kleśas* and dispelling the darkness of ignorance,
> The brilliance of *prajñā* is a glorious torch.[6]

The offering of perfumed water represents kindness:

> Pure water mixed with perfume and herbal ingredients is the bathing water of the victorious ones . . .
> May kindness, raining continually from cloudbanks of wisdom, purify the multitude of foul odors.[7]

The offering of food represents *amṛta*:

> Though the victorious ones have no hunger,
> For the benefit of beings, I offer this divine *amṛta* food.[8]

The offering of musical instruments represents the melody of liberation:

> The gong and cymbals are the liberating melody of Brahmā.[9]

On the wall behind the shrine or on an adjacent wall is a *t'ang-*

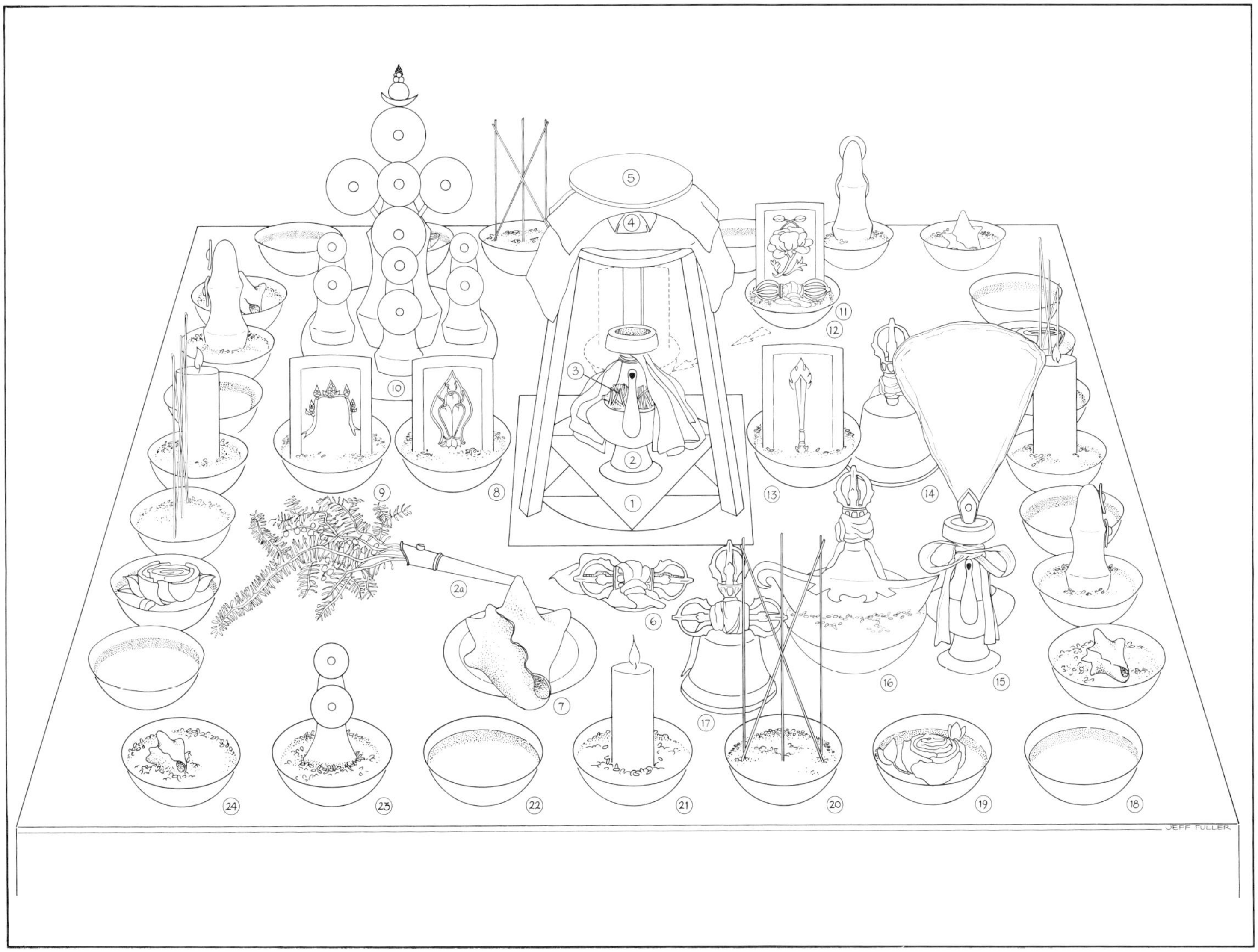

Ill. 4 — Shrine of Vajrayoginī.

ka, or painting, of Vajrayoginī. The *t'ang-ka* of Vajrayoginī is further tribute to her, and it is also an aid to visualization for the practitioner. In order to explain the iconography of Vajrayoginī as depicted in the *t'ang-ka*, it would be helpful to briefly discuss visualization practice itself, since a practitioner's connection to and understanding of the iconography come about from the visualization practice of Vajrayoginī.

VISUALIZATION

There are two stages of visualization practice: *utpattikrama* (*bskyed-pa'i rim-pa*) and *sampannakrama* (*rdzogs-pa'i rim-pa*). *Utpattikrama* literally means "developing stage," and *saṃpannakrama* means "fulfillment stage." *Utpattikrama* is the process of visualizing the *yi-dam*, in this case, Vajrayoginī. In the self-visualization, the practitioner visualizes himself as the *yi-dam*. The visualization arises from emptiness, from *śūnyatā*, as do all tantric visualizations. The text amplifies this concept:

> All the *dharmas* comprising grasping and fixation become empty. From within emptiness . . . arises the source of *dharmas*, a triangle . . . On that is the nature of my consciousness . . . like a fish leaping from water, I arise in the body of Jetsun Vajrayoginī.[10]

So the process of visualizing oneself as the *yi-dam* comes first from the experience of emptiness and egolessness. Out of that arises the source of *dharmas*, the abstract form of coemergence; and on that, the practitioner visualizes himself as the *yi-dam*. The visualization, therefore, is essentially empty as well. The practice of visualization is identifying oneself with the *yi-dam*, realizing the deity as the nonmanifested, or empty, manifestation of basic enlightened nature. The form of the *yi-dam*, her clothing, ornaments and stance, all represent aspects of the enlightened state of mind. So when one visualizes oneself as a blazing, youthful red lady decked with bone ornaments, one is not particularly trying to conjure up an exotic costume as the latest fashion, but one is identifying oneself with Vajrayoginī, the embodiment of wisdom and compassion.

The visualization of oneself as Vajrayoginī is called the *samayasattva*, the "sacred bondage of one's being." The *samayasattva* is basically the expression of the *samayas* of body, speech, and mind. It expresses one's commitment to the teacher and the teachings and one's trust in one's fundamental state of mind.

Having visualized the *samayasattva* of basic being, one invites what is known as *jñānasattva*. The *jñānasattva* is another level of being or experience. *Jñāna* is a state of wakefulness or openness, whereas *samaya* is an experience of bondage, of being solidly grounded in one's experience. *Jñāna* literally means "wisdom" or, more accurately, "being wise." One invites this state of wisdom, this level of wakefulness, into one's own imperfect visualization, so that the visualization comes alive with a feeling of openness and humor.

At the conclusion of the visualization practice, the visualization is dissolved back into emptiness and one meditates, or rests, in that nondual state of mind. This is the *saṃpannakrama* or fulfillment stage. It is said in the tantric texts that the proper understanding of visualization practice is that the *utpattikrama* and the *saṃpannakrama* stages are not fundamentally different; that is, in this case, that the *saṃpannakrama* experience of emptiness-emptiness and the *utpattikrama* experience of form-emptiness should not be seen as two things, but as one expression of the world of the Coemergent Mother.

Saṃpannakrama meditation is similar to the practice of *śamatha-vipaśyanā*; in fact, without prior training in these meditation practices, it is impossible to practice *saṃpannakrama*. *Saṃpannakrama* is an expression of vastness. Experiencing the *vajra* mind of Vajrayoginī is so deep and vast that if thoughts arise, they do not become a highlight: they are small fish in a huge ocean of space.

THE VAJRAYOGINĪ PRINCIPLE AND ITS ICONOGRAPHY

The major features of the iconography are identified in Ill. 4. An examination of the meaning of the following praise to Vajrayoginī from the *sādhana* may help us to understand the Vajrayoginī principle in relation to the iconography of Vajrayoginī. The praise begins:

> Bhagavatī Vajrayoginī
> Personification of *vajra* emptiness
> Blazing with the *kalpa*-ending fire, uttering the terrifying sound of *hūṃ*
> I prostrate to Vajra-caṇḍalī.[11]

Bhagavatī means "blessed one." This stanza refers first to Vajrayoginī as the anthropomorphic form of *śūnyatā*, the "personification of *vajra* emptiness." It then praises her fiery quality of passion and cosmic lust. In the iconography, Vajrayoginī's body is red and blazes with rays of light, which is described here as "blazing with the *kalpa*-ending fire." This is her *padma* family quality, which transmutes neurotic passion into all-consuming compassion. *Kalpa* means "an historical era." The "*kalpa*-ending fire" in Indian mythology is the explosion of the sun which burns up the solar system and brings an end to the *kalpa*. Vajrayoginī's passion is so bright and so consuming that it is likened to that fire. The "terrifying sound of *hūṃ*" expresses the wrath of her passion, which is terrifying to ego. *Caṇḍalī* (*gtum-mo*) in yogic practice is the yogic heat, cosmic heat, which is again the Vajrayoginī principle of passion arising free from habitual tendencies. Such passion is immensely powerful; it radiates its warmth in all directions. It simultaneously nurtures the welfare of beings and blazes to destroy the neurotic tendencies of ego. The praise continues:

> Your sow's face shows nonthought, the unchanging *dharmakāya*,
> You benefit beings with wrathful mercy
> Accomplishing their welfare with horrific accoutrements,
> I prostrate to you who benefit beings in nonthought.[12]

Nonthought is an important aspect of the Vajrayoginī principle. It is the experience of mind totally freed from the habitual chatter of ego, freed from the grasping and fixation that give rise to neurotic thought patterns. Until the aggression and wildness of mind are tamed through meditation practice, there is no possibility of experiencing the nonthought possibilities in one's mind.

Vajrayoginī is often depicted with a sow's head over her right ear. When she wears this ornament, she is referred to as Vajravārāhī, "*vajra* sow." The sow traditionally represents ignorance or stupidity. In this case, the sow's head symbolizes the transmutation of ignorance, or delusion, into the *vajra* ignorance, which is nonthought or complete spaciousness of mind.

This stanza equates nonthought with *dharmakāya* which, roughly translated, is the primordial mind of Buddha. The practice of the *Vajrayoginī sādhana* is very much connected with realizing this primordial space of nonthought, which could also be called the truth of complete nonreference point. The purpose of the *sādhana* practice is not so much to cut immediate thoughts as it is to cut the habitual tendencies that are the root of discursive thought.

The "horrific accoutrements" referred to in the stanza are the necklace of freshly severed heads that Vajrayoginī wears. It says in the *sādhana* that she wears this necklace because "the fifty-one *saṃskāras* are completely purified." *Saṃskāra* means "formations," which refers to concepts. Vajrayoginī's necklace of heads signifies that all habitual concepts are purified or destroyed in nonthought.

The praise continues:

> Terrifying heroine who annihilates the unsuitable,
> With three eyes, clenching your fangs, the absolute *trikāya*,
> Your terrifying cry cuts off the *kleśas*,
> I prostrate to you who subjugate and conquer the *māras*.[13]

Vajrayoginī is frequently called the conqueror of the *māras*. The *māras* are the forces of worldly confusion. In the stories of the Buddha's enlightenment, Māra, "the evil one," sends his daughters, the four *māras*, to tempt Śākyamuni and his armies to attack him. Vanquishing them, Śākyamuni becomes the Buddha, the Awakened One. Thus, the basic idea of Vajrayoginī as the conqueror of the *māras* is the conquest of ego. From ego's point of view, Vajrayoginī is "terrifying" because her wakefulness is so piercing and uncompromising. At another point in the *sādhana*, it says: "Grimacing wrathfully to subdue the four *māras*, she clenches her fangs and bites her lower lip."[14] This further explains the stanza's reference to Vajrayoginī's fierceness.

The reference to Vajrayoginī's three eyes means that nothing escapes the vision of Vajrayoginī; therefore, ego has nowhere to hide. The *sādhana* also says: "Because she is the knower of the past, present, and future, she rolls her three furious bloodshot eyes."[15]

The notion that Vajrayoginī is "the absolute *trikāya*" is that her wisdom and skillful means manifest on all levels of body and mind: the *dharmakāya* level of absolute, primordial mind; the *sambhogakaya* level of energy, emotions, and symbols; and the *nirmāṇakāya* level of manifested form, or body. The *trikāya* also refers to the levels of body, speech, and mind in one's practice, which are the levels of physical body, the emotions and concepts, and the basic spaciousness of mind. Vajrayoginī joins all of those levels together, and again leaves no place for the *māras* to hide.

The stanza also says that her terrifying cry "cuts off the *kleśas*." *Kleśas*, or obscurations, refer to conflicting emotions, neurotic emotion. The five *kleśas* are passion, aggression, delusion, jealousy, and pride, all of which are subjugated by the Vajrayoginī principle.

The next stanza reads:

> Naked, with loosed hair, of faultless and terrifying form
> Beyond the vice of the *kleśas*, you do benefit for sentient beings.
> You lead beings from the six realms with your hook of mercy,
> I prostrate to you who accomplish Buddha activity.[16]

Vajrayoginī is naked because she is completely untouched by the neurosis of the *kleśas*; therefore she has no armor of ego to clothe her. Because of this, she is able to "do benefit for sentient beings," to extend absolute compassion to them. The reference to her loosed hair signifies her compassion for beings. The "hook of mercy" refers to Vajrayoginī's hooked knife, with which she lifts beings out of the suffering of the six realms, *saṃsāra*, into the *vajra* world. Therefore, she completely accomplishes action which is free from karmic defilement, action which is completely awake, "Buddha activity."

The next stanza reads:

> Dwelling in the charnel ground, subjugating Rudra and his wife,
> Wrathful, fearsome, uttering the sound of *phaṭ*
> You do benefit for beings with the mercy of your skill,
> I prostrate to the wrathful one who subjugates the *māras*.[17]

The charnel ground refers to the basic space in which birth and death, confusion and wakefulness arise—the ground of coemergence. Vajrayoginī is not an ethereal principle; she dwells in the heart of saṃsāric chaos, which is also the heart of wisdom. "Rudra and his wife" refers to ego and its embellishments, which Vajrayoginī subjugates utterly. She is "the terrifying heroine who annihilates the unsuitable"; therefore, "she is wrathful and fearsome and utters the sound of *phaṭ*," a syllable associated with subjugation, destruction of ego-clinging, and the proclamation of *vajra* truth. At the same time, she is skilled and merciful. Combining these qualities, she is, again, the subjugator of the *māras*.

The next verse reads:

> You have realized ultimate *dharmatā* and abandoned death.
> On a seat of a corpse, sun, moon and lotus
> Your wrathful form, beautified with all the ornaments,
> I prostrate to you who have perfected all good qualities.[18]

The lotus, sun disk, and moon disk are the customary seats for both Buddhas and *yi-dams* in tantric iconography. The lotus is a symbol of purity and also signifies the birth of enlightenment amidst the world of confused existence. The sun symbolizes *jñāna*, or wisdom, while the moon is a symbol of *bodhicitta*, or compassion. The fact that Vajrayoginī also stands on a corpse signifies that she is a semiwrathful deity. There are peaceful, semiwrathful and wrathful *yi-dams* in tantric iconography. The peaceful deities represent the energy of pacifying and taming while semiwrathful and wrathful *yi-dams* work more directly and forcefully with passion, aggression, and delusion—conquering and trampling them on the spot.

The figure of the corpse symbolizes the death of ego and shows that Vajrayoginī has "abandoned death." "Ultimate *dharmatā*" in the stanza is a reference to Vajrayoginī's stance. In an earlier portion of the *sādhana*, it says: "Since she does not dwell in the extremes of *saṃsāra* or *nirvāṇa*, she stands on a seat of a lotus, corpse and sun-disk with her left leg bent and her right leg raised in dancing posture."[19] The idea of ultimate *dharmatā* is transcending the dualism, or extremes, of *saṃsāra* and *nirvāṇa* by realizing coemergent wisdom: seeing how confusion and enlightenment arise simultaneously. *Dharmatā* means "the state of *dharma*." It is complete realization of the *dharma*, which is seeing the "is-ness" or the "suchness" of reality.

This stanza also refers to the ornaments that beautify Vajrayoginī's wrathful form: her bone headdress, her bone earrings, her necklace, her girdle, and her anklets and bracelets. These represent her perfection of generosity, discipline, patience, exertion, and meditation—five of the six *pāramitās* or transcendent actions of the Mahāyāna. The perfection of the sixth *pāramitā, prajñā*, is not represented as an ornament because the being of Vajrayoginī is the epitome of *prajñā*. Thus she is called Prajñāpāramitā. *Prajñā* as the perception of *śūnyatā* was mentioned earlier. At the level of *prajñāpāramitā*, *prajñā* is complete nondual realization that cuts through any clinging to either existence or nonexistence. Prajñāpāramitā is called the mother of all the buddhas: all the buddhas of the past, present, and future are born from this stainless good knowledge which shows the nature of phenomena as *śūnyatā*. In an earlier section of the *sādhana*, Vajrayoginī is praised as Prajñāpāramitā:

> *Prajñāpāramitā*, inexpressible by speech or thought,
> Unborn, unceasing with a nature like sky
> Which can only be experienced by discriminating awareness wisdom,
> Mother of the victorious ones of the three times,
> I praise you and prostrate.[20]

The next stanza reads:

> Holding a hooked-knife, a *khaṭvāṅga*, and a skull cup in your hands,
> Possessing the light of wisdom, you cut off the *kleśas*.
> As the spontaneous *trikāya*, you cut off the three poisons,
> I prostrate to you who benefit beings.[21]

The second line: "Possessing the light of wisdom you cut off the *kleśas*," further emphasizes the Vajrayoginī principle as Prajñāpāramitā, the essence of discriminating awareness wisdom.

The hooked knife has been discussed as Vajrayoginī's "hook of mercy." It is also a weapon that is used to slice through the deceptions of ego. It is a symbol of the power and cutting quality of nonthought. In her left hand Vajrayoginī holds a skull cup, or *kapāla*, filled with *amṛta*, representing the principle of intoxicating extreme beliefs. The *kapāla* filled with *amṛta* is also a symbol of wisdom. The *khaṭvāṅga* is the staff that Vajrayoginī holds up against her shoulder. It represents her skillful means. The staff is also the secret symbol of Vajrayoginī's union with her consort, Cakrasaṃvara, who is the essence of skillful means.

On the *khatvānga* are three heads representing the *trikāya* principle mentioned in this stanza. The reference to Vajrayoginī as the spontaneous *trikāya* means that the brilliance of her wisdom applies equally to all levels of experience. Because of the universality of her wisdom, she utterly cuts off the three poisons: passion, aggression, and delusion. In doing so, she benefits beings.

The next stanza reads:

> The self-born great bliss, the Vajraḍākiṇī,
> You are the unchanging wisdom *vajra* of *dharmakāya*,
> The nonthought unconditioned wisdom, absolute *dharmadhātu*,
> I prostrate to your pure nondual form.[22]

Again, this stanza praises Vajrayoginī as the essence of wisdom, which is the primordial "wisdom *vajra* of *dharmakāya*," the even more primordial "unconditioned wisdom" of "absolute *dharmadhātu*" and is completely nondual. Beyond that, this stanza brings together the Vajrayoginī principle of wisdom with the principle of the great bliss, *mahāsukha*, which is self-born, that is, self-existing rather than created or manufactured by conceptual mind.

Mahāsukha is an actual experience of bliss, a physical, psychological, total experience of joy that comes from being completely without discursive thoughts, being completely in the realm of nonthought. It is uniting with the nondual, awake state of being. This experience is the fruition of the Vajrayoginī practice; it comes only from complete identification with the wisdom mind of the *yi-dam*. According to the scriptures, *mahāsukha* and wisdom are indivisible; therefore, the practice of Vajrayoginī leads to this experience of the self-born great bliss because she is the essence of wisdom.

In the next stanza of the praise, the third line reads:

> Self-born great bliss, the ultimate *mahāmudrā*[23]

This refers to Vajrayoginī. Experiencing *mahāsukha* or the wisdom of bliss and emptiness, is the realization of *mahāmudrā*, which is the pinnacle of the tradition of *anuttara-tantra*. *Mahā* means "great" and *mudrā* means "sign" or "gesture." *Mahāmudrā* experience is realizing that the literal truth and the symbolic truth and the absolute truth are actually one thing, that they take place on one dot, one spot. It is experiencing reality as the great symbol which stands for itself.

The bliss of *mahāmudrā* is not so much great pleasure, but it is the experience of tremendous spaciousness, freedom from imprisonment, which comes from seeing through the duality of existence and realizing that the essence of truth, the essence of space, is available on this very spot. The freedom of *mahāmudrā* is measureless, unspeakable, fathomless. Such fathomless space and complete freedom produce tremendous joy. This type of joy is not conditioned by even the experience of freedom itself; it is self-born, innate.

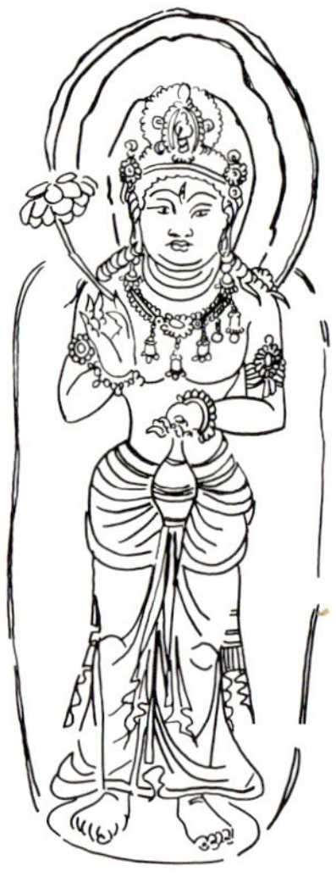

CONCLUSION

Some of what has been discussed here may be very difficult to grasp. In fact, it should be that way. If it were possible to experience the Vajrayāna simply by reading about it, it would cease to exist, because no one would practice it; one would simply study the texts. Luckily this does not work. The only way to gain the *vajra* freedom is to practice the *Buddhadharma* as it was taught by the Buddha and as it has been preserved and passed down for 2,500 years.

I am very happy that it has been possible to discuss the Vajrayāna and the Vajrayoginī tradition so genuinely and thoroughly. But the most important thing that one could ever do for oneself and others is to sit down and unravel the confusion in one's mind. This is a very, very simple thing to do, and because it is so simple, it is also very easy not to see this possibility.

It is my hope that this discussion will provide a glimpse of the Vajrayāna world: its grandeur and sacredness. Sacred possibilities always exist in our lives. The goodness and the gentleness of the world are always there for us to appreciate. This is not a myth; it is actual fact. We could experience Vajrayoginī at any time, if we have the courage to acknowledge our own wakeful nature and the greatness of our heritage as human beings.

> Eternally brilliant, utterly empty,
> *Vajra* dancer, mother of all,
> I bow to you.
> The essence of all sentient beings lives as Vajrayoginī.
> From the milk ocean of her blessing
> Good butter is churned
> Which worthy ones receive as glory.
> May everyone eternally enjoy
> The lotus garden of the Coemergent Mother.

Vajrācārya the Venerable
Chögyam Trungpa, Rinpoche

Notes

All passages quoted in this article are from the *sādhana* of Vajrayoginī written by the third Karmapa, Rangjung Dorje (1284–1339), at Tsurphu monastery in Tibet. The source used for the translation is a modern handwritten copy printed in India, which has sixty folios. All folio references given are to this printing.

1. ji-ltar bltams-pa tsam gyis ni/
lha-rnams-kyis-ni khrus gsol-ltar/
lha-yi chu-ni dag-pa-yis/
de-bźin bdag-gis dbaṅ-bskur-ro//
(44B: 4–5)

2. dpal-ldan lhan-cig-skyes-ma rdo-rje-rnal-'byor sgrub-thabs dkyil-'khor-gyi cho-ga gsaṅ-chen mchog-gi myur-lam gsal-ba'i 'dren-pa bźugs-so
(Title page 1A)

3. sems-can ñon-moṅs bag-chags sbyaṅ slad-du/
sku-gsuṅ-thugs-la khrus-chab'di gsol-bas/
(31A: 4–5)

4. dkyil-'khor kun-tu-rgyal-ba mñes gyur-pa'i/
lha-rdzas dbyibs-legs me-tog dam-pa'di/
(31B: 1)

5. tshul-khrims dri-ldan spos-mchog dam-pa'di/
(31B: 2–3)

6. ñon-moṅs dug-sreg ma-rig mun-sel-ba'i/
shes-rab gzi-ldan dpal-gyi sgron-me-'di/
(31B: 5)

7. spos-daṅ sman-sbyar chu-gtsaṅ rgyal-ba'i khrus/
(31B: 6–32A: 1)
mi-gtsaṅ dri-ma'i tshogs-rnams dag-gyur-cig/
(32A: 1–2)

8. rgyal-ba'i sku-la bkres-pa mi-mṅa' yaṅ/
'gro-ba'i don-du lha-rdzas bdud-rtsi'i bšas/
(32A: 2)

9. dril-chen sil-sñan rnam-grol tshaṅs-pa'i-dbyaṅs/
(32A: 3)

10. bzuṅ-ba daṅ 'dzin-pas bsdus-pa'i chos thams-cad stoṅ-pa-ñid-du gyur . . .stoṅ-pa'i ṅaṅ-las . . . chos-kyi 'byuṅ-gnas gru-gsum-pa . . . steng-du/
raṅ-gi rnam-par-śes-pa'i ṅo-bo . . . chu-la ña ldaṅ-ba'i tshul-du rje-btsun rdo-rje-rnal-'byor-ma'i skur gyur-pa ni/
(17B: 2–18A: 1)

11. bcom-ldan-'das-ma rdo-rje-rnal-'byor-ma/
stoṅ-ñid rdo-rje ldan-pa'i bdag-ñid-can/
bskal-pa'i me-'bar 'jigs-pa'i hūṃ sgra-sgrogs/
rdo-rje gtum-mo de-la phyag-'tshal-lo//
(32A: 5–32B: 1)

12. phag-gdoṅ rtog-med chos-sku 'gyur-med ston/
khro-mo'i thugs-rje 'gro-ba'i don-mdzad-ma/
'gro-don rdzogs-mdzad 'jigs-pa'i cha-lugs-can/
rtog-med 'gro-don mdzad-la phyag-'tshal-lo//
(32B: 1–2)

13. 'jigs-ruṅ dpa'-mo ma-ruṅ tshar-gcod-ma/
spyan-gsum mche-brtsigs sku-gsum don-daṅ-ldan/
ñon-moṅs gcod-mdzad 'jigs-pa'i ṅa-ro-can/
bdud-'dul 'joms-ma'i sku-la phyag-'tshal-lo//
(32B: 2–4)

14. bdud-bźi 'dul-ba'i khro-gñer daṅ mche-ba rnam-par-gtsigs śiṅ ma-mchu tshems-kyis mnan-pa
(18B: 1)

15. dus-gsum mkhyen-phyir rab-tu-gtum-pa'i spyan-gsum khrag-ltar dmar źiṅ zlum-la gyo-ba
(18A: 5–18B: 1)

16. skra-grol gcer-bu skyon-bral 'jigs-pa'i gzugs/
ñon-moṅs skyon-bral sems-can don-mdzad-ma/
thugs-rje'i lcags-kyu'i 'gro-drug gnas-nas 'dren/
phrin-las rdzogs-mdzad de-la phyag-'tshal-lo//
(32B: 4–5)

17. dur-khrod gnas-bźugs ru-dra pho-mo 'dul/
drag-mo 'jigs-tshul phaṭ-kyi sgra-sgrogs śiṅ/
thabs-mkhas thugs-rjes 'gro-ba'i don-mdzad-ma/
bdud-'dul drag-mo'i sku-la phyag-'tshal-lo//
(32B: 5–33A: 2)

18. chos-ñid don-rtogs 'chi-ba'i tshul spaṅs-ma/
ro daṅ ñi zla pad-ma'i gdan gyi tshul/
rgyan-rnams kun-gyis rab-mdzes khro-mo'i sku/
yon-tan rdzogs-mdzad de-la phyag-'tshal-lo//
(33A: 2–3)

19. 'khor-'das gñis-kyi mtha'-la mi-gnas-pa'i phyir gdan pad-ma ro daṅ ñi-ma'i dkyil-'khor-gyi steṅ-du źabs-brkyaṅ-bskum-gyi gar-stabs-su bźugs-pa'o
(18B: 4–5)

20. smra-bsam brjod-med śes-rab pha-rol-phyin/
ma-skyes mi-'gag nam-mkha'i ṅo-bo-ñid/
so-so-raṅ-rig ye-śes spyod-yul-ba/
dugs-gsum rgyal-ba'i yum-la phyag-'tshal-bstod//
(10A: 1–2)

21. gri-gug thod-pa kha-ṭvāṃ phyag na bsnams/
ñon-moṅs gcod-mdzad ye-śes 'od-daṅ-ldan/
dug-gsum gcod-mdzad sku-gsum lhun-gyis-grub/
'gro ba'i don-mdzad de-la phyag-'tshal-lo//
(33A: 3–4)

22. bde-chen raṅ-byuṅ rdo-rje mkha'-'gro-ma/
mi-'gyur ye-sés rdo-rje chos-kyi-sku/
rtog-med spros-bral ye-sés chos-dbyiṅs don/
yaṅ-dag gñis-med sku-la phyag-'tshal-lo//
(33A: 4–5)

23. bde-chen raṅ-byuṅ phyag-rgya-chen-mo'i don
(33B: 1)

ERRATA AND CORRIGENDA

Copyright page: ". . supported by a grant . ." should be changed to: ". . supported by grants."
List of Lenders:
Istituto Italiano per il Medio ed Estremo Oriente, Rome
Museum für Völkerkunde, Vienna
Table of Contents: ch. VI.(c): "Ta-pho" instead of "Ta-Pho".

P. 13, l.col., lines 18-19 f.a.: I.D.Mathur, Acting Director . .
P. 14, r.col., line 2 f.a.: Ye-śes 'Öd . .
R.col., line 8 f.b.: Kāśmīra, . .
P. 22, l.col., line 16 f.b.: Nicolas-Vandier 1976.
P. 21, r.col., line 6 f.a.: (Figs. 2, 3, 4, 5, 6, 6a).
P. 42, l.col., line 9 f.b.: . . Xuanzong (Hsüan-tsung) . .
P. 49, l.col., line 5 f.b.: . . Prajapati: . .
R.col., line 1 f.b.: (. . quoted from Hornbein 1968*).
P. 57, r.col., line 27 f.a.: . . pañcavarṣika . .
P. 73, Fig. 20, lines 5-6 f.a.: . . Tshul-khrims-Öd . .
P. 77, r.col., lines 27-28 f.a.: . . (Bhagavān)
P. 79, r.col., line 2 f.a.: . . Tsaparang, . .
R.col., line 2 f.b.: . . Sam-ye, . .
P. 80, l.col., line 7 f.a.: . . Jokhang . .
P. 83, l.col, line 31 f.b.: (Kosambi 1970: 133-76).
L.col., line 17 f.b.: (Kosambi 1970: 162-3).
L.col., line 9 f.b.: (Kosambi 1970: 159).
L.col., line 4 f.b.: (Francke 1907 . .)
R.col., lines 20-21: (. . Kosambi 1970 . .)
P. 84, r.col., line 3 f.a.: (Klimburg-Salter 1981a).
R.col., line 24 f.b.: (Jettmar 1980b).
P. 90, r.col., line 3-4 f.a.: . . is meaningless" (Kosambi 1970: 181).
R.col., line 2 f.b.: (Chavannes 1903b: 205-6).
P. 91, m.col., line 8: Kreitman Gallery, instead of: Neil Kreitman.
Ibid., r.col., line 7: Xuanzang (Hsüan-tsang).
P. 92, m.col., line 13 f.b.: (Pl.2) instead of: (Pl.1).
P. 95, l.col., line 37 f.b.: (Jettmar 1980b).
M.col., line 1 f.b.: (Taddei 1978b . .).
R.col., lines 6 and 16 f.a.: (Jettmar 1980b . .).
R.col., line 19 f.b.: (Jettmar 1977, 1980a, 1980b).
P. 97, m.col., line 13 f.b.: (Tucci 1977b . .).
P. 98, m.col., line 3 f.b.: (Pal 1975b:210; . .).
R.col., line 4 f.b.: . . Buddhas in Bāmiyān . .
P. 99, r.col., line 11 f.b.: (Pal 1975b . .).
P. 100, l.col., line 4 f.b.: (Pal 1975b . .).
P. 102, l.col., line 1 f.b.: (Taddei 1978a).
P. 105, r.col., line 5 f.b.: delete: Pal 1975a:36.
P. 107, l.col., line 2 f.b.: (Pal 1975b . .; . .).
P. 108, Pl. 39, line 12 f.b.: (Trans. by Beal 1884 . .).
Pl. 41, line 1 f.b.: (Granoff 1979, . .).
P. 109, Pl. 40, line 4 f.b.: (Pal 1975b . .).
P. 110, l.col., line 2 f.b.: (Pal 1973b . .).
R.col., line 17 f.a.: (Taddei 1978a . .).
P. 113, r.col., line 7 f.a.: (Klimburg-Salter 1981a).
P. 117, l.col., line 2 f.a.: (Klimburg-Salter 1981a . .).
P. 118, r.col., line 8 f.a.: (Pelliot 1920–24 . .).
P. 119, l.col., line 2 f.a.: (Kwanten 1980, Snellgrove . .).
P. 122, l.col., line 3 f.b.: (Klimburg-Salter 1976, 1981b).
P. 124, l.col., line 13 f.a.: (Pal 1975b . .).
L.col., line 16 f.b.: (Macdonald 1962).
L.col., line 11 f.b.: (. . Jones 1949–56)
R.col., line 17 f.a., and line 2 f.b.: (Stein 1921b . .).
P. 129, l.col., line 17 f.a.: Stein 1921b . .
L.col., line 18 f.a.: Soper 1965.
R.col., line 1 f.b.: Soper 1965.
P. 132, r.col., line 6 f.a.: (Klimburg-Salter 1981a).
R.col., line 12 f.a.: (Granoff 1970).
P. 133, line 4: Nicolas-Vandier . .
Line 2: . . Chinesische Malerei, Haus der Kunst, Munich 1959.
P. 136, m.col., line 3 f.b., and r.col., line 1 f.b.: Nicolas-Vandier . .
P. 137, r.col., line 12 f.a.: Stein 1921b . .
R.col., line 3 f.b.: to be added under "Previously published": Andrews 1935:232.
P. 140, line 11 f.b.: (Stein 1921b . .).
P. 141, l.col., line 18 f.a.: (Stein 1921b . .).
P. 144, l.col., line 18 f.a., and line 2 f.b.: Nicolas-Vandier.
P. 147, m.col., line 22 f.b.: (1921b . .).
P. 150, l.col., line 13 f.a., and r.col., line 3 f.b.: Stein 1921b.
P. 151, m.col., line 5 f.a.: Ca. eleventh-twelfth century.
P. 152, r.col., line 3 f.a.: (Yi Liang Chou . .).
P. 154, r.col., lines 30 and 36: Snellgrove.
P. 155, l.col., line 7 f.b.: . . foundation of the Sakya and . .
P. 156, l.col., line 23 f.b.: Lhakang Soma, Alchi.
P. 157, l.col., line 23 f.a.: Mang-nang.
L.col., line 36 f.a.: . . , and the 'du-khang at Sumda . .
P. 163, r.col., line 1 f.b.: (Klimburg-Salter . .).
P. 164, r.col., lines 19 f.b.: Gandhavyūha.
R.col., line 18 f.b.: Lokesh Chandra 1980.
P. 167, l.col., line 28 f.a.: (Pl. 128).
L.col., line 15 f.b.: . . Little painting remains . .
P. 168, l.col., line 13 f.a.: . . of the Ta-pho Avataṃsaka-sūtra . .
P. 169, line 12 f.a.: . . in the temple at Avantipur . .
Line 2 f.b.: Ohri 1975.
P. 179, r.col., to be added: Previously published: Pal 1982.
P. 180, Pl. 96, line 12 f.a.: . . : the pointed halo, . .
P. 183, r.col., line 4-5 f.b.: delete: Le Coq 1922–1933:I, pl.32,35.
P. 184, m.col., line 1 f.b.: . . Dhargyey 1975.
P. 185, Pl. 105, lines 7-8 f.a.: Istituto Italiano per il Medio ed Estremo Oriente.
P. 188, Pl. 106, lines 7-8 f.a., and Pl. 107, lines 7-8 f.a.: Istituto Italiano per il Medio ed Estremo Oriente.
P. 193, Pl. 111, line 11 f.a.: . . paintings in Pls. 109 and 110.
P. 201, Pl. 121, line 7 f.a.: Museo Nazionale d'Arte Orientale (no. 963/796).
Pl. 122, line 2 f.b.: Cheryl Snell.
P. 203, Pl. 123, to be added: Previously published (Tucci 1949:II, 542–543, III, Pl. 143; Musée Guimet 1977:161).
Pl. 126, line 1 f.b.: . . Dhargyey 1977.
P. 204, line 30 f.b.: . . of three Rigs-ldan kings . .
Line 3 f.b.: Béguin . .
P. 205, l.col., line 3 f.a.: . . brought Indian Buddhist monks, . .
P. 206, r.col., line 22 f.b.: (Ch. V), instead of: (Ch.III).
P. 207, l.col., lines 25 and 34 f.b.: the Sixteenth Gyalwa Karmapa . .
P. 243, l.col., line 1 f.b.: delete: Jina; . . ; Tathāgata;
P. 244, l.col., under Asher, Frederick: delete "L'Arte del Gandhara . . Bussagli 1958".
P. 249, l.col., to be added under Karmay, Heather: 1977 Tibetan costume, seventh to eleventh centuries. In Macdonald and Imaeda 1977:64–81.
L.col.: Lowry, John, instead of Loury, John.
R.col., under Mission Pelliot 1967: Douldour-Aqour.
P. 250, r.col., under Richardson 1977: Ariane Macdonald.
List of Photo Credits:
R.Datta Gupta, instead of: R.Gupta
Deborah Klimburg-Salter: Figs. 41-42, 45, 47-49, 51-60.
Maximilian Klimburg: Figs. 1-6a, 7a.
R.Datta Gupta: Figs. 43-44, 46, 50.
Elizabeth Goldblatt: Fig. 61.
Further Photo Credits:
G. Holmes and B. Hansen: Fig. 63.
Paul Kloppenburg: Fig. 62.
Illustration 3 is by Glen Eddy. Copyright 1976 by Shambhala Publ.

Numerous Tibetan and Sanskrit misspellings, which are still intelligible in their present form, and obvious typographical errors are not included in this list.

Abbreviations: f.a. = from above, f.b. = from below.

Glossary of Sanskrit and Other Names and Terms

abhiṣeka (Tibetan: *dbaṅ-skur*)
Literally "consecration by sprinkling"; a ritual initiation into tantric teachings and practices.

Akṣobhya (Tibetan: Mi-bskyod-pa)
"The Imperturbable"; one of the Five Buddhas, he presides over the *vajra* family and embodies the principle that wrath may be transmuted into the enlightened energy known as "Mirror-like Wisdom." He is blue in color.

Amitābha (Tibetan: Od-dpag-med)
"Boundless Light"; the Buddha who presides over the lotus *(padma)* family, his red color signifies the transmutation of desire into the discriminating awareness of enlightenment.

Amoghapāśa
A variant form of Avalokiteśvara equipped with multiple arms. *See also* Avalokiteśvara.

Amoghasiddhi (Tibetan: Don-yod 'grub-pa)
"Infallible Success"; one of the Five Buddhas, he is green in color and presides over the *karma* family.

arhat (Tibetan: *dgra-bcom-pa)*
Literally a "worthy"; one who attains liberation through meditation upon the fundamental Four Truths according to the system of the Disciples. *See also śrāvaka.*

Atīśa
A renowned Indian Buddhist master who visited Tibet in 1042 A.D. and made significant contributions to the form and content of Tibetan Buddhism. The Kadampa *(bka' -gdams-pa)* order, founded by his foremost disciple, Drom-tön, was based largely upon the teachings of Atīśa.

Avalokiteśvara (Tibetan: Spyan-ras-gzigs)
Most popular of the eight Bodhisattvas, he personifies the compassion of the Buddha for the suffering of beings and is regarded by Tibetans as the tutelary deity of their land.

bodhicitta (Tibetan: *byaṅ-sems)*
The resolve of a Bodhisattva to seek Buddhahood in order to become able to help other beings also to attain that state of liberation.

Bodhisattva (Tibetan: Byaṅ-chub sems-dpa')
Literally "enlightenment being"; any being who has vowed to achieve Buddhahood but, more specifically, one who has actually attained any of the ten stages of Bodhisattvahood.

Bön
The indigenous shamanistic religion that prevailed in Tibet prior to the introduction of Buddhism.

Buddha (Tibetan: Saṅs-rgyas)
"Enlightened One"; an enlightened sage, such as Śākyamuni, who has achieved the highest state of transcendence as a result of perfecting the spiritual qualities known as *pāramitās. See also* Five Buddhas, Jina, *pāramitās,* Tathāgata.

chöd (gCod) (Tibetan)
"Cutting off"; name of the principal ritual of the Źi-byed school introduced into Tibet by Pha-dam-pa Sangye. It stresses the overcoming of all opposites through awareness of the void *(śūnyatā). See also Machik Labdrön.*

dhāraṇi (Tibetan: *gzuṅs*)
A sacred formula, similar in form and function to a *mantra. See also mantra.*

dharma (Tibetan: *chos*)
The true state of affairs; also, a Buddha's statement on the real nature of things. Thus, the term connotes the whole of Buddhist doctrine as well as those realizations to which its various teachings refer.

dharmacakra (Tibetan: *chos-kyi 'khor-lo)*
"The Wheel of Dharma," a symbol of the universality of the Buddha's discourse.

dharmakāya (Tibetan: *chos-sku)*
"Body of Reality"; the formless "body" of a Buddha's transcendent gnosis.

dharmapāla (Tibetan: *chos-skyoṅ)*
"Guardian of the Teachings"; a class of deities, usuallly wrathful in form.

Faxien (Fa-hsien)
A Chinese pilgrim who recorded descriptions of Buddhist India in ca. 400 A.D.

Five Buddhas (Five Tathāgatas, Five Dhyani Buddhas, Five Jinas)
A pentad of cosmic Buddhas often portrayed in configurations on Vajrayāna *maṇḍalas.* For the ordering of the Five Buddhas according to the *yoga-tantras,* see Snellgrove, Ch. V; according to the *anuttara-tantras,* see Trungpa, Rinpoche, Ch. VII. Each Buddha represents an aspect of enlightened consciousness. *See also:* Akṣobhya (blue); Amitābha (red); Amoghasiddhi (green); Jina; Ratnasaṃbhava (yellow); Tathāgata; Vairocana (white).

Gelugpa (dge-lugs-pa)
The largest of the four major Tibetan Buddhist orders, it was founded in the fourteenth century by Tsong-kha-pa. The Dalai Lama is the head of this sect.

Huichao (Huie-Chao)
Korean pilgrim who left an important account of his travels to India, ca. 720 A.D.

Indra
In Vedic mythology, the king of the gods.

jātaka (Tibetan: *skye-rabs)*
A collection of "birth stories" relating the career of Śākyamuni in his previous lives.

Jina (Tibetan: *rgyal-ba)*
"Conqueror"; an epithet of Śākyamuni and other Buddhas, referring to their victory over the forces of delusion. It is also used as a synonym for each of the five cosmic Tathāgatas. *See also:* Five Buddhas, Tathāgatas.

Kagyu, Kagyud *(bka'-brgyud)*
A major Tibetan Buddhist order, founded by Marpa in the eleventh century.

Kālacakra (Tibetan: *Dus-kyi 'khor-lo)*
"Wheel of Time"; the principal deity of a major *tantra* introduced into Tibet during the early eleventh century.

Kanjur (bka-'gyur)
"The translated words (of the Buddha)"; the Tibetan version of the Buddhist canon, consisting of 108 volumes.

Liṅga
A representation of the Hindu deity, Śiva, in phallic form.

Ma-chik Labdrön, Machik Drönma (Ma-gcig bslab-kyi sgron-ma)
Most celebrated of the female Tibetan Buddhist teachers, she was a direct disciple of the Indian master, Pha-dam-pa Sangye, who introduced the *gCod* system of practice into Tibet in the eleventh century. *See also chöd (gCod).*

Mahāyāna (Tibetan: Theg-pa chen-po)
"The Great Vehicle"; a branch of Buddhism that espouses the Bodhisattva ideal. Vajrayāna is a branch of Mahāyāna.

Mahīśāsuramardinī
"Slayeress of the Buffalo Demon"; a multi-armed manifestation of the Hindu goddess, Durgā.

Maitreya (Tibetan: Byams-pa)
"Loving One"; one of the eight Bodhisattvas, he is often also designated as the "Future Buddha" since tradition holds that he will be Śākyamuni's successor.

maṇḍala (Tibetan: *dkyil-khor)*
A circular diagram, containing symmetrical configurations of tantric deities and symbols, which presents to the initiated a statement of sacred outlook.

Mañjuśrī (Tibetan: *'Jam-dpal)*
"Gentle Splendor"; one of the eight major Bodhisattvas, he embodies the "wisdom aspect" of Buddhahood.

mantra (Tibetan: *sṅags)*
A sequence of sacred syllables whose enunciation promotes a state of identification with the deity being invoked.

Marpa (1012-1096)
An eleventh-century Tibetan translator, he obtained tantric teachings from Nāropa, which became the basis of the Kagyu order's meditative system. *See also* Nāropa.

Milarepa
Poet and ascetic *sans pareil* of Tibet, he was the chief disciple of Marpa.

mudrā (Tibetan: *phyag-rgya)*
Literally a "seal"; in Buddhist usage, a stylized hand-gesture; e.g., *varada-mudrā,* the gesture of generosity.

Nāropa
One of the eighty-four great masters *(mahāsiddha)* of Indian Vajrayāna Buddhism, his tantric teachings were transmitted to Tibetan masters in the eleventh century and are important in the Sakya and Kagyu orders.

ngöndro (sṅon-'gro) (Tibetan)
A preliminary stage of meditation that precedes tantric initiation *(abhiṣeka).* (See Trungpa, Rinpoche, Ch. VII, for a complete description.)

Ngor
A monastery in southwestern Tibet, founded in 1429 by Ngorchen Kunga Zangpo, it

was the seat of the Ngor subsect of the Sakya order until its destruction after 1959.

Nirmāṇakāya (Tibetan: *sprul-sku)*
"Manifest Body," the form in which a Buddha appears among ordinary beings, e.g., Śākyamuni. *See also* Dharmakâya, Saṃbhogakāya, Trikāya.

nirvāṇa (Tibetan: *mya-ṅan-las 'das-pa)*
The state of liberation from the process of birth and death, attained through the elimination of that process's causes. *See also saṃsāra.*

Nying-ma (rñiṅ-ma)
Oldest of the four major Tibetan Buddhist orders, it traces its origins to Padmasaṃbhava.

Padmasaṃbhava
An Indian tantric master who was instrumental in establishing the Buddhist religion in Tibet during the eighth century. He is also regarded as the founder of the Nyingma order.

pāramitā (Tibetan: *pha-rol-tu-phyin-pa)*
A set of six (or ten) spiritual "perfections" (e.g., patience) that a Bodhisattva must accomplish in order to reach Buddhahood.

Pārvatī
"Lady of the Mountains"; the principal wife of Śiva. Umā is another name of this goddess, frequently paired with that of her consort in the compound Umā-Maheśvara.

prajñāpāramitā (Tibetan: *śes-rab-kyi pha-rol-tu-phyin-pa)*
The "perfection of wisdom"; most important of the Bodhisattva's transcendent virtues, it consists of insight into egolessness or the absence of an inherent identity in all phenomena. Also the name of a goddess who embodies this principle.

pratyeka-buddha (raṅ-saṅs-rgyas)
A "Solitary Buddha," one who achieves liberation by and for himself, and is not concerned with the salvation of others.

Ratnasaṃbhava (Rin-chen 'byuṅ-gnas)
"Source of Jewels"; one of the Five Buddhas, he presides over the jewel family and is yellow in color.

Rin-chen Zangpo (Rin-chen bZang-po)
"The "Great Translator," (958–1055) whose activities as a teacher in western Tibet and Kashmir exerted much influence on Tibetan Buddhism in its formative period.

Sachen Kunga Nyingpo (1093–?)
Second patriarch of the Sakya order, who was in large part responsible for the systematization of its doctrines and their propagation in Tibet.

sādhana (Tibetan: *sgrub-thabs)*
A meditative rite that, in tantric usage, enables the practitioner to invoke and achieve identification with a chosen deity.

Sakya (Sa-skya)
One of the four major Tibetan Buddhist orders, it was founded in the eleventh century by Khön Könchog Gyalpo.

Śākyamuni (Tibetan: *Śākya thub-pa)*
"Sage of the Śākya (clan)" (Prince Siddhārtha); an epithet of Gautama Buddha, who lived in India ca. 500 B.C. and founded the religion that bears his name. *See also* Nirmāṇakāya.

samādhi (Tibetan: *gtiṅ-ṅe-'dzin)*
A stage of meditation in which the mind's energies are concentrated in intense contemplation.

śamatha (Tibetan: *źi-gnas)*
The first stage of meditation in which the mind is single-pointedly focused upon an object in order to still thought formations.

Śambhala (Shambhala)
A legendary realm where the *Kālacakra-tantra* is claimed to have originated, usually placed to the north of Tibet, in Central Asia.

Saṃbhogakāya (Tibetan: *loṅs-sku)*
"Body of Bliss"; the communicative aspect of the Buddha's triune form, which he manifests to aspirants whose spiritual vision has been purified.

saṃsāra (Tibetan: *'khor-ba)*
The round of birth-and-death in which sentient beings remain involved so long as they fail to win liberation through recognition of their own Buddha-nature.

Saṃvara (Śamvara, Sambara; Tibetan: bDe-mchog)
One of the major Vajrayāna *yi-dams,* whose consort is the goddess Vajrayoginī.

saṅgha (Tibetan: *dge-'dun)*
The Buddhist order, or more generally, the community, of monks, nuns, and laity. *See also* Tri-ratna.

Śiva
A major Indian deity, he personifies the principle of creation and destruction.

śrāvaka (Tibetan: *sñan-thos)*
"Disciple"; the early followers of Śākyamuni.

stūpa (Tibetan: *mchod-rten)*
A reliquary mound; the Buddhist monument, symbolic of the Dharmakāya. *See also* Dharmakāya.

śūnyatā (Tibetan: *stoṅ-pa-ñid)*
"The Void"; the ultimate nature of all phenomena; i.e., the absence in them of any inherent nature whatsoever.

Sūrya
The Hindu sun god.

sūtra (Tibetan: *mdo)*
A class of Buddhist literature consisting of discourses attributed to Śākyamuni.

t'ang-ka (Tibetan)
A painted scroll, often hung in Tibetan and Nepalese temples.

Tanjur (bstan-'gyur) (Tibetan)
A Tibetan collection of commentaries on the Buddhist canon *(Kanjur),* comprised of 225 volumes. *See also* Kanjur.

tantra (Tibetan: *rgyud)*
A class of Buddhist literature, usually consisting of discourses attributed to a tantric manifestation of the Buddha.

Tārā
"Savioress"; in Mahāyāna Buddhism, she is the most popular of female Bodhisattvas and is associated with the lotus family of Amitābha Buddha.

Tathāgata (Tibetan: de-bźin-gśegs-pa)
"Thus Gone"; an epithet of Śākyamuni and used especially in reference to the set of Five Buddhas. *See also* Five Buddhas.

trikāya (Tibetan: *sku-gsum)*
"Three Bodies" of Buddhahood; a Mahāyāna doctrine that posits a triune nature of Buddhas; i.e., that they are at once endowed with noetic, communicative, and manifest aspects. *See also* Dharmakāya, Nirmāṇakāya, Saṃbhogakāya.

Tripiṭāka (Tibetan: *sde-snod gsum)*
"Three Baskets"; the Buddhist canon consisting of three classes of literature: *vinaya; sūtra,* and *abhidharma.*

Tri-ratna (Tibetan: *dkon-mchog gsum)*
The three Buddhist refuges. *See also* Buddha, Dharma, Saṅgha.

Tsongkhapa (1357–1419)
Reformist founder of the Gelug-pa order, and author of several important works.

Tuṣita (Tibetan: *dga'-ldan)*
Name of the heaven whence Śākyamuni descended to our world. The Bodhisattva Maitreya resides in the outer court of the Tuṣita Heaven.

Uṣṇīṣavijayā
A popular goddess of the Mahāyāna pantheon who is associated with Vairocana Buddha.

Vairocana (Tibetan: rnam-par-snan-mdzad)
"The Illuminator"; one of the Five Buddhas, he presides over the *cakra* family. His color is white. In the *yoga-tantra* he is in the center (see Ch. V). Sometimes in the *anuttara-tantra,* he is located in other quarters (see Ch. VII). Another form is Sarvavid Vairocana, the Four-faced Vairocana; i.e., Vairocana facing in four directions simultaneously.

Vaiśravaṇa
Guardian deity of the northern quarter, he is associated with Kubera, the god of wealth.

vajra (rdo-rje)
"Diamond"; a scepter which, in Vajrayāna Buddhism, symbolizes the adamantine and indestructible nature of ultimate reality. *See also* Vajrayāna.

Vajrapāṇi (Tibetan: *phyag-na-rdo-rje)*
"Diamond Holder"; one of the eight Bodhisattvas, he personifies the tremendous power of Buddhahood.

Vajravārāhī (rdo-rje phag-mo)
"Diamond Sow"; a variant form of the goddess Vajrayoginī who, as an emanation of Vairocana, transforms passion into enlightened energy.

Vajrayāna (Tibetan: rdo-rje theg-pa)
"The Diamond Way," or tantric form of Buddhism, which bases its meditative practices upon the use of *maṇḍalas, mantras,* and *mudrās.*

Vighnāntaka
"Remover of Obstacles"; an emanation of Akṣobhya Buddha, he resembles the Hindu god Ganeśa.

vihāra (Tibetan: *dgon-pa)*
A monastery.

vipaśyanā (Tibetan: *lhag-mthong)*
"Insight"; the second stage in Buddhist meditation, in which understanding of the mind's nature is achieved.

Xuanzang (Hiuen-tsiang, Hsüan-Tsang)
A learned Chinese scholar-monk, whose pilgrimage to India in 631 A.D. is described in his *Buddhist Records of the Western World*

yi-dam (Tibetan)
In Vajrayāna Buddhism, a tutelary or personal deity whose invocation and intercession enable the practitioner to attain enlightenment. Some examples of *yi-dams* are Hevajra, Kālacakra, and Saṃvara.

Bibliography

Abhisamayālaṅkāra
1954 Translated by Edward Conze. Rome.

Agrawala, Vasudeva S.
1953 *India as known to Pāṇini: a study of the cultural material in the Ashṭādhyāyī.* Lucknow.

Ahmad, Zahiruddin
1968 "New light on the Tibet-Ladakh-Mughal war of 1679–1684." *East and West* 18:340–361.

Akiyama, Tarukaya, and Matsubara, Saburo
1969 *Arts of China II—Buddhist cave temples: new researches.* Translated by A. Soper. Tokyo and Palo Alto.

Al-Bīrūnī see Sachau 1910.

Alder, Garry J.
1963 *British India's northern frontier 1865–95.* London.

Allchin, F.R., and Hammond, N., eds.
1978 *The archaeology of Afghanistan, from earliest times to the Timurid period.* London.

Almgren, Bertil
1962 "Geographical aspects of the Silk Road, especially in Persia and East Turkistan." *Bulletin of the Museum of Far Eastern Antiquities* 34:93–106.

Alonso, Mary E., ed.
1979 *China's Inner Asian frontier: photographs of the Wulsin expedition to northwest China in 1923.* Cambridge.

Andrews, Frederick H.
1935 *Descriptive catalogue of antiquities recovered by Sir Aurel Stein in Central Asia, Kansu and Eastern Asia.* Delhi.
1948 *Wall paintings from ancient shrines in Central Asia; recovered by Sir Aurel Stein.* London.

L'Arte del Gandhara in Pakistan see Bussagli 1958.

Art Institute of Chicago
1965 *Master Bronzes of India.* Exhibition catalogue. Chicago.

Asher, Frederick
1980 *The art of eastern India, 300–800.* Minneapolis.

Asia Society, New York
n.d. *Handbook of the Mr. and Mrs. John D. Rockefeller 3rd Collection.* Asia Society, New York.

Auboyer, Jeannine
1968 *L'Afghanistan et son art.* Paris.

Avalon, Arthur (Sir John G. Woodroffe)
1927 *The Great Liberation (Mahānirvāṇa Tantra).* Madras.

Azarpay, Guitty
1981 *Sogdian painting.* Berkeley and Los Angeles.

Bacot, Jacques
1956 "Reconnaissance en Haute Asie septentrionale par cinq envoyés ouigours au VIIIe siècle." *Journal Asiatique* 244:137–153.
1962 *Introduction à l'histoire du Tibet.* Paris.

Bagchi, Prabodh C.
1931 "On foreign elements in the Tantra." *Indian Historical Quarterly* 7:1–16.
1950 *India and China; a thousand years of cultural relations.* 2nd ed, revised and enlarged. Bombay.
1955 *India and Central Asia.* Calcutta.

Bailey, H.W.
1936 "An itinerary of Khotanese Saka." *Acta Orientalia* 14:258–267.

Banerjea, Jitendra N.
1956 *The development of Hindu iconography.* 2nd ed. Calcutta.

Banerjee, P.
1968 "Painted wooden covers of two Gilgit manuscripts." *Oriental Art* 14:114–118.
1972 "Vairocana Buddha from Central Asia." *Oriental Art* 18:166–170.

Banerjee, P., and Agrawala, R.C.
1970 "Hindu sculptures in ancient Afghanistan." In *India's contribution to world thought and culture,* ed. Lokesh Chandra, pp. 215–228. Madras.

Bareau, André
1959 "Constellations et divinités protectrices des marchands dans le bouddhisme ancien." *Journal Asiatique* 247:303–309.

Bargar, E., and Wright, P.
1941 *Excavations in Swat and explorations in the Oxus territories of Afghanistan.* Memoirs of the Archaeological Survey of India, no.64. New Delhi.

Barrett, Douglas.
1957 "Sculptures of the Shahi period." *Oriental Art* III(2):54–59.
1960 "Gandhara bronzes." *The Burlington Magazine* 102:361–365.
1961 "Sculptures from Kashmir." *The British Museum Quarterly* XXIII(2):49–51.
1962 "Bronzes from northwest India and western Pakistan." *Lalit Kala* 11:35–44.

Barrett, Douglas, and Pinder-Wilson, Ralph
1967 *Ancient art from Afghanistan.* Catalogue of the Exhibition at the Royal Academy of Arts. London.

Barthold, W. W.
1956 *Four studies on the history of Central Asia.* Translated by V. and T. Minorsky. 3. vols. Leiden.
1968 *Turkestan down to the Mongol invasion.* Translated by T. Minorsky. 3rd ed. London.

Barthoux, Jules J.
1933 *Les fouilles de Hadda.* Mémoirs de la Délégation archéologique française en Afghanistan, Vol. 4. Paris.

Basham, Arthur L.
1954 *The wonder that was India. New York.*
1968 (ed.) Papers on the date of Kaniṣka. Leiden.

Bazin, Louis
1963 "Man and the concept of history in Turkish Central Asia during the eighth century." *Diogenes* 41:81–97.

Beal, Samuel, transl.
1884 *Si-yu-ki: Buddhist records of the western world, by Hiuen Tsiang.* 2 vols. London. Reprinted New York, 1968.
1911 *The Life of Hiuen-Tsiang, by Hwui Li.* London.

Beckwith, Christopher I.
1980 "The Tibetan empire in the west." In *Tibetan studies in honour of Hugh Richardson,* eds. M. Aris and Aung San Suu Kyi, pp. 30–38. Warminster.

Béguin, Gilles
1974 "Bronzes himâlayens." *La Revue du Louvre et des musées de France* 1974/4–5:333–344.
1979 *Musée Guimet. Arts du Nepal et du Tibet.* Paris.
1981 *Les mandalas himalâyens du musée Guimet.* Catalogue of the exhibition in Nice. Paris.

Belenitsky, Aleksandr M.
1968 *Central Asia.* Translated by James Hogarth. Geneva.

Belenitskii, A.M.; Boronina, V.L.; and Kostrov, P.I.
1959 *Skulptura i zhivopis drevnego Pyandzhikenta.* Moscow.

Bernard, Paul
1964 "Les fouilles de Kohna Masjid." *Academie des Inscriptions et Belles Lettres, Comptes Rendus* V:212–221.

Bernard, Paul, and Grenet, Franz
1981 "Découverte d'une statue du dieu solaire Surya dans la région de Caboul." *Studia Iranica* 10:127–146.

Beyer, Stephan
1973 *The cult of Tārā: magic and ritual in Tibet.* Berkeley.

Bhattacharya, Chhaya
1977 *Art of Central Asia (with special reference to wooden objects from the northern silk route).* Delhi.

Bhattacharya, Dipak C.
1974 *Tantric Buddhist iconographic sources.* New Delhi.
1980 *Iconology of composite images.* New Delhi.

Bhattacharya, G.
1980 "Stūpa as Maitreya's emblem." In *The stūpa: its religious, historical and architectural significance,* ed. A.L. Dallapiccola, pp. 100–111, Wiesbaden.

Bhattacharya, Narendra N.
1981 *History of researches on Indian Buddhism.* New Delhi.

Bhattacharyya, Benoytosh
1964 *An introduction to Buddhist esoterism.* 2nd rev. ed. Varanasi.
1968 *The Indian Buddhist iconography.* 2nd ed. Calcutta.

Biddulph, John.
1880 *Tribes of the Hindoo Kush*. Calcutta. Reprinted Graz, 1971.
Birnbaum, Raoul
1979 *The healing Buddha*. Boulder.
Bongard-Levin, G.M., and Stavinsky, B.Ya.
1970 "Central Asia in the Kushan period: archaeological studies by Soviet scholars." In *Kushan Studies in the U.S.S.R.*, ed. D. Chattopadhyaya, pp. 27–52. Calcutta.
Boulnois, Luce
1966 *The silk road*. Translated by D. Chamberlin. New York.
Boyer, A.M.; Rapson, E.J.; and Senart, E., eds.
1920–1929 *Kharoṣṭhī inscriptions discovered by Sir Aurel Stein in Chinese Turkestan*. 3 vols. Oxford.
Briggs, George W.
1938 *Gorakhnāth and the Kānphaṭa Yogīs*. London.
Brough, John
1964 "The Chinese pseudo-translation of Ārya-Śūra's Jātaka-mālā." *Asia Major* (n.s.) 11:27–53.
Buitenen, J.A.B. van
1973 *The Mahābhārata I: The book of the beginning*. Chicago.
Burlington Magazine
1966 "Golden anniversary acquisitions by the Cleveland Museum of Art." *Burlington Magazine* (Nov. 1966).
Burton, Richard
1966 "Fifty years of the Cleveland." *The Connoisseur* 163:128–135.
Bushell, S.W.
1880 "The early history of Tibet from Chinese sources." *Journal of the Royal Asiatic Society of Great Britain and Ireland* 12:435–541.
Bussagli, Mario
1958 *L'Arte del Gandhara in Pakistan e i suoi incontri con l'arte dell'Asia centrale*. Catalogue of the exhibition in Turin. ISMEO, Rome.
1979 *Painting of Central Asia*. Translated by L.Small. Geneva.
Bu-ston see Obermiller 1931–1932.
Caman, Schuyler
1950 "Suggested origin of the Tibetan mandala paintings." *Art Quarterly* 13:107–119.
Carter, Martha L.
1979 "An Indo-Iranian silver rhyton in the Cleveland Museum." *Artibus Asiae* 41:309–325.
Chandra, Moti
1977 *Trade and trade routes in ancient India*. New Delhi.
Chattopadhyaya, Alaka
1967 *Atīśa and Tibet*. Calcutta.
Chavannes, Édouard
1894 *Les religieux éminents qui allèrent chercher la loi dans le pays d'occident. Mémoire composé à l'époque de la grande dynastie T'ang. Par I-tsing*. Paris.
1903a "Voyage de Song Yun dans l'Udyāna et le Gandhāra (518–522 apr.J.-C.)". *Bulletin de l'École française d'Extrême Orient* 3:379–841.
1903b *Documents sur les Tou-kiue (Turcs) occidentaux*. St. Petersburg. Reprinted with Chavannes 1904, Paris, 1941.
1904 "Notes additionelles sur les Tou-kiue (Turcs) occidentaux." *T'oung Pao* (ser. 2) 5:1–11.
1905 "Les pays d'occident d'après le Wei-lio." *T'oung Pao* (ser. 2) 6:519–571.
1940 "Notes on ancient Chinese documents, discovered along the Han frontier wall in the desert of Tun-huang." Reprinted from the *New China Review*, 1921–1922.
1962 (1910–1953) *Cinq cents contes et apologues extraits du Tripitaka chinois*. 4 vols. Paris.
Ch'en, Kenneth K.S.
1946 "The Tibetan Tripitaka." *Harvard Journal of Asiatic Studies* 9:53–62.
1964 *Buddhism in China; a historical survey*. Princeton.
Ch'en Yuan
1940 *Ming-chi-Tien Ch'ien Fo-Chiao K'ao*. Beijing.
Clark, Walter Eugene
1937 *Two Lamaistic pantheons*. Cambridge, Mass.
Cleveland Museum of Art
1966 *Handbook of the Cleveland Museum of Art/1966*. Cleveland.
1975 *Indian art from the George P. Bickford collection*. Catalogue by Stanislaw Czuma. Cleveland Museum of Art, Cleveland.
1978 *Handbook of the Cleveland Museum of Art/1978*. Cleveland.
Conze, Edward
1949 "The iconography of the Prajñāpāramitā, Part 1." *Oriental Art* 2:47–52.
1954 See *Abhisamayālaṅkāra*.
1970 *Buddhist thought in India; three phases of Buddhist philosophy*. Ann Arbor.
1960 *The Prajñāpāramitā literature*. The Hague.
1961 *Prajñāpāramitās. The large Sūtra on perfect wisdom*. Translated by Edward Conze. London.
Conze, E.; Hormer, I.B.; Snellgrove, D.; and Waley, A., eds.
1954 *Buddhist texts through the ages*. Oxford. Reprint New York 1964.
Coomaraswamy, A.K.
1943 *Hinduism and Buddhism*. New York.
Copeland, Carolyn
1980 *Tangkas from the Koelz Collection*. Michigan papers on South and Southeast Asia, no. 18. Ann Arbor.
Cowell, E.B.
1901 *The Jatakas: stories of the Buddha's former births*. Cambridge.
Crosby, Oscar Terry
1905 *Tibet and Turkestan*. New York.
Crossley-Holland, Peter
1977 "Musical instruments in the legends of Tibet." In *Tribute volume to Professor Liang Tsai-Ping*. Taipei.
Cunningham, Alexander
1854 *Ladak: physical, statistical and historical*. London.
Curzon, George N.
1896 The Pamirs and the source of the Oxus. London.
Czuma, Stanislaw, see Cleveland Museum of Art.
Dagens, B.; Le Berre, M.; and Schlumberger, D.
1964 *Monuments préislamiques d'Afghanistan*. Mémoirs de la Délégation archéologique française en Afghanistan, vol. 19. Paris.
Dagyab, Loden S.
1977 *Tibetan religious art*. 2 vols. Wiesbaden.
Das, Asok K.
1979 "An interesting bronze from Ladakh." *Oriental Art* 25:227–230.
Daśabhūmikasūtra et Bodhisattvabhūmi
1926 Edited and with introduction by J. Rahder. Paris.
Dasgupta, Surendranath
1932 *A history of Indian philosophy*. Vol. II. Cambridge.
Decleer, Hubert
1978 "The Working of Sādhana: Vajrabhairava." In *Tibetan Studies*, eds. M. Brauen and P. Kvaerne, pp. 113–123. Zurich.
Demiéville, Paul
1937 "Byô." In *Hōbōgirin*, vol.III:224–265.
1952 *Le concile de Lhasa*. Paris.
1970 Recents traveux sur Touen-houang; apercu bibliographique et notes critiques. Leiden.
1973 *Choix d'études bouddhiques, 1919–1970*. Leiden.
Demiéville, Paul; Levi, S.; and Takakusu, J., eds.
1929– *Hōbōgirin: dictionnaire encyclopédique du bouddhism*. 4 vols. to date. Tokyo.
Denes, Françoise
1976 *Catalogue raisonné des objets en bois provenant de Dunhuang et conservés au musée Guimet*. Publications du musée Guimet. Paris.
Deshpande, M.N.
1973 "Buddhist art of Ajanta and Tabo." *Bulletin of Tibetology* 10:1–44.
Dey, Nuno Lal
1971 *The geographical dictionary of ancient and medieval India*. New Delhi.
Dhargyey, Ngawang
1975 "An introduction to and an outline of the Kalacakra initiation." *The Tibet Journal* 1:72–77.
Diakonova, N.
1962 *Masterpieces of eastern art in the Hermitage*. Exhibition catalogue. Leningrad.
Dohanian, D.K.
1961 *The art of India*. Exhibition catalogue. Memorial Art Gallery of the University of Rochester. Rochester.
Doris Wiener Gallery
1974 *Thangka art*. Exhibition catalogue. New York.
Douglas, Nik
1980 *The enlightened ones in sacred Buddhist art*. Kreitman Gallery, Los Angeles.
Drew, Frederic
1875 *The Jummoo and Kashmir territories*. London.
Dudbridge, Glen
1970 *The Hsi-yu chi: a study of the antecedents to the sixteenth century Chinese novel*. Cambridge.
Dunhuang Institute for Cultural Relics
1980 *Dunhuang caisu*. (Dunhuang painted sculptures.) Beijing.
1980 *Dunhuangdi yishu baocang*. (Art Treasures of Dunhuang.) Hong Kong and Beijing.
Dunhuang Qianfodong bihua jilan
n.d. (Frescoes from the Thousand-Buddha Caves, Dunhuang). Pan-keng Publishing Book House, Taipei.

Dutt, Nalinaksha
1930 *Aspects of Mahāyāna Buddhism and its relation to Hīnayāna*. London.
1939–1953 (ed.) *The Gilgit manuscripts*. 3 vols. Srinagar.
Dutt, Sukumar
1962 *Buddhist monks and monasteries of India*. London.
Earle, Timothy, and Ericson, Jon, eds.
1977 *Exchange systems in prehistory*. New York.
Eberhard, Wolfram
1968 *The local cultures of south and east China*. Revised and translated by Alide Eberhard. Leiden.
Eimer, Helmut
1978 "Life and activities of Atiśa (Dīpaṃkaraśrījnāna). A survey of investigations undertaken." In *Tibetan Studies*, eds. M. Brauen and P. Kvaerne, pp. 125–136. Zurich.
Eliade, Mircea
1958 *Rites and symbols of initiation*. Translated by Willard R. Trask. New York.
1969 *Yoga: immortality and freedom*. Translated by Willard R. Trask. 2nd ed. Princeton.
Elphinstone, Mountstuart
1815 *An account of the kingdom of Caboul and its dependencies in Persia, Tartary and India*. London.
Emmerick, R.E.
1967 *Tibetan texts concerning Khotan*. London.
1979 *A guide to the literature of Khotan*. Tokyo.
Enoki, K.
1959 "On the nationality of the Ephtalites." *Memoirs of the Research Department of the Toyo Bunko* 18:1–58.
Esin, Emel
1967 "Antecedants and development of Buddhist and Manichean Turkish art in eastern Turkestan and Kansu." In *Handbook of Turkish culture*, supplement to Vol.II. Istanbul.
Fabri, Charles
1939 "Buddhist baroque in Kashmir." *Asia Magazine* (Oct. 1939):592–598.
1955 "Akhnur terra-cottas." *Marg* 8(2):53–64.
Faccenna, Domenico
1962 *Sculptures from the sacred area of Butkara I (Swāt, Pakistan). Part 2 (plates)*. Reports and Memoirs of ISMEO, Vol. II,2. Rome.
Fairley, Jean
1975 *The lion river: the Indus*. London.
Faxian (Fa-hsien) see Beal 1884, Legge 1886, and Giles 1923.
Fields, Rick
1981 *How the swans came to the lake. A narrative history of Buddhism in America*. Boulder.
Filippi, Filippo de
1912 *Karakorum and western Himalaya 1909*. New York.
1923 *Storia della spedizione scientifica italiana nel Himàlaia Caracorùm e Turchestàn cinese (1913–1914)*. Bologna.
1934 *I viaggiatori italiani in Asia*. Rome.
Filliozat, Jean
1934 "La médecine indienne et l'expansion boddhique en Extrême-Orient." *Journal Asiatique* 224:301–307.
1937 *Le Kumāratantra de Rāvana et les textes parallèles indiens, tibétains, chinois, cambodgiens et arabes*. Paris.
1969 "Taoïsme et Yoga." *Journal Asiatique* 257:41–87.
Fisher, M.W.; Rose, L.E.; and Huttenback, R.A.
1963 *Himalayan battleground*. London and Dunmow.
Fogg Art Museum
1974 *The discerning eye: Radcliffe collectors' exhibition*. Fogg Art Museum, Cambridge, Mass.
Fong Chow
1971 *Arts from the rooftop of Asia*. Exhibition catalogue. The Metropolitan Museum of Art. New York.
Fontein, Jan
1967 *The pilgrimage of Sudhana*. The Hague.
Forstner, Martin
1970 "Ya'qūb b. al-Laiṯ und der Zunbīl." *Zeitschrift der Deutschen Morgenländischen Gesellschaft* 120/1:69–83.
Forte, Antonino
1976 *Political propaganda and ideology in China at the end of the seventh century*. Naples.
Foucher, Alfred
1905–1922 *L'Art gréco-bouddhique du Gandhāra*. 2 vols. Paris.
1942–1947 *La vieille route de l'Inde de Bactres à Taxila*. 2 vols. Mémoires de la Délégation archéologique française en Afghanistan, Vol. 1. Paris.
Francke, A.H.
1901 "A Ladakhi Bonpa hymnal." *The Indian Antiquary* 30:359–364.
1907 *A history of western Tibet*. Reprinted as *A history of Ladakh*, New Delhi, 1977.
1914a "Notes on Sir Aurel Stein's collection of Tibetan documents from Chinese Turkestan." *Journal of the Royal Asiatic Society of Great Britain and Ireland* 1914:37–59.
1914b *Antiquities of Indian Tibet*. 2 vols. Calcutta. Reprint New Delhi, 1972.
1929–1930 "Notes on Khotan and Ladakh (from an Indian point of view)." *The Indian Antiquary* 58:108–112, 146–152; 59:41–46, 62–72.
Franke, Otto
1930–1952. *Geschichte des chinesisches Reiches*. 5 vols. Berlin.
Fuchs, Walter
1938 "Huei-ch'ao's Pilgerreise durch Nordwest-Indien und Zentral-Asien um 726." *Sitzungsbericht der Preussischen Akademie der Wissenschaften, phil.hist. Klasse*, vol. 25:426–469.
Fujieda, Akira
1981 "Une reconstruction de la 'bibliothèque' de Touenhouang." *Journal Asiatique* 269:65–68.
Fussman, Gérard
1974 "Ruines de la vallée de Wardak." *Arts Asiatiques* 30:65–130.
1978 "Inscriptions de Gilgit." *Bulletin de l'École française d'Extrême-Orient* 65:1–64.
Fussman, Gérard, and Le Berre, Marc
1976 *Monuments bouddhiques de la région de Caboul: le monastère de Gul Dara, vol.1*. Mémoires de la Délégation archéologique française en Afghanistan, vol.22. Paris.
Fux, Herbert
1969 "Śambhala und die Geschichte des Kâlacakra—ein lamaistisches Than-ka aus dem österreichischen Museum für Angewandte Kunst." *Alte und Moderne Kunst* 107:18–24.
Gabain, Annemarie von
1954 "Buddhistische Türkenmission." In *Asiatica: Festschrift für Friedrich Weller*, ed. J. Schubert, pp. 161–173. Leipzig.
1961 "Der Buddhismus in Zentralasien." In *Handbuch der Orientalistik*, section VIII/2:496–514. Leiden.
Galerie, Robert Buraway
1978 *Peintures du monastére de Nor*. Paris.
Ganhar, J.N., and Ganhar, P.N.
1956 *Buddhism in Kashmir and Ladakh*. New Delhi.
Gaulier, Simone; Jera-Bezard, Robert; and Maillard, Monique
1976 *Buddhism in Afghanistan and Central Asia*. 2 vols. Leiden.
Gazetteer of Kashmir and Ladakh
1890 Calcutta. Reprint Delhi, 1974.
Gergan, S.S.
1976 *La-dvags rgyal-rabs 'chi-med gter*. Srinagar (Kashmir).
Gergan, S.S., and Hassnain, F.M.
1977 "Critical introduction and annotations." In reprint 1977 of Francke 1907.
Gernet, Jacques
1956 *Les aspects économiques du bouddhisme dans la société chinoise du Ve au Xe siècle*. Paris.
1966 "Location des chameaux pour les voyages à Touen-houang." *Mélanges de sinologie offerts à Monsieur P. Demiéville*, vol. I:41–51. Paris.
Getty, Alice
1974 *The gods of northern Buddhism*. 2nd. ed. Oxford.
Ghosh, Mallar
1980 *Development of Buddhist iconography in eastern India: a study of Tārā, Prajñās of Five Tathāgatas and Bhṛikuṭī*. New Delhi.
Ghurye, Govind S.
1953 *Indian Sadhus*. Bombay.
Giles, Herbert Allen
1923 *The travels of Fa-hsien (A.D. 399–414)*. Cambridge.
Giles, Lionel
1957 *Descriptive catalogue of the Chinese manuscripts from Tunhuang in the British Museum*. London.
"Gime Toyo bijutsukan"
1968 In *Sakai no bijutsukan* 14, Tokyo.
Glynn, C.
1972 *Aspects of Indo-Asian art from the Los Angeles County Museum of Art*. Exhibition catalogue. Peppers Art Gallery, University of Redlands.
Göbl, Robert
1967 *Dokumente zur Geschichte der iranischen Hunnen in Baktrien und Indien*. 4 vols. Wiesbaden.
Godard, André; Godard, Yvette; and Hackin, Joseph

1928 *Les antiquités bouddhiques de Bāmiyān, avec des notes additionnelles de M. Paul Pelliot.* Mémoires de la Délégation archéologique française en Afghanistan, Vol. 2. Paris.

Goetz, Hermann
1957 "Late Gupta sculpture in Afghanistan: the Scorretti marble and cognate sculptures." *Arts Asiatiques* 4:13–19.
1969 *Studies in the history and art of Kashmir and the Indian Himalaya.* Wiesbaden.

Gonda, J.
1963 "The Indian Mantra." *Oriens* 16:244–297.
1966 *Ancient Indian kingship from the religious point of view.* Leiden.

Govinda, Anagarika
1976 *Psycho-cosmic symbolism of the Buddhist stūpa.* Emeryville, Calif.
1977 *Foundations of Tibetan mysticism.* (English edition originally published in London, 1960.) New Delhi.

Granoff, Phyllis
1968 "A portable Buddhist shrine from Central Asia." *Archives of Asian Art* 22:80–95.
1970 "Tobatsu Bishamon: three Japanese statues in the United States and an outline of the rise of this cult in East Asia." *East and West* 20:144–167.
1979 "Maheśvara/Mahākala: a unique Buddhist image from Kashmir." *Artibus Asiae* 41/1.
1981 "A letter to the editor: Some remarks on the Fattehgarh Siva: a response to Dr. Pratapaditya Pal." *Art International* 24: 146–148.

Gray, Basil, and Vincent, J.B.
1959 *Buddhist cave paintings at Tun-huang.* London.

Gropp, Gerd
1974 *Archäologische Funde aus Khotan, Chinesisch-Ostturkestan. Die Trinkler-Sammlung im Übersee-Museum, Bremen.* Bremen.

Grünwedel, Albert
1912 *Altbuddhistische Kultstätten in Chinesisch-Turkistan.* Berlin.
1915 *Der Weg nach Sambhala.* Munich.

Gulik, R.H. van
1935 *Hayagrīva: the mantrayānic aspect of horse-cult in China and Japan.* Leiden.
1956 *Siddham—an essay on the history of Sanskrit studies in China and Japan.* Nagpur.

Gupta, S.; Hoens, D.J.; and Goudriaan, T.
1979 *Hindu Tantrism.* Leiden.

Hackin, Joseph
1911 "Asie centrale et Tibet, Missions Pelliot et Bacot." *Bulletin archéologique du Musée Guimet,* fasc. 2, no. 8:9–20.
1928 "Mythologie du bouddhisme en Asie centrale." In *Mythologie asiatique illustrée.* Paris.
1932 (ed.) *Asiatic Mythology.* New York.
1936 *Recherches archéologiques au Col de Khair Khaneh près de Kābul.* Mémoires de la Délégation archéologique française en Afghanisan, vol. 8. Paris.
1939 *Recherches archéologiques à Begram.* Mémoires de la Délégation archéologique française en Afghanistan, vol. 9. Paris.

Hackin, J., and Carl, J.
1933 *Nouvelles recherches archéologiques à Bāmiyān.* Mémoires de la Délégation archéologique française en Afghanistan, vol. 3. Paris.

Hackin, J.; Carl, J.; and Meunié, J.
1959 *Diverses recherches archéologiques en Afghanistan (1933–1940).* Mémoires de la Délégation archéologique française en Afghanistan, vol. 8. Paris.

Hajime, Nakamura
1964 "A critical survey of Mahayana and esoteric Buddhism." *Acta Asiatica* VI:57–58; VII:36–94.

Hallade, Madeleine
1968 *Gandhāran art of north India.* Translated by D. Imber. New York.

Hallade, M., and Hambis, L.
1956 *Sculptures et peintures de l'Asie centrale: inédits de la mission Paul Pelliot.* Exhibition catalogue. Musée Guimet, Paris.

Haloun, G., and Henning, W.B.
1952 "The compendium of the doctrine and styles of the teaching of Mani, the Buddha of Light." *Asia Major* (n.s.) 8:184–212.

Hambis, Louis, ed.
1977 *L'Asie centrale: histoire et civilisation.* Paris.

Hambly, Gavin, ed.
1969 *Central Asia.* New York.

Hamilton, James
1958 "Autour du manuscrit Staël-Holstein." *T'oung Pao* 46:115–153.

Harcourt, A.F.P.
1874 *The Himalayan districts of Kooloo, Lahoul and Spiti.* Government of the Punjab. Reprint Delhi, 1972.

Harper, Prudence O.
1978 *The royal hunter: art of the Sasanian empire.* Exhibition catalogue. The Asia Society, New York.

Hatt, Robert T.
1980 "A thirteenth century Tibetan reliquary." *Artibus Asiae* 42:175–220.

Haus der Kunst, Munich
1959 *Tausend Jahre chinesische Malerei.* Exhibition catalogue. Munich.

Hedin, Sven A.
1909 *Trans-Himalaya.* 2 vols. London.

Henderson, George
1873 *Lahore to Yarkand.* London.

Herrmann, Albert
1910 *Die alten Seidenstrassen zwischen China und Syrien.* Berlin.

Hillebrandt, Alfred
1980 *Vedic mythology.* (English transl., originally published in Breslau, 1891–1902.) 2 vols. New Delhi.

Ho, Wai-Kam
1968 "Notes on Chinese sculpture from northern Ch'i to Sui, Part I: Two Seated Buddhas in the Cleveland Museum." *Archives of Asian Art* 22:7–55.

Hoernle, A.F. Rudolf
1916 *Manuscript remains of Buddhist literature found in Eastern Turkestan.* Oxford. Reprint Amsterdam, 1970.

Hoffmann, Helmut
1961 *The religions of Tibet.* Translated by E. Fitzgerald. New York.
1969. "An account of the Bon religion in Gilgit." *Central Asiatic Journal* 13:137–145.

Honkō, Yaritomi
1981 "Some of the controversial points concerning the iconographic paintings of Lamaism." (In Japanese). *Ars Buddhica* 134–69–83.

Hopkirk, Peter
1980 *Foreign devils on the silk road.* London.

Huc and Gabet
1928 *Travels in Tartary, Thibet and China.* I–II. London.

Hudūd al'Ālam
1937 *The regions of the world; a Persian geography, 372 A.H./982 A.D.* Translated and explained by V. Minorsky. Oxford.

Hulsewé, A.F.P.
1974 "Quelques considérations sur le commerce de la soie au temps de la dynastie des Han." In *Mélanges de sinologie offerts à Monsieur Paul Demiéville,* vol.2:117–135. Paris.

Hulsewé, A.F.P., and Loewe, M.A.N.
1979 *China in Central Asia—the early stage: 125 B.C.–A.D. 23.* Leiden.

Hummel, Siegbert
1953 *Geschichte der tibetischen Kunst.* Leipzig.
1958 *Ammerkungen zur Apokalypse der Lamaismus (Apokalypse Chambhala).* Archiv orientálni 26/2.

Huntington, J.C.
1968 *The style and stylistic sources of Tibetan painting.* Ph.D. diss. Los Angeles.
1970 "Avalokiteśvara and the Namaskāra mudrā in Gandhāra." *Studies in Indo-Asian art and culture* 1:91ff.
1972 "Gu-ge bris: a stylistic amalgam." In *Aspects of Indian Art,* ed. P. Pal, pp. 105–117. Leiden.
1975 *The phur-pa, Tibetan ritual daggers.* Ascona.

Imperial Gazette
1908 *The imperial gazette of India.* 26 vols. Oxford. Reprint Faridabad, 1972.

Ishida Mosaku
1964 *Japanese Buddhist prints.* Translated by Charles S. Terry. New York.

I Tsing
1896 *A record of the Buddhist religion.* Translated by J. Takakasu. Oxford.

Jao Tsong-yi and Demièville, Paul
1971 *Airs de Touen-houang: airs à chanter des VIIIe-Xe siecles.* Paris.

Jao Tsong-yi; Ryckmans, Pierre; and Demiéville, Paul
1978 *Peintures monochromes de Touen-houang/Dunhuang baihua.* 3 vols. Paris.

Jera-Bezard, Robert
1976 "La représentation de Vaiśravana dans l'Asie centrale; son rapport possible avec le monde Kusana." In *Actes du XXIXe Congrès international des Orientalistes,* 1973. Paris.

Jera-Bezard, Robert, and Maillard, Monique
1976 "Un paradis d'Amitabha de la collection Aurel Stein conservé au Musée Nationale de New Delhi." *Arts Asiatiques* 32:269–285.
1980 "Une peinture murale d'un sanctuaire bouddhique d'Asie centrale." *La Revue du Louvre et des Musées de France* 30:38–44.

Jettmar, Gabriele
1964 *Die Holztempel des oberen Kulutales in ihren historischen, religiösen und kunstgeschichtlichen Zusammenhängen.* Wiesbaden.

Jettmar, Karl
1974 (ed.) *Cultures of the Hindu Kush: Selected Papers from the Hindu Kush*

cultural conference held at Moesgård 1970. Wiesbaden.
1975 *Die Religionen des Hindukusch.* (With contributions by S. Jones and M. Klimburg.) Stuttgart.
1977 "Bolor: a contribution to the political and ethnic geography of north Pakistan." *Zentralasiatische Studien* 11:411–448.
1980a. "Bolor—zum Stand des Problems." *Zentralasiatische Studien* 14/2:115–132.
1980b. "Neuentdeckte Felsbilder und -inschriften in den Nordgebieten Pakistans" (with English resumé). *Allgemeine und vergleichende Archäologie, Beiträge* 2:151–199.
Jones, J.J., transl.
1949–1956 *Mahāvastu.* 3 vols. London.
Joshi, Lalmani
1967 *Studies in the Buddhist culture of India.* Delhi.
Journal Asiatique
1981 *Manuscrits et inscriptions de Haute Asie du Ve au XIe siècle.* Journal Asiatique, 269, fasc.1–2.
Kak, Ram Chandra
1925 "Ancient and medieval architecture of Kashmir." *Rupam* 24:86–96.
Kalhaṇa
See Stein 1900.
Kane, Pandurang V.
1930–1962 *History of Dharmaśāstra.* 5 vols. Poona.
Karmay, Heather
1975 *Early Sino-Tibetan art.* Warminster.
Karmay, Samten G.
1980 "The ordinance of Lha bla-ma ye-shes'od." In *Tibetan studies in honour of Hugh Richardson,* eds. M. Aris and Aung San Suu Kyi, pp. 150–162, Oxford.
1972 *The treasury of good sayings; a Tibetan history of Bon.* London.
Kaufmann, Walter
1975 *Tibetan Buddhist chants.* Bloomington.
Keay, John
1977 *When men and mountains meet: the explorers of the western Himalayas 1820–75.* London.
1979 *The Gilgit game: the explorers of the western Himalayas 1865–95.* London.
Khosla, Romi
1979 *Buddhist monasteries in the western Himalaya.* Kathmandu.
Khosla, Sarla
1972 *History of Buddhism in Kashmir.* New Delhi.
Kiang, Chao-yuan
1937 *Le voyage dans la Chine ancienne, consideré principalement sous son aspect magique et religieux.* Shanghai. Reprint Vientiane, 1975.
Kitagawa, Joseph M., ed.
1967 *The history of religions; essays on the problem of understanding.* Chicago.
Klimburg, Maximilian
1966 *Afghanistan: das Land im historischen Spannungsfeld Mittelasiens.* Vienna.
1970 *Der 2. indo-iranische Stil von Kutscha.* Doctoral dissertation. University of Vienna, Vienna.
1974 "Die Entwicklung des 2. indo-iranischen Stils von Kutscha." In *Sprache, Geschichte und Kultur der Altaischen Völker,* eds. G. Hazai and P. Zieme. Berlin.
1975 "Male-female polarity symbolism in Kafir art and religion. New aspects in the study of the Kafirs of the Hindu-Kush." *East and West* 26:479–488.
1981 "A collection of Kafir art from Nuristan: a donation by the Federal Republic of Germany to the National Museum of Afghanistan." *Tribus* 30:155–202.
Klimburg-Salter, Deborah
1976 *The Buddhist painting of the Hindu Kush: Bamiyan, Foladi, Fondukistan, and Kakrak.* Doctoral dissertation. Harvard University, Cambridge, Mass.
1981a "Vaiśravana in north-west India." In *Madhu: Recent researches in Indian archaeology and art history,* ed. Shri M.N. Deshpande. New Delhi.
1981b "Ritual as interaction at Bāmiyān." In *Systems of communication and interaction in South Asia,* ed. P. Gaeffke and S. Olekiw. Pp. 65–69. Philadelphia.
n.d. *The kingdom of Bāmiyān.* Boulder. (In press).
n.d. "Dukhtar-i Nushirwan: an ideology of kingship." In *Festschrift for S. Sivaramurti* (forthcoming).
n.d. "A note on the formation of esoteric Buddhist iconography." In *Kunst und Kultur Ostasiens,* ed. R. Goepper. Cologne (forthcoming).
Kljaštornyj, S.G., and Livšic, V.A.
1972 "The Sogdian inscription of Bugut revised." *Acta Orientalia* 26:69–102.
Kobayashi, T.
1980 "The Mandala of Tibet." (In Japanese.) *Mizue* 1980/8(905):3–79.
Kosambi, D.D.
1965 *The culture and civilization of ancient India in historical outline.* London.
1970 Reprint of 1965. New Delhi.
1975 *An introduction to the study of Indian history.* Bombay.
Kozlov, P.K.
1911 *Russkii putesestvannik v Tsentral'noi Azii i mertvyi gorod Khara-Khoto.* St. Petersburg.
Kramrisch, Stella
1964 *The art of Nepal.* Catalogue of the exhibition at the Asia House, New York.
Kreitman Gallery see Douglas 1980.
Kruglikova, Irina T.
1974 *Dil'berdzin (raskopki 1970–1972 gg.).* Moscow.
Kuwayama, Shoshin
1972 *Archaeological survey of Kyoto University in Afghanistan 1970.* Kyoto.
1974 "Kāpiśī Begrām III: renewing its dating." *Orient* 10:57–78.
1975 "Khair Khaneh and its Chinese evidences." *Orient* 11:93–107.
1976 "The Turki Śāhis and relevant Brahmanical sculptures in Afghanistan." *East and West* 26:375–407.
Kwanten, Luc
1978 "The role of the Tangut in Chinese Inner Asian relations." *Acta Orientalia* 39:191–198.
1979 *Imperial nomads: a history of Central Asia, 500–1500.* Leicester.
Kwanten, Luc, and Hesse, Susan
1980 *Tangut (Hsi Hsia) studies: a bibliography.* Bloomington.
Laing, Ellen J.
1981 "Evidence for two possible Sasanian rugs depicted in Tun-huang murals of A.D. 642." *Ars Orientalis* 12:69–71.
Lalou, Marcelle
1946 "Mythologie indienne et peintures de Haute-Asie I. Le dieu bouddhique de la fortune." *Arbitus Asiae* 9:97–111.
Lamotte, Étienne
1958 *Histoire du bouddhisme indien des origines à l'ère Saka.* Louvain.
1970–1976 *Le traité de la grande vertu de sagesse de Nāgārjuna, par S. Nāgārjuna.* Vol. 3 and 4. Louvain.
Lauf, Detlef Ingo
1976 *Tibetan sacred art: the heritage of Tantra.* Translated by Ewald Osers. Berkeley.
1979 *Eine Ikonographie des tibetischen Buddhismus.* Graz.
Lawrence, W.R.
1895 *The valley of Kashmir.* London.
Le Coq, Albert von
1913 *Chotscho.* Berlin.
1922–1933 *Die buddhistische Spätantike in Mittelasien.* 7 vols. (vols. 6–7 with E. Waldschmidt). Berlin.
1925 *Bilderatlas zur Kunst und Kulturgeschichte Mittelasiens.* Berlin.
Lee, Sherman E.
1967 "Clothed in the sun: a Buddha and a Surya from Kashmir." *Bulletin of the Cleveland Museum of Art* 54:42–64.
1954 "Some little-known Indian bronzes." *Art Quarterly* 17:16–29.
1970–1975 *Asian Art—selections from the collection of Mr. and Mrs. John D. Rockefeller 3rd.* 2 vols. New York.
Lee, Sherman, and Ho, Wai-kam
1959 "A colossal eleven-faced Kuan-yin of the T'ang dynasty." *Artibus Asiae* 22: 121–137.
Legge, James
1886 *A record of Buddhistic kingdoms etc.* Oxford. Reprint New York, 1965.
Leitner, G.W.
1868–73 *Results of a tour in Dardistan, Kashmir, Little Tibet, Ladak, etc.* 5 vols. London.
1877 *The languages and races of Dardistan.* Lahore.
Lemoine, Jacques
1982 *Yao ceremonial paintings.* Bangkok.
Lerner, Martin
1975 *Bronze sculptures from Asia.* Metropolitan Museum of Art, New York.
Lessing, Ferdinand D., and Wayman, Alex
1968 *Mkhas grub rje's fundamentals of the Buddhist tantras.* Translated from the Tibetan. The Hague.
Lévi, Sylvain
1902–1905 "Notes chinoises sur l'Inde." *Bulletin de l'École française d'Extrême Orient,* 2 (1902):246–255; 3 (1903):38–53; 4 (1904):543–579; 5(1905):253–305.
1925 "Le sūtra du sage et du fou dans la littérature de l'Asie centrale." *Journal Asiatique* 207:305–332.
1929 "Les 'marchands de mer' et leur rôle dans le bouddhisme primitif." *Bulletin de l'association des amis de l'orient* 3.
1932 "Note sur des manuscrits Sanscrits provenant de Bamiyan (Afghanistan), et de Gilgit (Cachemire)." *Journal Asiatique* 220:1–45.
Lévi, Sylvain, and Chavannes, Édouard

1895 "Voyages des pèlerins bouddhistes: l'itinéraire d'Ou-k'ong (751–790)." *Journal Asiatique* (ser. 9)6:341–384.

Lewis, I. M.
1971 *Ecstatic religion: an anthropological study of spirit possession and shamanism*. Hammondsworth.

Liebert, Gösta
1976 *Iconographical dictionary of the Indian religions: Hinduism, Buddhism, Jainism*. Leiden.

Ligeti, Louis, ed.
1978 *Proceedings of the Csoma de Körös memorial symposium*. Budapest.

Litvinsky, B.A.
1970 "Outline history of Buddhism in Central Asia." In *Kushan studies in the U.S.S.R.*, ed. B.G. Gafurov, pp. 53–132. Calcutta.

Loehr, Max
1968 *Chinese landscape woodcuts: from an imperial commentary to the tenth century printed edition of the Buddhist canon*. Cambridge, Mass.

Loewe, Michael
1979 *Ways to paradise: the Chinese quest for immortality*. London.

Lokesh Chandra
1972 *The esoteric iconography of Japanese mandalas*. New Delhi.
1979 "Origin of the Avalokiteśvara of Potala." *Kailash* 7:5–25.
1980 "Borabudur as a monument of esoteric Buddhism." *The South East Asian Review* 5/1: 1–41.

Lokesh Chandra and Raghu Vira
1961–1972 *A new Tibeto-Mongol pantheon*. 20 vols. New Delhi.

Lokesh Chandra and Snellgrove, David L.
1981 *Sarva-Tathāgata-tattva-Saṅgraha*. New Delhi.

Los Angeles County Museum of Art
1975 *A decade of collecting*. Exhibition catalogue. Los Angeles.

Loury, John
1973 *Tibetan art*. London.

Macdonald, Alexander W.
1975 "On Prajāpati." In *Essays on the ethnology of Nepal and South Asia*, ed. A. Macdonald, pp.1–13. Kathmandu.

Macdonald, Ariane
1962 *Le mandala du Mañjuśrīmūlakalpa*. Paris.

Macdonald, Ariane, and Imaeda, Yoshiro
1977 *Essais sur l'art du Tibet*. Paris.

MacKenzie, D.N.
1976 *The Buddhist Sogdian texts of the British library*. Tehran and Liège.

Mahāvastu see Jones 1949–1956.

Mahāvastu Avadāna
1960 Edited by R. Basak. Calcutta.

Maillard, Monique
1973 "Essai sur la vie matérielle dans l'oasis de Tourfan pendant le haut moyen âge." *Arts Asiatiques* 29 (special issue).

Makita, Tairyo
1976 *Gikyō kenkyū*. Kyoto.

Mallman, Marie-Thérèse de
1948 *Introduction à l'étude d'Avaloketeçuara*. Paris.
1964 *Étude iconographique sur Mañjuśrī*. Paris.
1969 "Notes d'iconographie tantrique IV: à propos de Vajravāhārī." *Arts Asiatiques* 20:21–35.

Mañjuśrimulakalpa see Macdonald 1962

Maspero, Henri
1953 *Les documents chinois de la troisième expedition de Sir Aurel Stein en Asie centrale*. London.

Mathieu, Remi
1978 *Le 'mu tianzi zhuan.'* Paris.

Matsumoto, Eiichi
1937 *Tonkō-ga no kenkyū*. 2 vols. Tokyo.

Matsunaga, Alicia
1969 *The Buddhist philosophy of assimilation*. Rutland.

Mau-tsai, Liu
1969 *Kutscha und seine Beziehungen zu China vom 2.Jh. vor bis zum 6.Jh. nach Chr*. 2 vols. Wiesbaden.

Maxwell, T.S.
1980 "Lākhamaṇḍal and Trilokināth." *Art International* 24:9–74.

May, Jacques
1967 "Chinkiyaku (remède de déchets gâtés)." In *Hōbōgirin*, vol. 4:329–335.

Meisezahl, R.O.
1967 "Die Göttin Vajravāhārī. Eine ikonographische Studie nach einem Sādhana-Text von Advayavajra." *Oriens* 18–19:228–303.

Metropolitan Museum of Art
1980–81 "Linga with one face (Ekamukhaliṅga)." In *Notable Acquisitions 1980–1981*, p.77.

1982 *Along the ancient silk routes: Central Asian art from the West Berlin State Museums*. New York.

Meunié, Jacques
1942 *Shotorak*. Mémoires de la Délégation archéologique française en Afghanistan, vol. 10. Paris.
1943 "Le couvent des otages chinoises de Kaniṣka au Kāpiśa." *Journal Asiatique* 234:151–162.

Miller, Robert J.
1961 "Buddhist monastic economy and the Jisa mechanism." *Comparative Studies in Society and History* 3:427–438.

Ministry of Culture, Beijing
1953 *Binglingsi shiku (Ping-ling ssu shih k'u)*. Publication of the Bureau of Social and Cultural Affairs, no. 80.

Ministry of Information and Broadcasting, New Delhi
n.d. *The Way of the Buddha*. Published on the occasion of the 2500th anniversary of the Mahaparinirvana of Buddha.

Minorsky. See Hudūd

Mission Paul Pelliot
1947 *Manuscrits et peintures de Touen-houang, Mission Paul Pelliot 1905–1909*. Collections de la Bibliotheque Nationale et du Musée Guimet. Paris.
1961–1964 *Toumchouq*, ed. Louis Hambis. Documents archéologiques, vols. I–II. Paris.
1967 *Koutcha, temples construits; Douldour-Agour et Soubachi*. Documents archéologiques, vol. III. Paris.

Mitra, Debala
1971 *Buddhist monuments*. Calcutta.

Mizuno, Seiichi and Nagahiro, T.
1951–1956 *Unkō sekkutsu*. (Yünkang, the Buddhist cave temples of the fifth century A.D. in north China.) 16 vols. Kyoto.

Monod, Odette
1966 *Le Musée Guimet I: Inde, Khmer, Tchampa, Java, Nepal, Tibet, Afghanistan, Pakistan, Asie Centrale*. Paris.

Montell, Gösta
1935–1938 "Sven Hedin's archaeological collections from Khotan." *Bulletin of the Museum of Far Eastern Antiquities* 7 (1935):145–221 and 10 (1938):83–113.

Moorcroft, William, and Trebeck, George
1841 *Travels in the Himalayan provinces of Hindustan and the Punjab*. 2 vols. Edited by H.H. Wilson. London. Reprint 1971, New Delhi.

Morgenstierne, George
1931 "The name *Munjān* and some other names of places and peoples in the Hindu Kush." *Bulletin of the School of Oriental Studies* 6:439–444.
1973 *Irano-Dardica*. Wiesbaden.

Moses, Larry W.
1976 "T'ang tribute relations with the Inner Asian barbarians." In *Essays on T'ang society*, eds. J.C. Perry and B.L. Smith. Leiden.

Müller, F.W.K.
1925 "Eine soghdische Inschrift in Ladakh." *Sitzungsberichte der Preussischen Akademie der Wissenschaften* 1925:371–372.

Müller-Stellrecht, Irmtraud
1978 *Hunza and China (1761–1891)*. Wiesbaden.

Murti, T.R.V.
1970 *The central philosophy of Buddhism*. 2nd ed. London.

Mus, Paul
1935 *Barabuḍur: esquisse d'une histoire du bouddhisme fondée sur la critique archéologique des textes*. 2 vols. Hanoi.
1939 *La lumière sur les six voies*. Paris.
1948 "Le Buddha paré, son origine, Ćakyamūni dans le Mahāyānisme moyen." *Bulletin de l'École française d'Extrême-Orient* 28:153–278.

Musée Guimet, Paris
1966 See Monod, Odette.
1976 *La route de la soie*. Exhibition catalogue. Paris.
1977 *Dieux et démons de l'Himâlaya*. Catalogue of the exhibition in the Grand Palais. Paris.
1979 *Arts du Nepal et du Tibet*. Paris.

Museum of Art and Archaeology, University of Missouri
1969 "Hayagriva, a minor incarnation of Vishnu." *Annual of the Museum of Art and Archaeology, University of Missouri, Columbia*, 46–47.

Museum of Fine Arts, Boston
1966 *The arts of India and Nepal: the Nasli and Alice Heeramaneck collection*. Boston.

Nagai, Evelyn H.
1977 *Iconographic innovations in Kuchean Buddhist art*. Ph.D. dissertation, University of California, Berkeley.

Nāgārjuna, Siddha, see Lamotte 1944.

Nagatomi, M., and contributors, eds.
1980 *Sanskrit and Indian studies: essays in honour of Daniel H.H. Ingalls*. Dordrecht and Boston.

Naitō Tōichiro
1943 *The wall paintings of Hōryūji*. Edited and translated by W.R.B. Acker and B. Rowland, Jr. 2 vols. Baltimore.
Narain, A.K., ed.
1979 *Studies in Pali and Buddhism*. New Delhi.
National Museum, Tokyo
1969 *Exhibition of Scythian, Persian and Central Asian art from the Hermitage Collection, Leningrad*. (In Japanese.) Tokyo.
National Museum of Western Art, Tokyo
1976 *Masterpieces of world art from American museums; from ancient Egypt to contemporary*. Exhibition catalogue. Tokyo.
Naudou, Jean
1980 *Buddhists of Kaśmīr*. Delhi.
Nebesky-Wojkowitz, René de
1956 *Oracles and demons of Tibet. The cult and iconography of the Tibetan protective deities*. London.
Needham, Joseph
1956 *Science and civilization in China*. Vol.II. Cambridge.
Newark Museum
1950–1971 *Catalogue of the Tibetan collection and other Lamaist articles in the Newark Museum*, by Eleanor Olson. 5 vols. Newark.
Nicolas-Vandier, Nicole
1954 *Sàriputra et les six maîtres d'erreur*. Paris.
1976 *Bannières et peintures de Touen-Houang conservées au Musée Guimet*. Part 2 (planches). Mission Paul Pelliot. Paris.
Obermiller, E., transl.
1931–1932 *History of Buddhism (Chos-hbyung) by Bu-ston*. 2 vols. Heidelberg.
Ogawa Kan'ichi
1973 *Bukkyō bunkashi kenkyū*. Kyoto.
Ohri, Vishṇa Chandra, ed.
1975 *Arts of Himachal*. Simla (Himachal Pradesh).
Ol'denburg, S.F.
1914 *Buddiiskoi ikonografii Khara-Khoto*. St. Petersburg.
Olschak, Blanche C., with Geshe Thupten Wangyal
1973 *Mystic art of ancient Tibet*. London.
Olson, E., see Newark Museum
Omura, Seigai
1915–1920 *Shina bijutsu shi chōso hen*. 2 vols. Tokoyo.
Oyama Kojun
1961 "Abhiṣeka." In *Encyclopedia of Buddhism*, ed. G.P. Malalasekera, vol. I:125–130. Colombo.
Padoux, André
1963 *Recherches sur la symbolique et l'énergie de la parole dans certains textes tantriques*. Paris.
Pal, Pratapaditya
1967 "Iconography of Cintāmani-cakra Avalokiteśvara." *Journal of the Indian Society of Oriental Art*, n.s. 2:39–48.
1969 *The art of Tibet*. Exhibition Catalogue. The Asia Society, New York.
1972 "A note on the mandala of the Eight Bodhisattvas." *Archives of Asian Art* 26:71–73.
1973a "Bronzes of Kashmir: their sources and influences." *Journal of the Royal Society of Arts* 121:726–749.
1973b "A brahmanical triad from Kashmir and some related icons." *Archives of Asian Art* 27:33–45.
1975a *Nepal—where the gods are young*. Exhibition catalogue. The Asia Society, New York.
1975b *Bronzes of Kashmir*. Graz.
1978 *The sensuous immortals: a selection of sculptures from the Pan-Asian collection*. Exhibiton catalogue. Los Angeles County Museum of Art, Los Angeles.
1978 *The arts of Nepal*. 2 vols. Leiden.
1981 "An addorsed Śaiva image from Kashmir and its cultural significance." *Art International* 24:6–61.
1982 "Cosmic vision and Buddhist images." *Art International* 25:8–39.
Panday, Deena B.
1973 *The Shāhis of Afghanistan and the Punjab*. New Delhi.
Paquier, J.-B.
1876 *Le Pamir—étude de géographie physique et historique sur l'Asie centrale*. Paris.
Pelliot, Paul
1905 "Review of On Yuan Chwang's travels in India, 629–645 A.D., by Thomas Watters." *Bulletin de l'École française d'Extrême-Orient* 5:423–457.
1912 "Autour d'une traduction sanscrite du Tao-tö-king." *T'oung Pao* 13:351–430.
1920–1924 *Les grottes de Touen-houang*. 6 vols. Paris.
1961 *Histoire ancienne du Tibet*. Paris.
Perry, John C., and Bardwell, L.S., eds.
1976 *Essays on T'ang society: the interplay of social, political and economic forces*. Leiden.
Petech, Luciano
1939 *A study on the chronicles of Ladakh*. Calcutta.
1950 *Northern India according to the Shui-ching-chu*. Rome.
1952–1956 (ed.) *I missionari italiani nel Tibet e nel Nepal*. 7 vols. Rome.
1966 "La 'Description des pays d'Occident' de Che Tao-ngan." *Melanges de sinologie offerts a Monsieur Paul Demieville* I:167–190. Paris.
1977 *The kingdom of Ladakh*, c. 950–1842 A.D. Rome.

Polo, Marco
1958 *The travels of Marco Polo*. Translated by R. Latham. London.
Pott, P.H.
1966 *Yoga and Tantra: their interrelation and their significance for Indian archaeology*. The Hague.
1976 "Tibet." In *Kunst der Welt: Burma, Korea, Tibet*, pp. 143–218. Baden-Baden.
Pranavānanda, Swami
1949 *Kailās-Mānasarōvar*. Calcutta.
Puech, Henri-Charles
1979 *Sur le manichéism et autres essais*. Paris.

Rāmakṛishṇa, Sri
1947 *The Gospel*. Mylapore, Madras.
Rau, Wilhelm
1957 *Staat und Gesellschaft im alten Indien*. Wiesbaden.
Ray, Hem Chandra
1931 *The dynastic history of northern India*. Vol. I. Calcutta.
Raza, Moonis; Aijazuddin, Ahmad; and Ali Mohammad
1978 *The valley of Kashmir: a geographical interpretation*. New Delhi.
Renou, Louis
1960 *Le destin du Veda dans l'Inde*. Paris.
Renou, Louis, and Filliozat, Jean
1947–1953 *L'inde classique*. 2 vols. Paris and Hanoi.
Reynolds, Valrae
1978 *Tibet: a lost world*. The Newark Museum collection of Tibetan art and ethnography. Bloomington.
Rhie, Marylin M.
1974 "A T'ang period stele transcription and cave XXI at T'ien-lung Shan." *Archives of Asian Art* 28:6–34.
1976 "Some aspects of the relation of 5th-century Chinese Buddha images with sculpture from N. India, Pakistan, Afghanistan, and Central Asia." *East and West* 26:439–461.
Riboud, Krishna
1975 "Further indications of changing techniques in figured silks of the post-Han period." *Bulletin de liaison du CIETA*, no. 41. Lyon.
Riboud, Krishna and Vial, Gabriel with Hallade, Madeleine
1970 *Tissus de Touen-Houang* conserves au Musée Guimet et à la Bibliothèque Nationale. Paris.
Richardson, Hugh E.
1949 "Three ancient inscriptions from Tibet." *Journal of the Royal Asiatic Society of Bengal* 15/1:45–64.
1952 *Ancient historical edicts at Lhasa and the Mu Tsung/khri Gtsug of A.D. 821–822 from the inscription at Lhasa*. London.
1962 *A short history of Tibet*. New York.
1977 "The Jo-Khang 'cathedral' of Lhasa." In *Essais sur l'art du Tibet*, eds. Ariane MacDonald and Yoshiro Imaeda. Paris.
Roerich, George N.
1931 *Trails to inmost Asia. Five years of exploration with the Roerich Central Asian Expedition*. New Haven.
1949–1953 *The Blue Annals*. 2 vols. Calcutta. Reprinted as 1 vol. in Delhi, 1976.
Rosenfield, John M.
1967 *The dynastic arts of the Kushans*. Berkeley.
Rosenfield, John M., and ten Grotenhuis, Elisabeth
1979 *The journey of the three jewels*. New York.
Ross, E. Denison
1895 *A history of the Moghuls of Central Asia, being the Tarikh-i-Rashidi of Mirza Muhammad Haidar, Dughlát*. London. Reprint London, 1972.
Rowland, Benjamin
1934 "A Buddhist relief of the Udayana type from Turkestan." *Bulletin of the Fogg Art Museum* 4:4–10.
1947 "Indian images in Chinese sculpture." *Artibus Asiae* 10:5–20.
1963 *The evolution of the Buddha image*. Exhibiton catalogue. The Asia Society, New York.

1970 *The art and architecture of India: Buddhist-Hindu-Jain.* 3rd ed. London.
1971 "Wall paintings of Bāmiyān." In *The wall-paintings of India, Central Asia, and Ceylon,* by B. Rowland and A.K. Coomaraswamy, Boston, 1938. Reprinted in *Marg* 24/2:25–43.
1974 *The art of Central Asia.* New York.
Ruegg, D. Seyfort
1964 "Sur le rapport entre le bouddhism et le substrat religieux indien et tibétain." *Journal Asiatique* 252:77–95.
1978 "The study of Tibetan philosophy and its Indian sources." In Ligeti 1978.
Russell, Bertrand
1953 *Mysticism and logic.* London.
Sachau, Edward C.
1910 *Alberuni's India.* 2 vols. London. Reprinted Delhi, 1964.
Sasaguchi, Rei
1972 "A dated painting from Tun-huang in the Fogg Museum." *Archives of Asian Art* 26:26–49.
Sato, Chisui
1978 "The character of Yun-kang Buddhism." *Memoirs of the Research Department of the Toyo Bunko* 36:39–83.
Saunders, E.D.
1960 *Mudrā: a study of symbolic gestures in Japanese-Buddhist sculpture.* London.
Schafer, Edward H.
1963 *The golden peaches of Samarkand: a study of T'ang exotics.* Berkeley and Los Angeles.
1977 *Pacing the void: T'ang approaches to the stars.* Berkeley.
Scherman, Lucian
1932 *Buddha im Fürstenschmuck: Erläuterung hinterindischer Bildwerke des Münchener Museums für Völkerkunde.* Munich.
Schlumberger, Daniel
1955 "Le marbre Scorretti." *Art Asiatiques* 2:112–119.
Schmidt, Hanns-Peter
1968 *Brhaspati und Indra: Untersuchungen zur vedischen Mythologie und Kulturgeschichte.* Wiesbaden.
Schopen, Gregory
1975 "The phrase 'sa pṛthivīpradeśaś caityabhūto bhavet' in the Vajracchedikā: notes on the cult of the book in Mahāyāna." *Indo-Iranian Journal* 17:147–181.
Schroeder, Ulrich von
1981 *Indo-Tibetan bronzes.* Hong Kong.
Schuh, Dieter
1976 *Urkunden und Sendschreiben aus Zentraltibet, Ladakh und Zanskar.* Bonn.
Schwartzberg, J.E., ed.
1978 *Historical Atlas of South Asia.* Chicago.
Seckel, Dietrich
1964 *The art of Buddhism.* Translated by Ann E. Keep. New York.
Seibu Department Store, Tokyo
1963 *Silk road Bijutsu ten.* (Exhibition of the Silk Road.) Tokyo.
Seiiki Bunka Kenkyūkai
1958–1963 *Monumenta Serindica.* 6 vols. Kyoto.
Sekai no Bijutsukan
1968 "Gime Toyo Bijutsukan." In *Sekai no Bijutsukan,* vol. 14. Tokyo.
Sekine, Daisen
1968 *Mainōkyō no kenkyū.* Tokyo.
Shanhai J'ing
n.d. *Book of Mountains and Seas.* (In Chinese.)
Sharma, Brijendra N.
1979 "Sculptures and bronzes from Kashmir in the National Museum, New Delhi." *East and West* 29:131–137.
Sherpherd, Dorothy G.
1966 "Two silver Rhyta." *Bulletin of the Cleveland Museum of Art* 53:289–311.
Shuttleworth, H.L.H.
1923 "An inscribed metal mask discovered on the occasion of the Bhunda ceremony at Nirmand." *Acta Orientalia* 1:224–229.
Singh, Mandanjeet
1968 *Himalayan art.* Greenwich.
Sinor, Denis
1963 *Introduction à l'étude de l'Eurasie centrale.* Wiesbaden.
Sivaramamurti, Calambur
1977 *The art of India.* New York.
Skorupski, Tadeusz
1981 *Sarva-durgati-pariśodhana-tantra.* New Delhi.
1982 "Tibetan Homa rites." In Staal 1982a.
Smith, Gene E.
1970 "Introduction to Kontrul's encyclopaedia of Indo-Tibetan culture, Shes-bye Kun-khyab." In *Śata-Pitaka* 80, pp. 1–87. New Delhi.
Snellgrove, David L.
1954 "The Tantras." In Conze et al. 1954.
1957 *Buddhist Himālaya.* Oxford.
1959a *The Hevajra Tantra: a critical study.* 2 vols. London.
1959b "The notion of divine kingship in Tantric Buddhism." In *Sacral Kingship,* vol. IV of *Studies in the history of religions,* supplement to *Numen* 4. Leiden.
1961 *Himalayan pilgrimage.* Oxford.
1978 *Image of the Buddha.* London and Paris.
Snellgrove, David L., and Richardson, Hugh
1968 *A cultural history of Tibet.* London.
Snellgrove, David L., and Skorupski, Tadeusz
1977–1980 *The cultural heritage of Ladakh.* 2 vols. Warminster.
Soper, Alexander
1959 *Literary evidence for early Buddhist art in China.* Ascona.
1965 "Representations of famous images at Tun-huang." *Artibus Asiae* 27:349–364.
Soymié, Michel
1961 "Sources et sourciers en Chine." *Bulletin de la Maison Franco-Japonaise* 7/1.
Spanien, A., and Imaeda, Y.
1979 *Choix de documents tibétains conservés à la Bibliothèque Nationale.* Vol. II. Paris.
Spooner, D.B.
1908–1911 "Excavations at Shāh-jī-kī-Dhēri." *Archaeological Survey of India: Annual Report 1908–1909:* 38–59; 1910–1911:25–32.
Staal, J. Frits
1963 "Sanskrit and Sanskritization." *The Journal of Asian Studies* 22:216–275. Reprinted in J.A. Harrison, ed., *Enduring scholarship selected from the Far Eastern Quarterly - The Journal of Asian Studies,* Tucson, 1972.
1979a "Oriental ideas on the origin of language." *Journal of the American Oriental Society* 99:1–14.
1979b "The meaninglessness of ritual." *Numen: International Review for the History of Religion* 26:2–22.
1980 "Ritual syntax." in Nagatomi et al. 1980: 119–142.
1982a *Agni: the Vedic ritual of the fire altar.* 2 vols. Berkeley.
1982b *The science of ritual.* Poona.
1982c The stamps of Jammu and Kashmir. New York.
Stein, M. Aurel
1896 "Notes on Ou-k'ong's account of Kaçmīr." *Sitzungsberichte der phil.-hist. Classe d. kaiserl. Akad. d. Wissenschaften,* vol. 135:1–32. Vienna.
1900 (transl.) *Kalhaṇa's Rājataraṅgiṇī: a chronicle of the kings of Kashmir.* 2 vols. Westminster. Reprint New Delhi, 1961.
1901 *Archaeological and topographical exploration in Chinese Turkestan.* London.
1904 *Sand-buried ruins of Khotan.* London.
1907 *Ancient Khotan: detailed report of archaeological explorations in Chinese Turkestan.* Oxford.
1912 *Ruins of desert Cathay.* 2 vols. London.
1915 "Excavations at Sahri-Bahlol." *Archaeological Survey of India, Annual Report 1911–1912.* Calcutta.
1917 "On some river names in the Ṛgveda." *Journal of the Royal Asiatic Society of Great Britain and Ireland,* 1917/1:91–99.
1921a "La traversée du desert par Hiuan-tsang en 630 ap.J.C." *T'oung Pao* 20:332–354.
1921b *Serindia: detailed report of explorations in Central Asia and westernmost China.* 5 vols. Oxford.
1921c " A Chinese expedition across the Pamirs and Hindukush A.D. 747." *New China Review* 2:47–69.
1921d *The thousand Buddhas: ancient Buddhist paintings from the cave temples of Tun-huang on the western frontier of China.* 3 vols. London.
1923 *Memoir on maps of Chinese Turkestan and Kansu, from surveys made during Sir Aurel Stein's explorations 1900–1901, 1906–1908, 1913–1915.* Dehra Dun.
1928 *Innermost Asia.* 3 vols. Oxford.
1929a *On Alexander's track to the Indus.* London.
1929b *An archaeological tour in Waziristān and northern Balūchistān.* Memoirs of the Archaeological Survey of India, no. 37, Calcutta.
1930 *An archaeological tour in upper Swat and adjacent hill tracks.* Memoirs of the Archaeological Survey of India, no. 42. Calcutta.
1931 *An archaeological tour in Gedrosia.* Memoirs of the Archaeological Survey of India, no. 43, Calcutta.
1932 "On ancient tracks past the Pamirs." *The Himalayan Journal* 4:1–26.
1937 *Archaeological reconnaissances in north-western India and south-eastern Iran.* London.
1940 *Old routes of western Iran.* London.
1942 "From Swat to the Indus gorges." *Geographical Journal,* 1942 (August):49–56.

1944 "Archaeological notes from the Hindukush region." *Journal of the Royal Asiatic Society of Great Britain and Ireland,* 1944:5–24.
1964 *On ancient Central-Asian tracks.* New York.
1973 "A contribution to the history of the Shāhis of Kabul." (English translation.) *East and West* 23:13–20.

Stein, R.A.
1972 *Tibetan civilization.* London.

Strickmann, Michel
1977 "A survey of Tibetan Buddhist studies." *The Eastern Buddhist,* n.s. 10:128–149.
1980a "History, anthropology, and Chinese religion." *Harvard Journal of Asiatic Studies* 98:467–475.
1980b *Tun-huang studies: the manuscript tradition in mediaeval China.* Berkeley.
1982a "Homa in East Asia." In Staal 1982a.
1982b "Apocrypha and apocalyptic: two neglected aspects of Chinese Buddhism." In *Tantric and Taoist studies in honor of R.A. Stein,* II. Brussels.

Taddei, Maurizio
1962 "An Ekamukhaliṅga from the N.W.F.P. and some connected problems; a study in iconography and style." *East and West* 13:288–310.
1965 "A Liṅga-shaped portable sanctuary of the Śāhi period." *East and West* 15:24–25.
1968 "Tapa Sardār: first preliminary report." *East and West* 18:109–124.
1970 "Inscribed clay tablets and miniature stupas from Ghazni." *East and West* 20:70–86.
1971 "The Mahisamardini image from Tapa Sardār, Ghazni, Afghanistan." In *South Asian archaeology,* ed. N. Hammond, pp. 203–213. London.
1972 "Report on excavations at Tapa Sardār." *East and West* 22:379–384.
1974 "Appunti sull'iconografica di alcune manifestazioni luminose dei Buddha." In *Gururājamañjikā: Studi in onore di Giuseppe Tucci.* Vol. II:435–449. Naples.
1978a *India: monuments of civilization.* New York.
1978b "Tapa Sardār: second preliminary report" (with G. Verardi). *East and West* 28:33–157.

Taisho shinshu daizokyo
1924–1934 Revised, collated, augmented and rearranged by Takakusu, Junjiro, and Watanabe, Kaigyoku. Tokyo.

Tajima, R.
1936 *Étude sur le Mahāvairocana-sūtra.* Paris.
1959 *Les deux grands mandalas et la doctrine de l'esoterism Shingon.* Paris.

Takaaki, Sawa
1972 *Art in Japanese esoteric Buddhism.* Honolulu.

Takakusu, Junjiro
1947 *The essentials of Buddhist philosophy.* Honolulu.

Tāranātha
1970 *Tāranātha's history of Buddhism and India.* Translated by Lama Chimpa and Alaka Chattopadhyaya, edited by D. Chattopadhyaya. Simla.

Ta'rīkh-i-Ferishta
1873–1874 A.H.1290, Kanhpur.

Tarzi, Zemaryalai
1976 Hadda à la lumière des trois dernières campagnes de fouilles de Tapa-e-Shotor (1974–1976)." *Comptes rendus de l'Académie des Inscriptions et Belles Lettres,* 1976:381–410.
1977 *L'Architecture et le décor rupestre des grottes de Bāmiyān.* 2 vols. Paris.

Thapar, Rommila
1961 *Aśoka and the decline of the Mauryas.* London.
1972 *History of India I.* Harmondsworth.

Thomas, Edward J.
1960 *The life of Buddha as legend and history.* 3rd ed. New York.
1971 *The history of Buddhist thought.* 2nd ed. London.

Thomas, F.W.
1935 *Tibetan literary texts and documents concerning Chinese Turkestan. Part 1: Literary Texts.* London.

Thomas, F.W., and Konow, S.
1929 "Two medieval documents from Tun-huang." In *Indian and Central Asian miscellanies,* Etnographiske Museums Skrifter III:121–130. Oslo.

Thomson, Thomas
1852 *Western Himalaya and Tibet.* London.

Tokei, F.
1966 *Sur le mode de production asiatique.* Budapest.

Tonkō Bumbutsu Kenkyū, eds.
1980 *Chūgoku Sekkutsu-Tonkō Bakukō Kutsu.* (Caves of China: the Mugao caves of Dunhuang.) 2 vols. Tokyo.

Trubner, Henry
1950 *The art of greater India.* Exhibition catalogue. Los Angeles County Museum of Art, Los Angeles.

Trungpa, Chögyam
1975a *Empowerment.* Discography, Vajradhatu Recordings. Boulder.
1975b *Visual Dharma: the Buddhist art of Tibet.* Berkeley and London.

Tsuda, Shinichi
1978 "A critical Tantrism." *Memoirs of the Research Department of Toyo Bunko* 36:167–231.

Tucci, Giuseppe
1932–1941 *Indo-Tibetica.* 7 vols. Roma.
1937 "Indian paintings in western Tibetan temples." *Artibus Asiae* 7:191–204.
1949 *Tibetan painted scrolls.* 3 vols. Rome.
1951 "Buddhist notes: à propos Avalokiteśvara." *Mélanges chinoises et bouddhiques* 9(1948–51): 173–219.
1956 *To Lhasa and beyond.* Rome.
1958 "Preliminary report on an archaeological survey in Swat (Pakistan)." *East and West* 9:279–328.
1959 "A Tibetan classification of Buddhist images, according to their style." *Artibus Asiae* 22:179–187.
1963 "An image of a Devi discovered in Swat and some connected problems." *East and West* 14:146–182.
1966 *Tibetan folk songs from Gyantse and western Tibet.* Ascona.
1967 *Tibet—land of snows.* London.
1971a *The theory and practice of the mandala.* New York.
1971b *Deb-t'er dmar po gsar ma Tibetan chronicles by bSod-nams-grags-pa.* Rome.
1973 *Transhimalaya.* London.
1975 *On some aspects of the doctrines of Maitreya (nātha) and Asaṅga.* (Originally published in Calcutta, 1930.) San Francisco.
1976 *Pre-Diṅnāga Buddhist texts on logic from Chinese sources.* (Originally published in Baroda, 1929.) San Francisco.
1977a *Journey to Mustang, 1952.* Kathmandu.
1977b "On Swat. The Dards and connected problems." *East and West* 27:9–103.
1980 *The religions of Tibet.* Berkeley.

Uhlig, H., and Schroeder, U. von
1976 *Buddhistische Kunst aus dem Himalaya.* Exhibition catalogue. Kunst am Tempelhof. Berlin.

Utz, David A.
1978 *A survey of Buddhist Sogdian studies.* Tokyo.

Uyeno, Aki
1980 "Preaching scene murals of the cave of Māyā, the third area, Kizil (Part I) - Study of Central Asian murals collected by A. von Le Coq (Part II)." (In Japanese, with English resumé. Bijutsu Kenkyū 312: 12–25; 313: 19–25.

Varenne, Jean
1976 *Yoga and the Hindu tradition.* Chicago.

Varma, K.M.
1970 *The Indian technique of clay modelling.* Calcutta.

Vigne, G.T.
1842 *Travels in Kashmir, Ladak, Iskardo etc.* 2 vols. London.

Visser, M.W. de
1935 *Ancient Buddhism in Japan.* 2 vols. Leiden.

Vostrikov, A.I.
1970 *Tibetan historical literature.* Calcutta.

Waddell, L. Austine
1895 *The Buddhism of Tibet, or Lamaism.* London. Reprint New York, 1971.

Waley, Arthur
1931 *A catalogue of paintings recovered from Tun-huang by Sir Aurel Stein.* London.

Warner, Langdon
1926 *The long old road in China.* Garden City.
1938 *Buddhist wall-paintings.* Cambridge.
1966 *Langdon Warner through his letters,* ed. Theodore Bowie. Bloomington.

Watson, William
1971 "Styles of Mahāyānist iconography in China." In *Mahayanist art after A.D. 900. Colloquies on Art and Archaeology in Asia,* no. 2:1–9. London.

Watters, Thomas
1904–1905 *On Yuan Chwang's travels in India (A.D. 629–645).* 2 vols. London. Reprinted as 1 vol. in Delhi, 1973.

Wayman, Alex
1971 "Contributions on the symbolism of the mandala palace." In *Études tibétaines, dediées à la mémoire de Marcelle Lalou,* pp. 557–566. Paris.
1973 *The Buddhist tantras. Light on Indo-Tibetan esotericism.* New York.

Wessels, C.
1924 *Early Jesuit travelers in Central Asia, 1603–1721.* The Hague.

Whitfield, Roderick
1982 *The Stein collection at the British Museum. I: Art of Central Asia. II: Paintings from Dunhuang.* Tokyo.

Williams, Joanna
1973 "The iconography of Khotanese painting." *East and West* 23:109–154.

Wood, John
1872 *A journey to the source of the river Oxus*. London.
Woodman, Dorothy
1969 *Himalayan frontier; a political review of British, Chinese, Indian, and Russian rivalries*. London.
Woods, John E.
1976 *The Aqquyunlu—clan, confederation, empire*. Minneapolis.
Wylie, Turrell V.
1962 *The geography of Tibet according to 'Dzam-Gling-Rgyal-Bshad*. Rome.
Xuanzang (Hsüan-tsang) see Beal 1884 and 1911, and Watters 1904–1905.
Yamada, Ryujo
1959 *Daijō Bukkyō seiritsuron josetsu*. Kyoto.
Ye Xinshen
1981 "Evolution of style in Tibetan wall painting." *Meishuyanjiu* 3:64–72.
Yi-Liang, Chao
1944 "Tantrism in China." *Harvard Journal of Asiatic Studies* 8:241–332.
Young, Mahonri S.
1975 "The second seventy." *Apollo*, 1975 (February):136–139
Younghusband, F.E.
1890 *Report of a mission to the northern frontier of Kashmir in 1889*. Calcutta.
Zelliot, Eleanor
1979 "The Indian rediscovery of Buddhism 1855–1956." In Narain 1979:389–406.
Zimmer, Heinrich R.
1955 *The art of Indian Asia, its mythology and transformations*. 2nd ed. 2 vols. Completed and edited by Joseph Campbell. New York.
Zürcher, Erik
1959 *The Buddhist conquest of China*. 2 vols. Leiden.

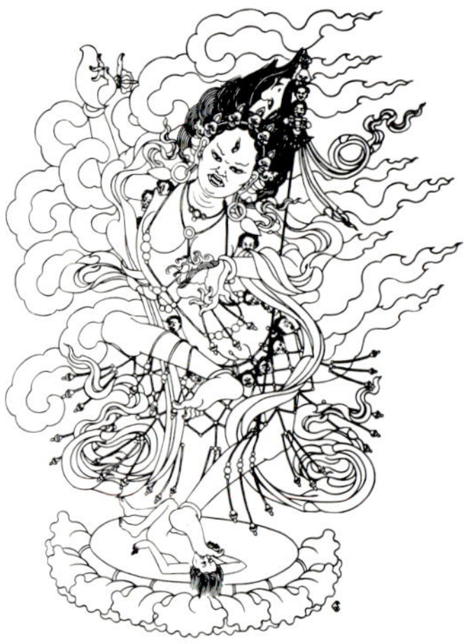

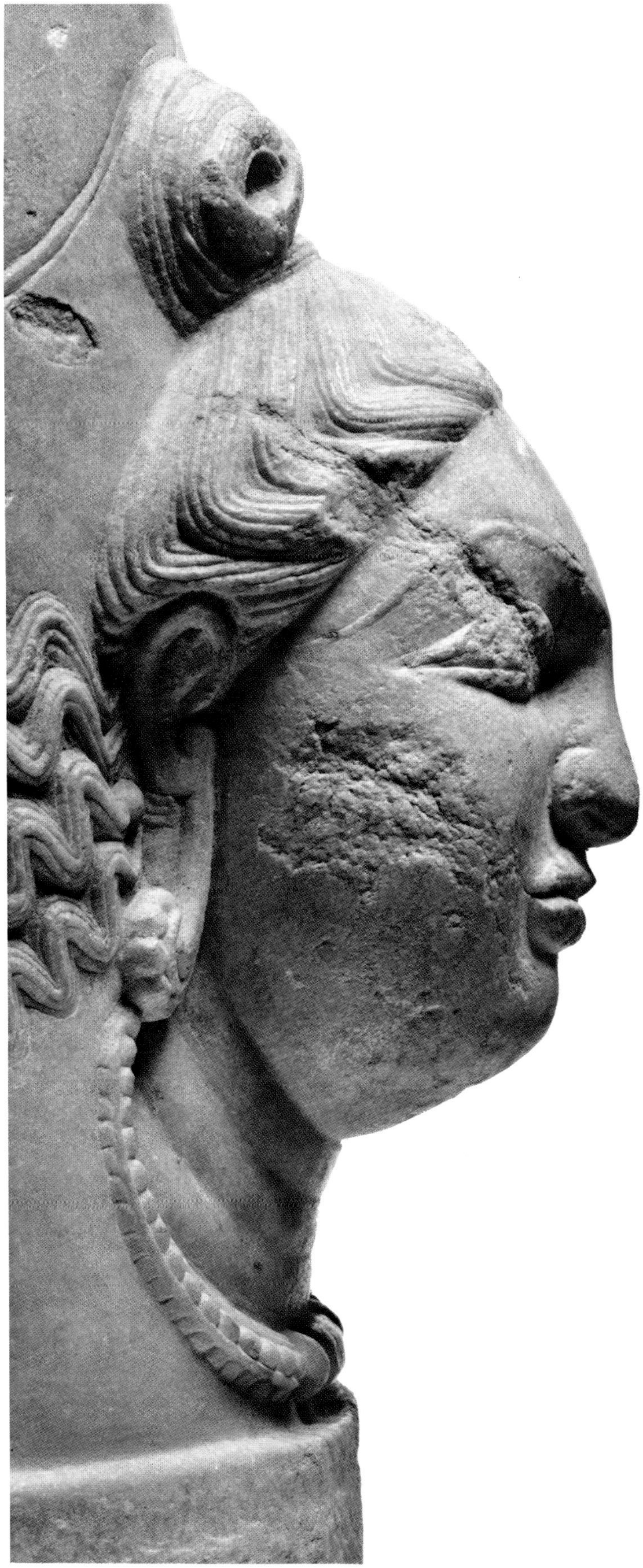

Exhibition Staff

Director: Edith Tonnelli
Associate Director: Jack Carter
Curator: Deborah E. Klimburg-Salter
Assistant Curator: Sarah Handler
Director of Audiovisual Components: Maximilian Klimburg
Administrative Assistant: Etsu Garfias
Fiscal Officer: Glynn Davies
Director, Educational Programs: Vickie Lockwood Joralemon
Special Educational Programs: Cheryl Snell
Museum Interns: Mollie Alexander, Elsie Ritchie
Research Assistants: Elizabeth Goldblatt, Chandra Reedy, Audrey Spiro, Jared Rhotan
Installation Technicians: David Paley, Will Reigle, Gene Riggs, Milt Young
Installation Assistants: Grace Barnes, Charles Enjaian, Laurie Livingston, Robert Jessup, Donald Olstad, Susan Shutt, David Singer
Administrative Analyst: Marian Eber
Secretary: Jan Keller

AFA/DC
2-07
5-

List of Photo Credits

PLATES:

O. E. Nelson
9, 30, 78, 79
Nathan Rabin
13,122
Patrick Young
108
R. Gupta
55, 56, 58, 62, 63, 64, 65, 66, 67, 71, 72, 73, 74, 75, 76, 77
British Museum
6, 31, 40, 43, 57, 69, 85, 90
Musées Nationaux de France
59, 60, 61, 68, 70, 92, 110
Russell Windman
97, 112

FIGURES

Bohung Jin
Fig. 34
Fogg Art Museum
Figs. 36, 37, 38, 39
David L. Snellgrove
Figs. 17, 18, 22, 23, 24, 25, 26
Adelaide de Menil
Figs. 7, 8
Deborah Klimburg-Salter
Figs. 28, 29
Maximilian Klimburg
Fig. 60
Musée Guimet
Fig. 60
Datta Gupta
Fig. 46

All other color transparencies and all other black and white photographs appear by courtesy of the lenders.

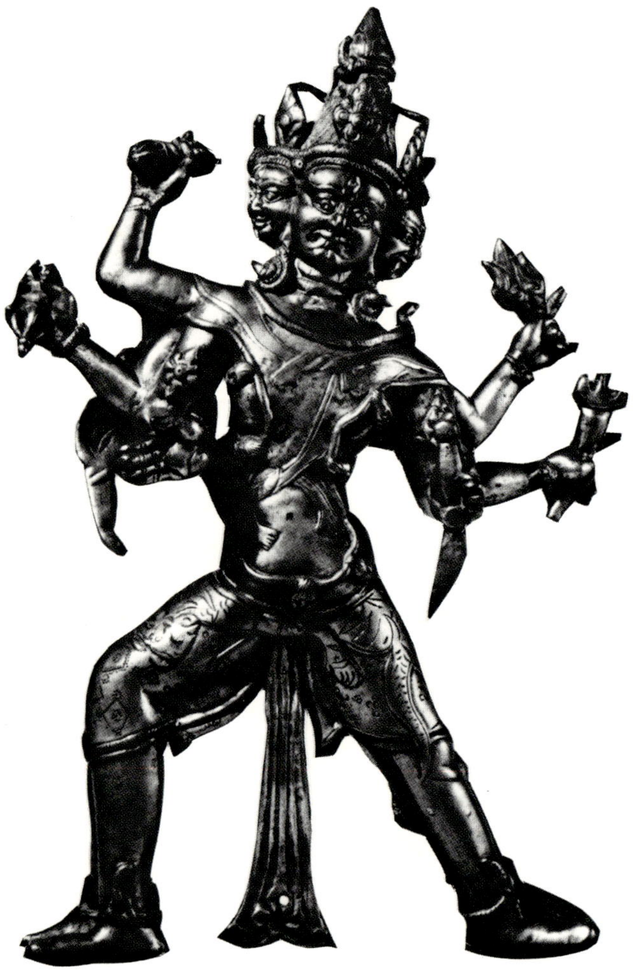

Credits for Catalogue

Publication Director: Kim Lockard
Designer: Jack Carter
Maps and Production: Roberta Roberts
Copy Editor: Ruth Hoover
Linguist/Proofreader: Jared Rhotan
Editorial Assistants: Sarah Handler, Vickie Joralemon, Molly Alexander, Elsie Ritchie, Jan Keller, Audrey Spiro
Administrative Coordinator: Etsu Garfias

This catalogue is printed on 80 lb. Quintessence Dull Book and 100 lb. Quintessence Dull Cover (soft edition). Composition by Graphic Typesetting Service. Color separations by Graphic Arts Systems. Printing by Alan Lithograph. 4,500 copies soft edition and 500 copies hard edition. Bound by Roswell Bookbinding Co.